OXFORD MEDICAL PUBLICATIONS

Cunningham's Manual of Practical Anatomy

Cunningham's Manual of Practical Anatomy

Fifteenth edition

G. J. ROMANES C.B.E.,
B.A., Ph.D., M.B., Ch.B., F.R.C.S.Ed., F.R.S.E., Hon. D.Sc.
Emeritus Professor of Anatomy in the University of Edinburgh

Volume Two
Thorax and abdomen

Oxford New York Tokyo
OXFORD UNIVERSITY PRESS

OXFORD
UNIVERSITY PRESS

Great Clarendon Street, Oxford OX2 6DP

Oxford University Press is a department of the University of Oxford.
It furthers the University's objective of excellence in research, scholarship,
and education by publishing worldwide in

Oxford New York

Auckland Bangkok Buenos Aires Cape Town Chennai
Dar es Salaam Delhi Hong Kong Istanbul Karachi Kolkata
Kuala Lumpur Madrid Melbourne Mexico City Mumbai Nairobi
São Paulo Shanghai Taipei Tokyo Toronto

Published in the United States
by Oxford University Press Inc., New York

First published 1893
Fifteenth edition 1986
Reprinted 1987 (with corrections), 1989, 1992, 1993, 1996,
1998, 1999, 2000 (three times), 2002 (twice), 2003 (twice), 2004 (five times),
2005 (twice), 2006, 2007, 2008, 2009 (twice), 2010.

British Library Cataloguing in Publication Data

Cunningham, D.J.
Cunningham's manual of practical anatomy.—
15th ed.—(Oxford medical publications)
1. Anatomy, Human
I. Title II. Romanes, G. J.
611 GM23.2

ISBN 978-0-19-922909-3 v. 1
ISBN 978-0-19-956533-7 v. 2
ISBN 978-0-19-922908-6 v. 3

Library of Congress Cataloging in Publication Data

Cunningham, D. J. (Daniel John), 1850-1909.
Cunningham's manual of practical anatomy.
(Oxford medical publications)
Includes index.
Contents: v. 1. Upper and lower limbs—v. 2. Thorax
and abdomen—v. 3. Head and neck and brain.
1. Anatomy, Human—Collected works. 2. Dissection—
Collected works. I. Romanes, G. J. (George John), 1916–
II. Title. III. Series.
[DNLM: 1. Anatomy. 2. Dissection. QS 130 C793d]
QM23.2C915 1986 611 86-16313
ISBN 978-0-19-956533-7

Printed by Thomson Press (India) Ltd.

Contents

Preface to the Fifteenth Edition

This edition has been extensively revised with a view to reducing the length of the text as far as possible commensurate with retaining the type of information which is necessary for an understanding of the structure of the human body at least sufficient to permit the intelligent examination of patients. In spite of this the length of the volumes has been increased principally by the introduction of many new figures which should assist the student without increasing the amount of reading matter. In addition and because shorter courses in anatomy make it increasingly difficult for the student to encompass several books, the introduction (Volume 1) has been expanded to cover a number of important items and there is a brief introduction to development in Volume 2 together with additional sections on the embryology of some of the parts of the trunk where a knowledge of development helps to clarify and is of importance to an understanding of the anatomy and of the clinically important anomalies which may arise. These sections are extensively illustrated with new diagrams intended to help the student to gain an appreciation of a complex subject with the minimal amount of extra reading matter. For the same reason and because of its importance for an appreciation of the new imaging techniques, an atlas of transverse sectional anatomy has been included together with similar scans produced by computerized tomography. These increase the sectional illustrations which have always been a feature of the book and are of particular importance to clinical work because they show the close packing of organs in a manner which is difficult to appreciate by dissection alone. Examples are also given of ultrasound and nuclear magnetic resonance scans so that the student may be aware of the type of information which modern imaging techniques can supply and which make a knowledge of sectional anatomy of increasing importance to clinical work.

The number of more conventional radiographs has also been increased to show the detail which more recent techniques (e.g. double contrast) can demonstrate and which permit the visualization of early pathological changes, e.g. in the mucosa of the gastro-intestinal tract.

The author is particularly indebted to Professor Emeritus Eric Samuel, C.B.E., for supplying most of the new radiographs and CT scans and to the Department of Medical Radiology of the University of Edinburgh for the CT scans of the head and the NMR scan of the author's cranium.

It is hoped that these many additions will increase the usefulness of the *Manuals* and help to make them a more complete text for the overburdened medical and dental students as well as serving the purposes of many of the students in the professions allied to medicine.

Edinburgh G. J. R.
January 1986

The thorax

Introduction

The thorax is that part of the trunk which extends from the root of the neck to the abdomen. The thorax contains the lungs which are separated from one another by a bulky, movable, median septum—the **mediastinum**. The main structures in the mediastinum are the heart and the great vessels which connect the heart to the body and lungs. In addition it transmits structures from the neck to the thorax, e.g. the trachea or windpipe, or to the abdomen, e.g. the oesophagus or gullet, or in the opposite direction, e.g. the thoracic duct.

The **movements of the thorax** are primarily concerned with increasing or decreasing the intrathoracic volume. In this way the pressure in the thorax is changed so that air is alternately drawn into the lungs (inspiration) and expelled from them (expiration) through the respiratory passages. To achieve these movements and to overcome the effects of atmospheric pressure, the walls of the thorax are strengthened by the movable thoracic cage. This consists of the **thoracic vertebrae,** the 12 pairs of **ribs** which articulate with these vertebrae, and the flexible **costal cartilages** which unite the ribs to the **sternum** (breast bone) or to each other. Layers of intercostal muscles fill the spaces between the ribs and between their cartilages. When they contract, these muscles move the ribs and cartilages and make the spaces rigid so that the intercostal tissues do not move out and in as the intrathoracic pressure alters.

The thoracic cavity is separated from the abdominal cavity by the musculo-aponeurotic **diaphragm**. This is attached to the lower margin of the thoracic cage (**inferior aperture of the thorax**) and bulges upwards inside it so that the upper abdominal organs lie under cover of the lower part of the thoracic cage. The diaphragm acts like a piston. When it contracts, it descends and increases the intrathoracic volume (inspiration). When the diaphragm relaxes, the contracting muscles of the abdominal wall force the abdominal contents and the overlying diaphragm upwards inside the thoracic cage,

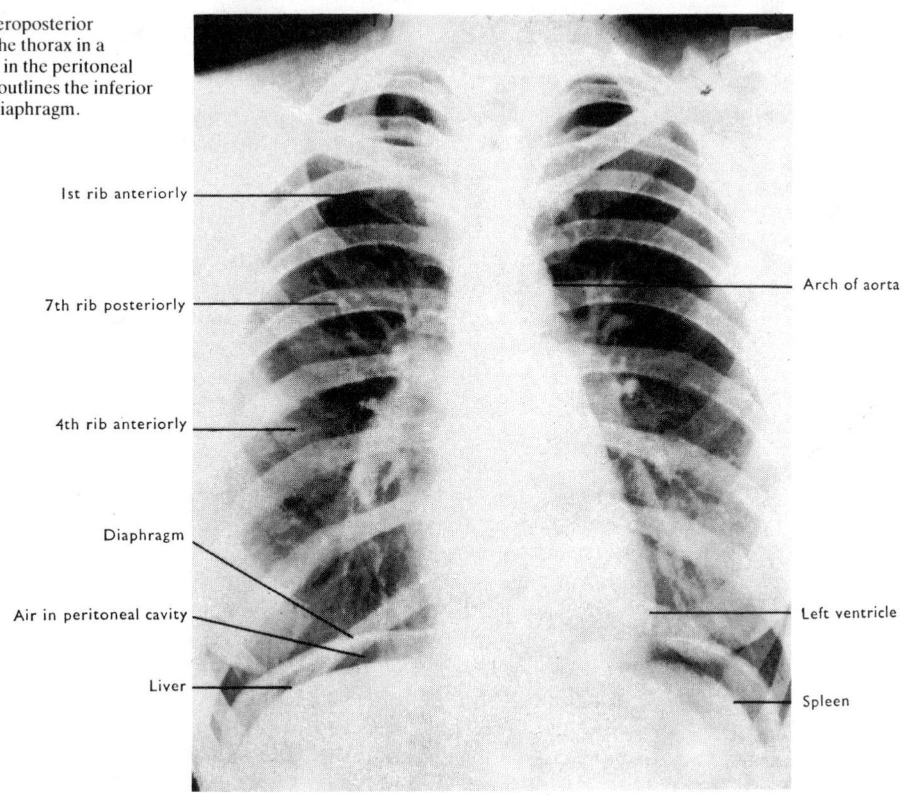

Fig. 1. An anteroposterior radiograph of the thorax in a patient with air in the peritoneal cavity. The air outlines the inferior surface of the diaphragm.

thereby decreasing the intrathoracic volume (expiration). These are the main movements in quiet respiration.

The small **superior aperture of the thorax** abuts on the solid tissues of the neck. It is formed by the internal margins of the first ribs, their cartilages, the sternum, and the first thoracic vertebra. This aperture is sealed by a rigid layer of fascia (**suprapleural membrane**) which extends from the vertebral column to the inner margin of the first rib on each side.

The changing pressure in the thorax produced by the respiratory movements alternatively assists and impedes the return of venous blood to the heart. Thus the volume of blood which the heart receives and transmits increases during inspiration and decreases during expiration with corresponding alterations in the volume of the heart itself [Figs. 13, 14] and of the blood pressure. Thus forced expiration against resistance, as in straining or blowing up a column of mercury, causes the veins to be distended and lowers the blood pressure because of the consequent reduction in output of the heart. This may be sufficiently severe to cause fainting as a result of reduced blood supply to the brain.

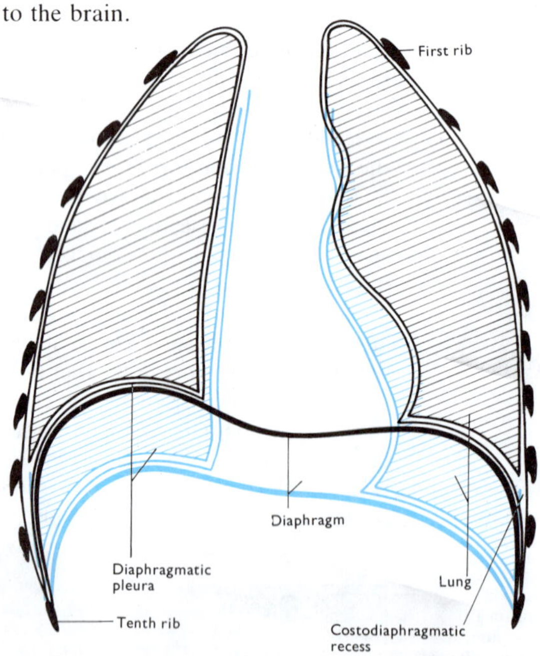

Fig. 2. An outline drawing to show the change in shape of the thoracic contents resulting from contraction of the diaphragm alone. The contracted positions are shown in blue. Note that the lungs and mediastinal structures are elongated, and that the lungs expand to fill the space vacated by the mediastinal structures and to enter the costodiaphragmatic recesses of the pleura. The movements which the ribs undergo in respiration are not shown.

Shape and framework of thorax

The thorax has the shape of a truncated cone. It expands inferiorly to surround the upper part of the abdominal cavity. It is flattened anteroposteriorly to fit the scapulae on its posterolateral aspects and to withstand the pull of the powerful upper limb muscles which overlap it anteriorly and posteriorly.

Each **rib** articulates posteriorly with the vertebral column. Thence the rib sweeps backwards and laterally then obliquely downwards and forwards in the curve of the thoracic wall. It ends anteriorly by fusing with a costal cartilage.

The **costal cartilages** are flexible extensions of the ribs. The cartilages of the upper seven ribs (**true ribs**) pass on each side to the corresponding margin of the sternum. The upper cartilages are in line with their ribs; the lower cartilages become progressively more angulated, the medial part passing upwards to the sternum [Fig. 3]. The ribs inferior to the seventh become progressively shorter so that the anterior ends of each successive pair lie further and further apart. The upturned ends of the cartilages of ribs 8–10 (**false ribs**) fail to reach the sternum but articulate with the margin of the cartilage above. Thus they form a continuous cartilaginous margin which diverges from the lower part of the sternum on each side to form the **infrasternal angle** between right and left **costal margins**. These begin at the articulation of the seventh costal cartilage with the junction of the middle (**body**) and lowest (**xiphoid process**) parts of the sternum. The margins are completed inferiorly by the cartilaginous caps on the ends of the eleventh and twelfth ribs (**floating ribs**) and the lower border of the twelfth rib.

Fig. 3. Front of portion of skeleton showing thorax.

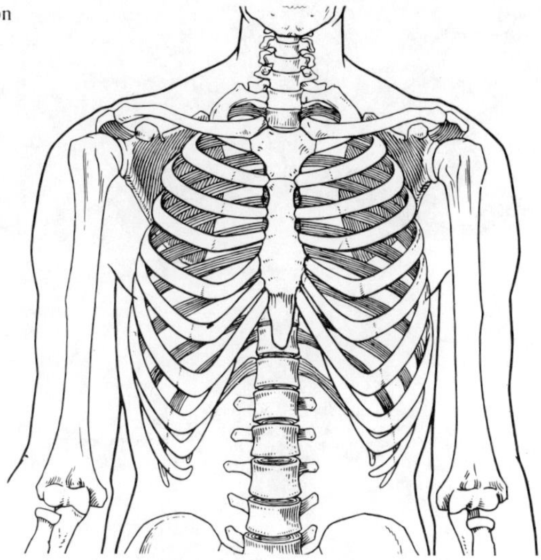

The flexibility of the costal cartilages, combined with their synovial joints with the sternum or with each other, permit the ribs to move relative to each other and to the sternum in respiration. The first costal cartilages differ from the others in that they are fused with the upper part (manubrium) of the sternum and are frequently calcified or ossified. This indicates that the first ribs and the manubrium move together as one piece. The other ribs have a greater degree of freedom of movement relative to the sternum and to each other, especially the floating ribs.

The progressive shortening of the lower ribs and consequent divergence of the costal margins inferior to the sternum make the anterior wall of the thoracic cage much shorter than the lateral or posterior walls. Thus the cage overlaps more of the abdominal contents laterally and posteriorly than it does anteriorly. This is shown by the levels of the parts of the inferior (costal) margin of the cage. These levels vary with the phases of respiration and with the position of the body, erect or recumbent [Table 1, p. 264]. However, the inferior end of the sternum (xiphoid process) lies approximately at the level of the ninth thoracic vertebra, and the lowest part of the costal margin (eleventh rib in the mid-axillary line) lies at the level of the third lumbar vertebra, close to the iliac crest [Fig. 3]. In elderly individuals, the costal margin may even touch that crest, so that the eleventh rib may be fractured against the crest in lateral flexion of the vertebral column.

In transverse section, the thorax is kidney-shaped because the vertebral bodies and the posterior parts of the ribs which articulate with them project anteriorly into it. This leaves a deep **paravertebral groove** on each side formed by the backwards and lateral sweep of the posterior parts of the ribs. The rounded posterior parts of the lungs lie in these grooves. The contents of the mediastinum for the most part lie anterior to the vertebral bodies [Fig. 12].

Bones and surface anatomy

Thoracic vertebrae

These vary in size and shape from above downwards. A middle, or typical thoracic vertebra has the following elements [Figs. 4, 5], but all can be recognized by the presence of at least one articular facet on the body for articulation with a rib.

The heart-shaped **body** lies anteriorly; the vertebral arch surrounds a circular **vertebral foramen** posterior to the body. The **vertebral arch** consists of a pedicle and a lamina on each side. The **pedicle** forms the lateral wall of the vertebral foramen. It extends backwards from the posterolateral surface of the body to the base of the stout transverse process [Fig. 4] where it also meets the **lamina**. The two laminae form the roof of the vertebral foramen. Each passes medially and backwards from the junction of the transverse process and the pedicle to join its fellow at the base of the spine. The **spine** projects downwards and backwards in the midline so that its palpable tip lies at the level of the upper part of the vertebral body two below the vertebra from which it originates. Thus the spines overlap each other like slates on a roof, effectively hiding the small intervals between the laminae of adjacent vertebrae.

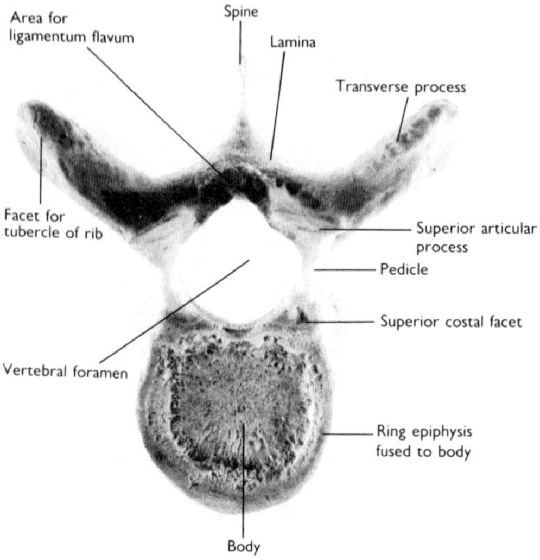

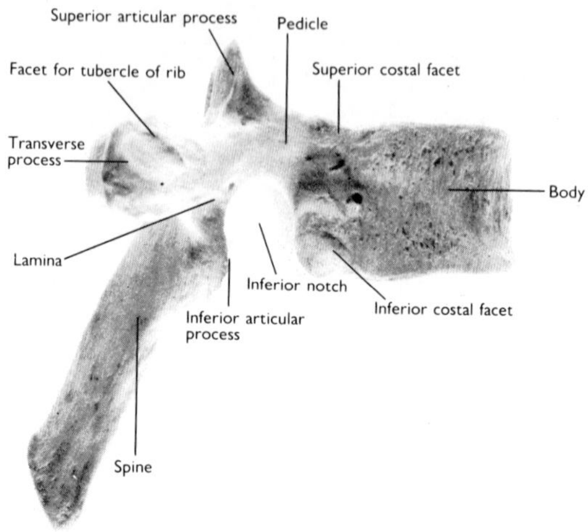

Fig 4 *(left)*. The superior surface of the seventh thoracic vertebra.

Fig 5 *(right)*. The right surface of the seventh thoracic vertebra.

The pedicle on each side is deeply notched inferiorly (**inferior vertebral notch**) to form the superior margin of an **intervertebral foramen**. The anterior margin of the foramen is formed by the posterolateral edge of the vertebral body and of the intervertebral disc between it and the body of the vertebra below. The remainder of the foramen is formed by the vertebra below: inferiorly, by the slightly notched margin of the pedicle; posteriorly, by the anterior surface of the wedge-shaped superior articular process. Each intervertebral foramen transmits the spinal nerve corresponding to the upper of the two vertebrae, large **intervertebral veins**, and a small spinal artery. It is the proximity of the spinal nerve to the disc that explains its involvement in rupture of the disc posterolaterally in the cervical and lumbar regions.

The **superior articular process** projects superiorly from the junction of the pedicle and lamina. It ends in a sharp margin superiorly. The smooth posterior surface of the process is covered with hyaline cartilage which articulates with the anterior surface of the **inferior articular process** of the vertebra above. In the thoracic vertebrae, the inferior process is the inferolateral angle of the rectangular lamina. The articulating surfaces of

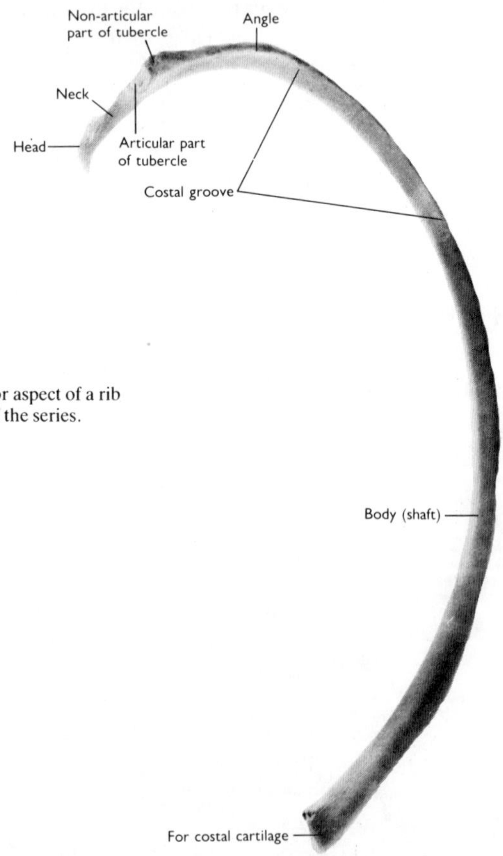

Fig. 6. The inferior aspect of a rib from the middle of the series.

these processes lie on an arc of a circle whose centre is in the vertebral body. Thus they permit slight rotatory movements of the vertebrae on each other around a vertical axis passing through the vertebral bodies [Fig. 93].

The stout **transverse processes** project posterolaterally. Each is grooved on the anterolateral surface of its tip by a concave smooth area which articulates with the tubercle of the corresponding rib. Medial to this, the anterior surface of the process gives attachment to the **costotransverse ligament** from the neck of the rib.

Immediately anterior to the lower part of the intervertebral foramen, the head of a rib articulates with the posterolateral surface of the intervertebral disc above its own vertebra and with the adjacent parts of both vertebral bodies. Hence the body of a typical thoracic vertebra has two articular facets on each side [Fig. 5]. The upper articulates with the lower facet on the head of the corresponding rib, the lower with the upper facet on the head of the rib below: an arrangement which places the head of the rib at a slightly higher level than the tubercle in the middle ribs of the series.

Variations

The first and the last two or three thoracic vertebrae differ from the remainder in having a complete facet for the head of the corresponding rib which articulates at a relatively lower level. This brings the articulations of the heads and tubercles of the first ribs on the two sides into the same horizontal plane and allows them to move together like a hinge with four bearings. The last two thoracic vertebrae have very small transverse processes which do not articulate with their ribs. This, combined with the failure of the costal cartilages of these ribs to articulate with those of other ribs, makes these ribs highly mobile (**floating ribs**). The **inferior articular processes** of the twelfth thoracic vertebra are lumbar in type, their convex articular surfaces facing laterally and anteriorly to fit within the concave, superior articular facets of the first lumbar vertebra. This sudden transition from thoracic intervertebral articulations, which permit slight rotation, to lumbar articulations, which effectively prevent it [Fig. 93], throws particularly heavy stresses on this region of the vertebral column which is frequently involved in fractures. The lower thoracic spines become progressively shorter and less oblique so that they approximate to the rectangular lumbar type of spine. The bodies of the thoracic vertebrae enlarge from above downwards in keeping with the increasing load which each has to carry.

Thoracic **intervertebral discs** are thin by comparison with the lumbar and cervical discs. This, together with the presence of the ribs and the overlapping spinous processes, greatly restricts movement in the thoracic region.

Ribs

These are curved strips of bone slightly twisted on their long axes. Posteriorly, they are more cylindrical and each ends in an expanded **head**.

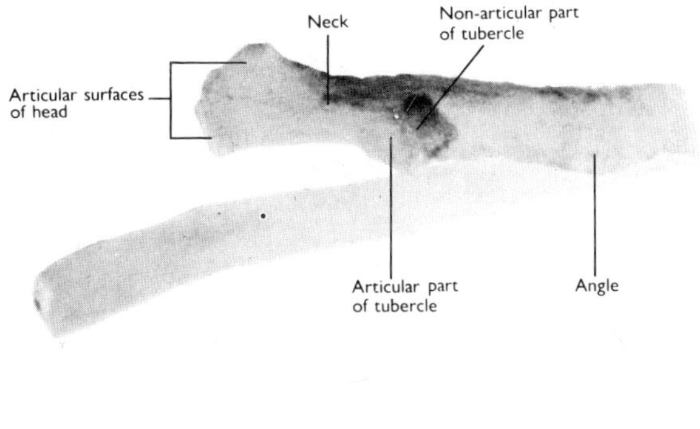

Fig. 7. The sixth right rib seen from behind.

This has the shape of a blunt arrow-head except in the first and the last two or three ribs where it is rounded. The apex of the head articulates with t[h]e intervertebral disc superior to its vertebra, while the sloping sides artic[ulate] with the adjacent vertebral bodies. The head is continuous with the slightly narrower **neck**. This extends to the tubercle. The **tubercle** is situated on the postero-inferior aspect of the rib and has two parts. The medial, rounded part articulates with the transverse process of the vertebra, the lateral part gives attachment to the **lateral costotransverse ligament** from the tip of that process. Lateral to this is the **body** of the rib. Posteriorly the external surface of the body is roughened by the attachment of the erector spinae muscles. This is limited laterally by a vertical ridge which marks the attachment of the **thoracolumbar fascia** which covers these muscles. Here the body of the rib is angled slightly forwards (**angle of the rib**) and continues antero-inferiorly in the curve of the chest wall. Anteriorly, it is fused to its costal cartilage which is inserted into a conical pit in the extremity of the rib.

Fig. 8. First and second right ribs as seen from above.

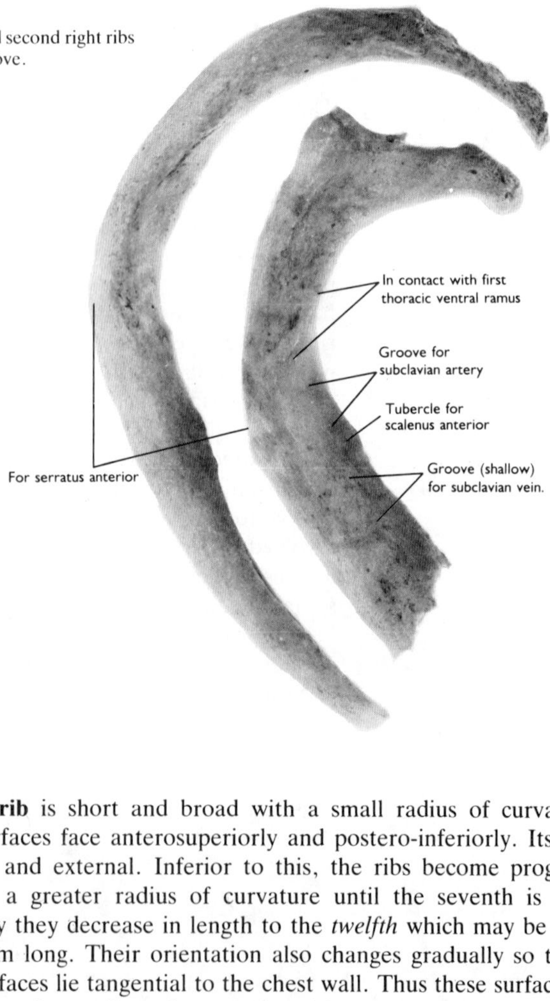

The **first rib** is short and broad with a small radius of curvature. Its flattened surfaces face anterosuperiorly and postero-inferiorly. Its margins are internal and external. Inferior to this, the ribs become progressively longer with a greater radius of curvature until the seventh is reached. Subsequently they decrease in length to the *twelfth* which may be no more than 7–10 cm long. Their orientation also changes gradually so that their flattened surfaces lie tangential to the chest wall. Thus these surfaces of the middle ribs face internally and externally, with superior and inferior margins, while those of the lowest ribs face upwards and inwards and downwards and outwards. The internal surfaces are smooth for they abut on the membrane (**pleura**) which lines the chest wall overlying the lungs. The external surfaces and margins are roughened by the attachment of muscles. The internal surface of most of the ribs is grooved (**costal groove**) posteriorly by the intercostal vessels and nerve. This makes the inferior margin sharp while the superior margin is rounded. Both margins give attachment to intercostal muscles except in the case of the first and twelfth ribs.

All ribs run downwards and forwards in the chest wall. The articulation of the tubercle is posterior to that of the head. These two features ensure that the anteroposterior and transverse diameters of the thorax are increased when the ribs are raised [Figs. 9, 10; p. 78]. The increase in transverse diameter is greater in those ribs in which the tubercle articulates at a lower level than the head.

Sternum

This is a flat bone which lies in the middle of the anterior surface of the thoracic wall. It consists of manubrium, body, and xiphoid process [Fig. 11].

The **manubrium** slopes downwards and forwards and is thicker and wider than the other two more vertical parts. The superior margin of the manubrium has three notches. In the midline, the **jugular notch** can be felt in the front of the root of the neck. On each side a clavicular notch articulates with the medial end of a clavicle which projects above the sternum. Immediately below each clavicular notch, the first costal cartilage (frequently ossified) fuses with the lateral margin of the manubrium. Then the manubrium narrows to the sternal angle where it articulates with the body of the sternum through the fibrocartilaginous disc of the manubriosternal joint. The second costal cartilages articulate with the sides of the disc and the adjacent parts of the manubrium and body by synovial joints.

The **sternal angle,** obtuse anteriorly, is readily palpable even in the obese. It forms a landmark for the **second costal cartilage** and rib and permits the identification of the other ribs by counting downwards from the second, the first rib being hidden by the clavicle. The angle also marks the horizontal level which separates the superior from the other parts of the mediastinum.

The **body of the sternum** is flat and widens from above downwards. It consists of four fused parts. The third to fifth **costal cartilages** articulate with the margins of the body at the junctions of these parts; the sixth articulates with the lowest part; the seventh with the junction of the lowest part and the xiphoid process. All these are synovial joints.

The thin **xiphoid process**—a cartilaginous plate, often perforated, that ossifies slowly throughout life—is fused with the postero-inferior margin of the body of the sternum (**xiphosternal joint**) leaving a depression, the **epigastric fossa** or 'pit of the stomach', anterior to the process. This lies in the infrasternal angle between the anterior ends of the costal margins.

The sternum, covered only by skin, superficial fascia, and periosteum, except where the pectoralis major muscles arise from its margins, is a readily accessible bone which contains red marrow. This may be obtained for study by perforating the cortex of the bone with a wide-bore needle and aspirating the soft tissue—sternal puncture.

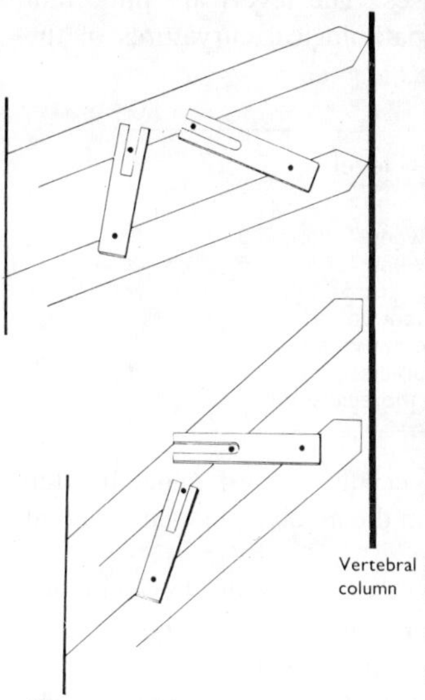

Fig. 9. A diagram to demonstrate that depression of the ribs decreases the anteroposterior diameter of the thorax. Note also that the internal intercostal muscle fibres are elongated in elevation of the ribs, while muscle fibres of the external intercostal muscle are shortened. The opposite occurs in depression of the ribs, i.e. on expiration.

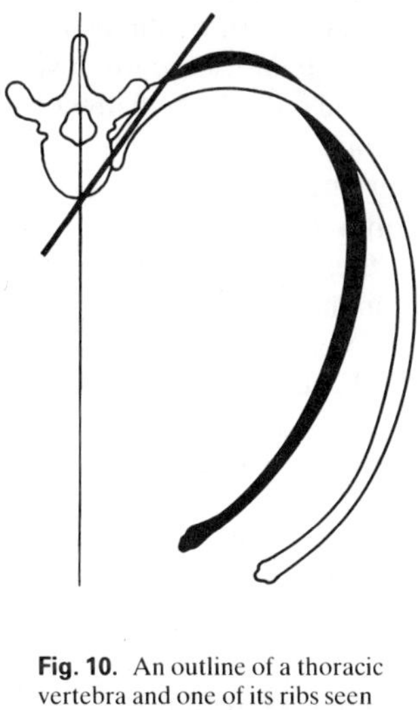

Fig. 10. An outline of a thoracic vertebra and one of its ribs seen from above. The rib is shown in the elevated (white) and depressed (black) positions. The axis of this movement is the solid line passing through the head, neck, and base of the tubercle of the rib. The diagram shows how the anteroposterior and transverse dimensions of the thorax are increased by elevation of the ribs.

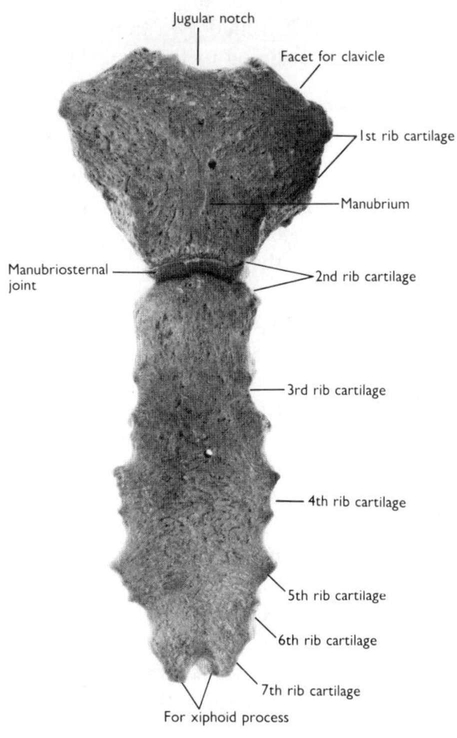

Fig. 11. Sternum (anterior view). The xiphoid process is missing.

Approximate vertebral levels

[Table 1, p. 264]

The levels given here and elsewhere are only approximate because of the movements of the thoracic cage and its contents. They also vary with the position of the body, standing or recumbent, and with the physical type and age of the individual. In the aged, the sternum tends to sag to a lower level and the thoracic vertebral curvature increases. The levels are important because they may be grossly disturbed by pathological curvatures of the vertebral column and by disease of the lungs.

Structure	Vertebral level
Jugluar notch	Disc between T.2 and T.3
Sternal angle	Disc between T.4 and T.5
Xiphosternal joint	Ninth thoracic vertebra
Tip of ninth costal cartilage	First lumbar vertebra
Lowest part of costal margin	Third lumbar vertebra
Root of spine of scapula	Third thoracic spine
Inferior angle of scapula	Seventh thoracic spine

The **nipple** is very variable in position, especially in the female. It often overlies the fourth intercostal space 10 cm from the median plane in the adult male.

All **thoracic vertebral spines** are palpable. The first is the lower of two knobs at the root of the back of the neck. The upper knob, the **vertebra prominens**, is formed by the spine of the seventh cervical vertebra.

The lateral surfaces of the upper **ribs** may be palpated by pressing the fingers upwards into the axilla with the arm by the side to relax the fascia of the axillary floor. The lower ribs are readily palpable except the twelfth which may not project beyond the lateral margin of the erector spinae muscle which covers the posteromedial parts of all the ribs. The posterolateral parts of the second to eighth ribs are covered by the scapula and so are not palpable.

Lungs

The lungs are a pair of sponge-like, elastic organs. They fill the greater part of the cavity of the chest, and consist of a myriad (approximately 300×10^6) of minute, air-filled cavities (**alveoli**). These are connected to the windpipe by the branching system of **bronchi** and **bronchioles**. The walls of the alveoli are formed by a thin layer of flattened epithelium which is continuous with the lining of the bronchial tree. This is all that separates the air in the alveoli from the pulmonary capillaries. Usually the alveoli abut on each other so that the pulmonary capillaries form a thin layer interspersed with **elastic tissue**, with alveolar epithelium on each side of them. The capillaries are often so close to the epithelium that blood and air are separated only by the flattened cytoplasm of the capillary endothelium and the alveolar epithelium, a barrier 0.002 mm thick. This permits rapid gaseous exchange between the blood and the alveolar air which is constantly changed by respiratory movements.

The total *area of the alveolar walls* in the two lungs is approximately 70 square metres. This, combined with alterations in the rate and depth of respiration, permits complete oxygenation and effective removal of carbon dioxide from the pulmonary blood even when the volume of blood traversing the lungs is greatly increased in exercise. Clearly, any disease process which reduces the area for gas transfer, e.g. any extensive lung infection or the breakdown of alveolar walls in emphysema, or which prevents the ready access of air to the alveoli, e.g. bronchial constriction or obstruction, will reduce the efficiency of the process. Even when transfer and ventilation are unimpaired, the same result may arise from a decrease in the flow of pulmonary blood, e.g. in heart failure, or of its oxygen-carrying capacity, e.g. in severe anaemia. Some of these conditions may require forced respiration even at rest to maintain minimal oxygen requirements.

The **mediastinum** is the broad septum which extends from the vertebral column to the sternum between the lungs. The medial surface of each lung is united to the mediastinum by a narrow **root** through which bronchi, blood and lymph vessels, and nerves enter or leave the lung. Elsewhere each lung is free to move on the surrounding tissues for it is separated from them by a narrow slit—the pleural cavity [Fig. 12].

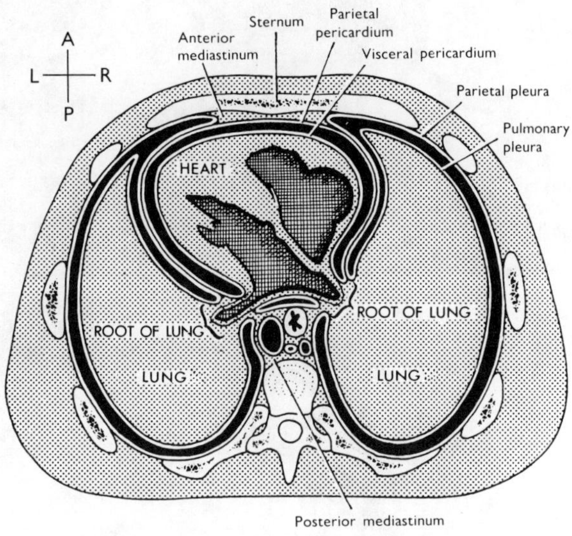

Fig. 12. A diagrammatic horizontal section through the thorax to show the positions of the major structures. The pleural and pericardial cavities are shown in black.

The **pleural cavity** is enclosed by a smooth, glistening membrane (**the pleura**) which covers the external surface of the lung (**pulmonary pleura**) and lines the internal surfaces of the structures which surround it (**parietal pleura**) except where the root of the lung is attached to the mediastinum. Here the pulmonary and parietal parts of the pleura become continuous as a short sleeve surrounding the lung root.

The lungs, and the mediastinum between them, are fitted to the convex upper surface of the diaphragm which separates them from the abdominal contents. Posteriorly and laterally, the periphery of the diaphragm extends downwards to its attachment to the internal surface of the costal margin. Near this attachment the pleura covering the superior surface of the diaphragm (diaphragmatic pleura) meets that lining the thoracic wall at an acute angle (**costodiaphragmatic recess of the pleura**). The sharp inferior margins of the lungs pass into the costodiaphragmatic recesses [Fig. 2] so that the pleural cavities and lungs overlap the contents of the upper abdomen. Thus penetrating wounds of the lower thorax frequently involve the abdomen, and this part of the abdomen is most easily approached by the surgeon through the pleural cavity and diaphragm.

The pleural cavity contains a small quantity of thin serous fluid which lubricates the pleural surfaces and allows them to slide freely on each other. This movement allows the sharp margins of the lungs to slide in and out of the recesses of the pleura, e.g. costodiaphragmatic, as these change in volume with respiration [Fig. 2]. The movement also equalizes pressure changes throughout the pleural cavity irrespective of the part of its wall (thoracic wall or diaphragm) which is moving, thus ensuring equal ventilation of all parts of the lung.

The lungs contain a large quantity of elastic tissue which permits the expansion of all parts of the lung on inspiration. This **elastic tissue,** drawing the lung inwards towards its root, is the main factor in expiration during quiet breathing, and being opposed by the rigid thoracic wall and the diaphragm, produces a subatmospheric pressure within the pleural cavity. Thus air flows into the pleural cavity through any hole in the chest wall or in the surface of the lung and continues to fill the expanding pleural cavity until the lung has completely collapsed on to its root (**pneumothorax**). If the hole is closed, the air in the pleural cavity is gradually absorbed by the pleural blood vessels and the lung expands again as the reduced intrapleural pressure is re-established. Similarly, if a bronchus is blocked, the air in the lung distal to the block is absorbed into the pulmonary blood vessels so that this part of the lung tends to collapse. Continuing respiratory movements cause the remainder of the lung to expand and fill the space vacated by the shrinking lobe or the mediastinum to shift towards that side as the opposite lung is expanded when a large part of one lung is involved. When a large bronchus is blocked and that part of the lung is unable to expand because air cannot enter it, the

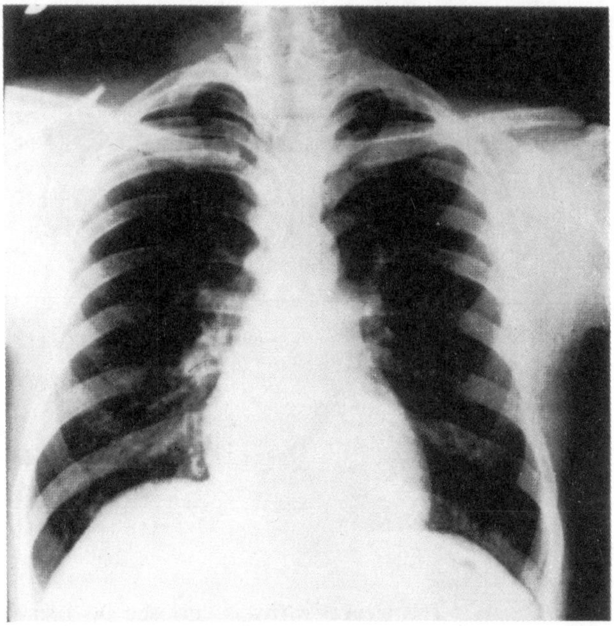

Fig. 13. An anteroposterior radiograph of the thorax in inspiration. Note that the right dome of the diaphragm lies below the level of the tenth rib posteriorly, and the outlines of the diaphragm and the costodiaphragmatic recesses are clear owing to the air content in the lungs.

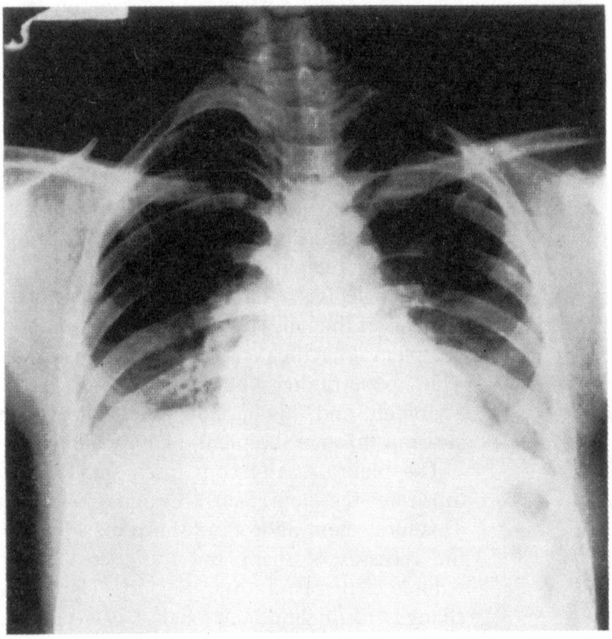

Fig. 14. An anteroposterior radiograph of the same individual as Fig. 13 but in expiration. Note that the right dome of the diaphragm reaches almost to the level of the eighth rib posteriorly, and that the shadow of the diaphragm and the costodiaphragmatic recesses are poorly defined because of the increased density of the basal parts of the lungs due to loss of air and their withdrawal from the recesses. Note also that the heart is shorter and broader in association with the raised diaphragm.

movement of the overlying chest wall is reduced and this can be seen or felt. Because of the clinical importance of these features, it is necessary to know the position of the pleural cavity and the distribution of the branches of the bronchial tree within the lung.

Apertures of the thorax

The **superior aperture** is the obliquely truncated apex of the thorax. The margins of the aperture are the body of the first thoracic vertebra, the first ribs and their cartilages, and the manubrium of the sternum. This aperture slopes steeply downwards and forwards [Fig. 19]. As a result, the apices of the lungs (each surrounded by a dome of parietal pleura) project through the lateral parts of the aperture to reach the level of the neck of the first rib, well above the first costal cartilage. These are separated by the structures which pass between the mediastinum and the upper limbs and neck.

The large **inferior aperture** slopes downwards and backwards. It is formed by the costal margins, the twelfth ribs, and the twelfth thoracic vertebra. It is closed by the diaphragm which is pierced by structures passing between the mediastinum and the abdomen.

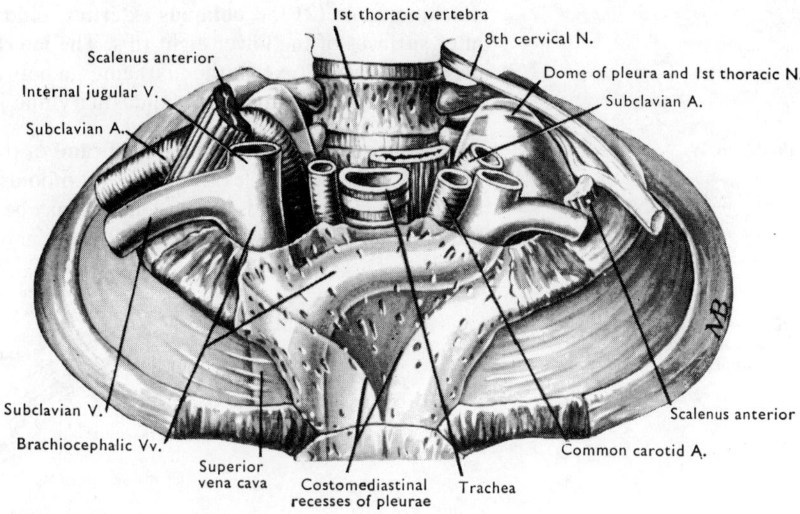

Fig. 15. The superior aperture of the thorax. The anterior margins (costomediastinal recesses) of the pleural sacs and the great veins are shown through the sternum. Cf. Fig. 23.

Respiratory movements

These have already been dealt with but are now summarized [Figs. 9, 10, 13, 14; Table 2, p. 265].

Inspiration

The anteroposterior and transverse diameters of the thorax are increased by raising the ribs. The contracting diaphragm [Fig. 2] lowers its dome. This increases the vertical diameter of the thorax, opens the costodiaphragmatic recesses, and elongates and narrows the mediastinum. Muscles of the posterior abdominal wall hold down the lower ribs to make the diaphragmatic contraction effective.

Expiration

This is the reverse movement. In quiet respiration, it is achieved by the *elastic recoil of the lungs*. In forced expiration, the ribs are pulled down mainly by contraction of the abdominal muscles which also increase the intra-abdominal pressure and force the relaxed diaphragm upwards.

If the elasticity of the lungs is lost, the thorax tends to remain permanently in a position of inspiration. There is also considerable expiratory difficulty and the tidal volume of air in each respiratory cycle is greatly reduced.

The walls of the thorax

Superficial structures

The greater part of the thorax is overlapped by muscles of the upper limb, the remainder by muscles of the abdomen. The **thoracic spinal nerves** supply the walls of the thorax and send cutaneous branches through or between these muscles to the overlying skin. These nerves innervate the thoracic and abdominal muscles but not the muscles of the upper limb. Only the first, or the first and second, thoracic spinal nerves supply muscles of the upper limb and then only through the fibres which they send to the limb through the brachial plexus.

Identify the remnants of the upper limb muscles still attached to the thorax and the blood vessels and nerves which pierce them.

Anteriorly

(1) **Pectoralis major** is attached to the margin of the sternum and the adjacent parts of the upper six costal cartilages. It is pierced near the sternum by the anterior cutaneous branches of the ventral rami (**intercostal nerves**; [Fig. 16]) of the second to fifth thoracic nerves (the first has no anterior cutaneous branch) together with branches of the internal thoracic artery. (2) The **rectus abdominis** is attached to the xiphoid process and the cartilages of the seventh to fifth ribs. (3) **Pectoralis minor** is attached to the third to fifth ribs near their costal cartilages.

Laterally

(1) **Serratus anterior** is attached to the upper eight ribs on the side of the thorax. Its lower four attachments interdigitate with the upper four

attachments of (2) the **obliquus externus abdominis** which arises from the outer surfaces of the lower eight ribs. The **lateral cutaneous branches** of the intercostal nerves (except the first) emerge between the attachments of these muscles a little anterior to the midaxillary line [Fig. 104].

Posteriorly

The cutaneous branches of the **dorsal rami** of the thoracic nerves have been removed with the muscles trapezius, rhomboids, and latissimus dorsi which they pierce. The cut ends of these nerves may be found where they pierce the thoracolumbar fascia which is deep to these muscles.

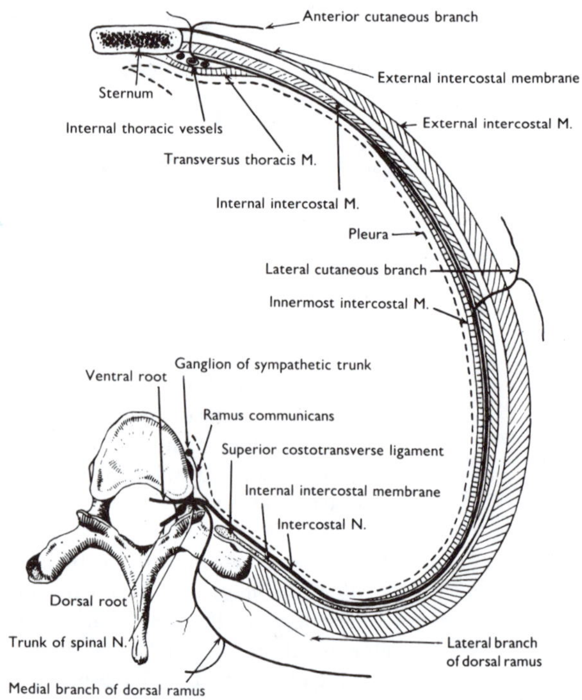

Fig. 16. A diagram of the upper thoracic spinal nerve in an intercostal space.

Dissection

Remove the remains of serratus anterior and the pectoral muscles from the upper ribs, but retain the cutaneous branches of the intercostal nerves. In two or more spaces, note the **external intercostal muscle**—its fibres run antero-inferiorly. Follow it forwards to the external intercostal membrane which replaces it between the costal cartilages.

Cut through the external intercostal membrane and muscle along the lower borders of two spaces. Turn them upwards to expose the **internal intercostal muscle**—its fibres run postero-inferiorly. Now follow the lateral cutaneous branch of one or more intercostal nerves to the parent trunk deep to the internal intercostal muscle. Follow the trunk of the **intercostal nerve** forwards and backwards with the accompanying vessels, cutting away as much of the lower margin of the rib and internal intercostal muscle as is necessary to expose them. Note the branches of the nerve to the intercostal muscles and its collateral branch lying along the upper margin of the rib below. The muscle which lies deep to the nerve and vessels is the **innermost intercostal muscle**. This muscle is absent anteriorly and posteriorly [Fig. 16]. Here the nerve and vessels lie on the parietal pleura except where transversus thoracis [Fig. 18] intervenes at the side of the sternum. The innermost intercostal muscles are supplemented internally by the subcostal muscles near the angles of the lower ribs.

Intercostal muscles

Three incomplete layers of muscle lie in each intercostal space—external, internal, and innermost intercostal muscles. In addition there are two small muscles deep to these which may cross more than one intercostal space—transversus thoracis and the subcostals.

The external intercostal muscle fibres run antero-inferiorly; those in the other two run postero-inferiorly. The innermost is differentiated from the internal intercostal only by the presence of the intercostal nerve and vessels between them. They pass, respectively, from the lower margin (external), costal groove (internal), and internal surface above the groove (innermost) of the upper rib to the rounded superior margin of the rib below.

The **external intercostal** extends from the tubercle of the rib almost to the costochondral junction. Anterior to this, it is replaced in the upper spaces by the **external intercostal membrane**. The **internal intercostal** muscle extends from the margin of the sternum to the angle of the rib. Posterior to this, it is replaced by the **internal intercostal membrane**. The **innermost intercostal** is variable. Usually it extends further posteriorly than the internal intercostal and not so far anteriorly as the external intercostal. **Nerve supply**: the intercostal nerves supply all three muscles. **Actions**: all three muscles prevent the intercostal spaces from being drawn in during inspiration or forced out during forced expiration. The external intercostal is active during inspiration and shortens [Fig. 9]. The internal and innermost intercostals shorten during expiration and are active during that movement.

Intercostal nerves

These are the ventral rami of the first to the eleventh thoracic spinal nerves. The twelfth (**subcostal nerve**) lies in the abdominal wall below the twelfth rib. The greater part of the first (and sometimes the second) passes to the brachial plexus.

Each intercostal nerve emerges from the intervertebral foramen inferior to the corresponding vertebra. The nerve then runs in the intercostal space. Here it is deep to the internal intercostal membrane and the internal intercostal muscle, and superficial to the innermost intercostal muscle in the subcostal groove of the corresponding rib. Where the innermost intercostal muscle is missing, it lies directly on the parietal pleura except where transversus thoracis and the internal thoracic vessels intervene close to the sternum [Fig. 16]. One centimetre from the sternum it turns forwards to end as the anterior cutaneous branch.

Branches

1. As it emerges from the intervertebral foramen it is connected to a ganglion of the sympathetic trunk by two branches (rami communicantes). One, the **white ramus communicans**, carries preganglionic nerve fibres from the nerve to the ganglion; the other, the **grey ramus communicans**, carries nerve fibres from the ganglion to the nerve for distribution through all the branches of that spinal nerve. These are **postganglionic sympathetic nerve fibres**.

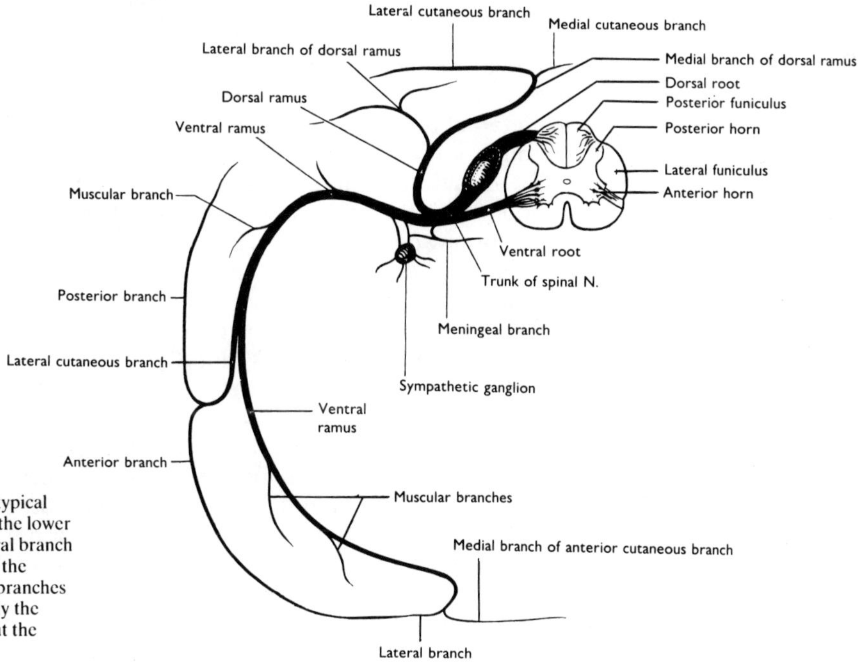

Fig. 17. A diagram of a typical thoracic spinal nerve. In the lower half of the trunk the lateral branch of the dorsal ramus gives the cutaneous branch. Both branches of the dorsal ramus supply the erector spinae throughout the trunk.

2. A **collateral branch** arises near the angle of the rib. It runs along the upper margin of the rib below to supply the intercostal muscles. It may rejoin the parent stem, or be absent.

3. The **lateral cutaneous branch** arises beyond the angle of the rib. It is thicker than the continuation of the nerve. It pierces the internal and external intercostal muscles obliquely about halfway round the chest and divides into anterior and posterior branches.

4. The **anterior cutaneous branch** pierces the internal intercostal muscle, the external intercostal membrane, and pectoralis major. It divides into medial and lateral branches.

5. **Muscular branches** supply the intercostal, subcostal, transversus thoracis, and serratus posterior muscles. *They do not supply any of the limb muscles which arise from the thorax.*

The above description applies only to the third to sixth intercostal nerves. The **first** and **second** run the early part of their course on the pleural surfaces of the corresponding ribs. The first has no lateral or anterior cutaneous branch. The second has a large lateral cutaneous branch to the floor of the axilla and the medial side of the arm (**intercostobrachial nerve**). The **seventh** to the **eleventh** intercostal nerves run an increasing part of their course in the abdominal wall and supply the skin and muscles of that wall. They enter it at the anterior ends of their intercostal spaces either directly (tenth and eleventh) or deep to the upturned end of the next costal cartilage. These lower thoracic ventral rami supply most of the skin and muscles of the abdominal wall. The anterior cutaneous branches of the fifth to twelfth pierce the rectus abdominis muscle and its sheath to reach the skin. Those of the ninth and tenth supply skin in the region of the **umbilicus**.

Intercostal arteries and veins

Each intercostal space receives three arteries. The largest is the single **posterior intercostal artery**. This accompanies the intercostal nerve and also gives a collateral branch along the superior margin of the lower rib. Both arteries end by anastomosing with the two smaller **anterior intercostal arteries**. These enter the space either from the internal thoracic artery [Fig. 18] in the upper six spaces, or from its musculophrenic branch in the seventh to ninth spaces. The corresponding **anterior intercostal veins** drain into the musculophrenic and internal thoracic veins. In the last two spaces there are no anterior intercostal arteries; the posterior intercostal artery and its collateral branch continue into the anterior abdominal wall. The arteries and veins which lie subjacent to the **mammary gland** and play a part in supplying it become greatly enlarged during pregnancy and lactation.

The remaining parts of the posterior intercostal arteries and veins will be seen later.

Dissection

Remove the intercostal muscles and membrane from the anterior parts of the first and second intercostal spaces. This exposes a part of the **internal thoracic artery** and veins about 1 cm from the side of the sternum.

Cut transversely through the manubrium of the sternum immediately inferior to its junction with the first costal cartilage. Take care not to carry the saw deeper than the bone. Cut through the parietal pleura in the first intercostal space on both sides. Carry this cut as far back as possible. Then cut inferiorly through the second and subsequent ribs and intercostal spaces from the posterior end of the pleural incision to the level of the xiphosternal joint. Cut through the internal thoracic vessels in the first intercostal space. Gently elevate the inferior part of the sternum with the costal cartilages and anterior parts of the ribs. Close to the midline, the parietal pleura passes from the back of the sternum on to the mediastinum on both sides. Cut through this pleura where it leaves the sternum. As the anterior part of the sternum is lifted away and hinged on the superior part of the abdominal wall, continue to cut through the pleura along the line of its reflexion from the sternum on to the mediastinum, to the level of the lower border of the heart. Note the position of this reflexion and its differences on the two sides [Fig. 25]. When the anterior thoracic wall has been hinged downwards, trace the cut edges of **parietal pleura** and note its smooth internal surface where it lines the thoracic wall and covers the lateral aspects of the mediastinum.

Strip the pleura and the endothoracic fascia external to it from the back of the sternum and costal cartilages. This exposes the transversus thoracis muscle and the internal thoracic vessels [Fig. 18]. If the line on which the thoracic wall is hinged downwards is lower than the inferior border of the heart, the anterior attachments of the diaphragm to the xiphoid process and costal cartilages will be stretched and torn. Note these attachments and divide them as necessary. This exposes the upper part of the transversus abdominis muscle and the posterior wall of the fibrous sheath of the rectus abdominis muscle.

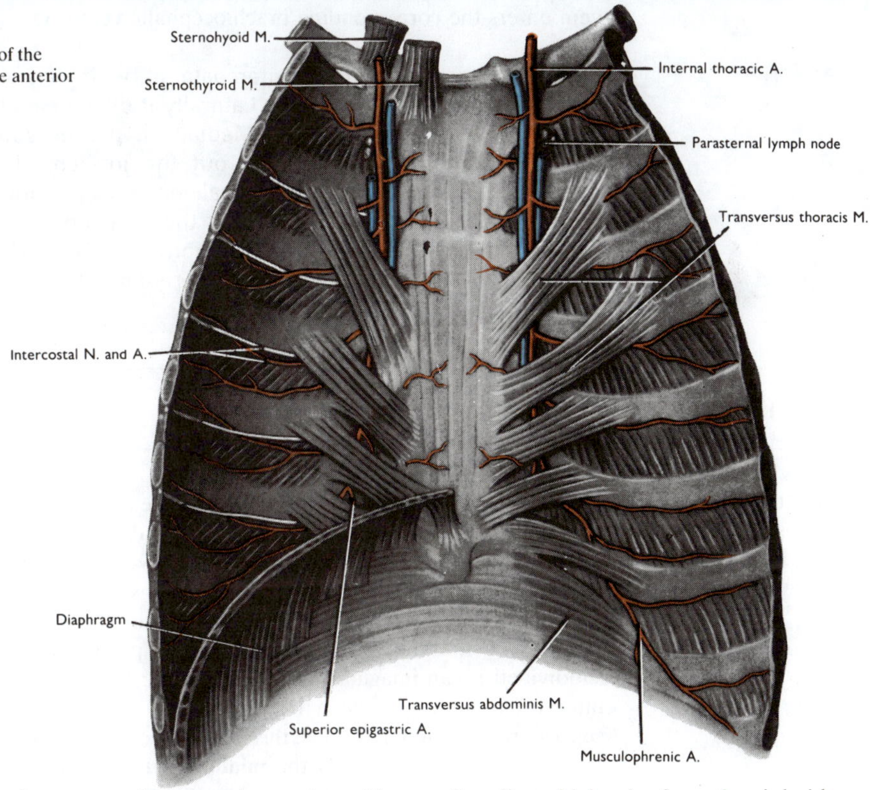

Fig. 18. A dissection of the posterior surface of the anterior thoracic wall.

Transversus thoracis

This muscle consists of four or five slips which arise from the xiphoid process and the lower part of the body of the sternum. They pass superolaterally to the second to sixth costal cartilages close to their junctions with the ribs. This muscle is continuous inferiorly with the deepest muscle of the anterior abdominal wall, the **transversus abdominis. Nerve supply**: the corresponding intercostal nerves. **Action**: a weak expiratory muscle.

Internal thoracic artery

This artery descends from the first part of the subclavian artery posterior to the medial ends of the clavicle and first costal cartilage. This part of its course can be exposed by dissecting upwards from the cut end of the artery to find the small pericardiacophrenic branch to the phrenic nerve [Fig. 22]. The internal thoracic artery descends about 1 cm from the margin of the sternum, anterior to the pleura and transversus thoracis and posterior to the upper six costal cartilages, the spaces between them, and the terminal parts of the intercostal nerves. It ends by dividing into superior epigastric and musculophrenic arteries at the sixth intercostal space [Fig. 18].

Branches

(1) Many small branches to the sternum, thymus, and pericardium. (2) The anterior intercostal arteries to the upper six spaces. (3) **Perforating branches** which accompany the anterior cutaneous branches of the intercostal nerves. These are large in the second, third, and fourth spaces in the female, for they help to supply the **mammary gland**. The corresponding veins and a number

of invisible **lymph vessels** run with these perforating branches. The lymph vessels drain the anterior thoracic wall and the medial part of the mammary gland. They pass to small **parasternal lymph nodes** which lie along the internal thoracic artery. (4) **Superior epigastric artery**. This branch passes between the sternal and costal origins of the diaphragm into the sheath of the rectus muscle in the anterior abdominal wall. Here it anastomoses with the inferior epigastric branch of the external iliac artery and thus unites the arteries of the upper and lower limbs. (5) **Musculophrenic artery**. This branch runs inferolaterally along the superior surface of the costal origin of the diaphragm deep to the costal cartilages. Near the eighth costal cartilage it pierces the diaphragm and runs on its abdominal surface to supply it.

Internal thoracic veins

Two venae comitantes of each internal thoracic artery drain the territory supplied by it and usually unite opposite the third costal cartilage. This single vein enters the corresponding brachiocephalic vein [Fig. 52].

Dissection

Find the anterior part of the intercostal nerve in one or more spaces. Trace it laterally and medially. Laterally it disappears external to the innermost intercostal muscle. Medially it passes superficial to the internal thoracic vessels. Clean out the intercostal spaces in the reflected flap of anterior thoracic wall leaving a part intact close to the cut ends of the ribs. The flap may then be replaced in its original position so that the relation between the ribs and the subjacent organs may be determined as these are dissected.

The cavity of the thorax

Mediastinum
[Figs. 276–282]

The mediastinum is the bulky septum between the pleural cavities and their contained lungs. Though it is thick and extends from the root of the neck to the diaphragm and from the sternum to the vertebral column [Fig. 20], it is relatively mobile in the fresh state. Thus it is elongated in inspiration and may be displaced to one side or the other if the pressures in the two pleural cavities are not the same. For descriptive purposes, the mediastinum is subdivided by an imaginary horizontal plane from the sternal angle to the intervertebral disc between the fourth and fifth thoracic vertebrae. The **superior mediastinum** lies above this plane. Below the plane, the mediastinum is further subdivided into: (1) the **middle mediastinum** which consists of the heart in the pericardial sac with a phrenic nerve on each side; (2) the **anterior mediastinum** between the pericardium and the sternum; (3) the **posterior mediastinum** between the pericardium and diaphragm anteriorly and the vertebral column posteriorly [Fig. 19].

The superior mediastinum has a smaller anteroposterior depth than the remainder; indeed the superior thoracic aperture is only 5 cm anteroposteriorly. The posterior mediastinum extends furthest inferiorly because it passes into the angle between the diaphragm and the vertebral column to reach down to the level of the twelfth thoracic vertebra [Fig. 19].

Lateral parts of thoracic cavity and pleura

On each side is a **pleural cavity** almost completely filled by a lung. Each lung is covered with a smooth, glistening layer of **pulmonary pleura** except on a limited part of its medial surface where the structures in the root of the lung are continuous with those in the medistinum. Here the pulmonary pleura which surrounds the root is continuous with the **parietal pleura** which covers the surface of the mediastinum (**mediastinal pleura**). The pleura which surrounds the root of the lung extends inferiorly as a narrow fold (the **pulmonary ligament**). This attaches the pleura on the medial surface of the lung below the root to the adjacent mediastinal pleura [Figs. 40, 41].

This arrangement arises because the embryonic lung grows laterally into the pleural cavity and carries the medial wall of that cavity with it as a covering (pulmonary pleura). The lung then expands outwards to fill the

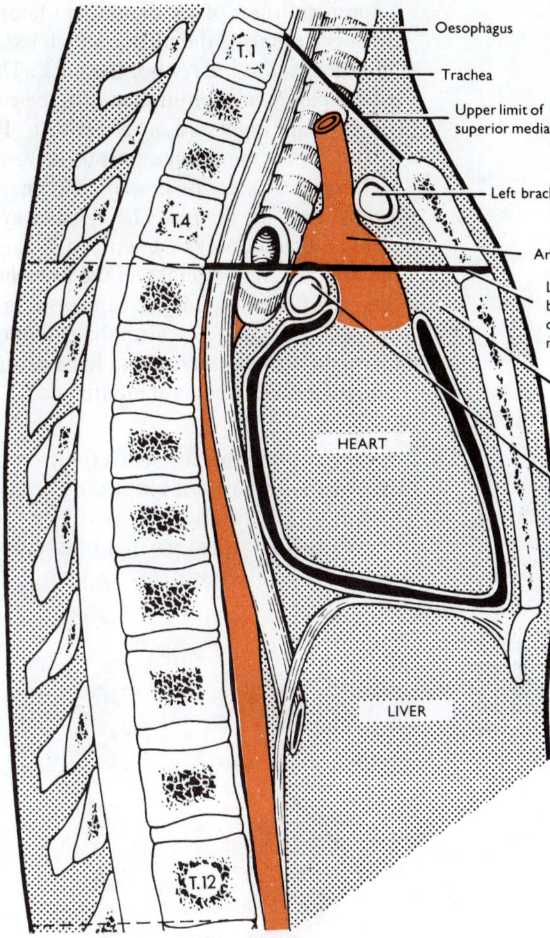

Fig. 19. A diagram of a median section through the thorax to show the general disposition of the ructures in the mediastinum. The art in the pericardium forms the ddle mediastinum, while the anterior and posterior mediastina lie between it and the sternum and vertebral column respectively; the posterior mediastinum also extends downwards behind the diaphragm.

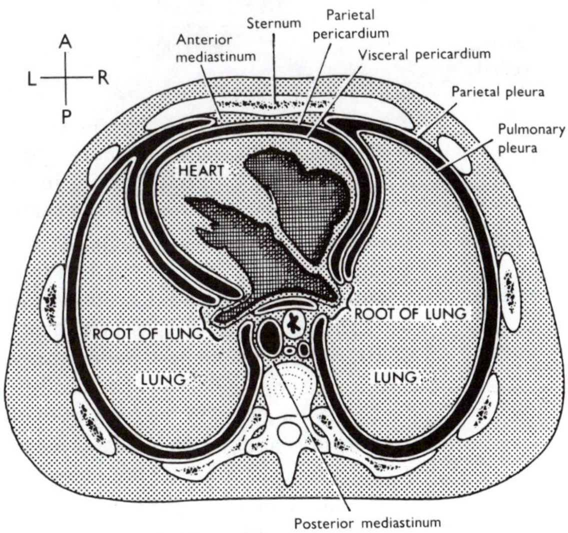

Fig. 20. A diagrammatic horizontal section through the thorax to show the positions of the major structures. The pleural and pericardial cavities are shown in black. See also Figs. 276–282.

cavity which is reduced to a mere slit between the outer wall of the cavity (parietal pleura) and the surface of the lung (pulmonary pleura). The original point of outgrowth from the mediastinum remains as the relatively narrow **root of the lung** around which the pulmonary and parietal parts of the pleura are continuous with each other. The same arrangement, which permits free movement of organs within the body, is found in the case of the heart in the pericardial cavity and the gut in the peritoneal cavity, though the method of development is not the same.

The **mediastinal pleura** is continuous with the other parts of the parietal pleura. (1) Anteriorly and posteriorly with the **costal pleura** which lines the thoracic wall. (2) Inferiorly, with the **diaphragmatic pleura** which covers the superior surface of the diaphragm lateral to the mediastinum. (3) Superiorly, with the **dome of the pleura** which extends through the superior aperture of the thorax into the root of the neck. The diaphragmatic pleura and the dome of the pleura are continuous with the costal pleura respectively at the margins of the diaphragm and of the first rib. Parietal pleura differs from pulmonary pleura in having a thick fibrous layer (endothoracic fascia) externally.

If the pleural cavity is opened in an individual who has suffered no disease of the lung, the lung may be lifted away from the parietal pleura except at the root and pulmonary ligament. In the aged it is common to find that the pulmonary and parietal pleurae are adherent at various points because of the spread of inflammatory or cancerous processes from the lung. Such adhesion makes it difficult to confirm the extent of the pleural cavity by dissection. Nevertheless, the cavity should be carefully explored and the root of the lung and pulmonary ligament identified.

Dissection

Pull the lung laterally from the mediastinum and find its root with the pulmonary ligament extending downwards from it. Cut through these structures from above downwards close to the lung. Remove the lung on each side and store in a plastic bag to prevent drying. Examine the extent of the pleural cavity.

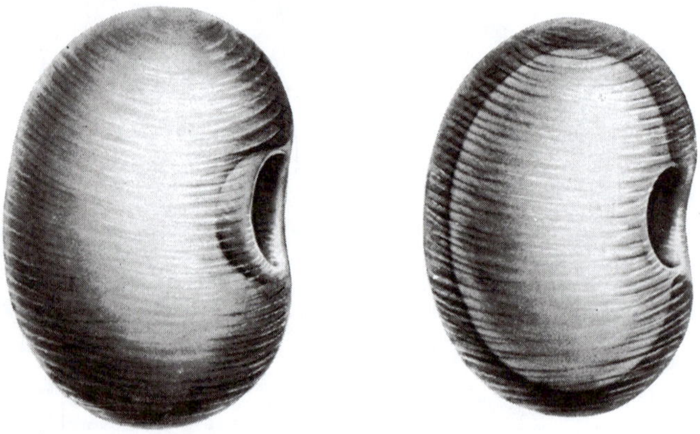

Fig. 21. A diagram to show how a structure may grow into a cavity carrying part of the wall in front of it as a covering. By expanding within the cavity the structure reduces it to a mere slit between the outer shell (parietal layer) and the layer intimately covering the structure (visceral layer). A thin film of fluid separates these two layers and allows free movement of the structure and the visceral layer within the parietal layer. This is the arrangement of the lung within the pleural cavity. The heart in the pericardial cavity and the gut in the peritoneal cavity are similarly placed, though the method of development is not exactly the same.

Dome of pleura

This part of the parietal pleura bulges up into the root of the neck from the internal margin of the first rib. Its apex rises to the level of the neck of the first rib, but is 3.5 cm above the anterior end of that rib and 1–2 cm above the medial third of the clavicle because of the obliquity of the first rib. The right and left domes are separated by the midline structures of the neck (trachea and oesophagus) and the blood vessels passing to and from the neck.

The **subclavian vessels** arch over the anterior surface of the dome, the artery near its highest point, the vein antero-inferior to the artery. The internal thoracic artery descends on the front of the dome from the subclavian artery to the back of the first costal cartilage. Between these two structures and the dome is a layer of dense fascia (**suprapleural membrane**) which spreads from the transverse process of the seventh cervical vertebra to the internal margin of the first rib. The membrane may contain some muscle fibres (**scalenus minimus**) which tighten it and so help it to maintain the pleural dome despite respiratory changes in intrapleural pressure.

Pleural recesses

These are the parts of the pleural cavity which are not occupied by the lung except in full inspiration. They lie where different parts of the parietal pleura meet at an acute angle and are in apposition except in deep inspiration. The **costomediastinal recess** lies along the anterior margin of the pleura. The **costodiaphragmatic recess** extends inferiorly between the thoracic wall and the lateral and posterior parts of the diaphragm [Figs. 24, 284]. Deep in this recess, where the costal and diaphragmatic parts of the pleura unite, they are bound down to the costal cartilages and diaphragm by a narrow thickening of the endothoracic fascia (**phrenicopleural fascia**).

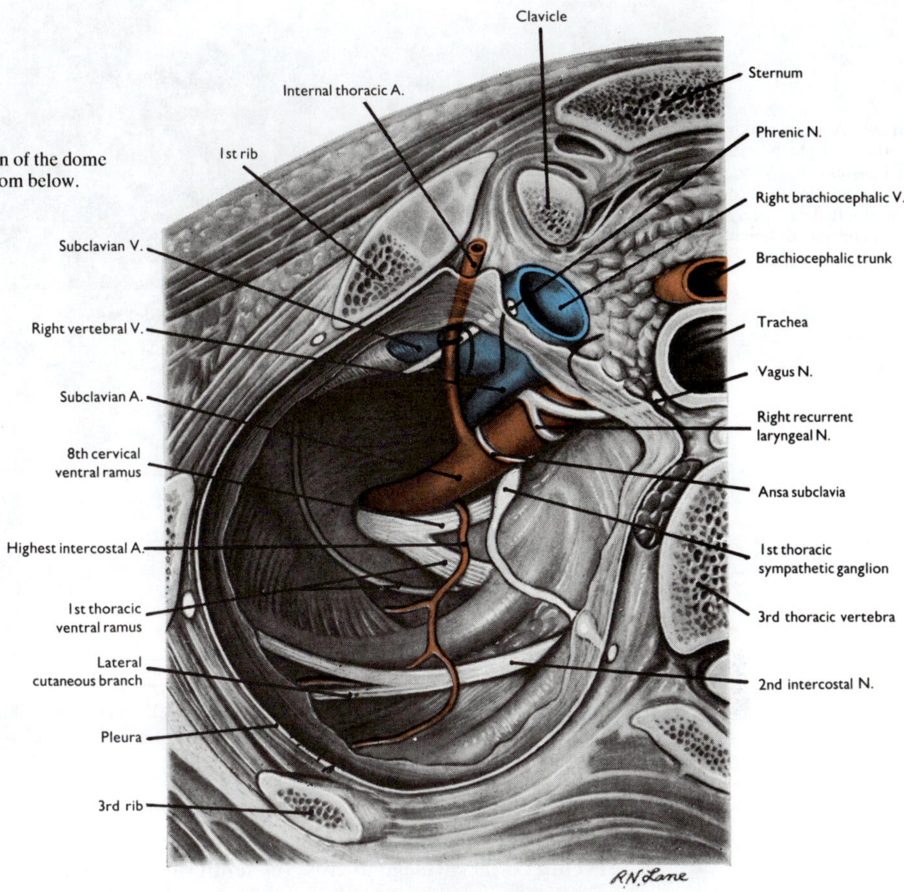

Fig. 22. A dissection of the dome of the pleura seen from below.

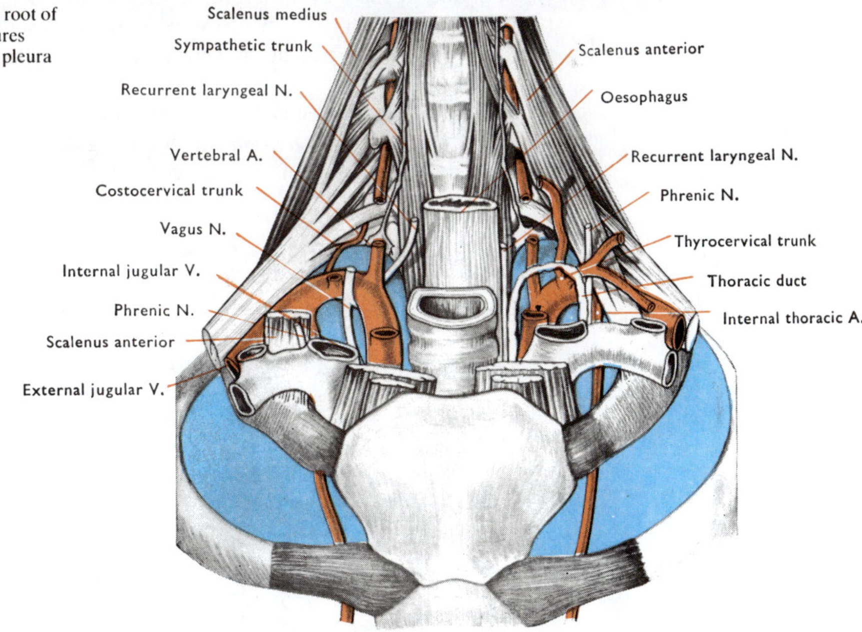

Fig. 23. A dissection of the root of the neck to show the structures adjacent to the dome of the pleura (blue).

Margins of pleural cavity

The *anterior margins* of the two parietal pleural sacs converge as they descend from the domes posterior to the sternoclavicular joints. They abut on each other at the sternal angle and below this remain in apposition to the level of the fourth costal cartilage [Figs. 25, 39]. Here the left pleural margin deviates to the left and descends posterior to the fifth and sixth costal cartilages close to the sternum because of the projecting heart and pericardium. The right pleural margin continues its vertical descent. Each anterior margin becomes continuous with the corresponding inferior margin at the level of the xiphosternal joint.

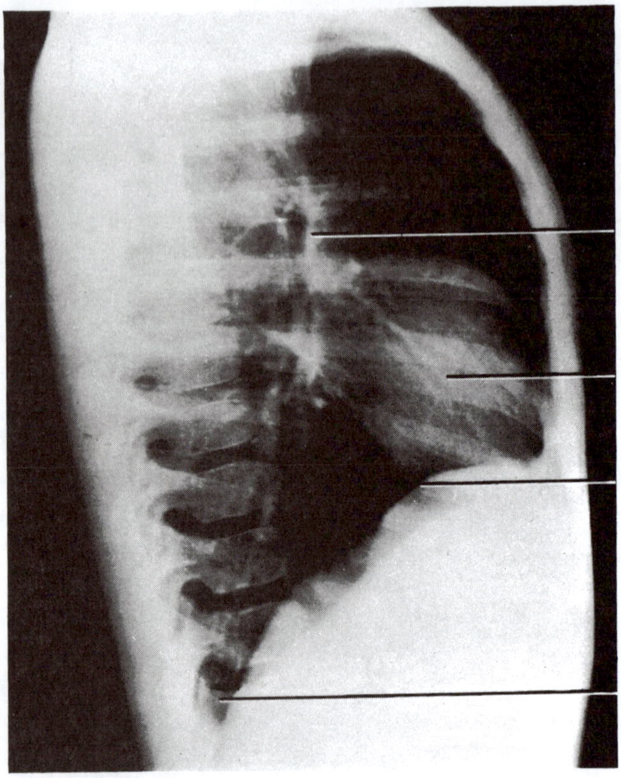

Fig. 24. A lateral radiograph of the thorax. Note the extension of the lung into the costodiaphragmatic recess posterior to the diaphragm and the upper abdominal contents.

Trace the *inferior margin* of each pleural cavity with a finger in the costodiaphragmatic recess. This margin passes postero-inferiorly deep to the seventh costal cartilage to cross the tenth rib in the mid-axillary line, about 5 cm superior to the costal margin. It then passes deep to the eleventh and twelfth ribs to reach the side of the vertebral column inferior to the medial part of the twelfth rib, at the level of the twelfth thoracic spine. It is important to remember that the pleural cavity reaches so far inferiorly, otherwise it may be damaged in clinical procedures on the upper abdomen.

The rounded *posterior margin* extends along the vertebral column from the dome to the end of the inferior margin.

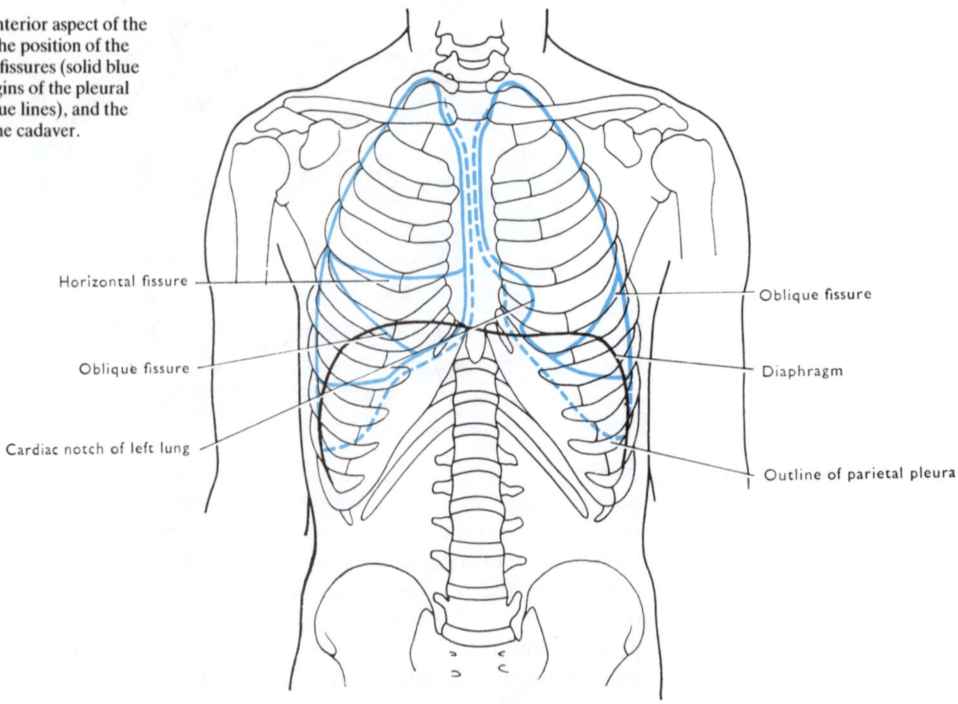

Fig. 25. The anterior aspect of the trunk to show the position of the lungs and their fissures (solid blue lines), the margins of the pleural sacs (broken blue lines), and the diaphragm in the cadaver.

The **inferior margin of the lung** does not extend deep into the costodiaphragmatic recess in quiet respiration. It follows a course from a point lateral to the xiphosternal joint to the eighth rib in the mid-axillary line, i.e. 10 cm above the costal margin, and the level of the tenth thoracic vertebral spine at the vertebral column.

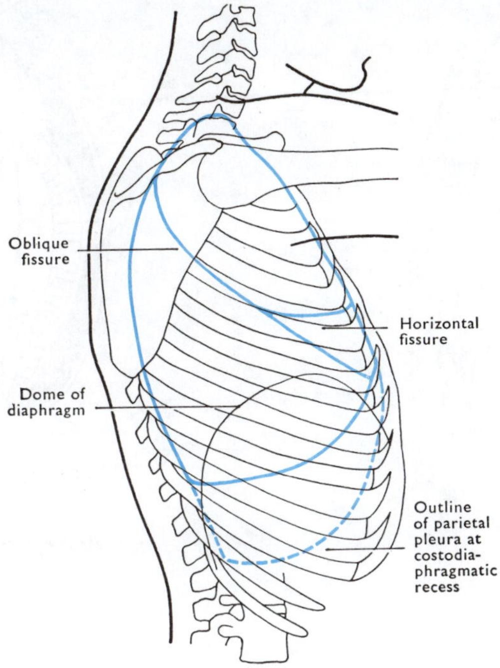

Fig. 26. The right lateral aspect of the trunk to show the position of the right lung and its fissures (solid blue lines), the inferior margin of the parietal pleura (broken blue line), and the diaphragm in the cadaver.

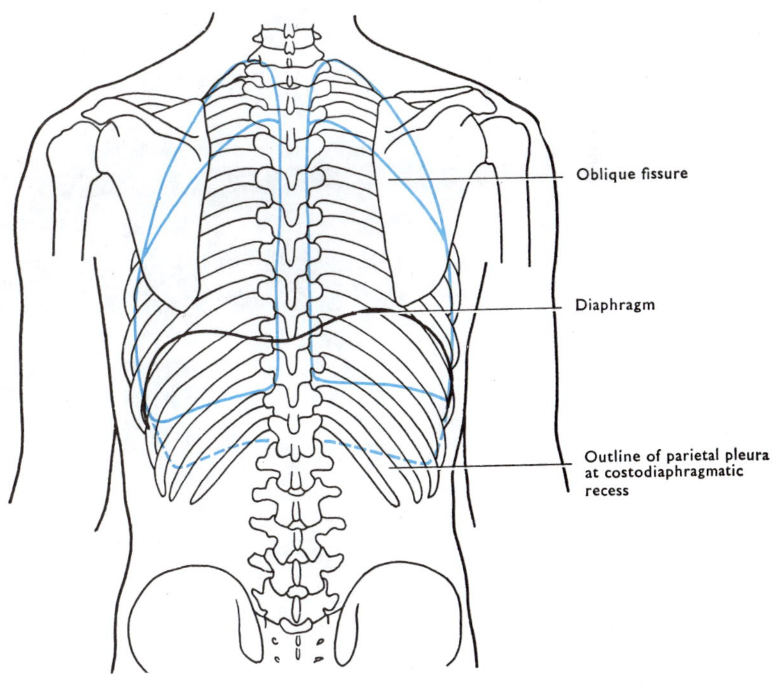

Fig. 27. The posterior aspect of the trunk to show the position of the lungs and their fissures (solid blue lines), the inferior margin of the parietal pleura (broken blue lines), and the diaphragm in the cadaver. In the living, the apices of the lower lobes lie at a lower level (T.5), and the oblique fissures are correspondingly lower.

General structure and position of heart

The human heart and the great arteries which arise from it form a U-shaped tube which lies obliquely across the thorax more or less in the sagittal plane [Figs. 31, 63]. The bend of the U lies antero-inferiorly (close to the sternum) while the ends of the two limbs are in a posterosuperior position (close to the vertebral column) one anterosuperior to the other. The tube is divided longitudinally by a continuous septum into right and left channels. Each channel is further subdivided by two transversely placed valves one of which lies approximately at the middle of each limb of the U. The **valves** in the postero-inferior limb (atrioventricular) separate the ventricles at the bend of

Figs. 28–31. Diagrams to show the folding of the heart during development, and the consequent change in position of its parts. The folding brings the venous and arterial ends of the heart into apposition posterosuperiorly, while the apex lies antero-inferiorly.

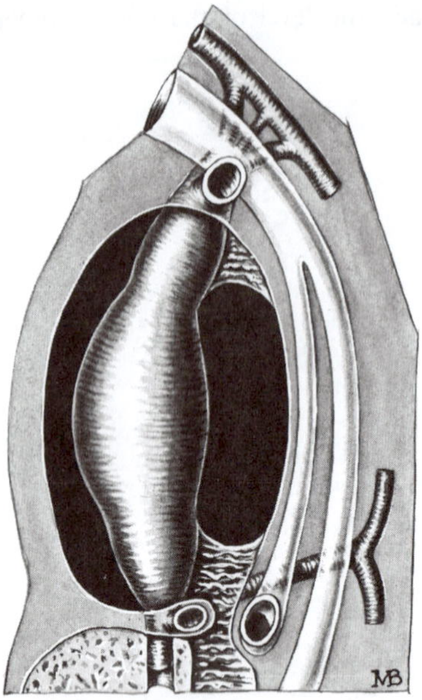

Fig. 28. A diagram of the early embryonic heart in the pericardial cavity. Cf. Fig. 29; see also p. 251.

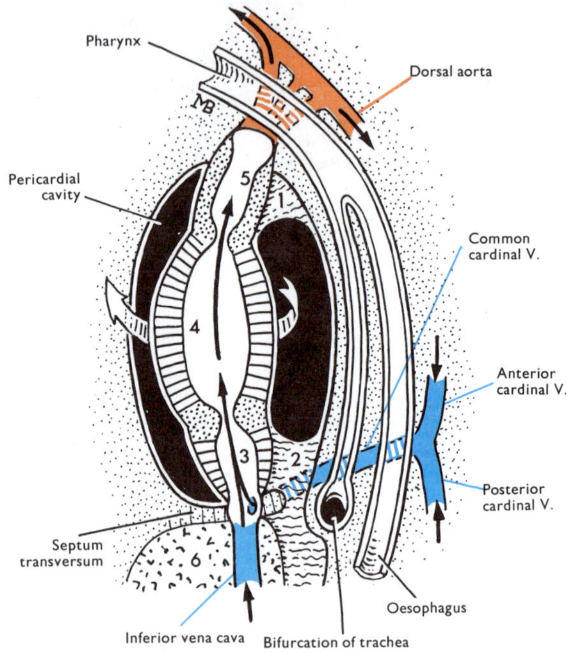

Fig. 29. A diagrammatic sagittal section through the heart shown in Fig. 28. The arrow passes through the transverse sinus of the pericardium.
1. } Remnants of the dorsal
2. } mesocardium.
3. Atrial chamber.
4. Ventricular chamber.
5. Bulbus cordis.
6. Liver in septum transversum.

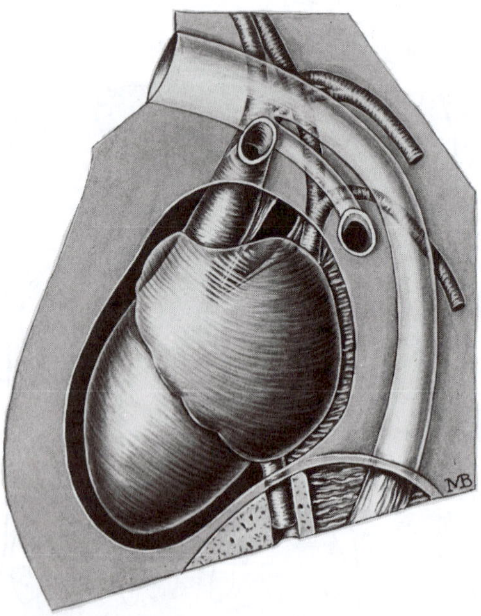

Fig. 30. A diagram of the embryonic heart in the pericardial cavity at a later stage of development than that shown in Fig. 28, to show the folding of the heart tube. Cf. Fig. 31.

the U from the atria; the valves in the anterosuperior limb (valve of aorta or of pulmonary trunk) separate the ventricles from the great arteries. The valves also ensure that the blood which enters the atria from the veins passes into the ventricles and emerges from them through the great arteries. The atria and ventricles are distended muscular chambers each of which shares one wall with the corresponding chamber of the other channel (the **interatrial septum** and the **interventricular septum**). The great arteries are parallel-sided, elastic tubes which are completely separate from each other [Fig. 66].

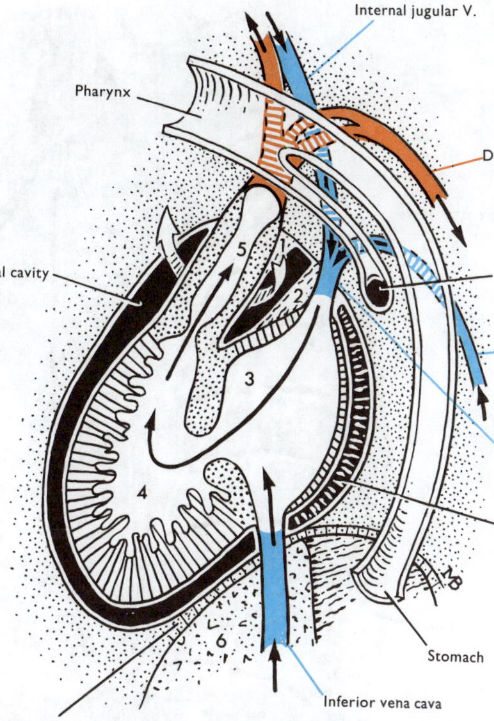

Fig. 31. A diagrammatic sagittal section through the heart shown in Fig. 30. The arrow passes through the transverse sinus of the pericardium.
1. } Remnants of the dorsal
2. } mesocardium.
3. Atrium.
4. Ventricle.
5. Bulbus cordis.
6. Liver.

The U-shaped heart lies in the pericardial cavity in the same manner as the lungs in the pleural cavities. The two ends of the U (veins entering the atria and the great arteries) correspond to the root of the lung and are relatively fixed. It is here that the **parietal pericardium** (the outer wall of the pericardial cavity) becomes continuous with the layer which immediately covers the heart (the **visceral pericardium**). The ventricles are fully surrounded by the pericardial cavity and have the greatest freedom of movement.

The **left atrium** is filled with oxygenated blood from the lungs through two pairs of pulmonary veins. The **right atrium** receives the deoxygenated blood from the rest of the body through the superior and inferior venae cavae and the main vein of the heart (coronary sinus). The thin-walled atria discharge into the corresponding thick-walled ventricles through the atrioventricular valves. The ventricles pump the blood either through the pulmonary trunk to the lungs (**right ventricle**), or through the aorta to the rest of the body (**left ventricle**).

In many quadrupeds, where the dorsoventral diameter of the thorax greatly exceeds its transverse diameter, the heart lies in the simple, sagittal position described above. In man, the thorax is flattened anteroposteriorly and the heart is rotated to the left with the bend of the U (**apex of the heart**) displaced to that side. As a result, the relative positions of the chambers of the heart are altered.

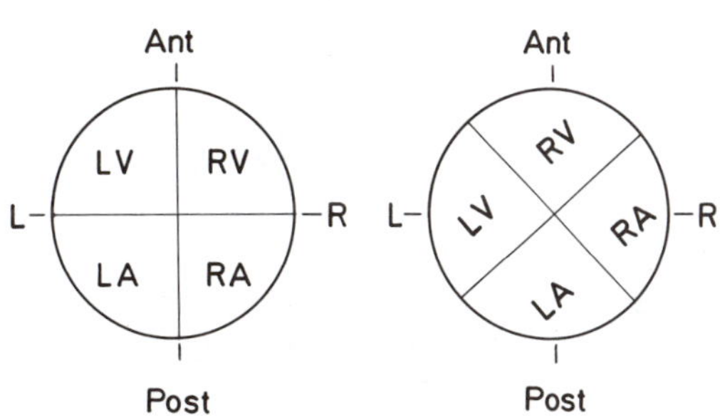

Fig. 32. A diagram to show the change in position of the various cavities of the heart as a result of its rotation. LV, RV = left and right ventricles; LA, RA = left and right atria. See also Figs. 281, 282.

(1) The longitudinal septum lies obliquely with the right chambers anterior and to the right of the left chambers. (2) The left atrium lies in a posterior

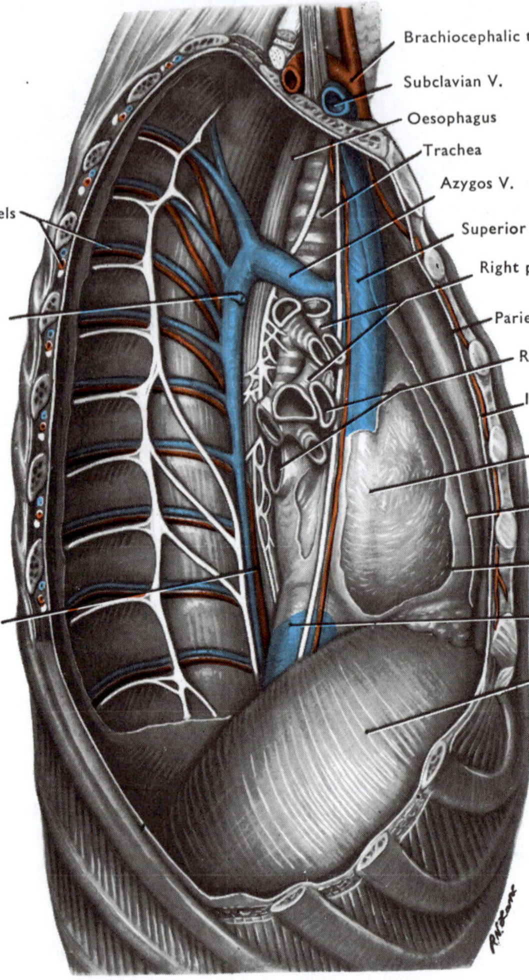

Fig. 33. The right side of the mediastinum and thoracic vertebral column. The pleura has been removed together with part of the pericardium. Pulmonary vessels uncoloured.

position against the vertebral column. It all but disappears from the left (pulmonary) surface of the heart, so that the left ventricle forms the greater part of this surface [Fig. 51]. Since the left atrium lies at the opposite end of the heart from the apex, it forms the **base of the heart** close to the vertebral column [Fig. 75]. (3) The displacement of the **apex** causes it to lie in the fifth left intercostal space just medial to a vertical line dropped from the midpoint of the clavicle (the **mid-clavicular line**). The displacement also removes the right ventricle from the **right margin** of the heart so that this margin is formed entirely by the right atrium. (4) The heart in its pericardial cavity bulges the left wall of the mediastinum far to the left, thus deeply indenting the pleural cavity and lung on that side. On the right, the gently convex surface of the right atrium indents the right pleural cavity and lung to a slight extent only.

Roots of lungs
[Figs. 33, 35, 40, 41, 278–280]

With the help of the above figures check the positions of the main structures in the sectioned roots of the lungs. Note the difference in the arrangement of the bronchi in the two lung roots due to the earlier division of the right principal bronchus. In addition there are a number of lymph nodes which are easily distinguished by the black carbon deposits in them. It may be possible to see the branches of the bronchial arteries on the posterior surfaces of the main bronchi.

Structures visible through pleura

The following structures are usually visible through the pleura unless it is thickened by disease or there is excessive deposition of fat. They should be identified before the pleura is removed.

On the *right side* [Fig. 33], identify the bulge of the heart and pericardium antero-inferior to the lung root. The **right brachiocephalic vein** down to the first costal cartilage and the **superior vena cava** inferior to this form a longitudinal ridge descending to the superior extremity of the bulge. The

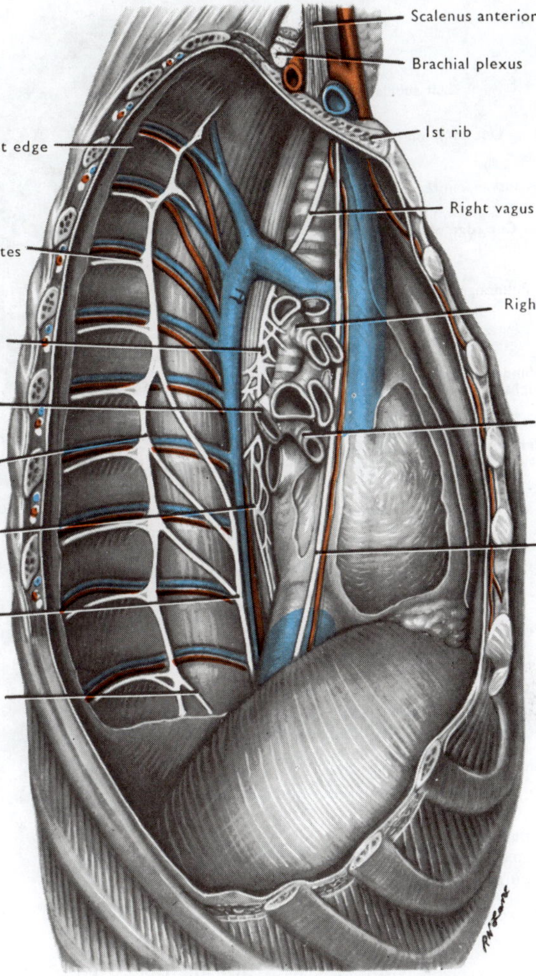

Fig. 34. The right side of the mediastinum and thoracic vertebral column. The pleura has been removed together with part of the pericardium. Pulmonary vessels uncoloured.

inferior vena cava forms a similar but shorter ridge ascending from the diaphragm to the postero-inferior extremity of the bulge. The **phrenic nerve** and its accompanying vessels form a vertical ridge on these vessels and on the pericardium, passing anterior to the lung root. The **vena azygos** arches over the lung root to enter the superior vena cava. Above this, the **trachea** and **oesophagus** may be seen or felt posterior to the phrenic nerve and superior vena cava. The **right vagus nerve** descends postero-inferiorly across the trachea to pass behind the lung root with the oesophagus. Posterior to the oesophagus are the thoracic vertebral bodies with the posterior intercostal vessels and the azygos vein lying on them. The **sympathetic trunk** may be seen or felt on the heads of the upper ribs and on the sides of the vertebral bodies below this anterior to the posterior intercostal vessels and the emerging intercostal nerves. The roots of the greater splanchnic nerve pass antero-inferiorly from the lower part of the trunk.

On the *left side* [Fig. 35], the large bulge of the heart in the pericardium and the lung root posterosuperior to it are separated from the vertebral column by the **descending aorta**. The **oesophagus** is hidden by the aorta except superior to the arch and inferiorly where it lies between the pericardium and the aorta. The **arch of the aorta** curves over the superior surface of the lung root. The left common carotid and subclavian arteries pass superiorly from the convex surface of the arch, anterior to the oesophagus. The phrenic and **vagus nerves** descend between these arteries on to the lateral surface of the aortic arch. The vagus passes to the posterior surface of the lung root, the phrenic nerve runs vertically over the pericardium to the diaphragm. The thoracic duct may be seen on the oesophagus superior to the aortic arch. The parts of the sympathetic system are arranged as on the right, though they may be partly hidden by the aorta.

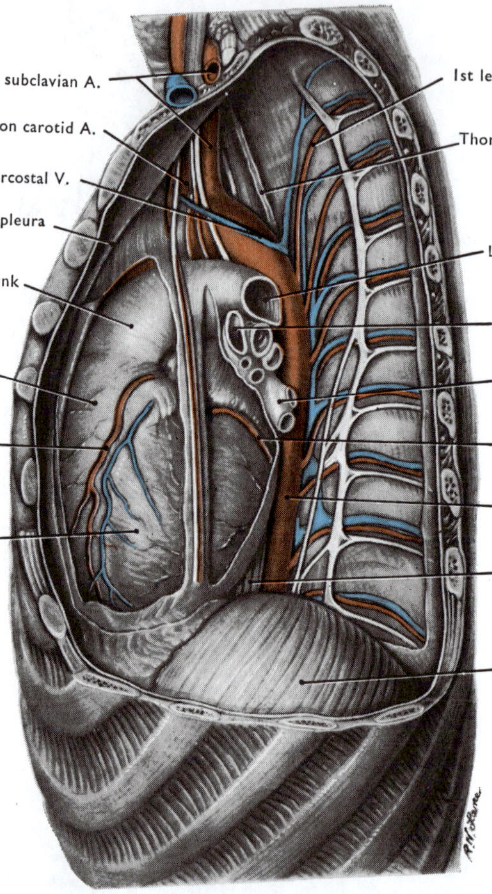

Fig. 35. The left side of the mediastinum and thoracic vertebral column. The pleura and part of the pericardium have been removed. Pulmonary vessels uncoloured.

Dissection

Make a longitudinal incision through the pleura parallel to and on each side of the phrenic nerve. Strip the pleura posterior to the nerve backwards to the intercostal spaces. Avoid injury to the underlying structures. Strip the anterior flap forwards to uncover the remainder of the pericardium and superior vena cava on the right and the arch of the aorta on the left.

Remove the fat and connective tissue from the sympathetic trunk and its anterior branches. Superiorly, these pass to the pulmonary plexus; inferiorly to the splanchnic nerves. In two or three ganglia, identify the **rami communicantes** which pass backwards to the corresponding intercostal nerve. Usually there are two to each nerve, but they may be combined, or one ganglion may send rami to two intercostal nerves [Figs. 17, 34, 36].

Follow the **posterior intercostal vessels** on the vertebral column and in the posterior parts of the intercostal spaces. Trace those in the first two spaces of each side to the neck of the first rib. On the right, the remaining veins pass to the **azygos vein**; on the left, they pass to the left superior intercostal and hemiazygos veins. The azygos and hemiazygos veins will be seen later, but the **left superior intercostal vein** may be followed obliquely across the arch of the aorta to the left brachiocephalic vein posterior to the manubrium of the sternum.

Find the vagus nerve on each side [Figs. 34, 36]. Trace it to the posterior surface of the corresponding lung root and its branches to the pulmonary plexus on that root.

On the right, identify and follow the trachea and oesophagus to the lung root and the superior and inferior venae cavae to the pericardium. Leave the phrenic nerve *in situ*. On the left, find the superior cervical cardiac branch of the left sympathetic trunk and the inferior cervical cardiac branch of the left vagus on the arch of the aorta between the vagus and phrenic nerves. Trace them superiorly. Inferiorly, they pass

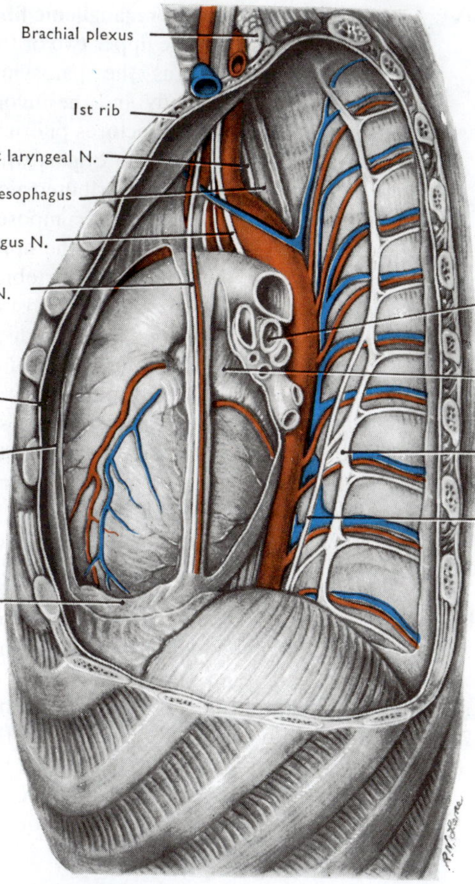

Fig. 36. The left side of the mediastinum and thoracic vertebral column. The pleura and part of the pericardium have been removed. Pulmonary vessels uncoloured.

medially under the concavity of the aortic arch. Trace the left subclavian artery and the oesophagus superior to the aortic arch. Avoid injury to the thoracic duct on the left surface of the oesophagus and to the recurrent laryngeal nerve on its anterolateral surface.

The autonomic nervous system

The sympathetic trunks are an important part of the autonomic nervous system. This system consists of peripherally situated groups (**ganglia**) of efferent nerve cells. These cells innervate involuntary structures, such as smooth muscle and glands, through the **postganglionic nerve fibres** which arise from them. All autonomic ganglion cells receive **preganglionic nerve fibres** which arise in the central nervous system and convey impulses to these cells for the purpose of controlling their activity. The system also transmits the processes of **sensory neurones** which are distributed in the visceral territory. These have no functional connexions with the autonomic ganglia but use the pathways of the preganglionic and postganglionic nerve fibres as a route to their sensory endings. The cell bodies of these sensory nerve fibres lie in the spinal or cranial ganglia and discharge into the central nervous system.

The autonomic nervous system has two divisions.

Parasympathetic part

This part is concerned with the innervation of the eye and of the gut tube and the structures developed in its wall, e.g. the heart, and of the respiratory and urogenital systems. It receives preganglionic fibres through certain cranial nerves and the second and third, or third and fourth, sacral spinal nerves. The parasympathetic ganglia lie in or near the structures which they innervate, so the preganglionic fibres end close to these organs. The parasympathetic nerves of the thorax are the **vagus nerves**. They are principally concerned with the innervation of the heart, lungs, trachea, and oesophagus.

Sympathetic part

This part receives **preganglionic fibres (white rami communicantes)** from all the thoracic and the upper two or three lumbar nerves. Its ganglia supply the same structures as the parasympathetic part and also blood vessels throughout the body and the involuntary structures in the body wall, e.g. sweat glands and arrectores pilorum. The sympathetic ganglia usually lie at some distance from the organs which they innervate. Their postganglionic nerve fibres are often distributed along blood vessels.

The sympathetic part is composed of two elements. (1) The **sympathetic trunks**. These extend from the upper cervical region to the coccyx, one on each side of the front of the vertebral column. The ganglia of the trunks send **postganglionic nerve fibres** to most of the cranial and all of the spinal nerves (**grey rami communicantes**) for distribution through these nerves mainly to the body wall. The trunks also transmit preganglionic fibres and send some postganglionic fibres through visceral branches, e.g. the splanchnic nerves, to the sympathetic plexuses. (2) The **sympathetic plexuses** are networks of fine nerve fibres containing scattered ganglia. They are principally associated with the arteries which supply the viscera. The chief plexuses are found in the thorax (cardiac and pulmonary), the abdomen, and the pelvis. These plexuses also transmit parasympathetic fibres.

Sympathetic trunk

In the thorax this trunk consists of approximately 11 ganglia joined by longitudinal bundles of preganglionic and postganglionic fibres among which are scattered a variable number of ganglion cells. In the superior part of the thorax the trunk lies on the necks or heads of the ribs. Inferiorly it passes on to the bodies of the vertebrae as these increase in width. The **first thoracic ganglion** is frequently fused with the inferior cervical ganglion to form the **cervicothoracic** (stellate) **ganglion** on the neck of the first rib. This ganglion may also include the second thoracic ganglion.

Branches in thorax

1. **Grey** and **white rami communicantes** join each ganglion to one (or two) intercostal nerves. The white rami (preganglionic fibres) pass from the nerves to the trunk. The grey rami (postganglionic fibres) pass to the nerves from the ganglion cells in the trunk. The nerve fibres in each grey ramus are distributed through every branch of the spinal nerve to which they pass.

2. **Visceral branches**. (a) **Aortic** and **oesophageal branches** pass to these organs from the upper five thoracic ganglia and from the greater splanchnic nerve.

(b) **Cardiac** and **pulmonary nerves** run antero-inferiorly on the vertebral bodies to the corresponding plexuses from the third and fourth ganglia.

(c) The **greater splanchnic nerve** is formed by branches which run antero-inferiorly on the vertebral bodies from the fifth to ninth ganglia. This nerve sends branches to the aorta and oesophagus. It has a small splanchnic ganglion on it just before it pierces the crus of the diaphragm to enter the abdomen.

(d) The **lesser** and **lowest splanchnic nerves** are formed by similar branches respectively from the ninth and tenth, and the last thoracic ganglia. They enter the abdomen together through the crus of the diaphragm.

Subcostal muscles

These irregular muscle slips lie near the angles of the lower ribs. When present, they cross the internal surface of two or three intercostal spaces, parallel to the internal intercostal muscle. They are part of an incomplete muscle layer formed by the transversus thoracis and innermost intercostal muscles.

Internal intercostal membranes

These fascial sheets extend from the internal intercostal muscles to the superior costotransverse ligament (q.v.) on the neck of each rib. They separate the intercostal vessels and nerve from the external intercostal muscle in the posterior part of the intercostal space.

Vena azygos
[Figs. 86, 277–282]

This vein arises in the abdomen from the posterior surface of the inferior vena cava and enters the thorax immediately to the right of the aorta and thoracic duct. It ascends in the same position in the thorax, posterior at first to the diaphragm and then to the oesophagus, on the anterior surface of the vertebral bodies. At the fourth thoracic vertebra, it arches anteriorly, superior to the root of the right lung and lateral to the oesophagus, vagus nerve, and trachea. It enters the superior vena cava medial to the phrenic nerve. Occasionally a part of the lung (**azygos lobe**), surrounded by pleural cavity, extends upwards between the arch of the vein and the structures medial to it. This is recognizable radiologically.

Tributaries

The azygos vein receives the second to eleventh **posterior intercostal veins**, the **subcostal vein**, and blood from the posterior abdominal wall through the **ascending lumbar vein** (q.v.) on the right side. It also drains the same territory on the left side through the **hemiazygos** [Fig. 86] and **accessory hemiazygos veins**, except for the drainage into the left superior intercostal vein. **Bronchial** and some **oesophageal veins** also enter the azygos vein. The oesophageal tributaries communicate through the oesophageal orifice in the diaphragm with **gastric veins**. This is one route of communication between the systemic (body wall) system of veins and the portal (gastro-intestinal) system in the abdomen. The azygos vein also forms a channel of anastomosis between the superior and inferior venae cavae: (a) through its connection with both; (b) through the origin of the hemiazygos vein in the left renal vein; (c) through the communications of the tributaries of the inferior vena cava and azygos veins with the valveless **internal vertebral venous plexus** [Fig. 205].

Left superior intercostal vein

This vein drains at least the second and third left posterior intercostal veins. It descends to the vertebral end of the aortic arch and runs forwards on the arch, lateral to the vagus and medial to the phrenic nerve. It enters the left brachiocephalic vein with the pericardiacophrenic vein. It corresponds to the arch of the azygos vein and the upper part of the superior vena cava on the right. It may drain the accessory hemiazygos vein.

Dissection

Remove the pleura covering the phrenic nerves. Trace the nerves and the vessels which accompany them as far as possible.

Phrenic nerves

These nerves are the sole motor supply to the diaphragm. They transmit sensory nerve fibres from it and from the other structures developed in or from the septum transversum [p. 254], i.e. pericardium, pleura (mediastinal and diaphragmatic), inferior vena cava, liver and biliary apparatus. The origin of the phrenic and supraclavicular nerves from the **third and fourth cervical** ventral rami accounts for the pain felt in the right shoulder in biliary disease.

The phrenic nerve arises from the ventral rami of the third, fourth, and fifth cervical nerves. It descends into the thorax posterolateral to the corresponding internal jugular vein and is joined by the **pericardiacophrenic branch** of the internal thoracic artery at the root of the neck. Each nerve descends on the side of the mediastinum a short distance anterior to the root of the lung, immediately medial to the mediastinal pleura to which it gives sensory twigs.

The **right phrenic nerve** lies posterolateral to the right brachiocephalic vein and superior vena cava. It then lies on the parietal pericardium covering the right atrium of the heart, and passes to the diaphragm on the inferior vena cava [Fig. 34].

The **left phrenic nerve** descends on to the left surface of the arch of the aorta between the left common carotid and subclavian arteries. It then lies on and supplies the pericardium superficial to the left auricle and left ventricle of the heart [Fig. 36].

Both nerves pierce the diaphragm and are distributed to its inferior surface and to the structures attached to that surface.

The lungs

[p. 8]

Each of these structures has the shape of a half cone. They are comparatively light because of their content of air (right, approximately 600 g: left, 550 g in a healthy adult) and they float freely in water unless filled with fluid, e.g. before birth, or consolidated by disease.

The lungs contain a high proportion of **elastic tissue**. The fresh lung will contract and expel most of the air within it. This elasticity is responsible for most of the expiratory force in quiet respiration. The loss of elasticity in disease, e.g. emphysema, leaves the lungs permanently distended unless expiratory muscles are brought into play—a situation causing expiratory embarrassment.

In children the lungs are yellowish pink. In the adult, deposition of carbon particles which are picked up by phagocytes leads to the surface becoming mottled with dark patches and lines. The lines indicate the position of lymph channels in the interlobular fibrous septa.

Each lung lies free in its own pleural cavity, attached only to the mediastinum by its root. In most dissecting room cadavers the pulmonary pleura is adherent to the parietal pleura at places as a result of old inflammation of the pleura (pleurisy). When the lungs are fixed *in situ*, their elasticity is destroyed and so they retain the shape of the structures to which they are moulded in the thorax.

Apex

The apex of the lung extends into the root of the neck 3–5 cm above the anterior part of the first rib and 1–2 cm above the medial third of the clavicle. The subclavian artery and vein cross the anterior surface of this part of the lung and may groove it. They are separated from the lung by pleura and the suprapleural membrane [p. 18].

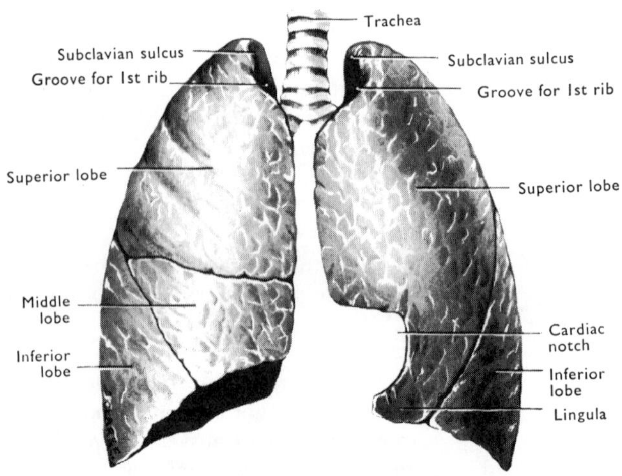

Fig. 37. The trachea, bronchi, and lungs of a child, hardened *in situ*.

Base

The base of the lung, semilunar in shape, is fitted to the dome of the diaphragm and is deeply concave, especially on the right side where the dome is higher [Fig. 13]. The concave base meets the costal surface of the lung at a sharp inferior margin which extends into the costodiaphragmatic recess but does not reach the lower limit of the recess except in deep inspiration. The inferior margin is blunt medially where it abuts on the pericardium.

Anterior margin

This thin margin extends into the narrow costomediastinal recess of the pleura. The margin passes posterior to the sternoclavicular joint from the apex to the middle of the lower border of the manubrium of the sternum. Thence it descends vertically to meet the inferior margin at the xiphosternal joint (right lung) but is deeply notched in the left lung posterior to the fifth costal cartilage by the bulging pericardium, and extends medially below this to form the **lingula** [Fig. 37]. This **cardiac notch** leaves part of the pericardium uncovered by lung. Percussion in this area gives a dull note (area of superficial cardiac dullness) in comparison with the resonant note obtained over the lung.

Posterior surface

This thick, rounded surface fits into the deep paravertebral gutter.

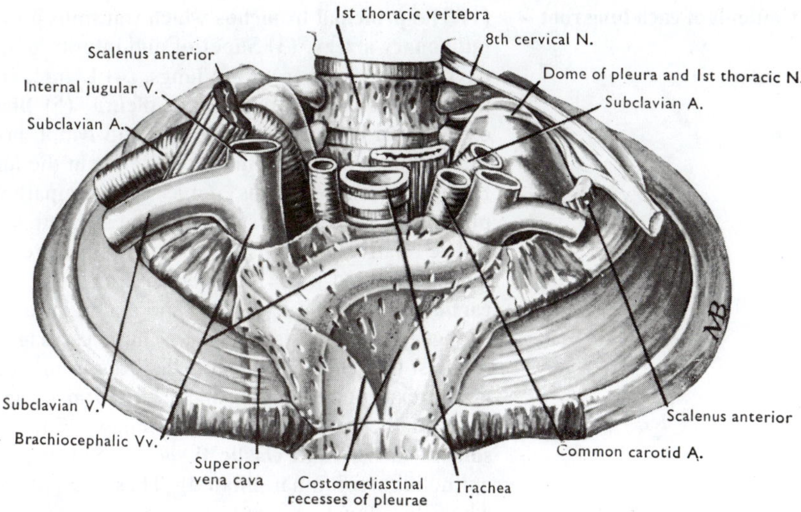

Fig. 38. The superior aperture of the thorax. The anterior margins (costomediastinal recesses) of the pleural sacs and the great veins are shown through the sternum.

Medial surface [Figs. 40, 41]

This surface is in contact with the vertebral column (vertebral part) and the mediastinum (mediastinal part) and is indented by the heart (cardiac impression) and great vessels especially on the left.

Hilus

The hilus of the lung lies near the centre of the medial surface. It is a large depressed area through which structures enter and leave the lung via its root.

Mediastinal surface of lung

This surface of the lung is indented by the larger structures projecting from the mediastinum. With the help of Figs. 33 and 41 and Figs. 35 and 40, identify these structures on the mediastinum and the grooves which they make on the lung. Smaller structures on the surface of the mediastinum leave no mark on the lungs. These are (1) the **phrenic nerve** and associated vessels on both sides; (2) the **right vagus** on the trachea and the **left vagus** on the aortic arch; (3) the **left superior intercostal vein** on the aortic arch; (4) the **thoracic duct** on the left side of the oesophagus [Figs. 59, 70].

Roots of lungs

All the structures which enter or leave the lung do so through its root. The root is enclosed in a short tubular sheath of pleura which joins the pulmonary and mediastinal parts of the pleura and extends inferiorly as a narrow fold—the pulmonary ligament [Figs. 40, 41].

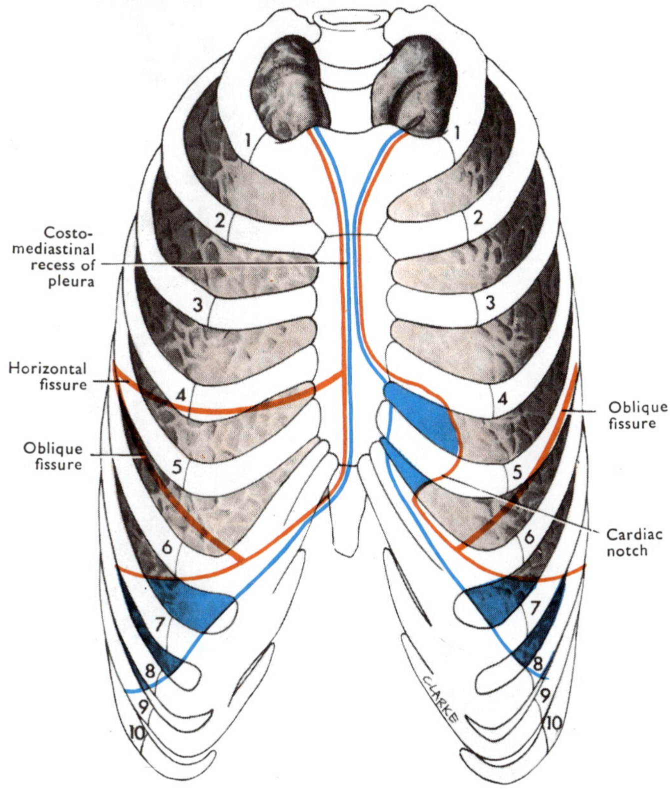

Fig. 39. A diagram to show the relation of the lungs (red) and parietal pleura (blue) to the anterior thoracic wall.

Contents of each lung root

(1) The **principal bronchus** which transmits air to and from the lungs. (2) A **pulmonary artery**. (3) Superior and inferior **pulmonary veins** which transmit oxygenated blood from the lungs. (4) **Lymph vessels** and **nodes** which drain the lung tissue and pulmonary pleura. (5) **Bronchial arteries** which carry oxygenated blood to the bronchi and lymph nodes. They anastomose with the branches of the pulmonary arteries in the lungs. (6) **Bronchial veins**. (7) Branches of the vagus nerve and sympathetic trunk which form the **pulmonary plexus** and supply all the structures in the lungs.

The relative positions of the larger structures in the lung roots can be seen in Figs. 40 and 41. The bronchus can be recognized by the firm, hyaline **cartilages** which lie in its wall and maintain the patency of its lumen despite changes in external pressure. These cartilages are found in all but the smallest branches of the bronchial tree (1 mm or less). They are incomplete in the extrapulmonary bronchi but form irregular encircling plates in the walls of the bronchi within the lungs. Within the lungs, spiral bundles of **smooth muscle** and **elastic tissue** lie between the cartilages and the lining epithelium (columnar ciliated). These permit the elongation of the bronchi when the lungs expand on inspiration and cause their shortening on expiration. The muscle can also reduce the diameter of the bronchial lumina sufficiently to embarrass respiration severely, e.g. asthma. Parasympathetic (vagus) nerves contract the muscle while the sympathetic nerves relax it. Hence the use of sympathomimetic drugs to control asthmatic attacks. The single pulmonary artery in each root may be differentiated from the two veins by its position and by the greater thickness of its wall.

Lobes of lungs
[Figs. 25–27, 277, 280]

The **left lung** is divided into two lobes by a deep **oblique fissure**. During life this fissure begins posteriorly at the level of the fifth thoracic vertebra. It passes antero-inferiorly in a spiral course, to meet the inferior margin close to the sixth costochondral junction. It extends into the lung almost to the hilus, and separates the inferior and superior lobes. After death, the lung collapses to a variable degree and the diaphragm rises. Thus the upper end of the oblique fissure is often at the level of the third thoracic vertebra in the cadaver [Fig. 27]. The **superior lobe** forms the apex and anterior margin of

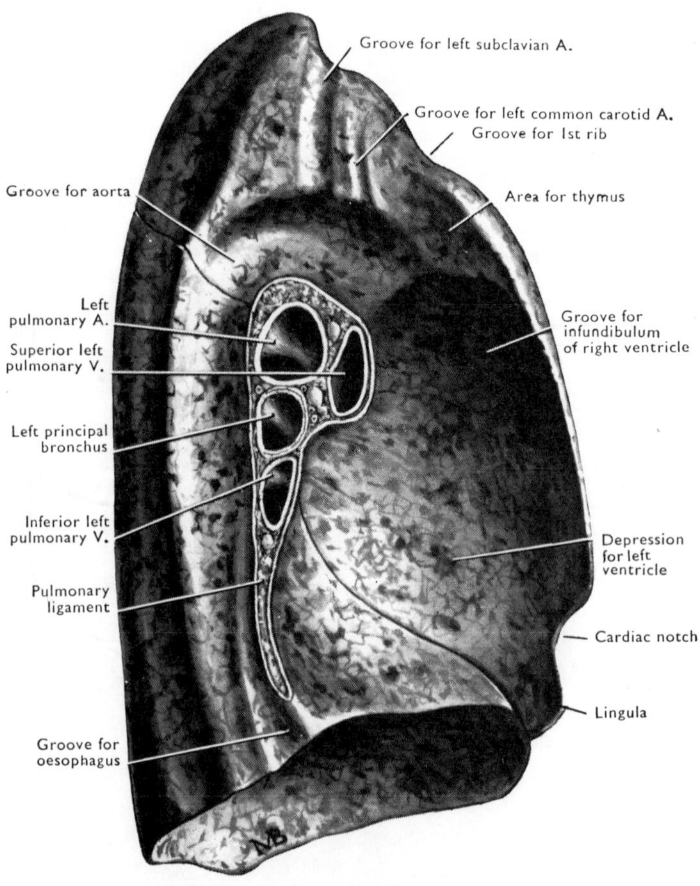

Fig. 40. The medial surface of the left lung hardened *in situ*.

the lung. The **inferior lobe** makes up the diaphragmatic and the greater part of the posterior surfaces.

The **right lung** is divided by a similar **oblique fissure**. This separates the **superior** and **middle lobes** from the **inferior lobe**. A second, **horizontal fissure** extends from the anterior margin (at the fourth costal cartilage) horizontally backwards to meet the oblique fissure in the mid-axillary line. This fissure separates the wedge-shaped **middle lobe** from the superior lobe.

Pulmonary pleura extends into the fissures of the lungs so that the lobes of the lungs can move on each other during respiration. The fissures may be obliterated by inflammation of the pleura (pleurisy) and an infection may become localized in the fissure to form an abscess between the lobes of the lung. In both cases the pleura in the fissure is thickened and may be visible in radiographs. Not all the fissures are constantly present. The horizontal fissure is commonly absent in whole or in part.

The right lung may be differentiated from the left because it has three lobes (usually), is shorter and broader, and has no cardiac notch. However, they cannot be confused because base, apex, medial aspect (root of lung), and thin anterior margin are unmistakable.

Intrapulmonary structures

Bronchi

A principal **bronchus** passes inferolaterally from the termination of the trachea to the hilus of each lung. A pulmonary artery passes transversely into each lung anterior to the bronchus. Two pulmonary veins pass from the antero-inferior part of each hilus directly into the left atrium [Figs. 40, 41, 71].

The bronchi divide in a tree-like fashion within the lung. Thus each branch supplies a clearly defined sector of the lung. Each **principal bronchus** divides into secondary, **lobar bronchi** (two on the left, three on the right) to the lobes of the lung. Each lobar bronchus divides into tertiary branches. These **segmental bronchi** supply sectors known as bronchopulmonary segments within each lobe of the lungs. Each of these bronchopulmonary segments is pyramidal in shape with its apex towards the root of the lung and its base at the pleural surface [Fig. 42].

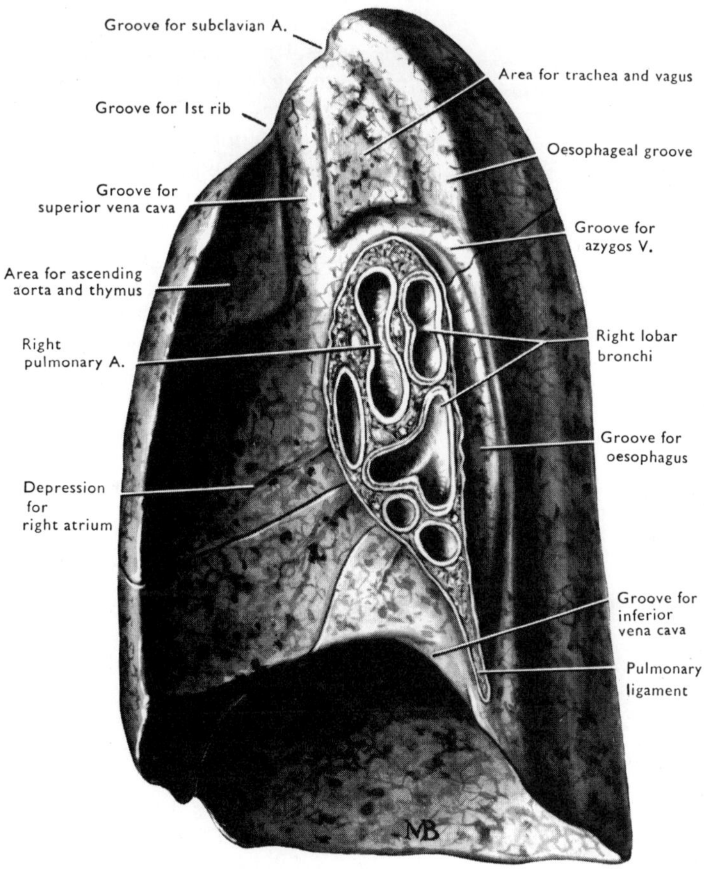

Fig. 41. The medial surface of the right lung hardened *in situ*.

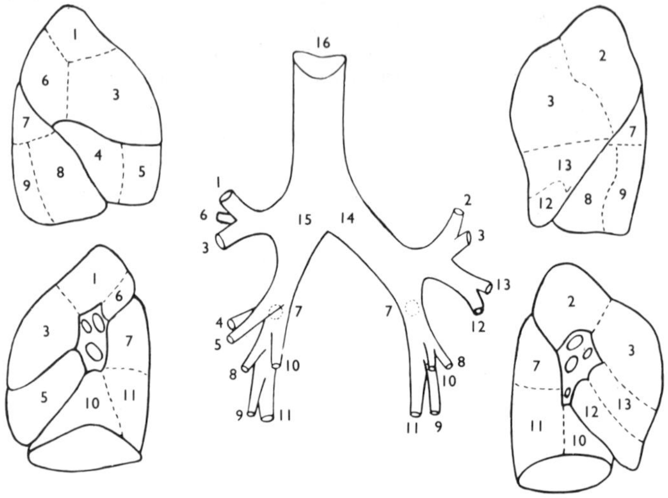

Fig. 42. The bronchi and bronchopulmonary segments. (After Jackson and Huber.) Each segmental bronchus has the same name as the subdivision of the lung supplied by it. The anterior and medial basal bronchi arise from a common stem in the left lung. This is often called the anteromedial basal bronchus.

1. Apical.
2. Apicoposterior.
3. Anterior.
4. Lateral. } Middle lobe.
5. Medial. } Middle lobe.
6. Posterior.
7. Apical (inferior lobe).
8. Anterior basal.
9. Lateral basal.
10. Medial basal.
11. Posterior basal.
12. Inferior lingular.
13. Superior lingular.
14. Left principal bronchus.
15. Right principal bronchus.
16. Trachea.

Bronchopulmonary segments

These are of considerable clinical significance because disease processes in the lung may be limited to one or more segments which can sometimes be identified by passing a bronchoscope down the trachea and examining the openings of the tertiary bronchi [Fig. 46]. These openings are the most distal which may be examined in this way. The arrangement of the segments also permits the surgeon to remove diseased parts of the lung with minimal disturbance to the surrounding lung tissue.

The general arrangement of the segments can best be understood by reference to Fig. 42 and by dissecting out the main branches of the bronchi and vessels close to the hilus of the lung. The arrangement of the tertiary bronchi to the inferior lobe is similar in both lungs, though a separate **medial basal bronchus** is not normally recognized in the left lung because it is usually a small branch of the anterior basal bronchus. There is a different pattern in the superior lobes of the two lungs because of the presence in the right lung of a middle lobe and the earlier division of the principal bronchus. Thus the **left superior lobar bronchus** is larger than the right because it supplies the entire upper lobe of the left lung which corresponds to the superior and middle lobes of the right lung. The upper main branch of the *left* superior lobar bronchus supplies two segments – **apicoposterior** and **anterior**. These correspond to the three segments of the *right* upper lobe—**apical, posterior**, and **anterior**. The lower main branch of the *left* superior lobar bronchus supplies **superior lingular** and **inferior lingular segments**. These pass to a sector which corresponds to but is smaller than the **lateral** and **medial segments** of the middle lobe of the *right* lung.

Blood vessels

The branches of the **pulmonary artery** distribute venous blood to the lungs. They follow the bronchi and lie mainly on their posterior surfaces. There is, therefore, a branch of the pulmonary artery to each lobe, bronchopulmonary segment, and lobule of the lung. These are centrally placed with the bronchi. The terminal capillaries lie in the walls of the alveoli and respiratory bronchioles where gaseous exchange takes place between the blood and the air.

The **pulmonary veins** drain oxygenated blood from the lungs to the left atrium of the heart. The lobular tributaries lie mainly in the interlobular

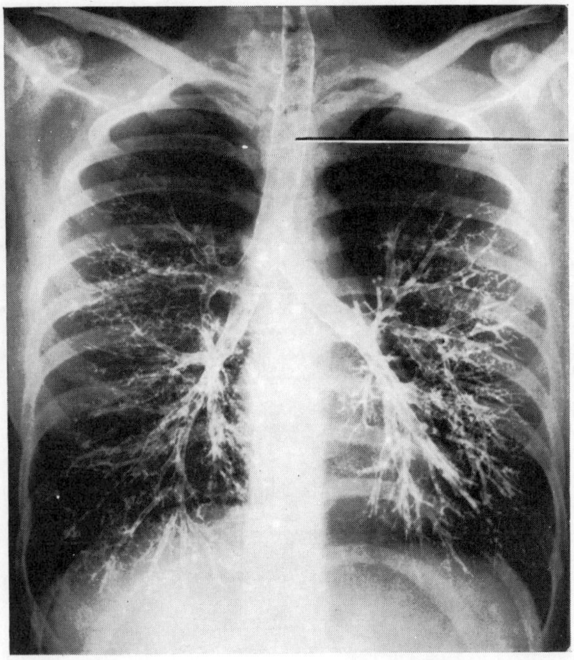

Fig. 43. An anteroposterior radiograph (bronchogram). The trachea and bronchi are outlined by the introduction of X-ray-opaque material. Cf. Fig. 42.

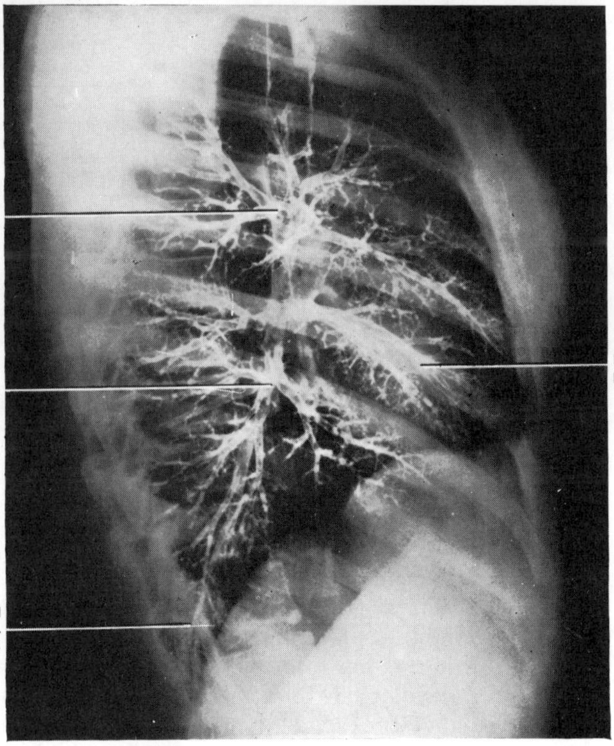

Fig. 44. A lateral radiograph to show the right bronchial tree by the introduction of X-ray-opaque material.

septa. One main vein drains each bronchopulmonary segment, usually on the anterior surface of the corresponding bronchus. Veins also run between the segments and on the mediastinal and fissural surfaces of the lungs. Some may even cross the line of a fissure when this is incomplete. The vessels of the right medial basal segment frequently arise from the vessels of the middle lobe. The **superior** right pulmonary vein drains the superior and middle lobes, and thus corresponds to the superior left pulmonary vein which drains the left superior lobe. The right and left **inferior** pulmonary veins drain the corresponding inferior lobes.

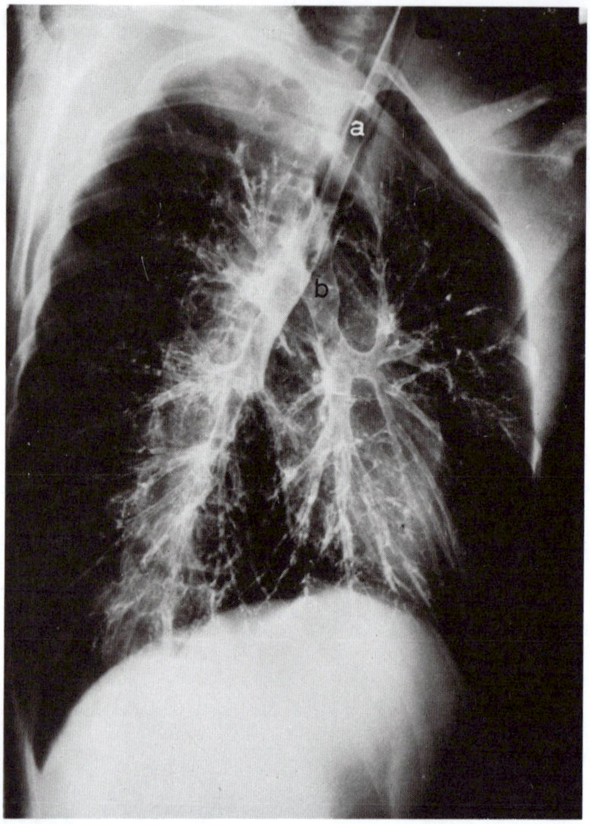

Fig. 45. An oblique radiograph of the thorax with a thin film of X-ray-opaque medium lining the larger bronchi (bronchogram) mainly to show the branching of the left principal bronchus (b) [cf. Figs. 42–44]. (a) Insufflation tube in trachea. Such radiographs can show blockage, compression, or dilatation of part of the bronchial tree and so can help to localize tumours, abscesses, etc. and determine whether they may be amenable to surgical intervention or other treatment.

Dissection

Begin by washing out the bronchi in the lungs as far as possible. Then shine a light into the main bronchus and attempt to see the apertures of its various branches. Compare these with Fig. 46 so that some idea of the view obtained by bronchoscopy can be appreciated.

When the surface of the lung has been broken at the hilus, it is simple to scrape away the alveolar tissue from the main veins, bronchi, and arteries. In both lungs, begin by cleaning the superior pulmonary vein and its tributaries. Then clean the corresponding bronchi posterior to the veins. Repeat this procedure with the inferior pulmonary vein and corresponding bronchi. Note the small, grey or black **pulmonary lymph nodes** which lie in the angles formed by the bifurcation of the bronchi. Now follow the branches of the pulmonary arteries. They follow the bronchi and lie mainly on their posterior surfaces.

As the principal bronchi are lifted forwards to expose the arterial branches, look for the **bronchial arteries** on their posterior surfaces. There are usually two bronchial arteries to the left lung and one to the right. The **left** bronchial arteries arise from the descending aorta, the **right** either from the first right aortic intercostal artery, or from the superior left bronchial artery. They are the nutrient arteries of the lung. The blood they transmit is returned either through the pulmonary veins or through the **bronchial veins** which enter the azygos and accessory hemiazygos veins on the vertebral bodies. In some congenital abnormalities of the heart and/or great vessels, the blood supply to the lungs through the pulmonary arteries is inadequate. In these cases, the bronchial arteries may enlarge to take over this function after birth [p. 257].

Lymph vessels and nodes of lung

The lymph vessels of the lung cannot be demonstrated in dissecting room specimens. The nodes are very obvious because of their black colour and the dense connective tissue which binds them to the bronchi. A **superficial plexus** of lymph vessels lies deep to the pulmonary pleura. It drains: (1) over the surface of the lung to the **bronchopulmonary lymph nodes** in the hilus, (2)

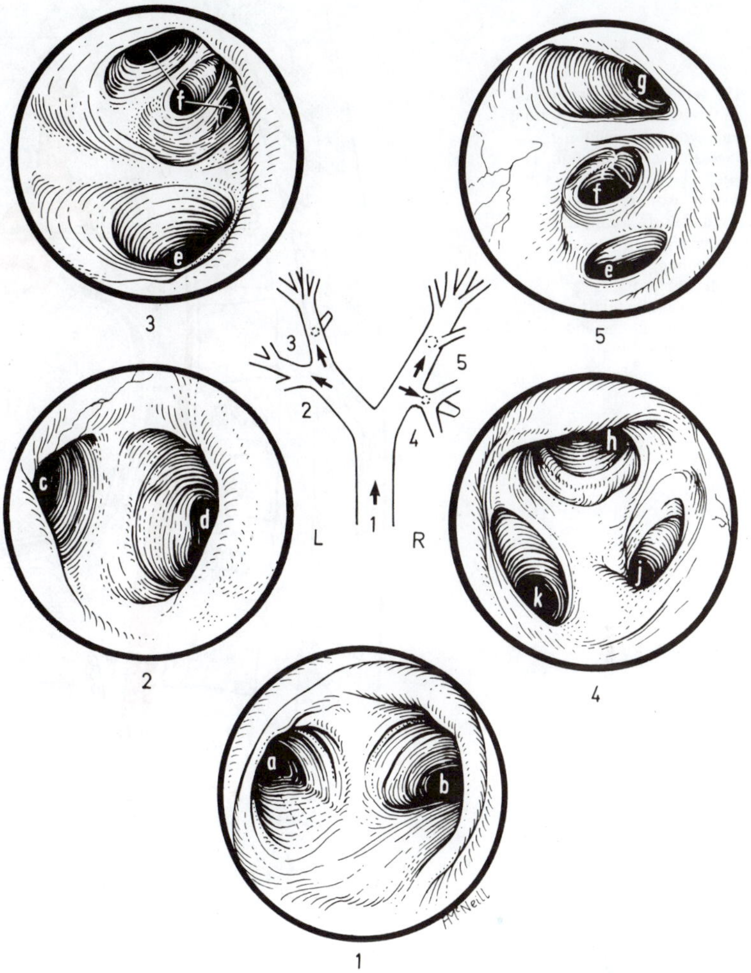

Fig. 46. Drawings of the bronchial tree as seen through the bronchoscope. Each view is numbered to correspond to the numbered arrows in the central drawing. Each arrow in the central drawing represents the position and direction of the tip of the bronchoscope when the particular view is obtained.

1. Tracheal bifurcation.
   a. Left principal bronchus.
   b. Right principal bronchus.
2. Left superior lobe bronchus.
   c. Common stem of apicoposterior and anterior bronchi.
   d. Common stem of superior and inferior lingular bronchi.
3. Left inferior lobe bronchus.
   e. Apical bronchus of lower lobe.
   f. Basal bronchi.
4. Right superior lobe bronchus.
   h. Anterior bronchus.
   j. Apical bronchus.
   k. Posterior bronchus.
5. Right middle (g) and lower lobe bronchi.
   e. Apical bronchus of lower lobe.
   f. Basal bronchi.

along the interlobular septa into deep lymph vessels. These drain along the bronchi and vessels and traverse **pulmonary nodes** to reach the bronchopulmonary nodes in the hilus of the lung. The bronchopulmonary nodes form the most lateral part of a mass of nodes stretching along the principal bronchus from the tracheal bifurcation to the hilus of the lung. The more medial nodes of this mass (superior and inferior **tracheobronchial nodes**) receive lymph from the bronchopulmonary nodes. They drain through the **bronchomediastinal trunk** of that side to the corresponding brachiocephalic vein, or through the thoracic duct on the left. Each bronchomediastinal trunk ascends lateral to the trachea and receives the efferent vessels from the **parasternal nodes**. Some of the lymph may drain to posterior mediastinal nodes or even to the lower deep cervical nodes.

When the bronchopulmonary nodes are enlarged by disease in the lung, they may be visible in radiographs as an increased density of shadow at the lung root.

Dissection

Find the left vagus on the aortic arch. Follow its **recurrent laryngeal** branch beneath the concavity of the arch. The nerve lies postero-inferior to a short fibrous cord (the **ligamentum arteriosum**) which unites the root of the left pulmonary artery to the aortic arch. Identify the cardiac nerves on the aortic arch. They turn medially under the arch to join a plexus of nerve cells and fibres—the superficial cardiac plexus. This is the left extremity of the extensive **cardiac plexus** which sends branches to the heart and great vessels.

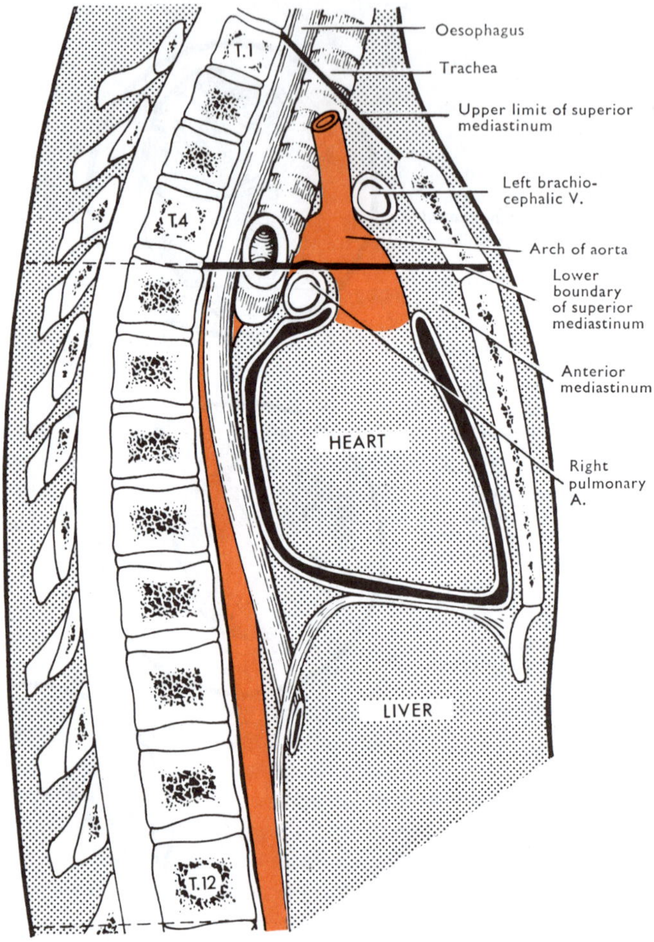

Fig. 47. A diagram of a median section through the thorax to show the general distribution of the structures in the mediastinum. The heart in the pericardium forms the middle mediastinum, while the anterior and posterior mediastina lie between it and the sternum and vertebral column respectively. Note that the posterior mediastinum also extends inferiorly between the diaphragm and the vertebral column.

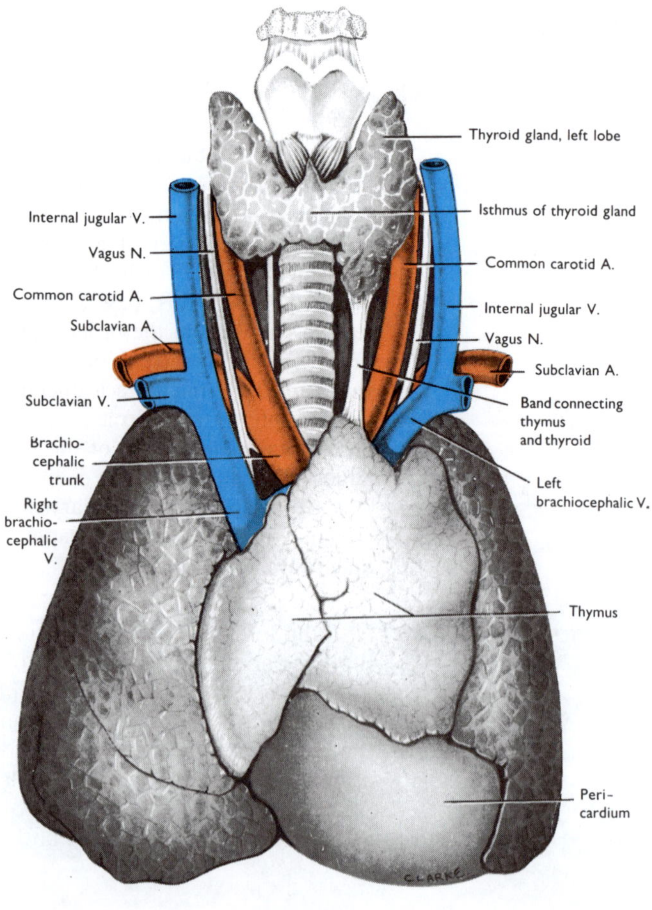

Fig. 48. The thyroid gland and thymus in a full-term fetus.

Superficial cardiac plexus

This is the left extremity of a complicated plexus of nerve cells and fibres which extends from the bifurcation of the trachea to the concavity of the arch of the aorta. It is continuous on the surface of the principal bronchi with the **pulmonary plexuses**. This combined mass sends nerve fibres to the heart and lungs. The superficial part receives nerve fibres through the superior cervical cardiac branch of the left sympathetic trunk and the inferior cervical cardiac branch of the left vagus. The deeper part receives the remaining cardiac branches from these two structures on both sides. All these **cardiac branches** descend obliquely from the neck as a result of the caudal displacement of the heart during development. Branches from the superficial part of the cardiac plexus pass to the heart predominantly on the pulmonary trunk, but it is virtually impossible to demonstrate the cardiac plexus satisfactorily by dissection.

The anterior mediastinum

This is a narrow cleft posterior to the body of the sternum. It contains the remains of the lower part of the thymus which descends to the level of the third or fourth costal cartilages. This and some loose fatty tissue separate the body of the sternum and costomediastinal recesses of the pleura from the great vessels and the pericardium [Figs. 49, 61].

Thymus

In the child this is a bilobed mass of lymph tissue. It develops as a bilateral structure from the third pharyngeal pouches of the embryo in common with the **inferior parathyroid glands**. Subsequently it descends with the pericardium from the neck into the thorax. Thus it may retain a fibrous connexion with one or both of the inferior parathyroid glands in the neck. In the fetus and new-born [Fig. 48] the thymus is nearly as large as the heart. It continues to grow until puberty but is progressively reduced in size thereafter. In dissecting room subjects it is usually reduced to two strips of lymph tissue infiltrated with fat and fibrous tissue, but the rate and extent of its involution are very variable.

The functions of the thymus are not entirely clear, but it is closely concerned with the development of immunity responses. It is responsible, especially in the young animal, for the proliferation and differentiation of lymphocytes produced in the bone marrow into T (thymus-dependent) lymphocytes which are essential for the development of immune responses including the stimulus to other (B) lymphocytes which are also produced in the bone marrow but pass directly to lymph tissues other than the thymus

Fig. 49. The thyroid gland and thymus in the adult.

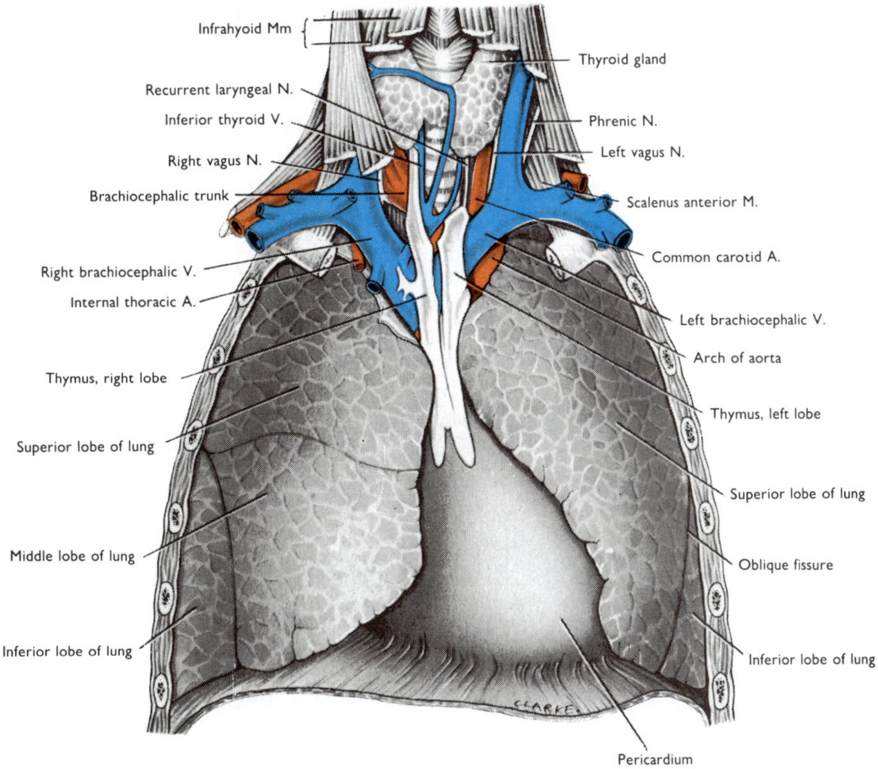

the thymus is removed from mice at birth, the animals fail to develop properly and die within a few weeks with a profound reduction in the number of circulating lymphocytes and a failure of the lymph tissues, e.g. lymph nodes, to develop. This is due to the absence of thymus lymphocytes, the consequent failure of the B lymphocytes to react, and to the absence of thymus hormones which stimulate the production of lymphocytes in the other lymph tissues. Thus it makes possible the production of cells which manufacture antibodies to foreign proteins and other antigens—an ability which only develops after birth.

Dissection

Remove the fat and fibrous tissue from the thymus as far as possible. Separate it from the pericardium and, turning it superiorly, note any blood vessels entering it. The **veins** pass superiorly on the deep surface of the thymus to the left brachiocephalic vein deep to the manubrium of the sternum. The **arteries** come from the internal thoracic vessels and occasionally from the arch of the aorta.

The middle mediastinum

Pericardium

The **pericardium** is a serous bag, akin to the pleura. The heart projects into it from above and behind. The pericardium consists of three layers: (1) an outer fibrous layer lined by (2) a parietal layer of serous pericardium and (3) a visceral layer of serous pericardium which covers the enclosed heart and adjacent parts of the great vessels. The two parts of the serous pericardium slide freely on each other when the heart moves within the pericardium.

As the great vessels enter and leave the heart they are surrounded by pericardium—the arteries together in one sheath, the veins in another [Fig. 52]. Here the fibrous pericardium fuses with the surfaces of the vessels and the two layers of serous pericardium become continuous deep to the fusion.

Inferiorly the **fibrous pericardium** is adherent to the central tendon of the diaphragm and both are pierced by the inferior vena cava posteriorly and to the right. The central tendon separates the pericardium from the liver and the fundus of the stomach in the abdomen. Superiorly, the aorta and pulmonary trunk pierce the pericardium together [Fig. 52]; the veins pierce it posteriorly and inferiorly. Within the fibrous sac, each of these sets of vessels is separately ensheathed in **serous pericardium**. On the right, the venous sheath surrounds the superior and inferior venae cavae with the right pulmonary veins between them. On the left, it encloses the two left pulmonary veins. Between these two parts is the **oblique sinus of the pericardium** [Fig. 71]. Between the arterial and venous sheaths of serous pericardium is the **transverse sinus of the pericardium**. This permits some movement between the arterial and venous ends of the heart.

The pericardium lies posterior to the body of the sternum and the cartilages of the second to sixth ribs. It is separated from these by the tissues of the anterior mediastinum and by the lungs and pleurae, except: (1) where two condensations of fibrous tissue (**sternopericardial ligaments**) connect it to the superior and inferior parts of the body of the sternum; and (2) where the left pleura deviates to the left and leaves the pericardium directly in contact with the sternum and transversus thoracis muscle. To the left of this, the pericardium is covered by the anterior extremity of the left plural sac which is filled by the cardiac notch of the left lung only in deep inspiration.

The lateral surfaces of the pericardium are in contact with the phrenic nerves and mediastinal pleura. The posterior surface is in contact with the oesophagus and descending aorta which separate it from the vertebral column. The pulmonary veins pierce the pericardium where the lateral and posterior surfaces meet [Fig. 74].

Dissection

Make a vertical cut through each side of the pericardium immediately anterior to the line of the phrenic nerve. Join the lower ends of these two incisions by a transverse cut approximately 1 cm above the diaphragm. Turn the flap of pericardium upwards and examine the pericardial cavity. Determine the attachment of the flap to the superior vena cava, aorta, and pulmonary trunk. Cut through these attachments, leaving a narrow strip of pericardium on the vessels so that its position may be determined later [Fig. 51].

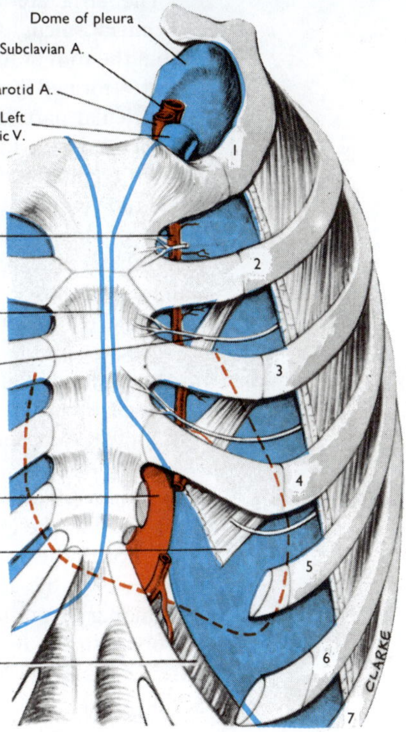

Fig. 50. A diagram to show the structures anterior to the pericardium and heart. Outline of pericardium and heart, broken red line; parietal pleura, blue. 1–7, ribs and costal cartilages.

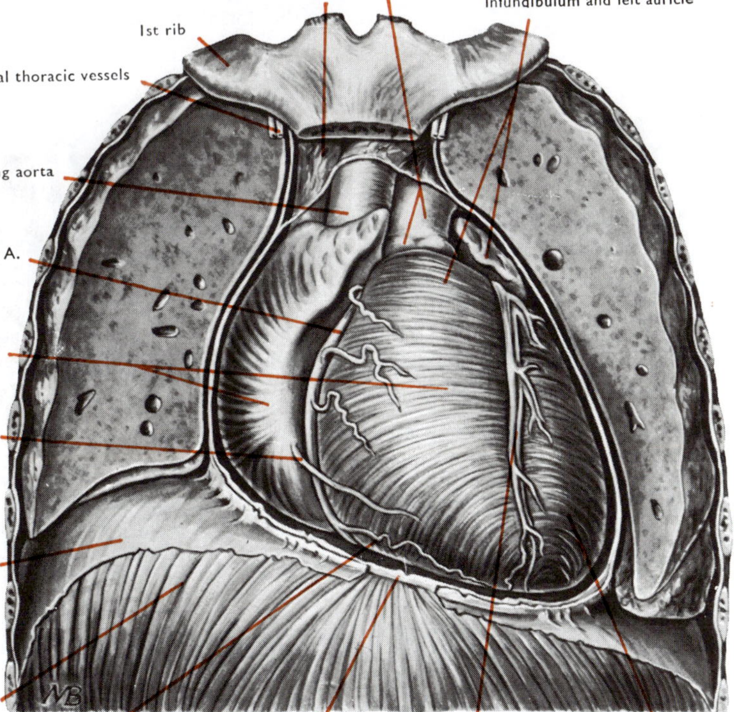

Fig. 51. The sternocostal surface of the heart *in situ*. The front of the pericardium has been removed together with the anterior parts of both lungs.

Sternocostal surface of heart [Figs. 281, 282]

The heart is rotated so that the **right ventricle** and **atrium** form the greater part of the sternocostal (anterior) surface with the left ventricle forming only a small strip which includes the apex pointing to the left and anteriorly.

The **atria** lie posterosuperior to the ventricles, and like them are completely fused though separated internally by a septum. The upper parts of the combined atria form a U-shaped structure the ends of which are the **auricles** of the atria. This U partly surrounds the ascending aorta and the pulmonary trunk, the auricles tending to overlap these anteriorly.

The atria are everywhere separated from the ventricles by the deep **coronary sulcus**. On the sternocostal surface, the sulcus passes obliquely from the root of the ascending aorta to the junction of the **right border** of the heart (formed by the right atrium) with the diaphragmatic surface. The ventricular part of the sternocostal surface lies to the left of this part of the sulcus and is divided by the **anterior interventricular sulcus** into a right two-thirds (right ventricle) and a left third (left ventricle). This sulcus marks the line along which the **interventricular septum** meets the sternocostal surface and contains the anterior interventricular branch of the left coronary artery and the great cardiac vein usually buried in fat. The sternocostal surface of the right ventricle narrows superiorly (**infundibulum** of the right ventricle) to become continuous with the pulmonary trunk. The continuity of the left ventricle with the aorta is not visible on this surface because it lies posterior to the infundibulum [Fig. 54].

The **left border** of the sternocostal surface is formed by the convex, bulging wall of the left ventricle with the **left auricle** superiorly.

Sinuses of pericardium

The **transverse sinus** of the pericardium lies between the pericardial sheath surrounding the great arteries and that enclosing the veins. Place your finger anterior to the lowest part of the superior vena cava and push it to the left, posterior to the ascending aorta. The finger appears on the left between the pulmonary trunk and the left auricle. With the finger in the sinus, pass a probe into the right pulmonary artery till it appears through the cut end of the left pulmonary artery. The probe lies posterosuperior to the finger in the sinus. Pass a blunt probe through one of the cut pulmonary veins to the upper limit of the left atrium. This probe will be felt postero-inferior to the finger in the transverse sinus. This demonstrates that the **pulmonary arteries** lie on the transverse sinus and the superior margin of the left atrium. The sinus is an aperture in the dorsal mesentery of the heart between its venous and arterial

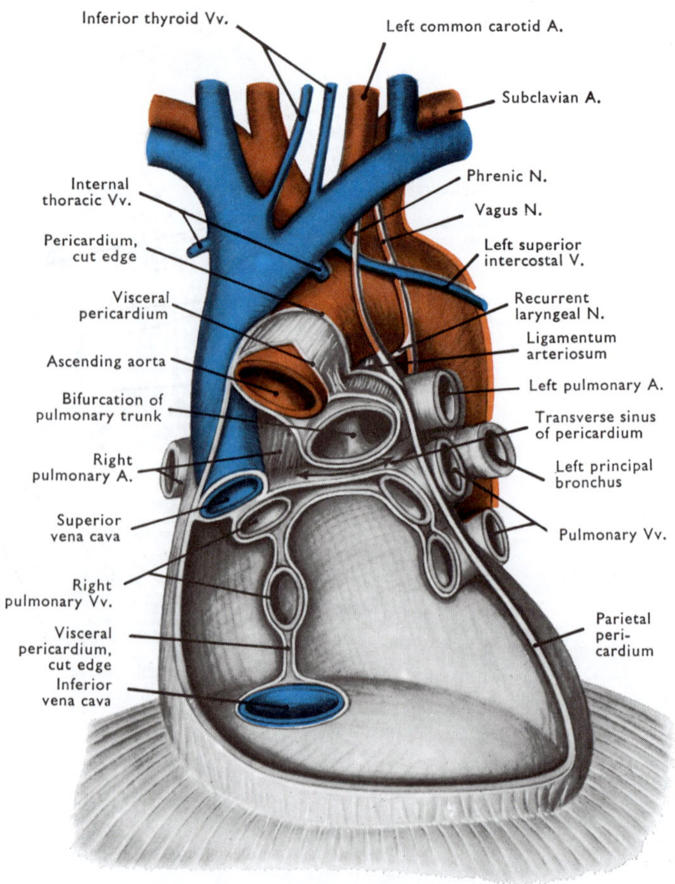

Fig. 52. The pericardium and great vessels after removal of the heart. The arrows lies in the transverse sinus of the pericardium, and the posterior wall of the oblique sinus lies between the right and left pulmonary veins. Pulmonary arteries and veins uncoloured.

ends. As the straight heart tube folds, the sinus is caught between these two ends of the heart tube as they come together [Figs. 29, 31].

The **oblique sinus** of the pericardium is a blind pocket of the pericardial cavity which lies posterior to the heart between the right and left pulmonary veins entering the left atrium [Figs. 52, 54, 71]. Lift the heart from the diaphragmatic pericardium and pass the fingers superiorly behind the heart into the sinus. A probe in any of the pulmonary veins may now be felt on the corresponding side of your fingers while their tips lie close to the finger in the transverse sinus [Fig. 54]. The left atrium lies immediately anterior to the fingers in the oblique sinus, but is separated from them by its covering of visceral pericardium.

Serous pericardium

This thin, elastic layer of tissue lines the fibrous pericardium (**parietal layer**) and covers the heart and the parts of the great vessels enclosed within the fibrous pericardium (**visceral layer**). The serous pericardium is more complex than the fibrous pericardium because of the presence of the oblique and transverse sinuses within it [Fig. 52].

Dissection

Strip the visceral pericardium from the sternocostal surface of the heart. Expose the **anterior interventricular branch of the left coronary artery** and the **great cardiac vein** by scraping the fat from the anterior interventricular sulcus. Note the branches of the artery to both ventricles and to the interventricular septum which lies deep to it. Trace the artery inferiorly to the diaphragmatic surface and superiorly to the left of the pulmonary trunk [Fig. 51].

Carefully remove the fat from the coronary sulcus. Avoid damage to the small **anterior cardiac veins** which cross it from the right ventricle to enter the right atrium directly. Find the **right coronary artery** in the depths of the sulcus. Follow the artery superiorly to its origin from the **right aortic sinus** (a swelling at the root of the ascending aorta deep to the right auricle) and inferiorly till it turns on to the posterior surface of the heart. Note the branches to the right ventricle and atrium. One of these passes over the left surface of the auricle towards the superior vena cava. It supplies part of the atrium and the sino-atrial node [p. 66].

Uncover the surface layers of the myocardium (muscle of the heart); note the general direction of its fibres and the depth of the coronary sulcus, the wall of the atrium passing deep to the bulging ventricular muscle.

Replace the anterior thoracic wall in position. Note the relation of the various parts of the sternocostal surface of the heart to the sternum and costal cartilages.

Surface anatomy of heart [Fig. 53]

The **superior border** of the heart is formed by the upper margins of the atria and is mainly hidden by the ascending aorta and the pulmonary trunk. The border extends from the upper part of the left second intercostal space (1–2 cm from the margin of the sternum) to the lower part of the same space on the right, close to the margin of the sternum. A line joining these points also marks the line of the pulmonary arteries which lie along this border of the heart.

The **right border** of the heart extends from the right end of the superior border to a point on the right sixth costal cartilage 1–2 cm from the margin of the sternum. This convex border is formed by the **right atrium** [Figs. 281, 282].

The **inferior border** extends from the lower extremity of the right border to the **apex of the heart**. This lies in the fifth left intercostal space immediately medial to a vertical line dropped through the midpoint of the clavicle (midclavicular line). This border, formed mainly by the right ventricle, lies at a lower level in the erect than in the recumbent posture and in inspiration than in expiration. It is normally slightly concave, but any condition leading to hypertrophy of the right ventricle, e.g. increased pulmonary arterial pressure, makes it convex, giving the heart a globular shape.

The **left border** is marked by a convex line joining the left ends of the superior and inferior borders. It is formed by the **left ventricle** except for a small part formed by the left auricle superiorly.

The **coronary sulcus** lies on a line joining the sternal ends of the third left and sixth right costal cartilages.

The great **orifices** of the heart and the **valves** which guard them lie on a line parallel and slightly inferior to the coronary sulcus. They will be seen when the heart is dissected. The **pulmonary orifice** lies posterior to the sternal end of the third left costal cartilage. The **aortic orifice** is posterior to the left margin of the sternum at the level of the third intercostal space. The **left atrioventricular** (mitral) **orifice** is posterior to the left half of the sternum at the level of the fourth costal cartilage. The **right atrioventricular** (tricuspid) **orifice** is posterior to the middle of the sternum at the level of the fourth intercostal space.

The positions given above are only approximate because the heart is a mobile organ whose shape and position varies with diaphragmatic movements and venous return. Thus if a deep breath is taken and expiration attempted against a closed mouth and nose, the heart is narrowed by the reduction in venous return caused by a high intrathoracic pressure and elongated by the lowering of the diaphragm. The converse effect is produced by attempting to inspire against a closed nose and mouth after full expiration [Figs. 13, 14].

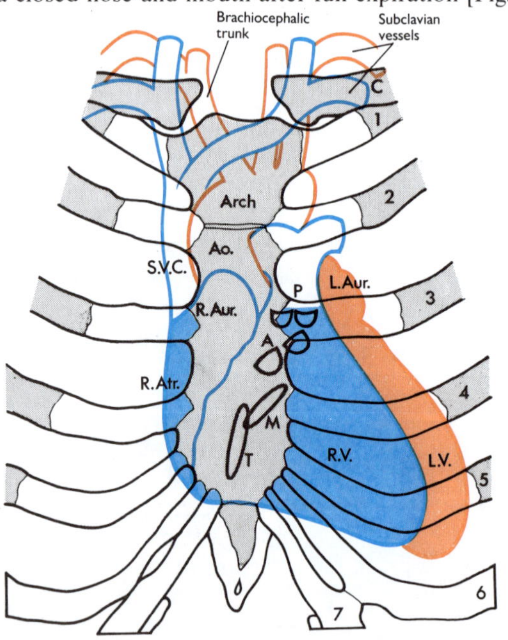

Fig. 53. The relation of the heart and the great vessels to the anterior wall of the thorax. The heart is shown in the high, cadaveric position.
1–7. Ribs and costal cartilages.
A. Aortic valve.
Ao. Ascending aorta.
C. Clavicle.
L.Aur. Left auricle.
L.V. Left ventricle.
M. Left atrioventricular (mitral) orifice.
P. Valve of pulmonary trunk.
R.Atr. Right atrium.
R.Aur. Right auricle.
R.V. Right ventricle.
S.V.C. Superior vena cava.
T. Right atrioventricular (tricuspid) orifice.

Diaphragmatic surface of heart

This slightly concave surface is formed entirely by the ventricles separated by the **posterior** (really inferior) **interventricular sulcus**, often visible as a line of fat. The sulcus contains the posterior interventricular branch of the right coronary artery and the middle cardiac vein. The left ventricle forms the left two-thirds of this surface [Fig. 76].

Base of heart [Fig. 281]

This is the posterior or vertebral surface. It is formed entirely by the **atria**, principally the left. The base is separated from the diaphragmatic surface by the posterior part of the **coronary sulcus**. This contains parts of the right and left coronary arteries and a large vein, the **coronary sinus**, which drains the heart and enters the right atrium to the left of the inferior vena cava [Figs. 71, 76, 282].

Coronary arteries [Figs. 51, 55, 66, 76]

These are the arteries of the heart. They are greatly enlarged vasa vasorum which arise from two of the three sinuses (dilatations) at the root of the aorta.

The **right coronary artery** arises from the right aortic sinus. It passes forwards between the auricle of the right atrium and the upper part of the infundibulum, and turns inferiorly in the coronary sulcus to the inferior border of the heart. Here it gives off the **marginal branch** [Fig. 51] and then turns to the left in the posterior part of the coronary sulcus where it gives off its largest, **posterior interventricular**, branch along the posterior inter-

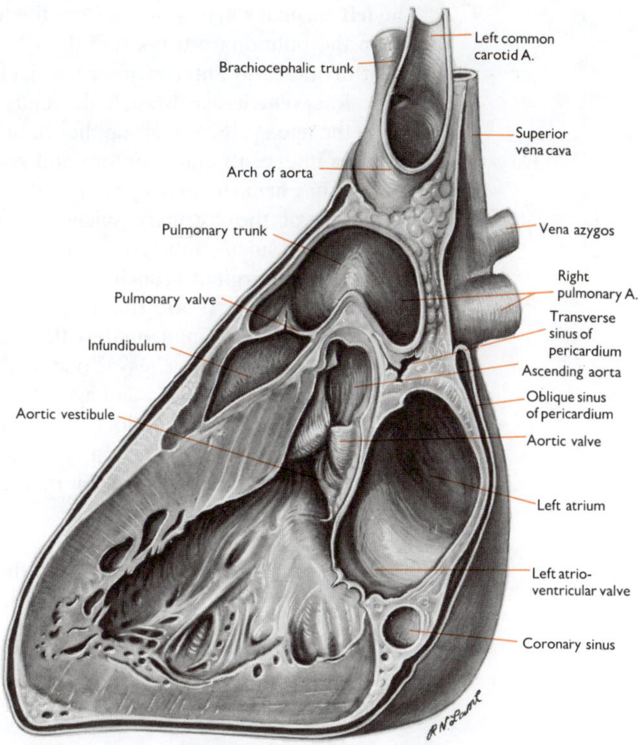

Fig. 54. A sagittal section through the heart and pericardium.

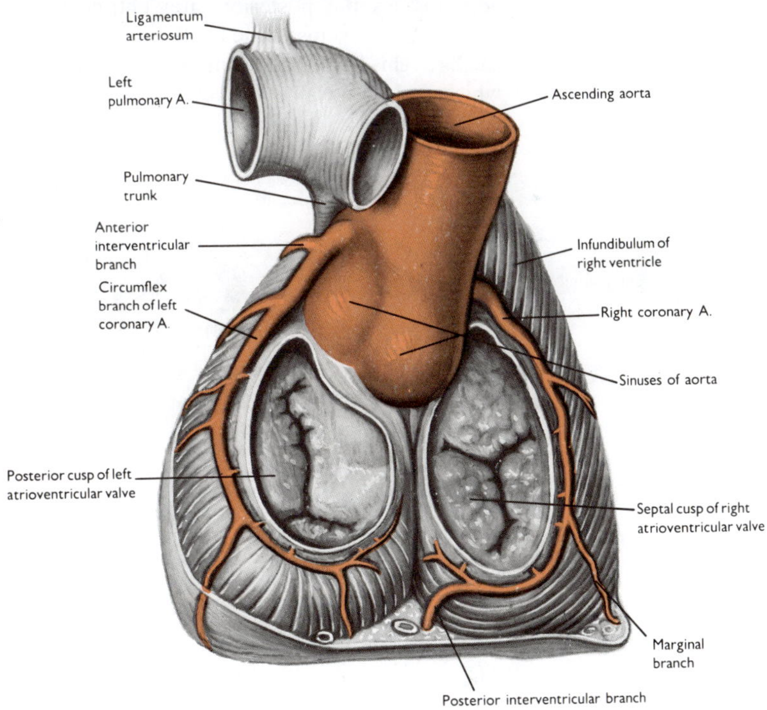

Fig. 55. The base of the ventricular part of the heart after removal of the atria. The right coronary artery usually extends further to the left than in this specimen; cf. Fig. 66. The sternocostal surface is to the right.

ventricular sulcus towards the apex [Fig. 76]. The right coronary artery continues in the coronary sulcus supplying a variable amount of the left ventricle and atrium. It ends *without anastomosing with the left coronary artery*. On the sternocostal surface, the right coronary artery supplies the right atrium and a large part of the right ventricle. While in the posterior part of the coronary sulcus, it supplies the remainder of the right atrium, all of the diaphragmatic part of the right ventricle, and a variable amount of the left atrium and ventricle. The posterior interventricular branch also supplies the postero-inferior part of the interventricular septum (including the atrio-ventricular node and bundle [p. 66]) and has small anastomoses with the anterior interventricular branch of the left coronary artery in the septum.

The **left coronary artery** arises from the left aortic sinus. It runs to the left between the pulmonary trunk and the left auricle. Emerging from between them, it divides into anterior interventricular and circumflex branches. The **anterior interventricular branch** descends in the anterior interventricular sulcus to the apex [Fig. 51]. It supplies both ventricles and the anterosuperior part of the interventricular septum and reaches the diaphragmatic surface. The **circumflex branch** curves postero-inferiorly with the great cardiac vein in the left part of the coronary sulcus. It ends to the left of the posterior interventricular sulcus and gives branches to the left atrium and ventricle, including a **left marginal branch**.

The coronary arteries are the only arterial supply to the heart. The two arteries anastomose so inadequately that blockage (coronary thrombosis) of any but the smallest branches of one artery usually leads to death of the muscle which it supplies. The damaged muscle is replaced by fibrous tissue if the individual survives the blockage. If the node or other parts of the conducting tissue of the heart [p. 65] are affected by the blockage, the ventricles may continue to contract at their own slow rate, independent of the atrial contractions (heart block).

Veins of heart

The coronary sinus will be seen later, but the main tributaries of this principal vein of the heart can now be seen [Fig. 56]. The **great cardiac vein** runs with the anterior interventricular and circumflex branches of the left coronary artery [Fig. 55] where it receives veins from the left ventricle. The **small cardiac vein** runs with the marginal branch of the right coronary artery and accompanies the right coronary artery in the posterior part of the coronary sulcus to the right extremity of the coronary sinus. The **middle cardiac vein** accompanies the posterior interventricular branch of the right coronary artery. All the veins of the heart enter the coronary sinus except the **anterior cardiac veins** [p. 43] and some small venous channels (**venae cordis minimae**) which lie in the walls of the heart and open directly into its chambers.

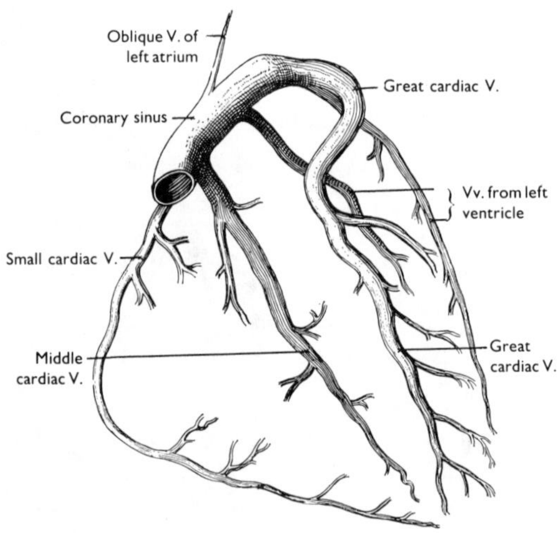

Fig. 56. A diagram of the tributaries of the coronary sinus viewed from in front.

Nerves of heart

The nerves are distributed to the heart from the cardiac plexuses which lie on the bifurcation of the trachea. They consist of sympathetic, parasympathetic, and sensory fibres. **Sympathetic fibres** come from the cervical and upper thoracic ganglia of the sympathetic trunk, and fibres transmitting pain run with these. **Parasympathetic fibres** arise in the cells of the cardiac plexuses and in ganglion cells scattered along the vessels of the heart. The preganglionic fibres reach these ganglion cells from the vagus which also transmits sensory fibres, mainly those concerned with recording pressure in the great veins and arteries. Stimulation of the sympathetic fibres dilates the coronary arteries and causes an increase in the rate and strength of cardiac contraction. Vagal stimulation slows or even stops the heart. The nerve fibres reach the heart along the great arteries (forming coronary plexuses on the coronary vessels) and veins. Many accompany the conducting tissue of the heart.

Chambers of heart

The chambers of the heart and the valves which separate them are best displayed by a series of coronal sections through the heart approximately parallel to the sternocostal surface [Figs. 57, 64, 73]. After each slice has been made, the sternum and costal cartilages can be folded back into position so that the relations of the parts of the heart to these structures can be determined. For development of the heart see p. 248.

Fig. 57. The heart *in situ*. A drawing of the parts of the heart exposed by the first coronal section. See dissection instructions, and Fig. 51.

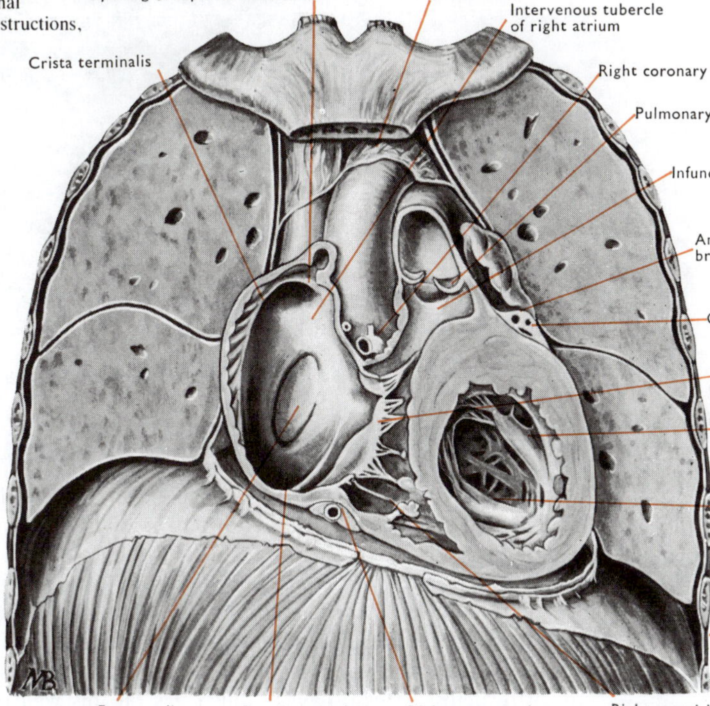

Dissection

The first coronal slice lies immediately anterior to the ascending aorta. Holding a knife in the coronal plane, lay it on the ascending aorta and cut towards the anterior part of the diaphragmatic surface of the heart. The knife should pass obliquely into the anterior surface of the pulmonary trunk and into the surface of the right atrium a short distance anterior to the entry of the superior vena cava. Continue the cut through the right surface of the right atrium to meet the diaphragmatic surface where the right coronary artery turns into the posterior part of the coronary sulcus. On the left side, carry the incision through the left surface of the heart to the apex in the same plane, passing immediately anterior to the left auricle. Lift the sternocostal surface of the heart anteriorly and divide the interventricular septum down to the anterior part of the diaphragmatic surface in the same plane. The two ends of the incision may now be joined, or the slice simply turned down on the diaphragmatic part of the heart. Remove any blood clot from the chambers of the heart without damaging the right atrioventricular valve or the valve of the pulmonary trunk. This exposes [Fig. 57] the right atrium, atrioventricular orifice and valve (tricuspid), and the right ventricle, infundibulum, pulmonary valve, and trunk and opens the left ventricle. Study all of these on both surfaces of the cut.

Right atrium
[Figs. 58, 281, 282]

The right atrium consists of (1) a smooth-walled posterior part which receives the superior and inferior venae cavae and the coronary sinus, and (2) an anterior part which is ridged by more or less parallel muscle bundles (**musculi pectinati**) which extend into the auricle. The two parts are separated on the

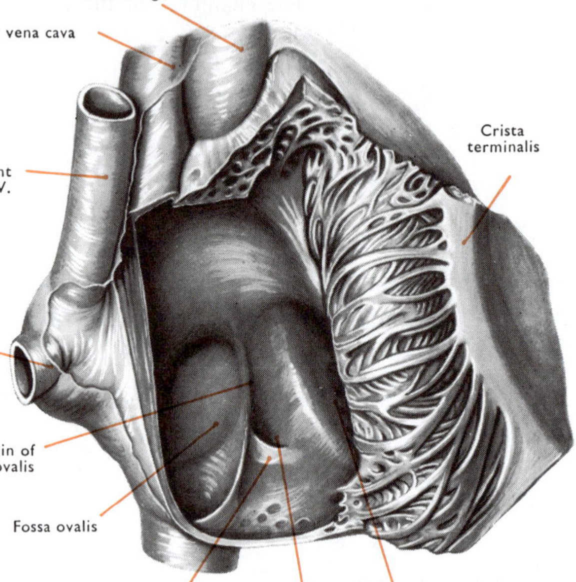

Fig. 58. The interior of the right atrium exposed by turning its right and anterior walls to the left.

right by an external groove (**sulcus terminalis**) and a corresponding internal vertical ridge (**crista terminalis**) which begins superiorly, anterior to the opening of the superior vena cava. It extends downwards and becomes continuous with a sharper ridge (valve of the inferior vena cava) which curves medially in front of the opening of the inferior vena cava and then ascends on the posteromedial wall of the atrium in line with the left wall of that vein. Here the ridge becomes continuous on its left with a small flap (**valve of the coronary sinus**) and superiorly with the curved margin (**limbus fossae ovalis**) of an oval fossa (**fossa ovalis**) which lies on this wall of the right atrium midway between the openings of the two venae cavae.

The crista terminalis and the valves of the inferior vena cava and coronary sinus together represent the remains of the right of two venous valves which guard the opening of the **sinus venosus** (smooth-walled part of the right atrium) into the right atrium (rough-walled portion of right atrium) in the embryo, before these two chambers coalesce to form the adult right atrium.

The posteromedial wall of the right atrium is the **interatrial septum** [Figs. 73, 281]. The fossa ovalis is the remnant of the **foramen ovale**—an oblique valvular opening which transmits the inferior vena caval blood (including the oxygenated blood from the placenta) from the right to the left atrium during intra-uterine life. Then the interatrial septum consists of two incomplete septa, each of which normally covers the aperture in the other. To the right lies the rigid septum secundum, the free margin of which becomes the limbus fossae ovalis. To the left lies the thin, flexible septum primum which is perforated above the upper limit of the limbus. During intra-uterine life, the septum primum balloons to the left, thus opening a channel (foramen ovale) which leads into the left atrium between the two septa. This channel remains open so long as the pressure in the left atrium is lower than that in the right atrium—a situation which is present before birth because of the small amount of blood traversing the lungs and entering the left atrium. After birth, the full pulmonary circulation is established. This raises the pressure in the left atrium so that the septum primum is forced against the septum secundum and closes the channel. Subsequently the two septa fuse, the septum primum forming the floor of the fossa ovalis and being adherent to the limbus fossae ovalis. Thus if the foramen ovale persists, it lies between the floor of the fossa and the upper margin of the limbus.

Note that the opening of the inferior vena cava into the right atrium faces directly towards the fossa ovalis on the sloping interatrial septum [Fig. 60] and that the valve of the inferior vena cava merely directs the blood towards

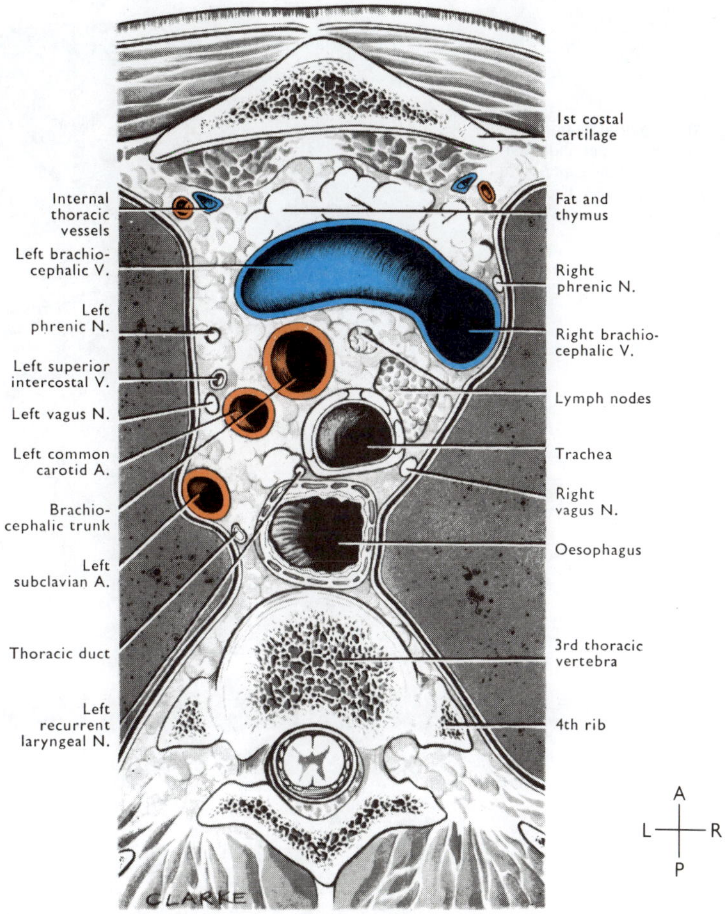

Fig. 59. A horizontal section through the thorax at the level of the third thoracic vertebra. See also Fig. 276.

the fossa. The opening of the superior vena cava into the right atrium lies on a more anterior plane and faces the right atrioventricular orifice—a feature marked by the **intervenous tubercle** [Figs. 57, 60]. This arrangement produces an almost complete separation of the two venous streams before birth.

Superior vena cava
[Figs. 277–280]

This vein is formed by the union of the right and left brachiocephalic veins behind the sternal end of the first right costal cartilage. It ends in the superior part of the right atrium at the level of the third right costal cartilage close to the sternum. The azygos vein arches over the superior surface of the right lung root [Fig. 33] and enters the posterior surface of the superior vena cava at its midpoint, just before it enters the pericardium. Thus the superior vena cava drains all the blood from the head and neck, upper limbs, and the walls of the thorax and upper abdomen (azygos vein).

The superior vena cava lies on the right partly in the superior and partly in the middle mediastinum. It is anterolateral to the trachea, anterior to the lung root, and lateral to the ascending aorta. The phrenic nerve and the right mediastinal pleura lie on its right surface, but are separated from its lower half by the pericardium. The close association of the superior vena cava with the right lung root and its contained pulmonary veins [Fig. 33] makes it possible for an abnormal pulmonary vein to drain directly into the superior vena cava from the right lung.

Inferior vena cava
[Figs. 60, 82]

The intrathoracic part of this vein is short. It pierces the central tendon of the diaphragm and pericardium approximately at the level of the eighth thoracic vertebra and immediately enters the inferior part of the right atrium at the level of the sixth chondrosternal joint. The right pleura and lung are wrapped round the right and posterior surfaces of the inferior vena cava and separate it from the vertebral column posteriorly. The right phrenic nerve descends on its right surface. For vein development see p. 249.

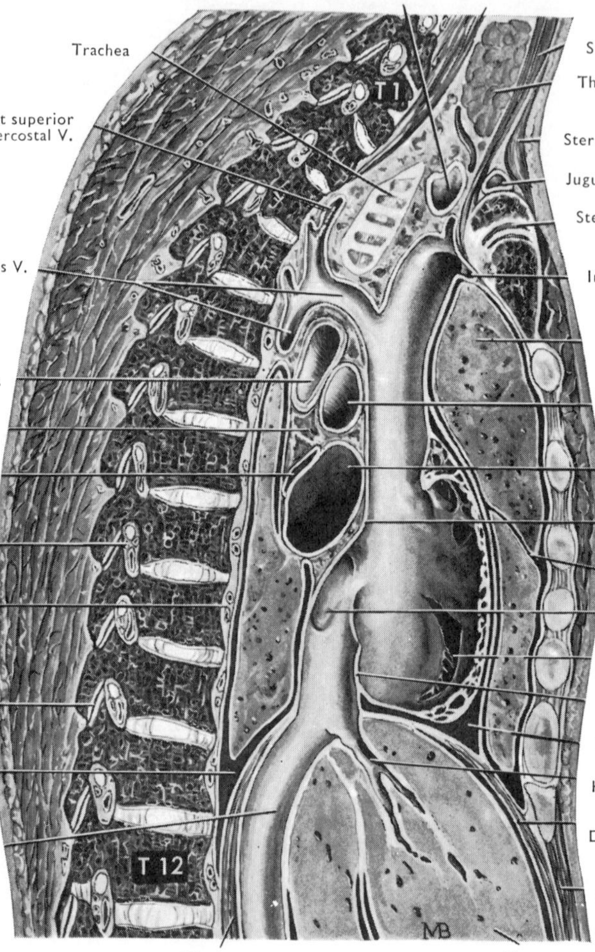

Fig. 60. A sagittal section through the thorax and upper abdomen along the line of the superior and inferior venae cavae. The remainder of this section is shown in Fig. 130.

Coronary sinus
[p. 64; Figs. 56, 58, 71, 76, 281, 282]

This main vein of the heart enters the right atrium immediately posterior to the right atrioventricular orifice and to the left of the valve of the inferior vena cava which separates it from the fossa ovalis. The **valve** of the coronary sinus lies to the right of its opening and directs its blood towards the atrioventricular orifice.

Veins of the heart which do not enter the coronary sinus are: (1) the **anterior cardiac veins** which pierce the anterior wall of the right atrium; (2) small **venae cordis minimae** which enter the right atrium through irregularly scattered openings which are difficult to identify.

The right atrioventricular orifice opens from the antero-inferior part of the right atrium into the postero-inferior part of the right ventricle. The orifice is guarded by the three cusps of the right atrioventricular (tricuspid) valve [Fig. 66].

Right ventricle
[Figs. 57, 62, 65, 78, 281, 282]

The cavity of the right ventricle is approximately triangular in shape when seen from the anterior surface [Fig. 62]. Blood enters through the **atrioventricular orifice** at the right inferior angle posteriorly, and leaves through the **pulmonary orifice** at the superior angle. The **infundibulum** (= a funnel) is the smooth-walled anterosuperior part of the ventricle which leads to the pulmonary orifice. The remainder of the ventricle has irregular muscle ridges (**trabeculae carneae**) projecting from its internal surface. In addition, a number of conical muscle masses project into the cavity of the ventricle. Each of these **papillary muscles** is inserted into the margins and ventricular surfaces of two adjacent cusps of the right atrioventricular valve by tendinous strands (**chordae tendineae**). When the papillary muscles contract, they draw the margins of adjacent cusps together and also prevent them from being forced back into the atrium as the intraventricular pressure rises. This increases the efficiency of the ventricular contraction and permits the atrium to fill completely while the ventricle is contracting.

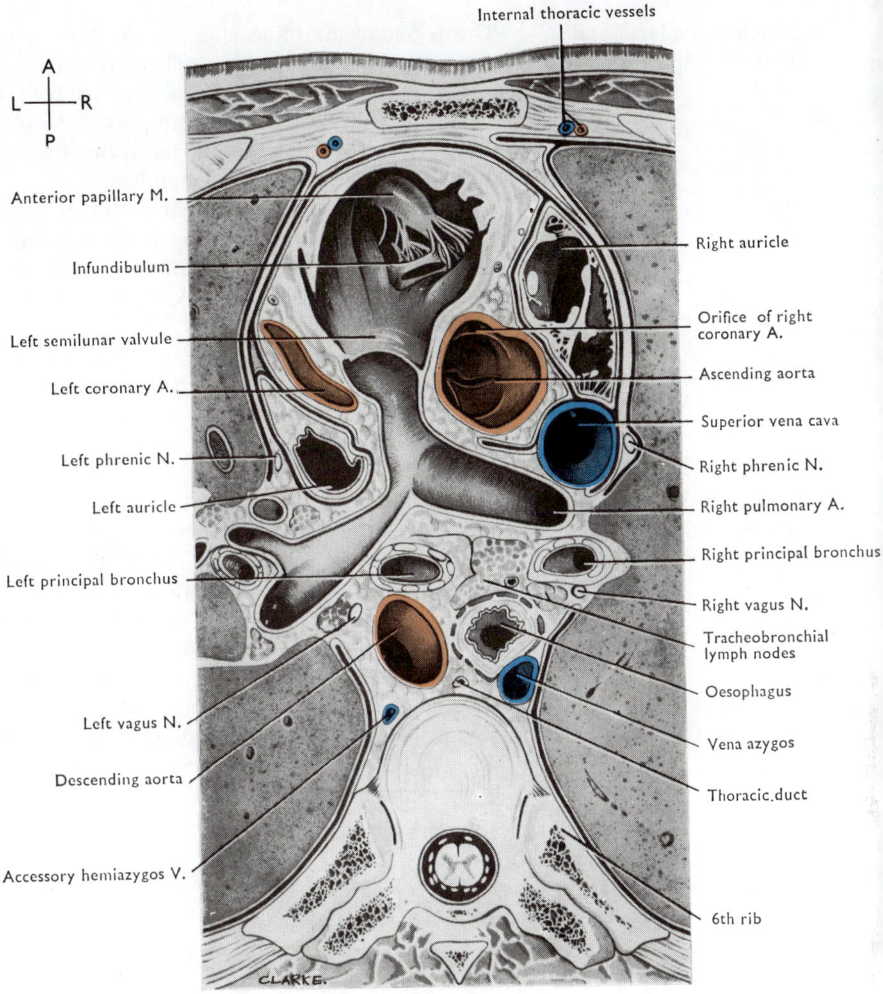

Fig. 61. A horizontal section through the thorax at the level of the intervertebral disc between the fifth and sixth thoracic vertebrae. See also Fig. 279.

Papillary muscles

There are usually three papillary muscles in the right ventricle. (1) A large posterior papillary muscle, attached to the inferior wall, sends chordae tendineae to the posterior and septal cusps of the valve. (2) A larger anterior papillary muscle, attached to the anterior wall, is distributed to the anterior and posterior cusps. (3) Several small septal papillary muscles, or simply chordae tendineae, pass from the septum to the anterior and septal cusps. The anterior and posterior muscles are occasionally divided into a number of smaller projections.

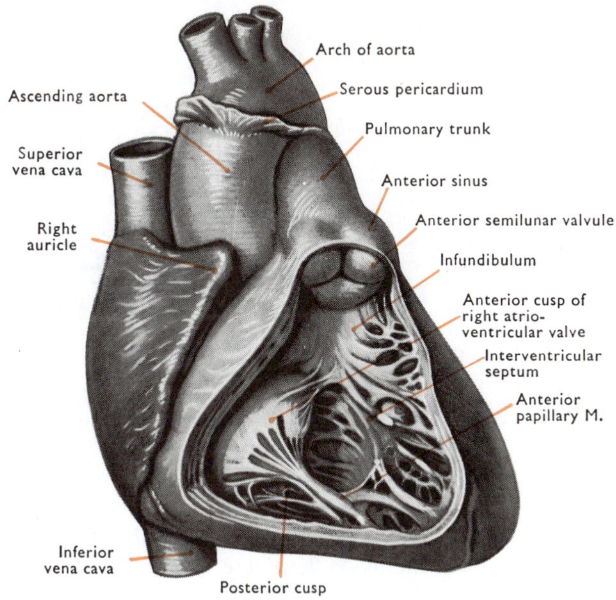

Fig. 62. The interior of the right ventricle exposed from in front.

Septomarginal trabecula [Figs. 62, 78]

This is one of the trabeculae carneae which passes from the septum to the anterior papillary muscle and carries part of the right crus of the **atrioventricular bundle** (conducting tissue of the heart, q.v.). This and similar parts of the bundle which pass to the other papillary muscles ensure early contraction of these muscles so that the chordae tendineae are already taut when ventricular contraction begins.

In transverse section, the right ventricle is crescentic in shape because the thick muscle of the interventricular septum bulges to the right. The difference in thickness of the muscle of the two ventricles is directly related to the work done by each in overcoming the low vascular resistance in the lungs (pulmonary systolic arterial pressure is 25–35 mm Hg) compared with the much higher pressure (120 mm Hg systolic) required to maintain the systemic circulation. Any condition which increases the pulmonary arterial resistance raises the right ventricular pressure and produces a compensatory hypertrophy of the right ventricular wall.

Right atrioventricular orifice [Figs. 57, 65]

This is approximately 2.5 cm in diameter. It is surrounded by a **fibrous ring** which gives attachment to the cusps of the right atrioventricular valve and the atrial and ventricular muscle. This ring is part of the **fibrous skeleton** of the heart which surrounds both atrioventricular orifices and also the pulmonary and aortic orifices. The cusps of all the valves are attached to the skeleton and its atrioventricular part interrupts the conduction of impulses from atrial to ventricular muscle except through the atrioventricular bundle. This special conducting bundle of muscle pierces the fibrous tissue at the postero-inferior part of the interventricular septum [Fig. 66]. This arrangement permits the delay which exists between atrial and ventricular contractions. The cut edge of the fibrous ring may be seen on the cut surface of the heart section [Fig. 67].

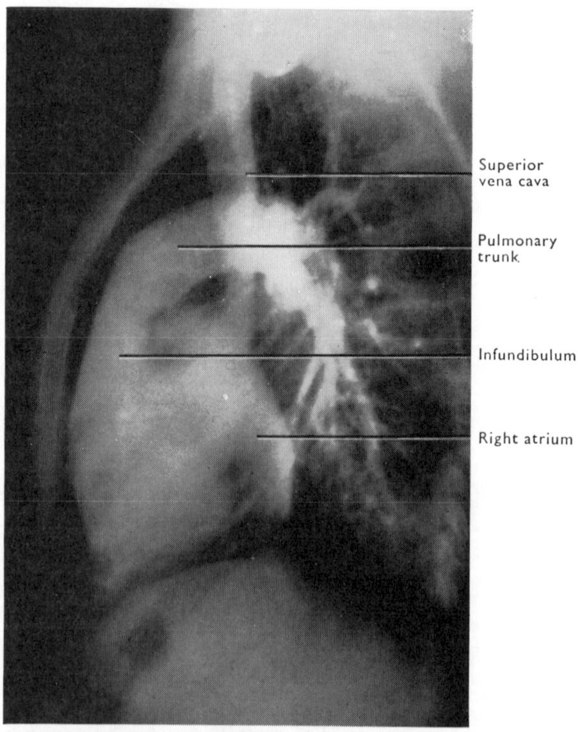

Fig. 63. A lateral radiograph of the thorax taken during the passage of a contrast material through the heart. In this phase the superior vena cava, right heart, pulmonary trunk, and pulmonary arteries are filled.

Right atrioventricular (tricuspid) valve

The three cusps of this valve are named from their position. The anterior separates the atrioventricular foramen from the infundibulum. The posterior lies on the inferior wall of the right ventricle. The septal lies on the interventricular septum. The anterior and posterior cusps are more nearly horizontal than vertical. The chordae tendineae are attached to the margins and ventricular surfaces of the cusps, while their atrial surfaces, over which the blood flows, are smooth.

Pulmonary orifice

This orifice lies at the apex of the infundibulum. It is surrounded by a slender fibrous ring which is continuous with the ventricular muscle and the pulmonary trunk and gives attachment to the valvules of the pulmonary valve internally.

Valve of pulmonary trunk

This has three **semilunar valvules** [Fig. 66]. Each is deeply concave on its arterial surface and is composed of a thin endothelial covered layer of fibrous tissue with a thickened free margin which forms the small, rounded **nodule** near the middle of that margin. The **lunules** are the thin, crescentic edges on each side of the nodule. The semilunar valvules are forced apart as blood is ejected from the contracting ventricle. As this ceases, the elastic recoil of the pulmonary trunk and arteries forces blood back towards the ventricle distending the semilunar valvules and forcing their margins together in the form of a Y with the nodules pressed together at the centre. The pulmonary valvules are named **anterior, right,** and **left** [Fig. 62]. The wall of the pulmonary trunk is slightly dilated opposite each valvule to form a **sinus**.

Pulmonary trunk
[Figs. 51, 54, 57, 63]

This great artery begins at the level of the pulmonary valvules, anterior and to the left of the ascending aorta, posterior to the sternal end of the third left costal cartilage. The trunk, approximately 5 cm long and 2 cm wide, winds round the left side of the ascending aorta to end in the concavity of the aortic arch posterior to the sternal end of the second left costal cartilage by dividing into right and left pulmonary arteries. The transverse sinus of the pericardium separates the trunk from the superior margin of the left atrium. The trunk and ascending aorta are enclosed in a single sheath of serous pericardium.

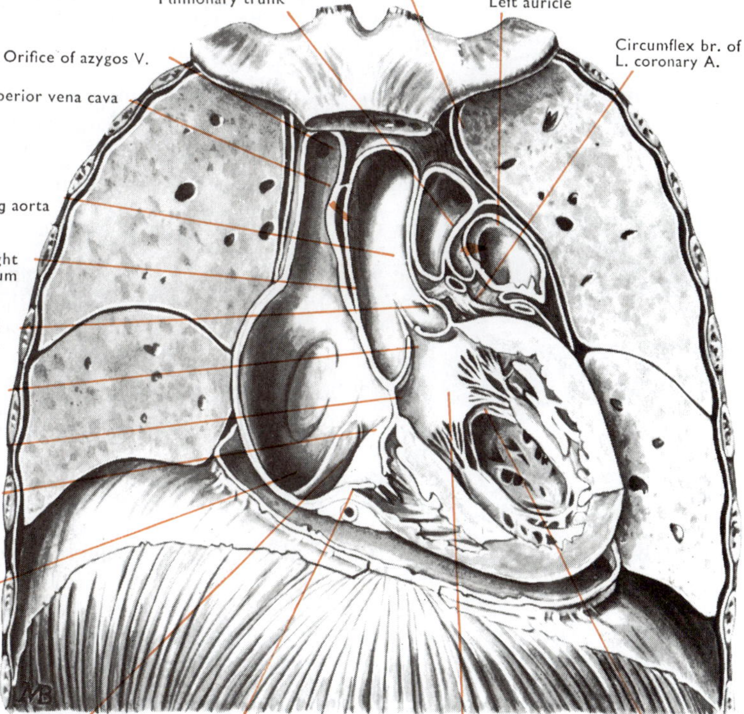

Fig. 64. The heart *in situ*. A drawing of the parts of the heart exposed by the second coronal section. See dissection instructions and Fig. 57. The arrow lies in the transverse sinus of the pericardium.

Dissection

Make the second slice through the heart [Fig. 64] by cutting transversely half through the superior vena cava and the aorta at the junction of the ascending part with the arch. Now turn the edge of the knife inferiorly, and cut longitudinally through the middle of both vessels parallel to the first slice. Carry this cut inferiorly through the right atrium, left auricle, and left ventricle as far as a horizontal line passing through the **membranous atrioventricular septum**. This can be identified as a small depression on the left wall of the right atrium approximately 1.5 cm anterior to the opening of the coronary sinus.

From the horizontal line, continue the cut downwards and forwards till it almost meets the first cut at the inferior surface of the heart.

Turn the slice forwards and remove any blood clot from the ascending aorta and the cavity of the left ventricle taking particular care not to damage the papillary muscles and chordae tendineae or fine strands which may be found passing from the interventricular septum to the papillary muscles. This exposes the ventricular end of the **left atrioventricular channel** and the smooth-walled **aortic vestibule** passing superiorly and to the right to the aortic valve. The vestibule is anterior to the anterior cusp of the left atrioventricular (mitral) valve and to the left of the membranous septum [below] which separates it from the right atrium and ventricle. In the posterior half of the aorta, find the orifice of the left coronary artery, and in its anterior half, find the orifice of the right coronary artery. Identify the opening of the azygos vein in the posterior wall of the superior vena cava.

In conjunction with the previous slice, the positions of all the valves of the heart can now be identified. Trace the left coronary artery. It lies posterior to the lowest part of the pulmonary trunk which has been removed. The anterior interventricular branch is divided at its origin by the last slice but the circumflex branch can be exposed by removing the fatty tissue between the root of the ascending aorta and the base of the left auricle.

Left ventricle
[Figs. 64, 65, 67, 282]

The cavity of the left ventricle is longer than that of the right. It is circular in transverse section, and its walls are very much thicker than those of the right ventricle. The trabeculae carneae are finer and more numerous than in the right ventricle. They are particularly marked at the apex, but the surfaces of the septum and upper part of the anterior wall are relatively smooth.

Papillary muscles
[Figs. 57, 64]

There are two large papillary muscles, anterior and posterior. The anterior is attached to the anterior part of the left wall. The posterior arises from the inferior wall further posteriorly. Each papillary muscle sends chordae tendineae to both cusps of the left atrioventricular (mitral) valve.

Aortic vestibule

The smooth walls of this part of the ventricle are mainly fibrous.

Aortic orifice

This orifice lies in the right posterosuperior part of the ventricle. It is surrounded by a fibrous ring to which the valvules of the aortic valve are attached. It is separated from the left atrioventricular orifice only by the anterior cusp of the mitral valve [Fig. 281]. Confirm this by passing a finger upwards between the cusps of the mitral valve. Thus the anterior cusp of the mitral valve separates the blood entering the ventricle from the atrium, from that leaving it to pass into the aorta. As a result the cusp is smooth on both surfaces. Note also that the aortic orifice is superior to the interventricular septum.

Aortic valve

This valve is the same as the pulmonary valve except that the valvules are thicker and differently placed (named right, left and posterior) and the **aortic sinuses** are larger [Fig. 65].

Interventricular septum

This septum is thick and muscular except posterosuperiorly where a thin membranous part [Figs. 64, 67] connects it with the fibrous rings which surround the atrioventricular and arterial orifices.

The interventricular septum is placed obliquely between the anterior and posterior interventricular sulci. The right surface faces forwards and to the right and bulges into the right ventricle [Fig. 57]. The **membranous part** extends from a point inferior to the right valvule of the aortic valve backwards to the anterior cusp of the mitral valve. The posterior part, which lies under the attachment of the septal cusp of the tricuspid valve, is very narrow and is continuous superiorly with the **membranous atrioventricular septum** which extends from it to the right wall of the aortic orifice and the muscular wall of the right atrium applied to the aorta. The interventricular and atrioventricular parts of the membranous septum together form the right wall of the aortic vestibule. The membranous interventricular septum is

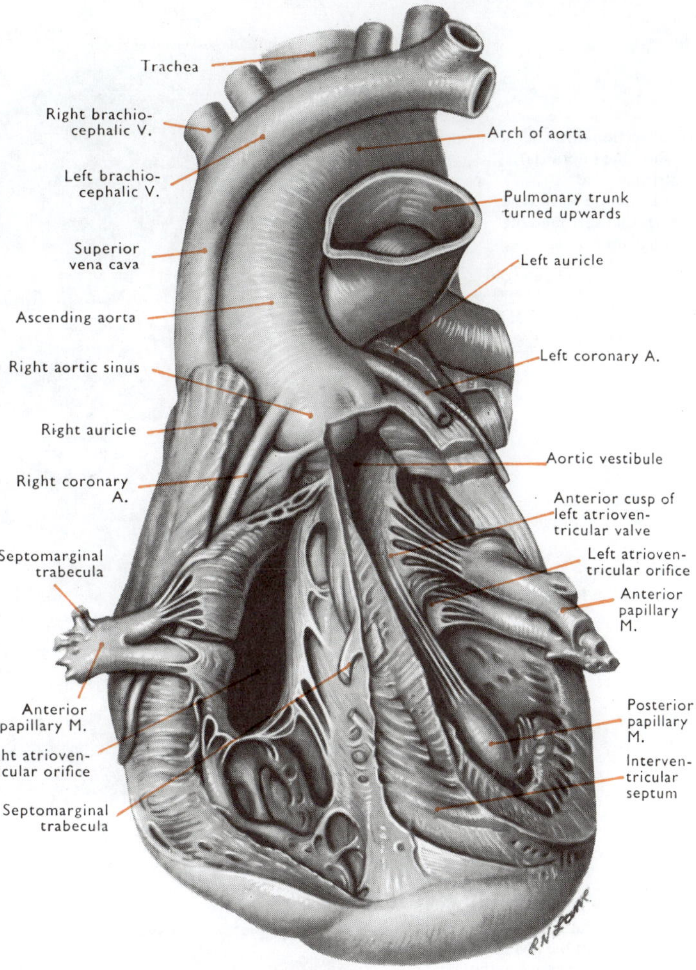

Fig. 65. A dissection of the ventricles of the heart. The root of the aorta has been exposed by separating the pulmonary trunk from the right ventricle and turning the trunk upwards.

developed from the same tissue which forms the valves of the heart. Since it develops separately from the muscular part of the septum, it may be deficient, thus leaving an interventricular foramen immediately inferior to the aortic orifice. The presence of such an **interventricular foramen** inevitably means that the pressures in both ventricles are the same—a situation which leads to hypertrophy of the right ventricular wall [p. 256].

The aorta

The aorta arises from the aortic orifice of the left ventricle behind the third left intercostal space at the margin of the sternum. It ends on the anterior surface of the fourth lumbar vertebra by dividing into right and left common iliac arteries.

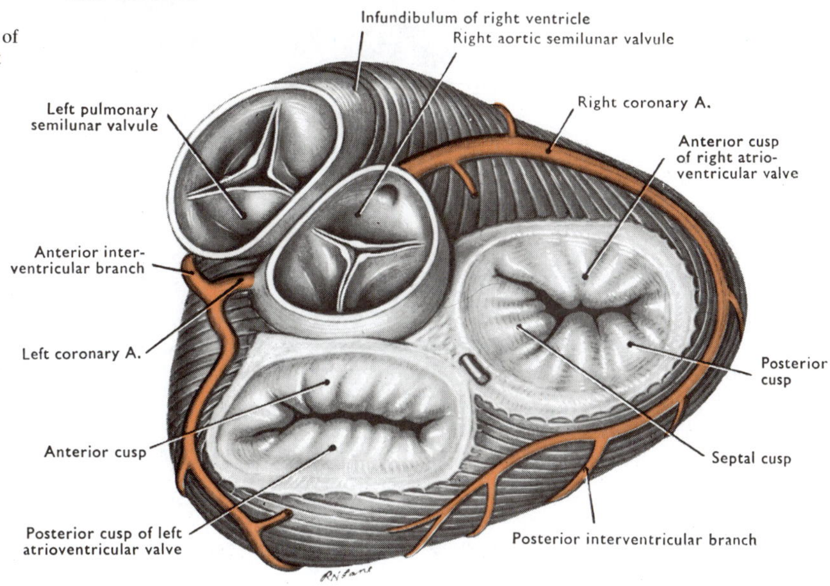

Fig. 66. A diagram of the base of the ventricular part of the heart with the atria and great vessels removed. The atrioventricular bundle is shown piercing the fibrous skeleton of the heart.

Fig. 67. A section through the heart to show the interatrial, atrioventricular, and interventricular septa, and the fibrous rings that surround the atrioventricular orifices.

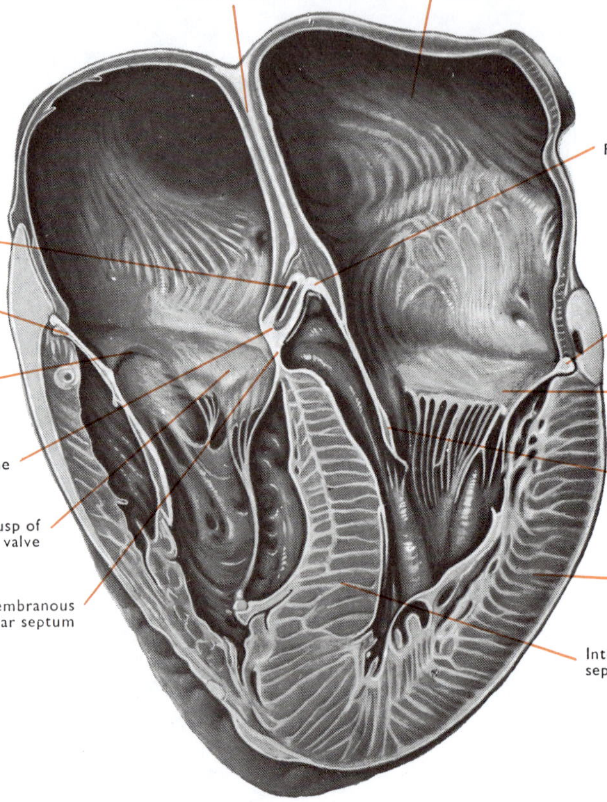

Fig. 68. A horizontal section through the thorax at the level of the intervertebral disc between the fifth and sixth thoracic vertebrae. See also Fig. 279.

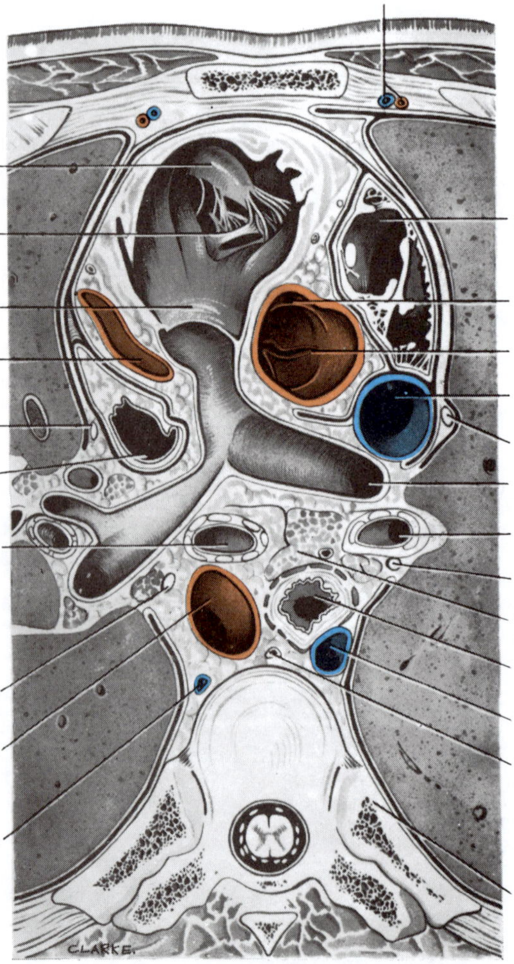

Ascending aorta
[Figs. 53, 57, 64, 65, 68, 75]

This is the first part of the aorta. It runs upwards, with a slight inclination forwards and to the right, to join the arch of the aorta behind the right half of the sternal angle. It is enclosed with the pulmonary trunk in a sheath of serous pericardium. The ascending aorta has four dilatations of its wall. (1) Three **aortic sinuses** at its root corresponding to the valvules of the aortic valve. (2) The **bulb of the aorta** is a swelling of the right border which receives the full thrust of the blood discharged from the left ventricle—a common site for the formation of an abnormal dilatation or aneurysm.

The ascending aorta begins between the left atrium and the infundibulum. The right atrium is on its right side. It then ascends anterior to the right pulmonary artery and right bronchus, with the superior vena cava to the right and the pulmonary trunk inclining posteriorly on its left surface [Fig. 68]. It is separated from the sternum by pericardium, pleura, lung, and remains of the thymus. The **vasa vasorum** of the ascending aorta arise principally from a branch of the left coronary artery which ascends on the left side of the aorta and sends circumferential branches at regular intervals. The right coronary artery may also send a branch.

The superior mediastinum

Dissection

If the upper limbs have been dissected and the clavicles divided, cut through the first ribs immediately anterior to the subclavian veins. Turn the manubrium of the sternum upwards to expose the superior mediastinum. If the upper limbs have not been dissected, make two drill holes through the middle of each clavicle approximately 1 cm apart. Cut through the clavicles between these holes with a fine saw, divide the first ribs as above, and turn the manubrium sterni upwards together with the medial parts of the clavicles and first costal cartilages. Later, the cut ends of the clavicles may be drawn together by a wire passed through the drill holes.

Identify the brachiocephalic veins and the upper part of the superior vena cava. Find the inferior thyroid, internal thoracic, and left superior intercostal veins and follow them into the brachiocephalic veins [Fig. 52]. Displace the veins and expose the remainder of the aortic arch and the branches which arise from its convex surface. Find the nerves which cross the left surface of the aortic arch and trace them superiorly between the left common carotid and subclavian arteries.

Find the left recurrent laryngeal nerve and the ligamentum arteriosum, anterior to the nerve, in the concavity of the aortic arch.

Brachiocephalic veins

Each of these veins is formed by the union of the internal jugular and subclavian veins posterior to the medial end of the corresponding clavicle. They unite to form the superior vena cava posterior to the lower border of the junction of the first right costal cartilage with the sternum [Figs. 38, 53, 59].

The **right brachiocephalic vein** has a short, vertical course. It is lateral to the brachiocephalic trunk and has the phrenic nerve posterolateral to it. The **left brachiocephalic vein** passes to the right and downwards, posterior to the upper part of the manubrium sterni. It lies anterior to the left common cartoid artery and the brachiocephalic trunk at their origins [Figs. 38, 47, 52, 59, 69].

Tributaries

Venous: the inferior thyroid, internal thoracic, vertebral, highest intercostal, and left superior intercostal veins. *Lymphatic: they are the only veins into which the lymph system of the body drains.* The right vein drains lymph trunks from the right side of head, neck, upper limb, and mediastinum. These combine in different ways before entering the vein. The left vein drains lymph from the remainder of the body through similar lymph trunks, but mainly through the thoracic duct.

Fig. 69. A horizontal section through the thorax at the level of the third thoracic vertebra. See also Fig. 276A.

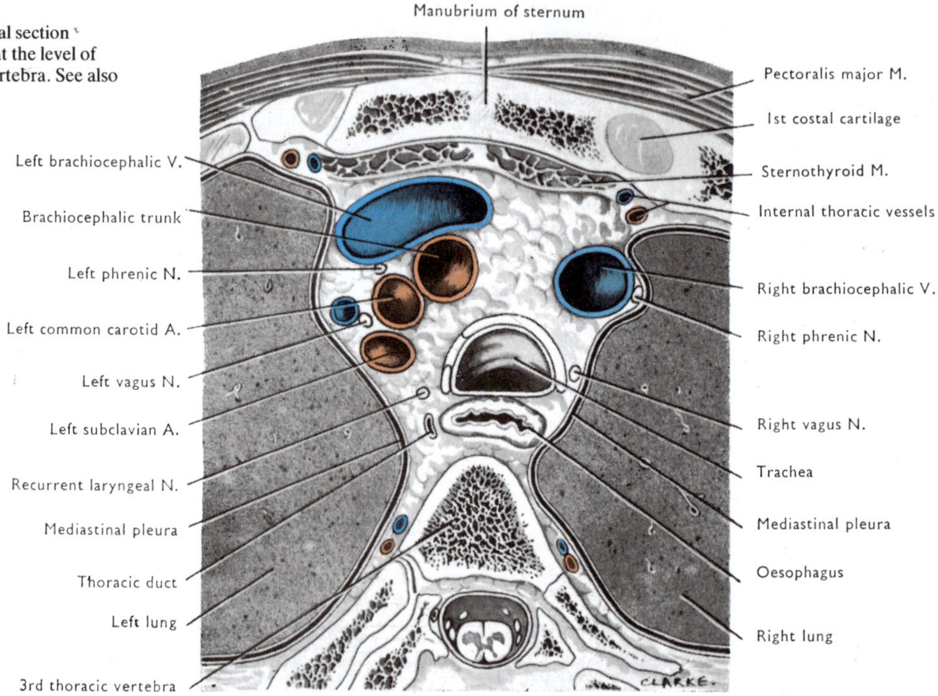

Fig. 70. A horizontal section through the thorax at the level of the fourth thoracic vertebra. See also Fig. 277.

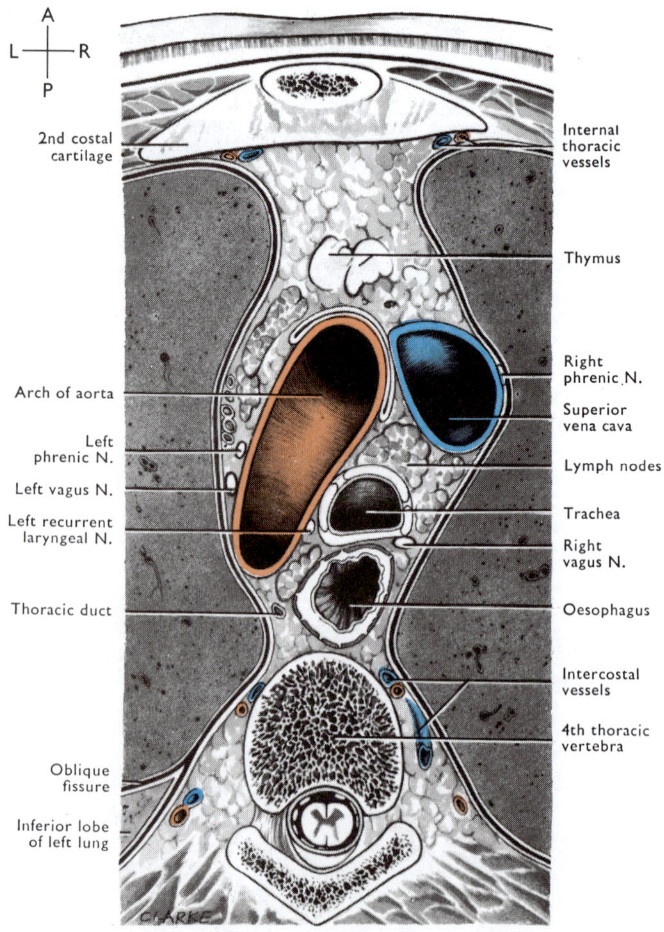

Arch of aorta

[Figs. 35, 52, 53, 70]

The arch begins posterior to the right half of the sternal angle. It passes posteriorly with a slight inclination and convexity to the left, while arching through the lower half of the superior mediastinum. The left convexity is where it crosses that side of the trachea and oesophagus [Fig. 70]. It joins the descending aorta on the left of the disc between the fourth and fifth thoracic vertebral bodies, in the same horizontal plane as its origin. Anteriorly it is in contact with remnants of the thymus and with the left brachiocephalic vein which crosses its upper part. Further posteriorly, the left surface of the arch is crossed by the phrenic nerve, the cervical cardiac branches of the left vagus (inferior) and sympathetic trunk (superior), the left vagus, and the left superior intercostal vein.

Inferior to the arch are the structures passing to the root of the left lung—the bifurcation of the pulmonary trunk, the left pulmonary artery, and the left bronchus [Figs. 73, 80]. The ligamentum arteriosum joins the arch to the root of the left pulmonary artery, with the left recurrent laryngeal nerve passing posterior to the ligament to the groove between the trachea and oesophagus, medial to the arch [Fig. 70]. The superficial cardiac plexus lies on the ligamentum arteriosum.

Branches of arch

Brachiocephalic trunk

This is the first and largest of the three branches. It arises behind the centre of the manubrium sterni [Fig. 53] anterior to the trachea and posterior to the left brachiocephalic vein. It passes superolaterally to reach the right side of the trachea, and ends posterior to the upper margin of the right sternoclavicular joint by dividing into right subclavian and right common carotid arteries, anterior to the dome of the pleura. The small **thyroidea ima artery** may ascend from it, on the front of the trachea, to the isthmus of the thyroid gland.

Left common carotid artery

This artery arises immediately to the left of the brachiocephalic trunk, and follows a similar course but on the left side. It is anterior to the left subclavian artery [Figs. 52, 59] with the left vagus and phrenic nerves between them, and enters the neck posterior to the left sternoclavicular joint.

Left subclavian artery

It arises from the arch or the aorta further to the left and more posterior than the other branches. It is in contact with the mediastinal pleura and ascends vertically. Thus it passes obliquely across the left side of the trachea, recurrent laryngeal nerve, oesophagus, and thoracic duct as they curve anteriorly with the vertebral column. It enters the neck some distance posterior to the sternoclavicular joint, and arches laterally, grooving the anterior surface of the cervical pleura and the apex of the lung [Figs. 35, 40].

Pulmonary arteries

These arteries will be seen more clearly in the next dissection, but their position should be confirmed now.

The **right pulmonary artery** [Figs. 68, 71, 73, 279, 280] begins in the concavity of the aortic arch anterior to the left bronchus. It passes to the right and slightly downwards, anterior to the oesophagus and right principal bronchus, posterior to the ascending aorta and superior vena cava. Close to the root of the lung it gives off the branch which accompanies the right superior lobar bronchus.

The **left pulmonary artery** lies inferior to the posterior part of the aortic arch [Fig. 73]. It passes posteriorly and to the left, crossing anterior to the left principal bronchus and the descending thoracic aorta [Fig. 68].

Ligamentum arteriosum

This short, fibrous band connects the superior surface of the root of the left pulmonary artery with the inferior surface of the arch of the aorta, distal to the origin of the left subclavian artery. The ligament lies between the left recurrent laryngeal nerve (posteriorly) and the superficial cardiac plexus (anteriorly). The ligament is the functionless remnant of a wide channel (the **ductus arteriosus** [Fig. 72]) which is of profound importance in fetal life.

During intra-uterine life, the lungs have no function because the fetal blood is oxygenated in the placenta and returned to the fetal heart through the umbilical vein and inferior vena cava. This blood, mixed with the venous blood from the lower limbs and abdomen in the inferior vena cava, passes

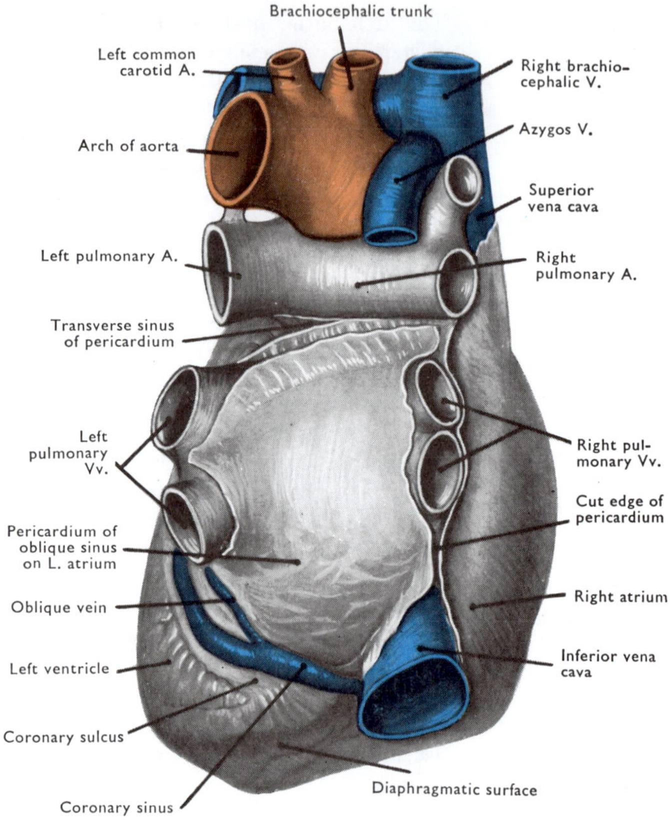

Fig. 71. The posterior surface of the heart and great vessels. The pulmonary vessels are not coloured.

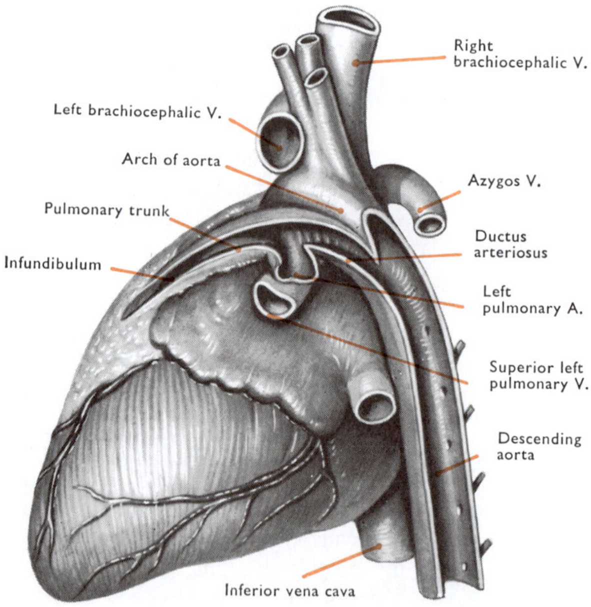

Fig. 72. A dissection of the heart and great vessels of a fetus. Note the direct connection of the pulmonary trunk with the aorta through the ductus arteriosus, a shunt which allows the blood in the pulmonary trunk to bypass the lungs in the fetus.

directly into the left atrium through the **foramen ovale** [p. 48] in the interatrial septum [Figs. 60, 270]. Thence it is passed to the left ventricle and pumped principally to the head, neck, and upper limbs through the branches of the aortic arch. A smaller quantity passes into the descending aorta.

The superior vena cava drains venous blood from the head, neck, upper limbs, and the walls of the thorax into the right atrium, and directs it through the right atrioventricular orifice into the right ventricle. Thence it passes through the pulmonary trunk and ductus arteriosus into the posterior part of the arch and descending aorta. Through this it is distributed to the remainder of the body and placenta, mixed with the smaller proportion of left ventricular blood. Thus none of the fetal tissues receive fully oxygenated blood—a feature which is compensated by an increased number of red blood corpuscles, a different haemoglobin, and more of it in each red cell.

That the blood in the pulmonary trunk enters the aorta indicates that the pressure is higher in the pulmonary trunk than in the descending aorta, and that the peripheral resistance in the lungs is greater than that in the territory of the descending aorta. This high pulmonary pressure accounts for the relatively thicker wall of the right ventricle in the fetus than in the adult.

The small amount of blood passing through the lungs accounts for the low pressure in the left atrium of the fetus. This permits the foramen ovale to remain open and the inferior vena caval blood to pass through it into the left atrium. At birth, the peripheral resistance in the pulmonary arteries drops suddenly by relaxation of their muscle, blood flows freely through the lungs from the pulmonary trunk to the left atrium raising the pressure in it and closing the foramen ovale. Subsequently the walls of the closed foramen fuse. The sudden drop in pulmonary arterial pressure causes blood to flow from the aorta to the pulmonary arteries along the ductus arteriosus. This is arrested by the contraction of the muscular wall of the ductus arteriosus which is usually complete within the first week after birth. Thus the pulmonary and systemic circulations are separated, and this becomes permanent with the obliteration of the lumen of the ductus arteriosus and the replacement of the ductus by fibrous tissue to form the ligamentum arteriosum by the end of the first year of life.

If the ductus arteriosus fails to close, the pressure in the pulmonary circulation remains as high as that in the systemic circulation. As a result the right ventricular wall hypertrophies and does not undergo the normal reduction in thickness which occurs in early postnatal life. The heart, therefore, becomes globular in shape, and the persistent high pulmonary pressure (pulmonary hypertension) has serious effects on the functions of the heart and lungs.

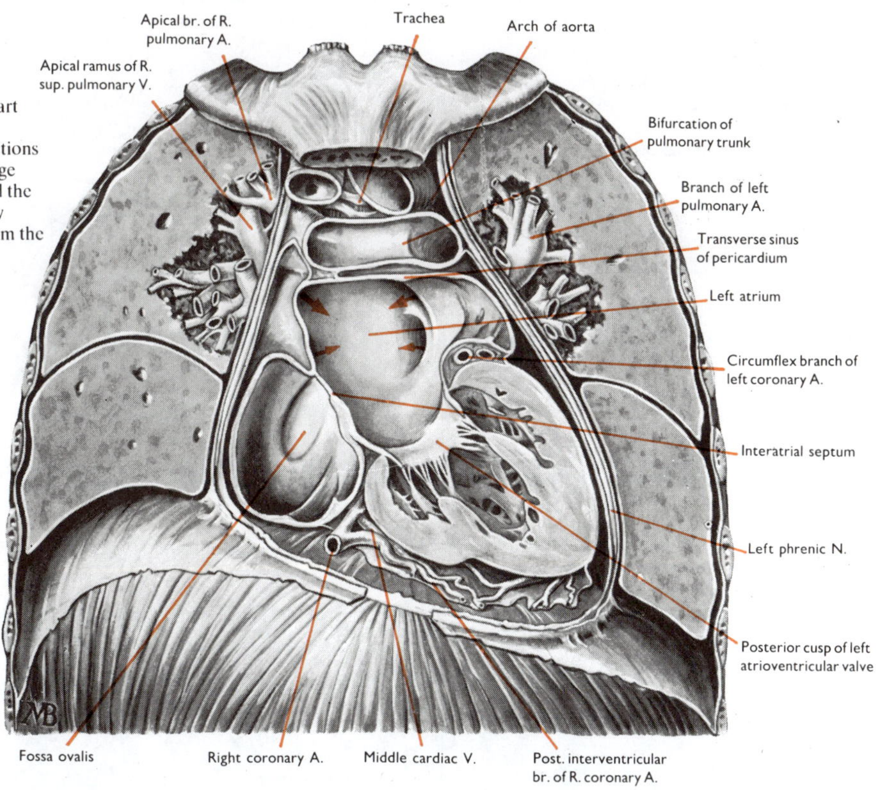

Fig. 73. The heart *in situ*. A drawing of the parts of the heart exposed by the third coronal section. See dissection instructions and Fig. 64. The arrows emerge from the pulmonary veins and the branches of the right coronary artery have been removed from the previous slice and left on the diaphragm.

Dissection

Turn the ventricular part of the heart anteriorly to expose the diaphragmatic surface. As far as possible define the vessels on this surface. In particular follow the **posterior interventricular artery** posteriorly and to the right to its origin from the right coronary artery. The **middle cardiac vein** runs a similar course to the right extremity of the coronary sinus.

The third slice through the heart [Fig. 73] is made parallel to the first. It exposes the left atrium, the left atrioventricular orifice, the posterior cusp of the left atrioventricular valve, the interatrial septum, and the pulmonary arteries. Begin at the apex of the heart 1–2 cm posterior to the previous section. Carry the knife posterosuperiorly through the left ventricular wall parallel to and between the cusps of the left atrioventricular valve, splitting the papillary muscles longitudinally and passing through the left atrioventricular orifice. Continue the incision through the left surface of the heart by passing through the base of the left auricle and the left pulmonary artery. Extend the cut in the artery to the right through the bifurcation of the pulmonary trunk and the root of the right pulmonary artery. Either cut through the arch of the aorta anterior to the ligamentum arteriosum, or leave the aorta intact. On the right side the cut should pass immediately anterior to the openings of the coronary sinus and inferior vena cava into the right atrium, and through the middle of the fossa ovalis. It should then pass posterior to the superior vena cava (leaving the phrenic nerve intact) to the level of the azygos vein. If the aorta has been divided, cut forwards through the superior vena cava and remove the slice, otherwise turn the slice forwards on the aorta and superior vena cava.

Remove the blood clot from the left atrium, pulmonary veins, and pulmonary arteries. Identify the cut ends of the right coronary artery, of the circumflex branch of the left coronary artery, and of the veins which accompany them in the right and left parts of the coronary sulcus. Confirm the arrangement of the pulmonary veins [Figs. 40, 41].

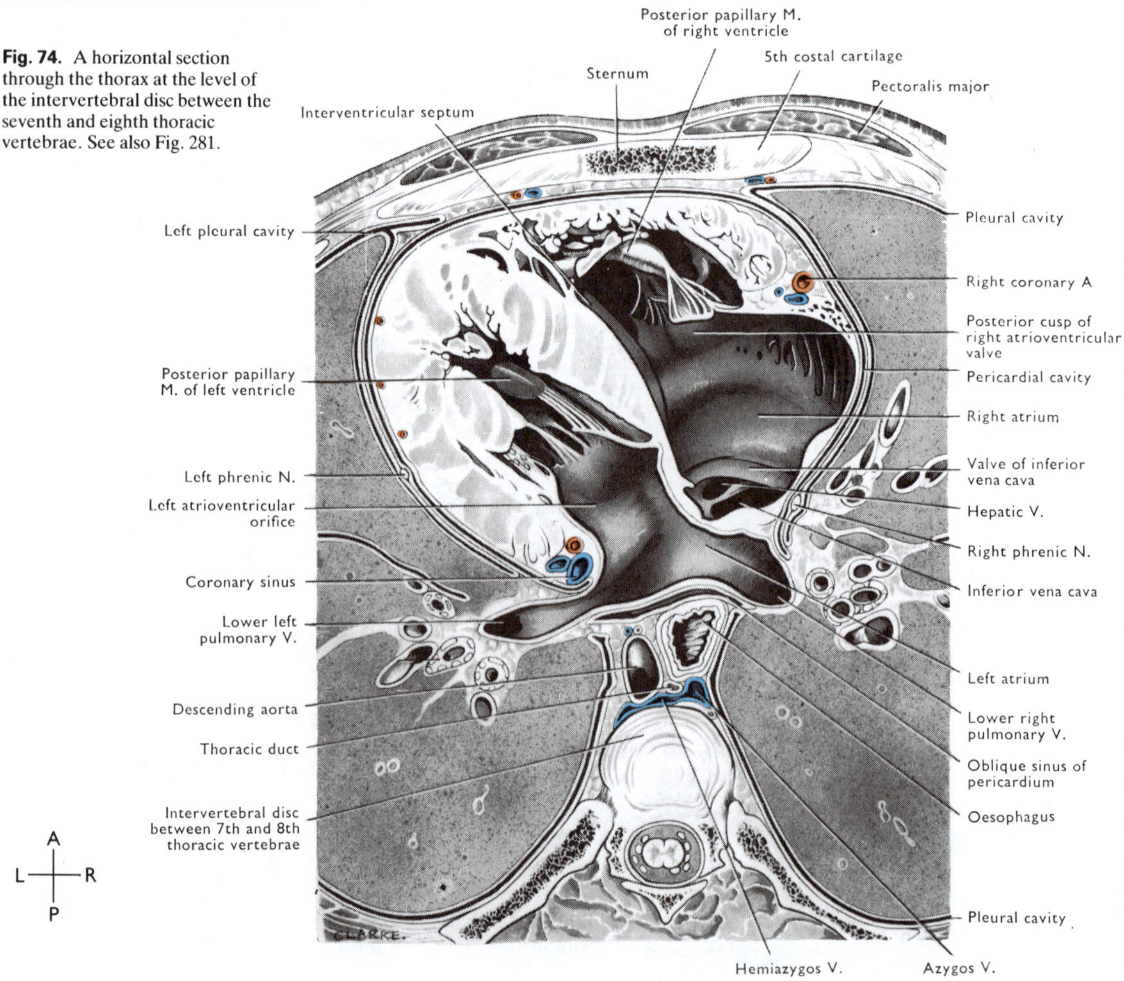

Fig. 74. A horizontal section through the thorax at the level of the intervertebral disc between the seventh and eighth thoracic vertebrae. See also Fig. 281.

Left atrium
[Figs. 54, 73–75, 281]

The left atrium lies posteriorly and forms the base of the heart. Anteriorly, the long narrow auricle projects forwards and partly overlaps the beginning of the pulmonary trunk. On each side, a **superior** and an **inferior pulmonary vein** enter the upper half of the atrium close to the lateral margins of the posterior surface. The superior veins are on a plane anterior to the inferior veins.

The upper part of the anterior surface of the left atrium is covered by the ascending aorta and the pulmonary trunk. The pulmonary arteries course along the superior margin. The coronary sinus runs transversely in the coronary sulcus along the inferior margin [Figs. 71, 76].

Interior of left atrium
[Figs. 54, 73, 74]

This is almost entirely smooth. Musculi pectinati are confined to the auricle. There is a prominent muscular ridge which projects into the atrium anterior to the left pulmonary veins, so that the orifices of these veins are not visible from in front.

The **interatrial septum** [Fig. 73] slopes posteriorly and to the right so that a considerable part of the left atrium lies posterior to the right atrium. Only the postero-inferior part of the right atrium, immediately superior to the entry of the inferior vena cava, forms part of the posterior surface of the heart.

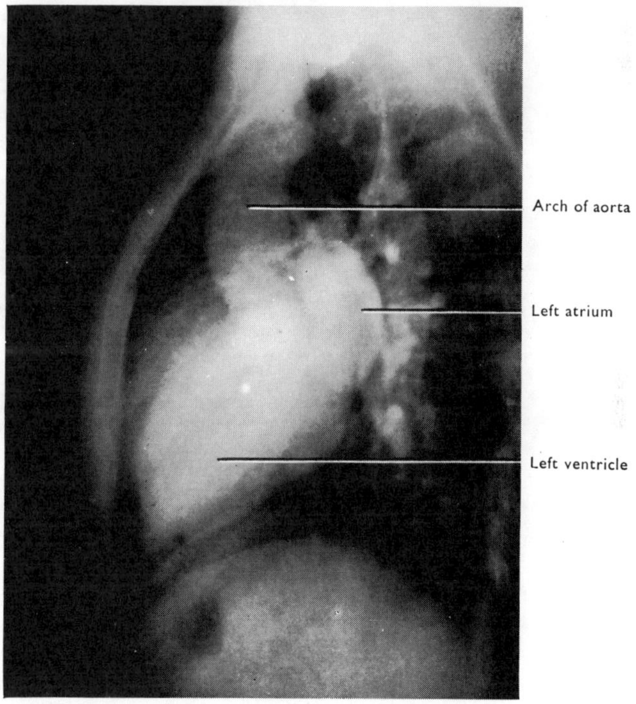

Fig. 75. A lateral radiograph of the thorax taken during the passage of contrast material through the heart. In this phase the left heart and part of the aorta are filled.

Orifices of left atrium

Neither the orifices of the pulmonary veins nor of the venae cordis minimae are guarded by valves.

The **left atrioventricular orifice** lies at the antero-inferior part of the left atrium. Through this orifice oxygenated blood is discharged into the left ventricle. The orifice is smaller (2 cm) than that of the right and usually admits the tips of two fingers only.

The **left atrioventricular** (mitral) **valve** has two obliquely set cusps. The larger anterior cusp lies anterior and to the right of the posterior cusp. The cusps are attached to the fibrous ring of the left atrioventricular orifice [Fig. 67] and they project into the ventricle. The **anterior papillary muscle** sends **chordae tendineae** to the ventricular surfaces and margins of the left or anterior halves of both cusps, while the **posterior muscle** is similarly attached to the posterior or right halves. The **anterior cusp** forms the anterior wall of the atrioventricular orifice and the posterior wall of the aortic vestibule. Thus it has blood flowing over both surfaces and has less extensive attachments of chordae tendineae to its smooth ventricular surface than the posterior cusp.

Dissection

Cut through the inferior vena cava and the pulmonary veins within the pericardial cavity including the pericardium which covers them [Fig. 52]. This pericardium and the contained veins form the walls of the oblique sinus of the pericardium posterior to the left atrium. Remove the remainder of the heart and examine its posterior surface.

Examine the coronary sulcus at the junction of the posterior and diaphragmatic surfaces of the heart. Remove the visceral pericardium which covers the sulcus and expose the vessels in it. First trace the **coronary sinus** to its opening into the right atrium, and then the branches of the right and left coronary arteries. Note that the right coronary artery supplies a considerable part of the diaphragmatic surface of the left ventricle, and that no large branches of the two coronary arteries anastomose in the coronary sulcus. Attempt to find the **oblique vein of the left atrium** [Fig. 76].

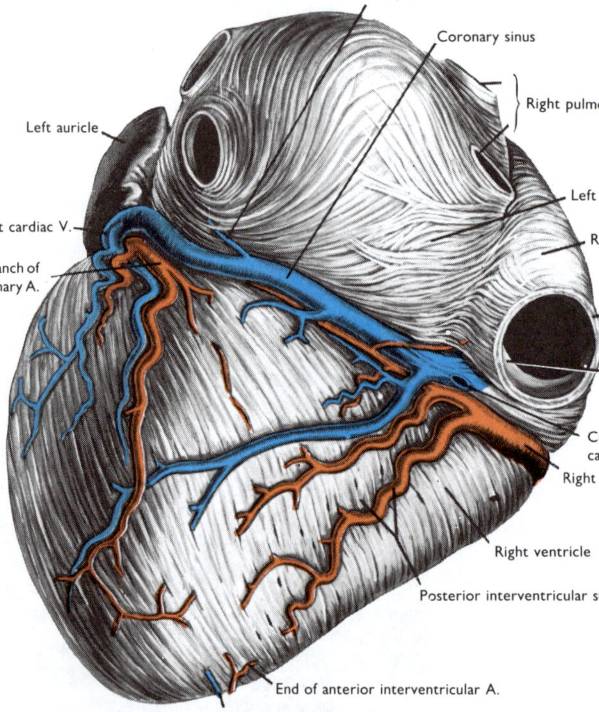

Fig. 76. A dissection of the diaphragmatic and posterior surfaces of the heart.

Coronary sinus

[Figs. 71, 76, 281, 282]

This large sinus drains all the venous blood from the heart except that carried in the anterior cardiac veins and the venae cordis minimae [p. 50]. The sinus formed by the junction of the great cardiac vein with the oblique vein of the left atrium [Fig. 71] runs from left to right in the posterior part of the coronary sulcus to the right atrium. The main *tributaries* of the coronary sinus [Fig. 56] are the **great cardiac vein** at its left extremity, and the **middle** and **small cardiac veins** at its right extremity. The great cardiac vein has a drainage corresponding to the left coronary artery while the middle and small cardiac veins drain most of the territory of the right coronary artery.

The **oblique vein of the left atrium** corresponds to the inferior half of the superior vena cava on the right. Thus a persistent left superior vena cava may replace the oblique vein and enter the coronary sinus. Both oblique vein and coronary sinus are partly covered by cardiac muscle on their posterior aspects.

Structure of walls of heart

The heart consists of a layer of cardiac muscle (**myocardium**) covered externally with serous pericardium (**epicardium**), and lined internally with **endocardium**. Both enclosing layers consist of connective tissue covered with relatively frictionless endothelium. The endocardium is continuous with the valve flaps and with the linings of the arteries and veins.

Myocardium

This is a striated type of muscle which consists of many short muscle cells joined end to end at intercalated discs. Many of the cells branch so that the whole forms a network over which electrical impulses can spread freely from cell to cell, except where the fibrous skeleton of the heart separates atrial and ventricular muscle.

Dissection of the muscle fibres is difficult once the heart has been sliced, but the general direction of the muscle fibres can be determined by stripping the muscle layer by layer.

Atrial muscle

(1) **Superficial fibres** run transversely round both atria. They are most easily seen close to the coronary sulcus. (2) A **deeper layer** runs anteroposteriorly across each atrium from the fibrous atrioventricular rings. (3) **Anular fibres** surround the orifices of the veins and extend a variable distance along the veins [Fig. 76]. All these layers merge with each other.

Ventricular muscle

(1) **Superficial fibres** arise from the atrioventricular fibrous rings and sweep spirally (clockwise as seen from the apex) towards the apex of the opposite ventricle. At the apex of each ventricle they form a whorl, and pass deeply to end in the **papillary muscles** of that ventricle. (2) The deeper layers consist of horizontal bundles which form S-shaped loops. These tend to begin and end in the papillary muscles. The intermediate part of each S lies in the interventricular septum with a loop in the wall of each ventricle. The loops are of unequal length in many bundles.

Conducting system of heart

[Figs. 77, 78, 269, 270]

This system consists of specialized muscle fibres. (1) It initiates the normal heart beat (**sino-atrial node**). (2) It delays the passage of the stimulating impulse from the atria to the ventricles (**atrioventricular node**) so that atrial contraction is complete before ventricular contraction begins. (3) It transmits the impulse through the fibrous skeleton of the heart to the ventricles (**trunk of the atrioventricular bundle**) and disseminates it rapidly throughout them (**crura of the atrioventricular bundle** and their branches).

Microscopically the nodes consist of fine, interlacing muscle fibres which are less heavily striated than normal cardiac muscle fibres. They are separated by a considerable amount of fibro-elastic tissue, and have a number of parasympathetic and sympathetic nerve cells and fibres associated with them.

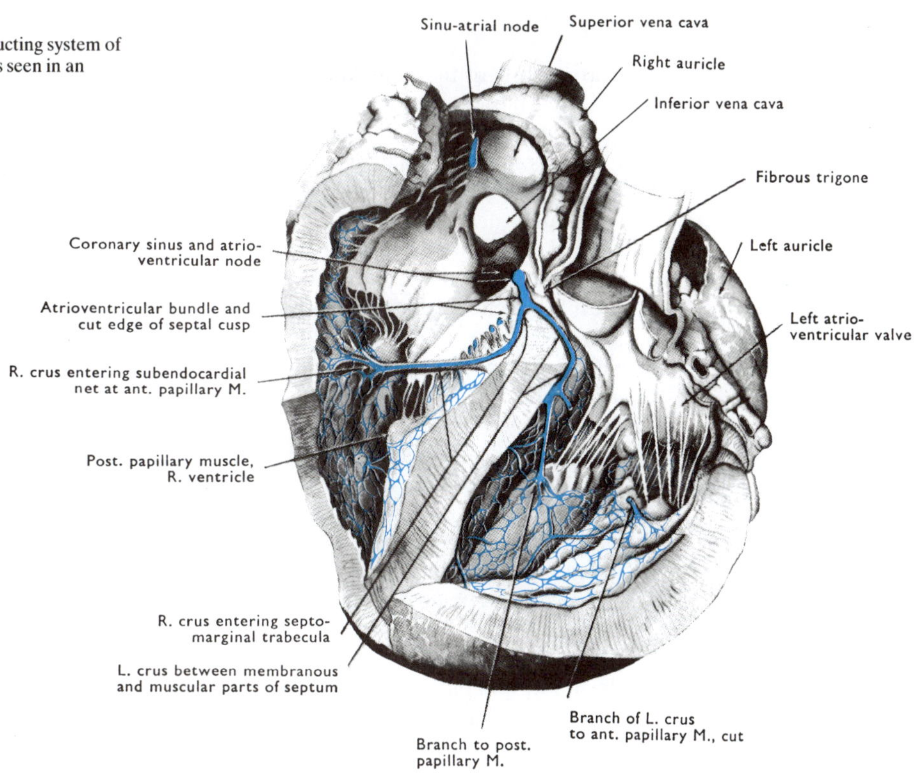

Fig. 77. The conducting system of the sheep's heart as seen in an injected specimen.

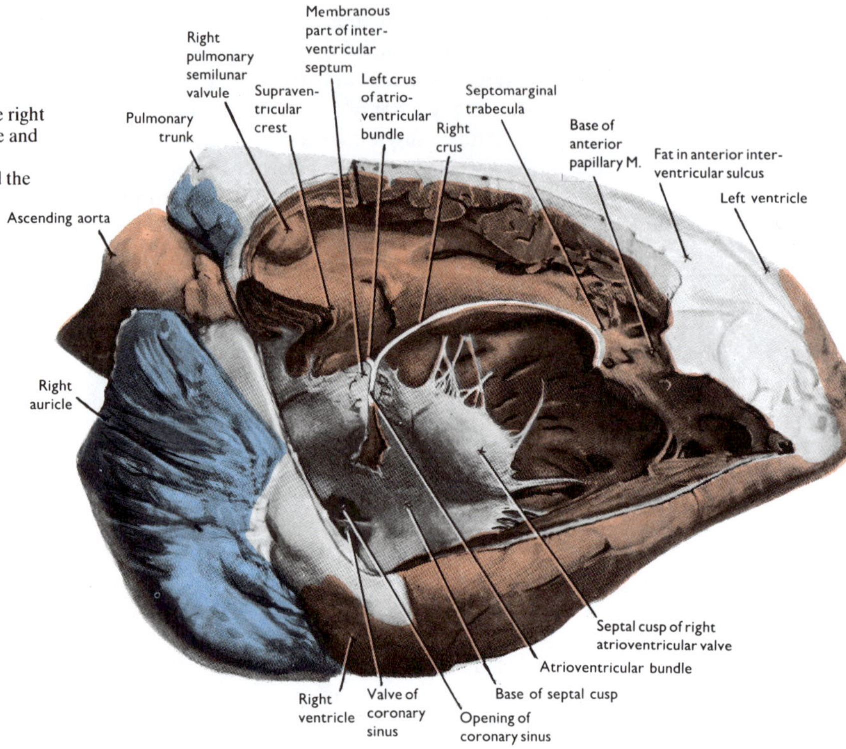

Fig. 78. A dissection of the right ventricle to show the course and division of the trunk of the atrioventricular bundle and the course of its right crus.

Sino-atrial node

This mass of nodal tissue lies in the superior end of the crista terminalis of the right atrium, anterior and to the right of the opening of the superior vena cava [Fig. 77]. It initiates the impulse which spreads through the atrial muscle and causes it to contract. The rate at which the node generates impulses can be altered by nervous stimulation. It is accelerated by sympathetic stimulation and slowed or even stopped by vagal stimulation. Both act through the cardiac plexuses. Cardiac muscle has the capacity for rhythmic contraction and its rate is normally dictated by the sino-atrial node. If that node is destroyed a slower heart rate is established which may be initiated by the atrioventricular node.

Atrioventricular node

This consists of the same kind of tissue as the sino-atrial node. It lies in the postero-inferior part of the interatrial septum, immediately above the opening of the coronary sinus. It receives impulses from the atrial muscle and transmits them to the atrioventricular bundle. The node conducts the impulses slowly, but sympathetic stimulation increases the rate and vagal stimulation decreases it.

Atrioventricular bundle

The trunk passes antero-inferiorly from the atrioventricular node. It pierces the fibrous atrioventricular tissue [Fig. 66] and passes along the postero-superior edge of the muscular interventricular septum at the attachment of the membranous interventricular septum. Here it lies inferior to the line of attachment of the septal cusp of the atrioventricular valve. The trunk divides into right and left **crura** which straddle the muscular interventricular septum [Fig. 77] beneath the endocardium.

The right crus passes towards the septal end of the septomarginal trabecula. It gives branches to the septum and posterior papillary muscle, and runs in the trabecula to the anterior papillary muscle. It supplies this muscle and spreads out on the wall of the right ventricle.

The left crus pierces the ventricular septum between its membranous and muscular parts. It descends on the left of the septum to the posterior papillary muscle, and gives fine strands across the cavity of the ventricle to the anterior papillary muscle. Branches of this crus also spread out to form a subendocardial net [Fig. 77].

The nodes, trunk, and crura cannot be demonstrated in fixed human hearts. Their fibres are not sufficiently different from the normal muscle fibres, though they are readily visible in the fetus and young child and in the calf and sheep. In the sheep the fibres of the subendocardial net are large and pale (**Purkinje fibres**) and contain glycogen. The entire extent of the ventricular conducting tissue has a connective tissue sheath which may be injected in the fresh ungulate heart to demonstrate the course of this system. In man the sheath is too weak to retain the injection. Both nodes and the bundle are supplied by the right coronary artery.

Dissection

Identify the septomarginal trabecula and the strands of conducting tissue which may be seen crossing the cavity of the left ventricle (occasionally the right also). Note the position of the muscular part of the interventricular septum and its relation to the membranous septum and the septal cusp of the right atrioventricular valve. Relate this to the position of the opening of the coronary sinus into the right atrium. This will give a reasonable impression of the position of the ventricular parts of the conducting tissue.

Action of heart

In the cardiac cycle, the **sino-atrial** node initiates the stimulating impulse which spreads rapidly over the atrial muscle and causes it to contract. The anular fibres around the veins partially constrict these orifices and reduce the reflux of blood into the veins. The impulse reaches the **atrioventricular node**, and is transmitted (with delay) through the trunk and crura of the **bundle** principally to the papillary muscles, but also throughout the ventricles. The early contraction of the papillary muscles ensures that the chordae tendineae are taut at an early stage in ventricular contraction so that the valve cusps are drawn together and prevented from ballooning into the atria. Much of the ventricular muscle arises from the papillary muscles, so the impulse spreads outwards from these to the rest of the ventricular muscle. Though the spread of the impulse through the ventricles is very rapid, and the subsequent contraction of the ventricular muscle begins at almost the same time throughout the ventricle, the septum and apex contract fractionally earlier than the base of the ventricles. This tends to give the contained blood a directional thrust towards the great arteries.

Dissection

Divide the ligamentum arteriosum and then remove the pulmonary arteries by separating them from the pleura. This exposes the tracheal bifurcation and the principal bronchi. Follow the **left recurrent laryngeal nerve** to the medial aspect of the arch of the aorta. Note the branches which the nerve gives to the **deep cardiac plexus** on the anterior aspect of the tracheal bifurcation. As the recurrent laryngeal nerve turns superiorly, medial to the aortic arch, it runs close to, or even in the same sheath as, the superior cervical cardiac branch of the left vagus and the middle and inferior cervical cardiac branches of the left sympathetic trunk. These are descending to the deep cardiac plexus. Note the branches which leave the deep cardiac plexus along the bronchi and towards the heart. The plexus itself cannot easily be differentiated from the connective tissue in which it lies. Expose the bronchi and the inferior part of the trachea.

Thoracic part of trachea

The trachea is a wide tube 10–12 cm long. It is kept patent by a series of U-shaped bars of **cartilage** embedded transversely in its fibro-elastic wall. The posterior surface is flat [Fig. 70] where the ends of the cartilage bars are united by plain muscle (trachealis) and fibro-elastic tissue. This surface is applied to the oesophagus. The thoracic part is 5–6 cm long and lies in the median plane of the superior mediastinum. It bifurcates approximately at the level of the sternal angle (level of third to fourth thoracic spines) but this level moves as the elastic trachea stretches on inspiration, so that the bifurcation may descend even to the level of the sixth thoracic vertebra.

The thoracic part of the trachea is nearly surrounded by blood vessels. Inferiorly, the **arch of the aorta** lies on the anterior and left surfaces of the trachea [Figs. 70, 79, 276–278]; the azygos vein arches forwards on the right

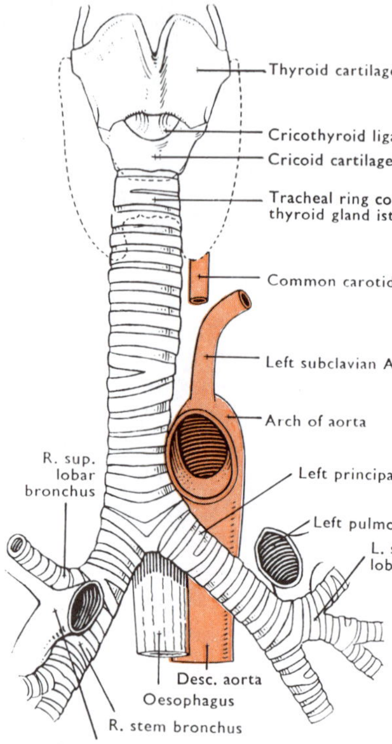

Fig. 79. The larynx, trachea, and bronchi. The thyroid gland is shown by a broken line.

surface. Superior to these vessels, the *anterior surface* of the trachea is in contact with the **brachiocephalic trunk** and the **left common carotid artery** [Fig. 69] and above these with the inferior thyroid veins and thyroidea ima artery [Fig. 49]. The *left surface* is in contact with the left subclavian and left common carotid arteries, with the left vagus and phrenic nerves between them [Fig. 35]. The *right surface* is covered with pleura except where the right vagus nerve intervenes [Fig. 34]. The *posterior surface* lies on the oesophagus and left recurrent laryngeal nerve which sends branches to both oesophagus and trachea.

Bronchi [Figs. 43, 278, 279]

Each principal bronchus passes inferolaterally into the hilus of the corresponding lung in line with the inferior lobar bronchus. The extrapulmonary parts of the principal bronchi contain U-shaped cartilaginous bars similar to those in the trachea. Hence they are flattened posteriorly, while the intrapulmonary parts of the bronchial tree are supported by irregular cartilage plates and so tend to be cylindrical in shape.

Right principal bronchus

Approximately 2.5 cm long, this bronchus is wider and more vertical than the left. Hence foreign bodies which enter the trachea tend to fall into it and lodge in one or other of its branches, most usually the right inferior lobar bronchus [Fig. 43]. When this happens, the air distal to the block is rapidly absorbed and that part of the lung collapses and becomes solid [p. 9].

The right principal bronchus passes posterior to the ascending aorta, superior vena cava, and the right pulmonary artery. It begins anterior to the right margin of the oesophagus and has the azygos vein posterior and superior to it. The **right superior lobar bronchus** is the first branch. It arises immediately medial to the hilus of the lung posterior to the right pulmonary artery.

Left principal bronchus

This bronchus is more horizontal and longer (approximately 5 cm) than the right because the distance from the tracheal bifurcation to the hilus of the left lung is greater, and because the **left superior lobar bronchus** (first branch) arises within the lung substance [Fig. 43].

Anterior to the bronchus are the left pulmonary artery (which separates it from the left atrium) and the upper left pulmonary vein at the hilus [Fig. 80].

The arch of the aorta is superior, and the descending aorta and oesophagus are posterior to it.

Both bronchi have the corresponding bronchial vessels and pulmonary plexus on their posterior surfaces.

Deep cardiac plexus

This interlacing plexus of parasympathetic (vagus) and sympathetic nerve fibres lies on the lowest part of the trachea, posterior to the arch of the aorta. It contains scattered groups of ganglion cells which are mainly parasympathetic.

Nerve fibres reach it: (1) from the sympathetic trunk by way of the cervical cardiac branches (except the left superior) and the cardiac branches of the second to fourth thoracic ganglia, and (2) from the vagi through their cervical cardiac branches (except the inferior left), the right thoracic cardiac branch, and branches of both recurrent laryngeal nerves.

The deep and **superficial** [p. 39] cardiac plexuses form a single mass. Together they send **efferent fibres**: (1) directly to the atria and great vessels, and to the rest of the heart through the **coronary plexuses**; (2) to the lungs through the anterior parts of the lung roots (**anterior part of pulmonary plexus**).

The cardiac plexuses are the pathways through which the central nervous system controls the action of the heart and monitors blood pressure and respiration. In addition to efferent fibres, the plexuses transmit afferent fibres to the vagus from the great arteries, veins, and the lungs, and through the upper thoracic ganglia of the sympathetic trunk the fibres responsible for producing the pain of ischaemic disease of the heart (angina pectoris).

Dissection

Remove the posterior surface of the parietal pericardium between the right and left pulmonary veins. This uncovers the anterior surface of the oesophagus in the posterior mediastinum. On each side of the oesophagus, and posterior to the corresponding bronchus find a vagus nerve leaving the pulmonary plexus as one or more trunks [Fig. 81]. Follow the vagi on to the oesophagus where their branches unite to form the oesophageal plexus. Follow the plexus anterior and posterior to the oesophagus.

Find the azygos vein and its tributaries on the vertebral column to the right of the oesophagus. To the left of this vein, find and follow the thoracic duct. Lift the left side of the oesophagus forwards and uncover the anterior surface of the descending aorta. As far as possible follow all these structures upwards and downwards. Turn the trachea upwards to expose the oesophagus in the superior mediastinum, and lift the diaphragm forwards to expose the aorta in the inferior part of the posterior mediastinum.

Thoracic parts of vagus nerves

Right vagus

The **right vagus** runs postero-inferiorly on the right surface of the trachea, at first medial to the pleura and then to the arch of the azygos vein. Posterior to the right bronchus, it divides into a number of branches (**posterior part of the pulmonary plexus**) which pass towards the lung and also link the right and left pulmonary plexuses anterior and posterior [Figs. 81, 82] to the oesophagus.

Branches

(1) A **cardiac branch** arises on the right of the trachea and descends on it to the cardiac plexus. (2) To the bronchi and lung through the **pulmonary plexus**. (3) To the oesophagus and pericardium through the **oesophageal plexus**.

Left vagus

It descends to the left side of the arch of the aorta between the left common carotid and subclavian arteries. At the inferior border of the arch it curves medially, gives off the left recurrent laryngeal nerve [Fig. 81], and breaks up into the left pulmonary plexus posterior to the left bronchus. It continues as several branches which pass on to the oesophagus (**oesophageal plexus**).

The **left recurrent laryngeal nerve** curves medially round the inferior surface of the aortic arch, posterior to the ligamentum arteriosum, sending branches to the cardiac plexus. The nerve then ascends in the groove between the left sides of the trachea and oesophagus, giving branches to both.

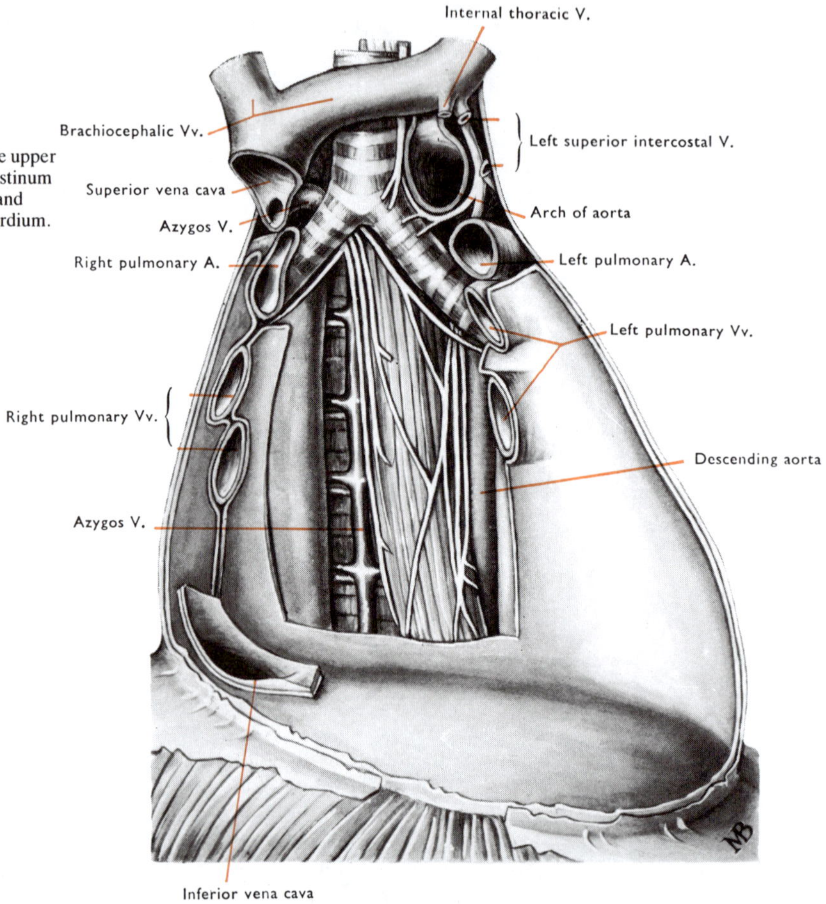

Fig. 80. A dissection of the upper part of the posterior mediastinum after removal of the heart and posterior wall of the pericardium. See also Fig. 81.

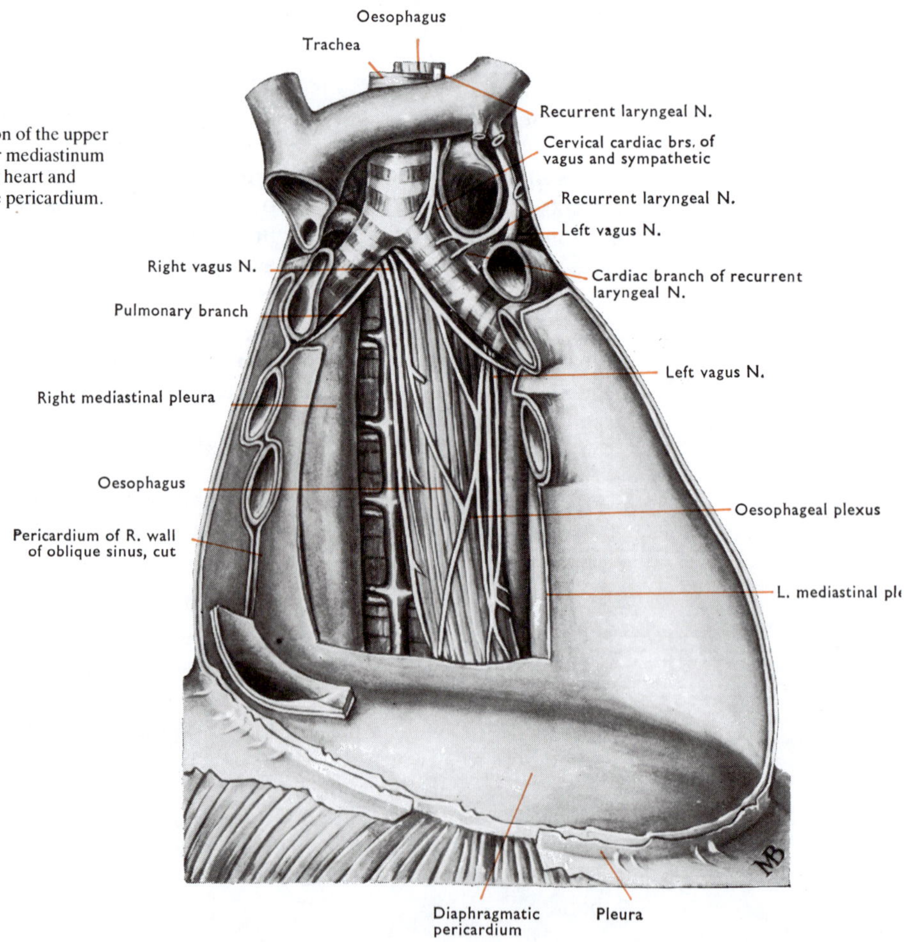

Fig. 81. A dissection of the upper part of the posterior mediastinum after removal of the heart and posterior wall of the pericardium. See also Fig. 80.

Pulmonary plexus

The major, posterior part of this plexus lies behind each lung root. Nerve fibres enter it from both vagus nerves and from the second to fourth thoracic ganglia of the sympathetic trunk. The smaller, anterior part is an extension of the cardiac plexus. It is joined by branches of the corresponding vagus nerve which arise above the lung root. Both parts supply the lung root, the lung (including the smooth muscle of the bronchi), and the visceral pleura.

Oesophageal plexus

This plexus surrounds the oesophagus. It contains nerve fibres from both vagi and sympathetic fibres which join it from the **greater splanchnic nerve**. It supplies the oesophagus, pericardium, and adjacent parietal pleura. Inferiorly, the plexus condenses into **anterior** and **posterior vagal trunks** which descend on the oesophagus and become the anterior and posterior gastric nerves on the stomach. Each of these trunks and nerves contains fibres from both vagi and from the sympathetic.

Oesophagus

[Figs. 33, 36, 59, 68, 70, 74, 81, 84, 276–283]

The oesophagus extends from the pharynx in the neck through the superior and posterior mediastina to pierce the diaphragm at the level of the tenth thoracic vertebra (ninth thoracic spine) 2–3 cm to the left of the median plane. In the superior mediastinum it lies between the trachea and the vertebral column, slightly to the left of the median plane. It enters the posterior mediastinum posterior to the **left principal bronchus** and right pulmonary artery, and descends posterior to the **left atrium**, separated from it by the oblique sinus of the pericardium [Fig. 74]. It then inclines to the left behind the posterior part of the diaphragm and in front of the descending

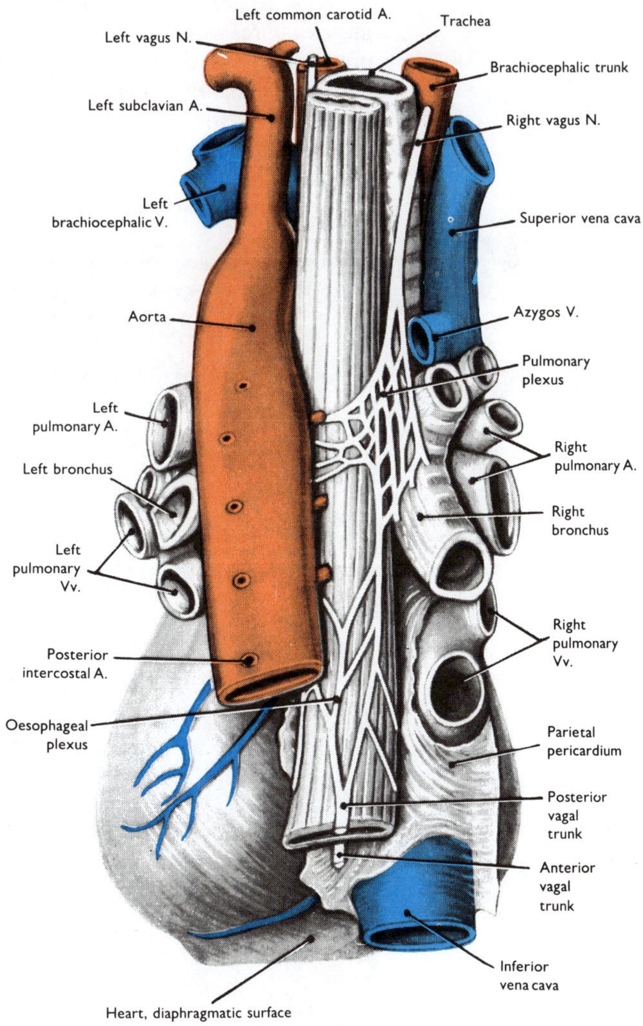

Fig. 82. The posterior aspect of the heart and of the structures in the superior mediastinum and the upper part of the posterior mediastinum.

thoracic aorta which passes to the median plane before entering the abdomen.

The oesophagus is separated from the vertebral column sequentially by the longus colli [Fig. 23], the thoracic duct, azygos vein, and upper six or seven right posterior intercostal arteries, and by the descending thoracic aorta.

The *right side* of the oesophagus is close to the right pleura, except where the arch of the azygos vein intervenes and where the oesophagus deviates to the left inferiorly and indents the left pleura and lung [Fig. 40].

The *left side* of the oesophagus is close to the left pleura above the arch of the aorta, but the thoracic duct and upper part of the left subclavian artery intervene. The arch and the descending part of the aorta lie to the left of the oesophagus from the fourth to the seventh thoracic vertebrae. The left recurrent laryngeal nerve is anterior to the oesophagus in the superior mediastinum.

The oesophageal plexus surrounds the oesophagus in the posterior mediastinum.

The oesophagus is compressed: (1) by the arch of the aorta; (2) by the left principal bronchus; (3) by the diaphragm. These sites may be shown as narrowings of the lumen in oblique radiographs taken while barium is being swallowed [Fig. 83]. If the left atrium is dilated, it forms a large, smooth indentation of the shadow of the oesophageal lumen inferior to that produced by the left principal bronchus.

Structure

The lining of the oesophagus is the mucous type of **stratified squamous epithelium**. It lies on a thick layer of areolar tissue containing longitudinal bundles of **muscularis mucosae**. The other **muscle** layers (outer longitudinal and inner circular) are mainly longitudinal in the superior part and are entirely **striated muscle fibres**. In the middle third, striated and smooth muscle fibres are mixed and the number of circular fibres increases progressively. In the lower third, the fibres are exclusively of **smooth muscle** and predominantly circular in direction. There is no special development of circular fibres to form a sphincter either at the level of the diaphragm or at the entry into the stomach. The striated muscle in the upper part ensures rapid transport of the bolus through that part which is applied to the trachea.

The human oesophagus contains very few glands except some of the

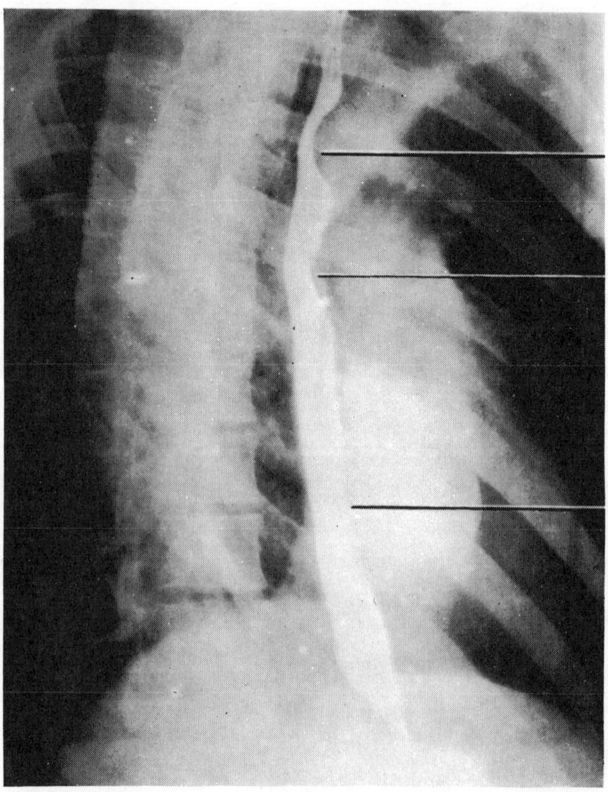

Fig. 83. A right oblique radiograph of the thorax with the oesophagus filled with barium.

mucous type which lie in the submucosa close to the diaphragm. There may be islands of gastric type mucous membrane in the inferior part of the oesophagus.

The oesophagus is surrounded by loose areolar tissue which allows it to expand freely during swallowing.

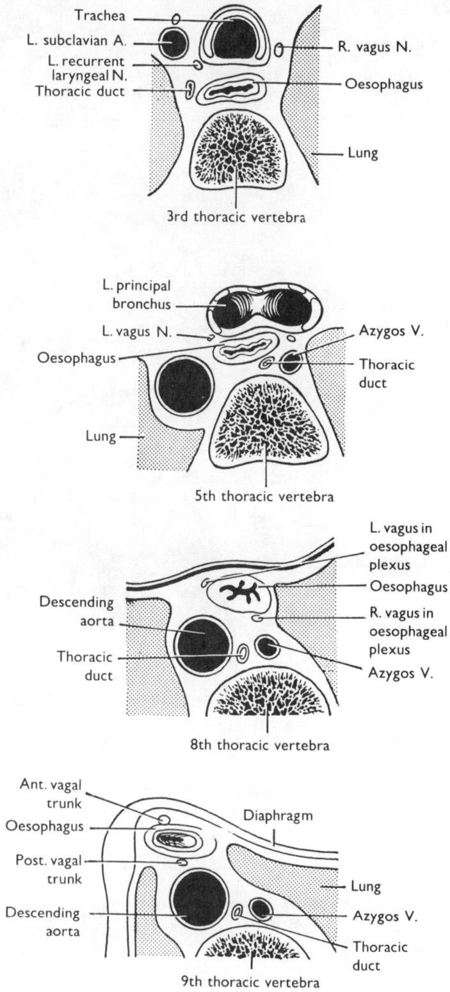

Fig. 84. Outline drawings of four sections through the oesophagus at different thoracic levels.

Descending aorta
[Figs. 35, 61, 74, 82, 84, 277–283]

It begins on the left side of the fourth thoracic intervertebral disc and oesophagus and descends through the posterior mediastinum between the left pleura and the thoracic duct and azygos vein. At first posterior to the left lung root and then to the pericardium, it inclines anteriorly and to the right behind the oesophagus to reach the anterior surface of the vertebral column behind the inferior part of the diaphragm. It enters the abdomen posterior to the dorsal edge of the diaphragm (**median arcuate ligament**) at the level of the twelfth thoracic vertebra. It lies on the vertebral column, the hemiazygos veins, and its own intercostal and subcostal branches.

Branches

From the anterior surface. (1) Two **left bronchial arteries**. The superior of these may give rise to the right bronchial artery [p. 75]. (2) Several **oesophageal branches**. (3) Small branches to the fat and lymph nodes of the mediastinum, the pericardium, and the diaphragm. *From the posterior surface.* Nine pairs of **posterior intercostal arteries** and one pair of **subcostal arteries**.

Thoracic duct
[Figs. 68–70, 84, 86]

This small, vein-like structure conveys most of the lymph of the body to the blood stream. It drains the lower limbs, pelvis, abdomen, and posterior thorax; and frequently receives lymph from the left side of the head and neck and left upper limb near its termination. Yet half the lymph it contains is said to come from the liver. The lymph in the thoracic duct often has a milky appearance because of the fine droplets of fat which enter it in the intestinal lymph (**chyle**).

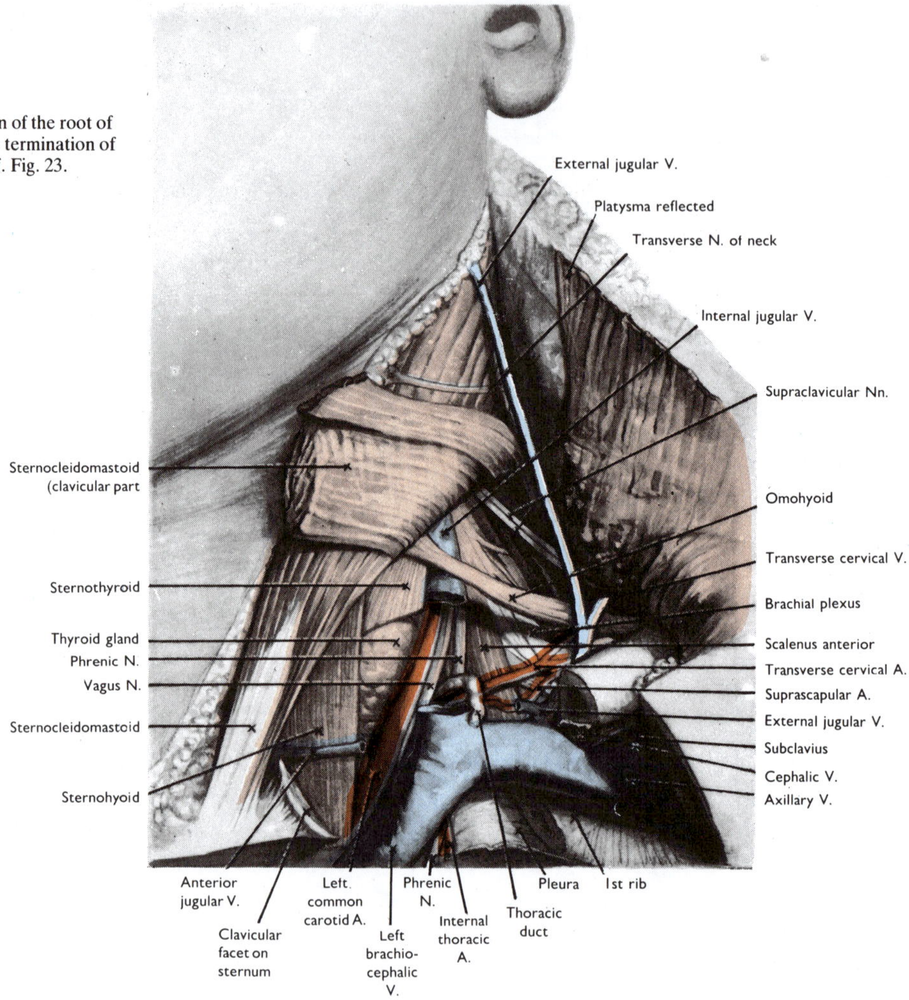

Fig. 85. A dissection of the root of the neck to show the termination of the thoracic duct. Cf. Fig. 23.

Dissection

Trace the upper part of the thoracic duct to its termination in the junction of the left subclavian and internal jugular veins.

The thoracic duct arises from an elongated lymph sac (**cisterna chyli**) which lies on the first and second lumbar vertebrae between the aorta and the right crus of the diaphragm. A similar sac often lies posterior to the aorta [Fig. 86]. This drains the left side, and joins the thoracic duct where it leaves the cisterna chyli to enter the thorax on the right of the aorta. In the posterior mediastinum the thoracic duct lies between the aorta and the azygos vein, at first posterior to the diaphragm and then to the oesophagus. At the arch of the aorta, the duct passes obliquely behind the oesophagus to reach its left side. The duct then ascends between the oesophagus and the left pleura to the root of the neck. Here it arches laterally and downwards (between the carotid sheath anteriorly and the vertebral vessels posteriorly) to enter the *junction of the internal jugular and subclavian veins* [Fig. 85].

The thoracic duct is frequently double in part of its course. It contains many valves. The last is a short distance from the end of the duct which may be filled with blood.

Tributaries

The cisterna chyli receives: (1) the right and left **lumbar lymph trunks** which drain the lower limbs, the lower part of the anterior abdominal wall, the pelvis, and the posterior abdominal wall (including gonads, kidneys, and suprarenal glands; (2) the **intestinal lymph trunks** which drain the abdominal contents (the superior part of the liver drains through the diaphragm to mediastinal or parasternal lymph nodes); (3) the lower **posterior intercostal lymph vessels.**

The thoracic duct receives: (1) the remaining posterior intercostal lymph vessels; (2) vessels from the oesophagus and the posterior parts of the diaphragm and pericardium; (3) the left jugular and subclavian trunks (which drain the left side of the head and neck and the left upper limb), though these may enter the left brachiocephalic vein independently. The **left bronchomediastinal trunk** drains the left lung, the left side of the heart, and a large part of the mediastinum to the left brachiocephalic vein or rarely the thoracic duct.

Right lymph duct

This vessel is occasionally formed by the union of the right jugular, right subclavian, and right bronchomediastinal trunks. It is more usual for the jugular and subclavian trunks to unite and enter the right veins at the same position as the thoracic duct on the left.

The **right bronchomediastinal trunk** corresponds to the left vessel but also drains the upper part of the right lobe of the liver and usually enters the right brachiocephalic vein.

Lymph nodes of thorax
[Figs. 278–280]

1. The **parasternal nodes** lie along the internal thoracic vessels. They drain an area corresponding to the distribution of the internal thoracic artery with the addition of lymph from the upper part of the liver. N.B. drainage from the mammary gland.

2. **Intercostal lymph nodes** lie in the posterior parts of the intercostal spaces and drain to the thoracic duct or cisterna chyli [Fig. 86].

3. **Phrenic nodes**. Some lie on the diaphragm near the entry of the phrenic nerves, others near its attachment to the anterior thoracic wall.

4. **Posterior mediastinal lymph nodes** lie along the descending aorta. They drain the posterior mediastinum (including the diaphragm, pericardium, and oesophagus) to the thoracic duct.

5. **Tracheobronchial lymph nodes** lie on the thoracic trachea and principal bronchi. They drain these structures and receive lymph from the lungs.

6. **Bronchopulmonary lymph nodes** lie in the hilus of the lung and in the angles of bifurcation of the larger bronchi. They drain the lung (pulmonary nodes) and visceral pleura.

7. **Anterior mediastinal lymph nodes** lie beside the left brachiocephalic vein. They drain the heart, pericardium, and thymus.

The **bronchomediastinal lymph trunks** receive efferent vessels from the bronchopulmonary, tracheobronchial, parasternal, and anterior mediastinal lymph nodes and ascend either over the arch of the aorta (left) or azygos vein (right).

Lymph from the lungs carries phagocytes which have ingested carbon particles deposited on the walls of the alveoli from the inspired air. Many phagocytes remain in the interlobular septa of the lung giving it its mottled appearance. Others reach the lymph nodes which become black with carbon particles.

Dissection

Complete the exposure of the posterior intercostal vessels and the intercostal nerves. Follow the left posterior intercostal veins to the hemiazygos and accessory hemiazygos veins. Expose these veins and their communications with the azygos vein.

Posterior intercostal arteries

One of these passes to each intercostal space. The first two spaces are supplied from the costocervical trunk by the **highest intercostal artery**. This descends anterior to the ventral rami of the eighth cervical and first thoracic nerves and the necks of the first two ribs [Fig. 22].

The remaining posterior intercostal and subcostal arteries arise from the posterior surface of the descending thoracic aorta. Because the aorta is displaced downwards and to the left, the right vessels are longer than the left and the upper four aortic posterior intercostal arteries ascend to reach spaces three to six. The first right aortic intercostal usually gives the **right bronchial artery**. The aortic intercostal arteries lie on the periosteum of the vertebral bodies and are posterior to the azygos or hemiazygos vein, the thoracic duct right arteries), and the sympathetic trunk. Each artery enters the intercostal space between the vein (superior) and the intercostal nerve (inferior) and reaches the costal groove near the angle of the rib [Fig. 6].

The **dorsal branch** passes posteriorly with the dorsal ramus of the spinal nerve and has a distribution corresponding to that of the nerve. A **spinal branch** passes through each intervertebral foramen to supply the contents of the spinal canal.

The **subcostal arteries** accompany the ventral rami of the twelfth thoracic (subcostal) nerves. They pass along the inferior borders of the twelfth ribs and enter the abdomen posterior to the lateral arcuate ligaments (q.v.).

Intercostal nerves

These are the ventral rami of the upper 11 thoracic spinal nerves which pass laterally posterior to the sympathetic trunk to enter the intercostal spaces [p. 13] inferior to the intercostal vessels.

The greater part of the **first thoracic ventral ramus** passes up across the neck of the first rib to join the eighth cervical ventral ramus in the brachial plexus. The small **intercostal branch** runs across the inferior surface of the first rib to enter the first space close to the costal cartilage. *It has no cutaneous branches*. The ventral ramus of the **second thoracic nerve** usually sends a small branch to the brachial plexus. When this branch is large, the lateral cutaneous branch of the second intercostal nerve (intercostobrachial) is small or absent.

The **subcostal nerve** passes into the abdominal wall with the subcostal artery. The lateral cutaneous branch of this nerve crosses the iliac crest to supply skin in the gluteal region.

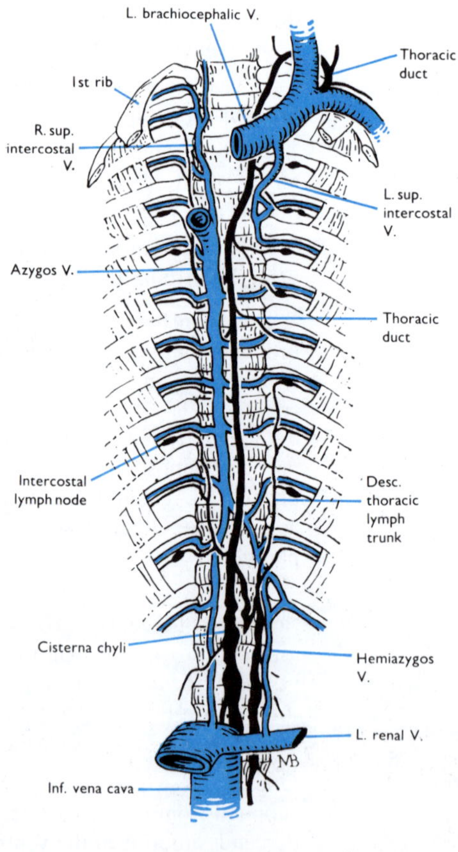

Fig. 86. The thoracic duct and posterior intercostal veins. In this case no accessory hemiazygos vein is present and the number of venous communications across the midline is greater than usual.

Posterior intercostal veins

The **highest** crosses the neck of the first rib to join the corresponding brachiocephalic vein. The second and third unite in the right and left **superior intercostal veins**. The right descends to enter the azygos vein. The left passes anterosuperiorly across the arch of the aorta to the left brachiocephalic vein, or descends to the accessory hemiazygos vein.

Of the remaining veins those *on the right* enter the azygos vein. *On the left*, the arrangement is variable. Commonly the fourth to eighth left posterior intercostal veins enter the **accessory hemiazygos vein**. This descends with the aorta to cross the midline and enter the azygos vein at the eighth thoracic vertebra. It may be replaced by a number of veins entering the azygos vein separately [Fig. 86].

The **hemiazygos vein** arises in the abdomen from the posterior surface of the left renal vein. It pierces the left crus of the diaphragm, receives the subcostal and remaining left posterior intercostal veins, and crosses the vertebral column, posterior to the aorta and thoracic duct, to join the azygos vein.

The joints of the thorax

Dissection

Identify the sternal, sternocostal, interchondral, and costochondral joints in the anterior shield of chest wall which was reflected downwards. Identify the ligaments on the surfaces of these joints, and then remove a thin slice from the anterior surface of each to expose the interior.

Sternal joints

The **manubriosternal joint** lies at the sternal angle. The cartilage-covered ends of the manubrium and body of the sternum are united by a **fibrous disc** in which there may be a cavity. It is strengthened anteriorly and posteriorly by longitudinal fibres from the periosteum. This joint moves in respiration and so rarely ossifies even in old age unlike the hyaline cartilage uniting the four pieces of the body of the sternum which ossifies between childhood and 21 years. The cartilaginous xiphosternal joint ossifies in middle life.

Sternocostal joints

Seven costal cartilages on each side articulate with the margins of the sternum. The **first costal cartilages** are fused with the manubrium and begin to calcify and ossify at the end of growth. Hence the first ribs, their costal cartilages, and the manubrium become a rigid structure which moves as one piece on its costovertebral joints.

The **second** to **seventh** sternocostal joints are synovial in type. Each has a fibrous capsule which is strengthened anteriorly and posteriorly by a **radiate sternocostal ligament** passing from the costal cartilage to the two pieces of the sternum with which each (except the sixth) articulates. The second sternocostal joint is divided into two by the **intra-articular sternocostal ligament** which passes from the costal cartilage to the fibrous disc of the manubriosternal joint. Some of the other joints may also be double. The seventh costal cartilage may have no synovial joint with the sternum.

Interchondral joints

These small synovial joints between the adjacent margins of the costal cartilages of the sixth to ninth ribs and the fibrous joint with the tenth increase the strength of the costal margin while maintaining its flexibility.

Costochondral joints

At these joints the cartilage fits into a conical pit on the end of the bony rib and is fused with it.

Dissection

Expose the ligaments which unite the heads of the ribs to the vertebral bodies and intervertebral discs [Fig. 87] and those that join the ribs to the transverse processes. Remove the anterior parts of the capsules of the joints of one or more heads of the middle ribs, and identify the intra-articular ligament, if present. Remove ribs at various levels by cutting the ligaments. Compare the articulations of the heads and tubercles at different levels.

Costovertebral joints
[Figs. 10, 87]

Most of these are complex joints. (1) The **head of the rib** articulates with the adjacent parts of its own vertebral body [Fig. 5], the vertebra above, and the intervertebral disc between. (2) The articular part of the **tubercle of the rib**

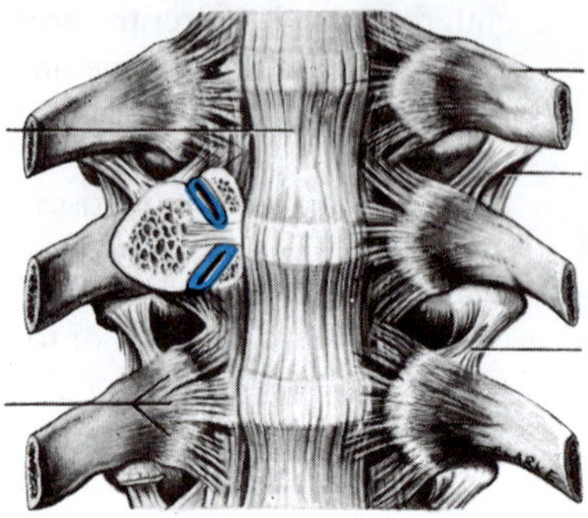

Fig. 87. The anterior longitudinal ligament and costovertebral joints from in front. One joint has been opened by an oblique slice through the head of the rib.

articulates with the transverse process of its own vertebra. The presence of these two separate articulations forces the rib to move round an axis which passes posterolaterally and downwards through both of them like a hinge. The axis can only be changed if the tubercle can slide supero-inferiorly on the transverse process. In the upper thoracic vertebrae the articular surfaces on the transverse processes are spherical and prevent such sliding. In the lower vertebrae they are flatter and allow this movement to a slight degree.

There are two exceptions to this general arrangement. (1) The heads of the *first* and of the *last three ribs* articulate only with their own vertebral bodies. (2) The *last two ribs* do not articulate with the transverse process and so have a much freer range of movement.

The heads of the ribs which articulate with two vertebrae do so by two bevelled facets each forming a separate synovial joint with the posterolateral surface of a vertebral body [Fig. 5]. The two joints are separated by the intra-articular ligament attached to the intervertebral disc. The joints are surrounded by an articular capsule and are strengthened anteriorly by the **radiate ligament** of the head [Fig. 87].

The **costotransverse joint** is surrounded by an articular capsule. This is strengthened laterally by the **lateral costotransverse ligament** passing from the non-articular part of the tubercle to the tip of the transverse process. In addition, (a) the **costotransverse ligament** unites the back of the neck of the rib to the anterior surface of the transverse process, and (b) the **superior costotransverse ligament** joins the crest of the neck of the rib to the transverse process above. The aperture between this ligament and the vertebral column transmits the dorsal ramus of the spinal nerve and the dorsal branch of the intercostal artery.

Movements of ribs

[Figs. 9, 10]

These have been described already [pp. 6, 11]. The salient points are: (1) The **two first ribs**, together with the manubrium sterni move as one piece on the first thoracic vertebra. These ribs slope downwards and forwards, so that raising the manubrium increases the anteroposterior diameter of the superior aperture of the thorax, and the pure vertical movement produces no lateral pressure on the structures which pass over the first rib into the upper limb. (2) Raising the **true ribs** increases the anteroposterior diameter of the thorax and carries the body of the sternum anteriorly as in the movements of the first ribs. However, the true ribs also move outwards on their obliquely placed posterior hinge [Fig. 10] and so increase the transverse diameter. This is allowed for in the true ribs by the angulation of the flexible costal cartilages. (3) The **false ribs** also move upwards and outwards and resist the tendency of the diaphragm to draw the costal margin inwards. (4) The **eleventh** and **twelfth ribs** are held down by the muscles of the abdominal wall (posterior part of external oblique and quadratus lumborum). Thus they increase the efficiency of the diaphragmatic contraction and prevent it from raising the costodiaphragmatic recess of the pleura.

Joints and ligaments of vertebral column

If the head and neck has been dissected and the spinal medulla removed, it is possible to see all the features of the vertebral ligaments. If this has not been done, display of these structures should be delayed since a clear picture can be obtained from the following description and illustrations, provided that the appropriate macerated vertebrae are studied at the same time.

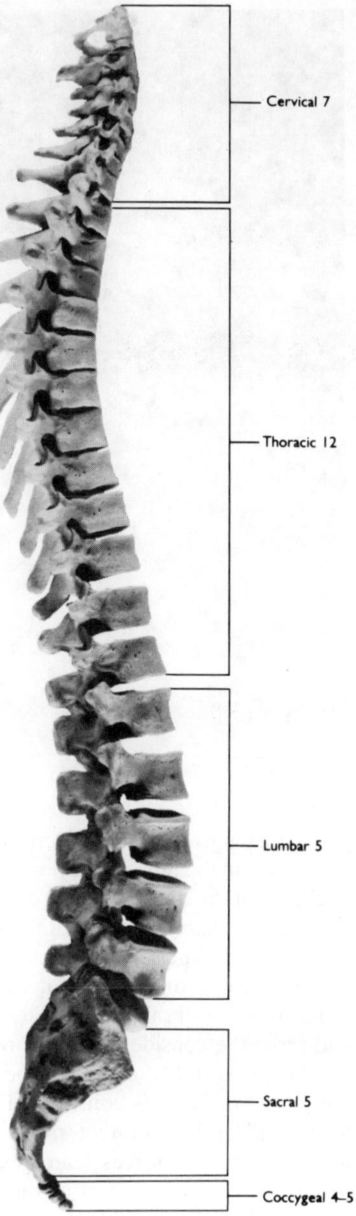

Fig. 88. The right surface of the vertebral column.

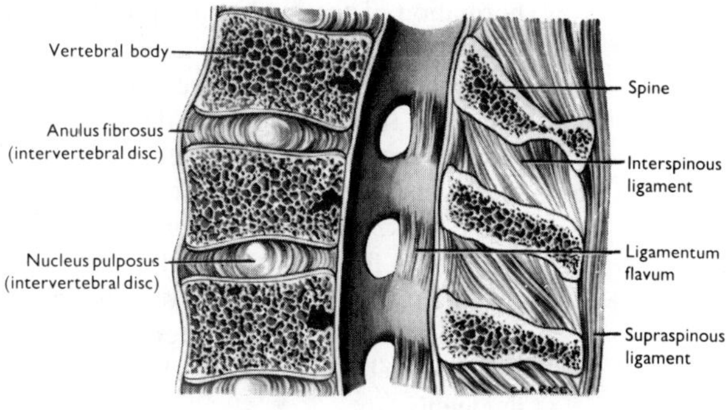

Fig. 89. A median section through part of the lumbar vertebral column.

Intervertebral discs

These discs lie between the vertebral bodies. They consist of many concentric layers of strong collangeous fibrous tissue (**anulus fibrosus**) that run between the cartilage-covered ends of the vertebral bodies. The alternate layers of collagen run at an angle to each other, and together surround an internal mass of gelatinous material (**nucleus pulposus**). This is held under pressure by the anulus and lies slightly nearer the posterior than the anterior surface of the disc [Fig. 89]. The discs confer flexibility on the vertebral column by

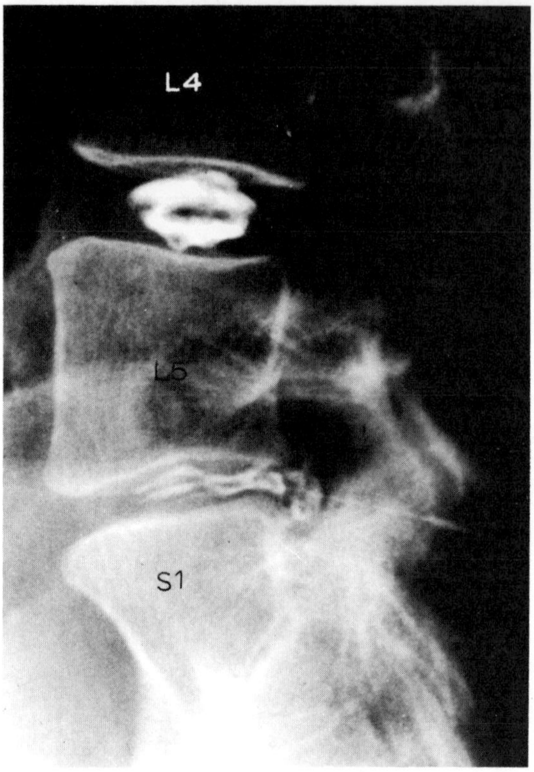

Fig. 90. Lateral radiograph of the intervertebral discs between the fourth and fifth lumbar and the fifth lumbar and first sacral vertebrae after injection of the nucleus pulposus with X-ray-opaque material. The disc between L4 and L5 is normal, that between L5 and S1 has torn permitting the nucleus pulposus to pass backwards into the intervertebral foramen. Note the collapse of the L5/S1 [cf. Fig. 260] disc, the narrowing of the intervertebral foramen, and the demonstration of how the contained, normal nucleus pulposus acts as a ball-bearing between the vertebrae.

The protruded nucleus pulposus usually compresses the fifth lumbar nerve or its ventral ramus and, by irritating the nerve fibres, causes severe pain referred to the area of its skin distribution (lateral side of the leg and dorsum of the foot [Fig. 219, Vol. 1]) especially when the disc is compressed in standing or lifting weights when more nuclear material is forced backwards. If the compression is severe, it also causes weakness of the muscles principally supplied by the fifth lumbar nerve (dorsiflexors of the ankle and evertors of the foot [Table 11, Vol. 1]). This type of investigation or a myelogram [Fig. 178, Vol. 3] can confirm this as the cause of the 'sciatica' and show that it is amenable to surgical treatment.

permitting movement between adjacent vertebrae. This movement takes place around the nucleus pulposus and its range is directly proportional to the thickness of the disc, while the direction of the movement is controlled by the articular facets on the vertebral arches. The discs are thickest in the lumbar region and thinnest in the thoracic region where movement is necessarily limited because of the effect it would have on the ribs.

The intervertebral discs also absorb shocks applied to the vertebral column and resist the considerable compression forces produced by the contraction of the powerful erector spinae group of muscles. The load on the intervertebral discs is considerable, e.g. when an 80 kg man jumps from a height and lands on his feet, or when he lifts a 50 kg sack. It is not uncommon to find that such forces lead to extrusion of the nucleus pulposus either through the posterior part of the disc (especially when this is stretched by flexion of the vertebral column—the reason for lifting weights with an extended vertebral column) or into the adjacent vertebral body. This herniation of the nucleus pulposus markedly interferes with the function of the intervertebral disc because of the loss of pressure in the disc and its consequent narrowing. Progressive narrowing of the discs from this and other causes is seen with increasing age. It causes a decrease in height and a reduced mobility of the vertebral column. Herniation of the nucleus pulposus may occur at any age in the cervical or lumbar regions. It is one cause of pain in the back. When herniation occurs posteriorly through the thinnest part of the anulus fibrosus, the nucleus may press on the spinal medulla (cervical region) or on one of the corresponding spinal nerves where it lies in the intervertebral foramen posterior to the disc.

The vertebral bodies are also united by anterior and posterior longitudinal ligaments.

The **anterior longitudinal ligament** stretches from the atlas vertebra to the sacrum. It is firmly attached to the anterior surfaces of the intervertebral discs and vertebral bodies. Its lateral margin is difficult to define as it fades into the periosteum [Fig. 87].

The **posterior longitudinal ligament** lies in the vertebral canal. It is attached to the posterior surfaces of the intervertebral discs and the adjacent margins of the vertebral bodies, but not to their posterior surfaces. Here the ligament is narrowed to permit the escape of the **basivertebral veins** [Fig. 91] from

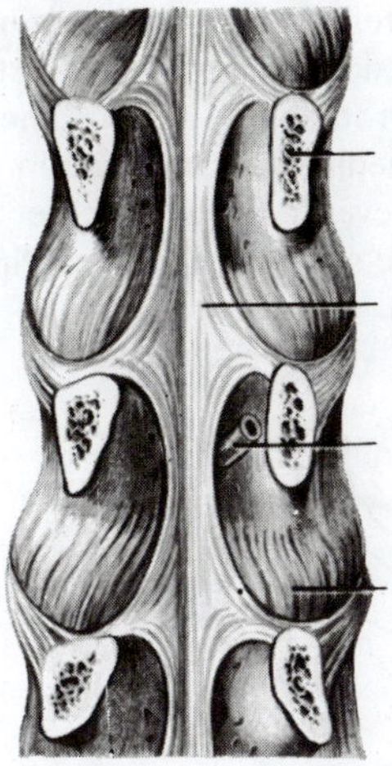

Fig. 91. The posterior longitudinal ligament of the vertebral column. The vertebral arches have been removed.

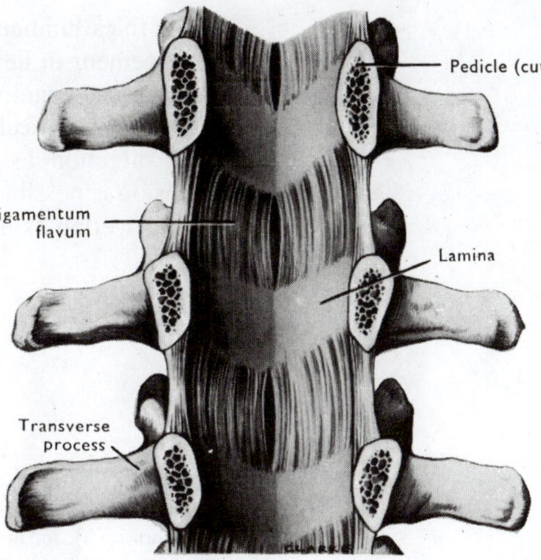

Fig. 92. The lumbar vertebral arches and ligamenta flava seen from in front after removal of the vertebral bodies.

the back of the vertebral bodies into the internal vertebral venous plexus [Fig. 205].

The **ligamenta flava** are strong, yellow, elastic ligaments which unite the laminae of adjacent vertebrae. They are relatively short and are limited on each side by the articular processes. With the laminae they form a smooth posterior surface to the vertebral canal [Fig. 92].

A thin **interspinous ligament** passes posteriorly from each ligamentum flavum. It unites the adjacent margins of the spines and is continuous posteriorly with a strong **supraspinous ligament**. This is attached to the posterior aspects of the spines throughout the length of the thoracic and lumbar parts of the vertebral column. All these ligaments are sufficiently elastic to allow separation of the laminae and spines on flexion of the vertebral column. They also help to return the vertebral column to its resting position when flexion ceases.

Dissection

If the spinal medulla has been removed, cut out a length of the thoracic vertebral column and split it with a saw in the median plane. Identify the parts of the intervertebral discs and their relation to the vertebral canal and intervertebral foramina.

Check the attachments of the ligaments of the vertebral column by the ridges which they make on macerated specimens of vertebrae from the various regions of the vertebral column. Note the positions and orientation of the articular facets.

Articular facets

These facets lie at the junction of the pedicle, lamina, and transverse process on each side. The orientations of the facets determines the type of movements which are possible between adjacent vertebrae. This is because the tight union of the vertebral bodies by the intervertebral discs forces all the *axes of movement* to pass through the nucleus pulposus [Fig. 93]. In the thoracic region, the plane of the articular facets is approximately on the arc of a circle with its centre at the nucleus pulposus. Hence rotation can take place in addition to flexion and extension, though all are limited by the thin intervertebral discs. In the lumbar region, the inferior facets of one vertebra fit between the superior facets of the vertebra below. This effectively prevents rotation but permits free flexion and extension. In the cervical region, the right and left facets are further apart and lie parallel to each other in an oblique coronal plane sloping upwards and forwards. They also prevent rotation, except in the special joints between the first and second cervical vertebrae [see Vol. 3] which permit rotation of the head on the neck.

The thick **lumbar intervertebral discs** give this region the maximum range of movement in flexion, extension and lateral flexion. The range is least in the thoracic region and consists principally of rotation. The movements between the typical cervical vertebrae are intermediate in range and in the same direction as in the lumbar region. However a greater degree of extension is possible in the cervical region because of the small spines which do not overlap as in the thoracic region [Fig. 88].

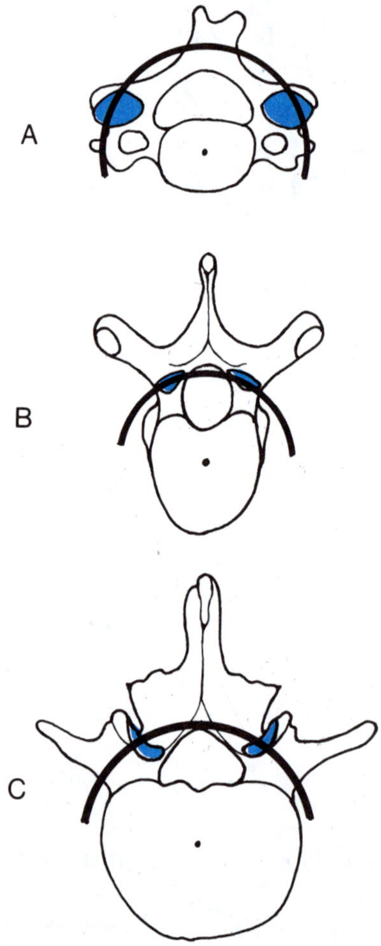

Fig. 93. Outline drawings of the superior surfaces of typical cervical (A), thoracic (B), and lumbar (C) vertebrae. In each case an arc of a circle, with its centre at the nucleus pulposus of the intervertebral disc, has been drawn through the articular facets. Only in the thoracic region is the arc parallel to the articular surfaces of the facets. Hence they permit free rotation only in this region. Blue = cartilage of the facets.

The abdomen

Before any dissection is begun, it is important to appreciate the position of the abdomen in relation to the other parts of the body. This is best achieved by examining the bony points in a living individual while relating these to the bones of a mounted skeleton. The cadaver is usually too firm to allow satisfactory palpation unless it is very thin and the bony points can be seen.

The relative positions of the various structures described in the following section are only approximations. This is because there is considerable individual variation and also because the positions alter in the same individual with age and posture. Thus the distance between the iliac crest and the costal margin is greater in infants and children (where the ribs are more horizontally placed) than it is in adults. The distance is still further reduced in old age by the progressive narrowing of the intervertebral discs and by the tendency to stoop. It is also less in the standing position (because of the lower position taken up by the ribs) than it is when lying supine, and it is greater in inspiration than in expiration.

Anteriorly, the **abdominal wall** extends from the surface of the **xiphoid process** (level of the ninth thoracic vertebra) to the **pubic symphysis** (level of **coccyx**). Laterally and posteriorly, the abdominal cavity is overlapped by the

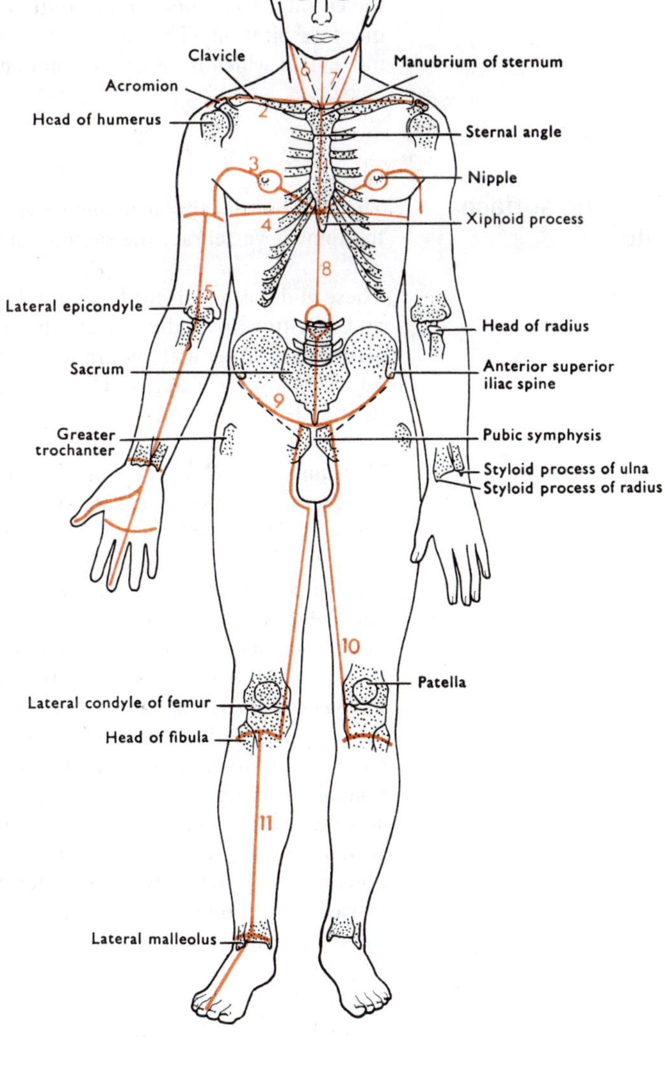

Fig. 94. Landmarks and incisions.

thorax superiorly and by the gluteal region of the lower limb inferiorly. The upper abdominal contents fill the concavity of the **diaphragm** and so lie internal to the lower parts of the thoracic cage, pleura, and lungs, but are separated from them by the diaphragm. These abdominal contents reach up to the level of the eighth thoracic vertebra in the median plane and to the level of the fifth rib in the right mid-clavicular line (right dome of the diaphragm) in full expiration. On the other hand, the **costal margin** lies at the level of the first lumbar vertebra in the mid-clavicular line (ninth costal cartilage) and the level of the third lumbar vertebra in the mid-axillary line (eleventh costal cartilage). Here the costodiaphragmatic recess of the pleura is only a short distance superior to the costal margin (level of tenth rib) and the superior limit of the gluteal region (the highest point on the **iliac crest**) is at the level of the fourth lumbar vertebra, less than 4 cm inferior to it. Posteriorly, the **costodiaphragmatic recess of the pleura** crosses the twelfth rib to reach the upper part of the first lumbar, vertebra in the paravertebral line. (*N.B.* the **mid-clavicular, mid-axillary**, and **paravertebral lines** are three imaginary vertical lines which pass respectively through the middle of the clavicle, midway between the anterior and posterior axillary folds, and at the sides of the vertebral column. They are used for descriptive purposes.)

This overlapping of the abdominal cavity by the lower thorax and gluteal regions means that penetrating wounds of these regions frequently involve the abdominal cavity also. It also makes it simpler for the surgeon to reach the upper abdominal cavity through the thorax and diaphragm than through the anterior abdominal wall. Because the mobile diaphragm forms the upper limit of the abdominal cavity, the abdominal contents descend with it on inspiration. This is made use of in the clinical examination of certain organs, e.g. liver or enlarged spleen, which may be exposed to palpation inferior to the costal margin on deep inspiration, though hidden by the thoracic cage in quiet respiration. The kidney may also be identified in the loin by the movement which it undergoes on deep inspiration.

Bones and surface anatomy

The bones of the abdomen and pelvis are the lower ribs and costal cartilages, the lumbar vertebrae, the sacrum and coccyx, and the hip bones.

Lower ribs

These and the costal cartilages are described on pages 2 and 5. The eleventh and twelfth ribs differ from the remainder in being shorter and not articulating either with the transverse processes of their vertebrae or with the adjacent costal cartilages. They are capable, therefore, of moving independently of the other ribs.

Lumbar vertebrae

The lumbar vertebrae have the same elements as the thoracic vertebrae [p. 3] but are more massive in keeping with the greater load which they have to transmit. The large kidney-shaped **bodies** have flat upper and lower surfaces. As in all other vertebrae, these surfaces show a large, centrally placed, rough area surrounded by a raised, smooth margin. This margin is formed by the **ring epiphysis** which has fused with each of these surfaces. These surfaces are nearly parallel to each other, except in the fifth lumbar vertebra where the body is much deeper anteriorly than posteriorly. This helps to produce the **lumbosacral angle** together with the wedge-shaped **lumbosacral intervertebral disc**. Elsewhere the anteroposterior **curvatures of the vertebral column** (convex anteriorly in the lumbar and cervical regions, concave in the thoracic region) are produced mainly by the intervertebral discs. These curvatures and the discs confer a degree of resilience on the vertebral column.

In the lumbar region, the circumference of the body is concave from above downwards, particularly on the lateral sides, and is perforated by a number of vascular foramina. These are particularly large on the posterior surface where one or two **basivertebral veins** emerge anterior to the posterior longitudinal ligament and pass round its margins to join the internal vertebral venous plexus [Fig. 205]. These veins drain the **red marrow** in the cancellous bone of the vertebral body.

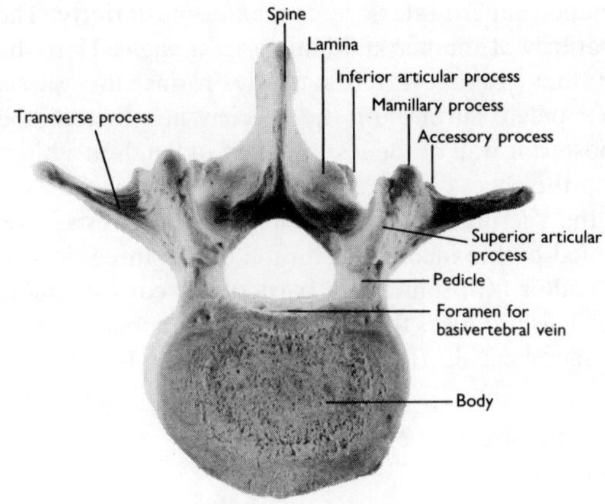

Fig. 95. The superior surface of the third lumbar vertebra.

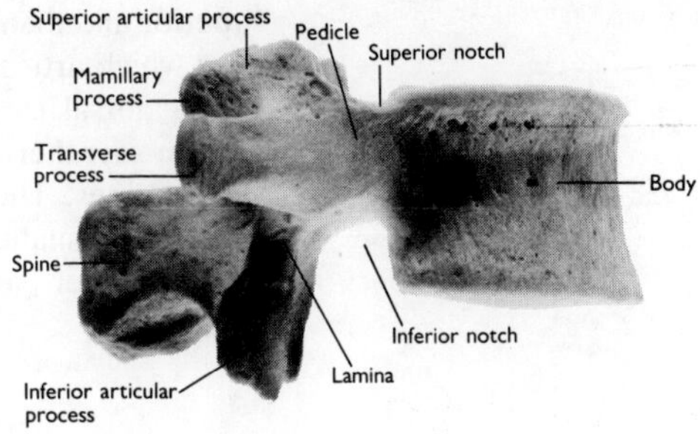

Fig. 96. The right surface of the third lumbar vertebra.

The thick **pedicles** arise from the upper two-thirds of the posterolateral surfaces of the body, superior to a deep **inferior vertebral notch**. The pedicles join relatively narrow **laminae** which pass downwards and backwards to meet in a thick rectangular **spine**. This projects backwards posterior to the lower two-thirds of the vertebral body and the intervertebral disc inferior to it. The laminae and pedicles surround a large, triangular **vertebral foramen**.

The inferior **articular processes** project inferiorly from the laminae with a V-shaped gap between them. This gap is wider in the lower than the upper lumbar vertebrae. The curved facets on the anterolateral surfaces of these processes fit between the blunt superior articular processes which project upwards from the junction of each pedicle and lamina of the vertebra below [Fig. 95]. This interlocking of the articular processes effectively prevents rotation [Fig. 93]. When two adjacent lumbar vertebrae are articulated, the V-shaped gap between the inferior articular processes faces a similar gap between the laminae of the vertebrae below. Together they form a diamond-shaped deficiency in the posterior wall of the vertebral canal. This is filled by the **ligamenta flava** through which a needle may be introduced into the lumbar vertebral canal—*lumbar puncture*, cf. the overlapping laminae in the thoracic region.

The **transverse processes** are thin and spatulate in the upper lumbar vertebrae, but thicker in the fourth and fifth. In the fifth, the bases of these processes extend forwards on to the vertebral body, further thickening the pedicles. In an articulated vertebral column, the lumbar transverse processes can be seen to lie in series with the ribs. They represent lumbar ribs fused to the vertebrae. Their extension forwards in the fourth and fifth lumbar vertebrae represent an increase in size of these costal elements which reaches its maximum in the fused vertebrae of the sacrum. The true lumbar transverse process is represented by the small **accessory process** on the dorsal surface of the transverse process at its base. The accessory process is immediately inferior to the rounded **mamillary process** which projects posteriorly from the superior articular process [Fig. 95]. Both of these processes give attachment to the erector spinae muscle.

Sacrum

The sacrum together with the two hip bones and the coccyx forms the skeleton of the pelvis. The sacrum consists of five fused vertebrae. It is concave anteriorly. The bodies of the sacral vertebrae are separated on the pelvic surface by the presence of ridges which have the remnants of intervertebral discs deep to them. Lateral to each of these ridges is a **pelvic sacral foramen**. This is directly continuous posteriorly with a dorsal sacral foramen and medially with a sacral intervertebral foramen which leads into the sacral canal. The **sacral canal** is the continuation of the vertebral canal posterior to the sacral vertebral bodies. It contains the caudal parts of the coverings (meninges) of the central nervous system, and transmits the sacral nerves and branches of the internal vertebral venous plexus to the sacral intervertebral foramina. Here the nerves divide into ventral and dorsal rami which emerge through the pelvic and dorsal foramina respectively.

The sacrum is wedge-shaped supero-inferiorly and anteroposteriorly. The broad **base** lies anterosuperiorly at the marked lumbosacral angle. Here the anterior margin of the first sacral vertebral body forms the **sacral promontory**. The concave pelvic surface of the sacrum lies first in the superior and then in the posterior wall of the lesser pelvis and ends in a blunt **apex** which articulates with the coccyx [Figs. 206, 236].

The dorsal surface of the sacrum shows three longitudinal crests. The **median sacral crest** is formed by the incomplete fusion of the three or four sacral spines. The fourth and/or fifth spines and parts of the corresponding lamina are usually missing. This produces the **sacral hiatus**—a dorsal opening into the lower part of the sacral canal. The hiatus is of variable length. The

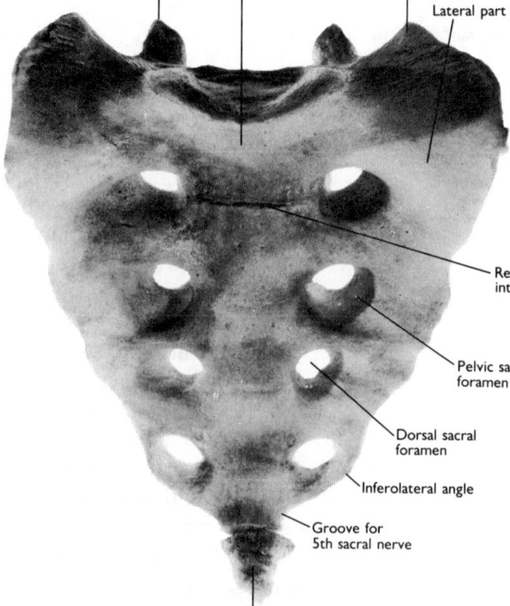

Fig. 97. The sacrum and coccyx (pelvic surface).

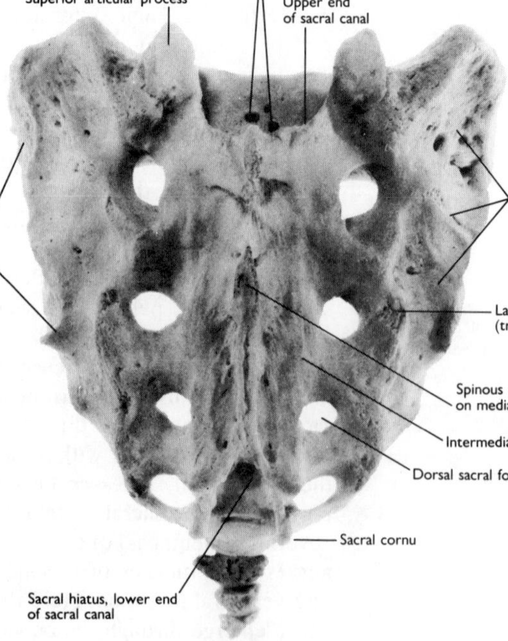

Fig. 98. The sacrum and coccyx (dorsal surface).

intermediate and **lateral sacral crests** lie respectively medial and lateral to the dorsal sacral foramina. The intermediate crests are formed by the fused articular processes. They are in line with the large, widely set, superior articular processes of the sacrum which articulate with the inferior processes of the fifth lumbar vertebra. The lateral crests correspond to the transverse processes and form a portion of the **lateral part** of the sacrum. This includes the costal elements which are greatly expanded in the first two or three sacral vertebrae and carry the curved **auricular surfaces** for articulation with the corresponding surfaces of the iliac bones (sacro-iliac joints). On the sacrum and both ilia, the rough areas (**tuberosities**) posterior to the auricular surfaces are for the powerful **interosseous sacro-iliac ligaments**. The auricular surfaces slope upwards and medially so that this almost horizontal part of the sacrum [Figs. 99, 289] is wedged between the hip bones and slung from them by the ligaments. The weight of the body transmitted to the sacrum tends to drive it downwards. This tightens the posterior sacro-iliac ligaments and draws the two hip bones firmly against the sacrum, increasing the rigidity of the sacro-iliac joints by tight fitting of their irregular surfaces.

The surface of the sacrum which articulates with the lumbosacral intervertebral disc slopes downwards and forwards. Thus there is a tendency for the fifth lumbar vertebra to slip forwards on the sacrum. This is prevented, in part, by the large superior articular processes of the sacrum. Occasionally the laminae, spine, and inferior articular processes of the fifth lumbar vertebra may be fractured from or ossify separately from the remainder. When this happens, the fifth lumbar vertebral body may slip forwards and downwards on the sacrum (spondylolisthesis). The large transverse process of the fifth lumbar vertebra may articulate with or be fused to the lateral part of the sacrum. This may be unilateral or bilateral. Indeed the fifth lumbar vertebra may be completely fused with the sacrum—**sacralization of the fifth lumbar vertebra**, or the first sacral vertebra may be partly or completely separated from the remainder of the sacrum (**lumbarization**).

Coccyx

This small, triangular mass of bone consists of four more or less fused rudimentary vertebrae. It articulates with the apex of the sacrum and is palpable in the natal cleft. The tip of the coccyx lies at the level of the upper border of the pubic symphysis.

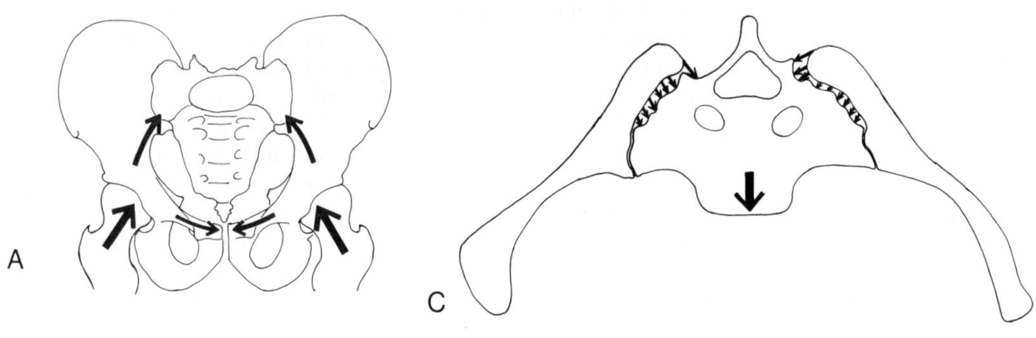

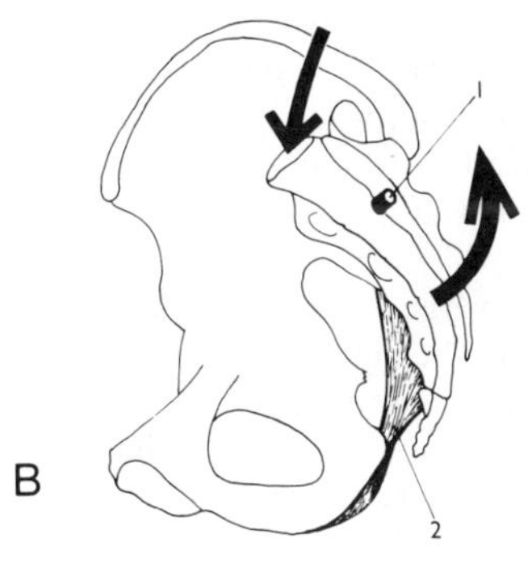

Fig. 99. Three diagrams to show the forces to which the pelvis is subjected and the structures which bear these forces or fracture when they are excessive. (A) shows forces transmitted to the trunk from the lower limbs, (B) and (C) the effects of the load of the body weight (static and dynamic) on the pelvis. Fractures due to overloading are partly obviated by the resilience conferred on the pelvis by the sacro-iliac joint and sacrotuberous ligament (B) and the interpubic disc of the pubic symphysis (A). In (C), the wedge of sacrum would appear to permit it to descend into the pelvis when loaded by the weight of the trunk (large arrow) but this is resisted by the posterior and interosseous sacro-iliac ligaments (small arrows) which draw the ilia inwards tightening the sacro-iliac joints. From (A) it is easy to see how the pelvis would deform if the bones soften as in rickets. This can cause serious problems in childbirth much later in life even in cases of mild and unnoticed rickets in childhood where the deformity is minimal.

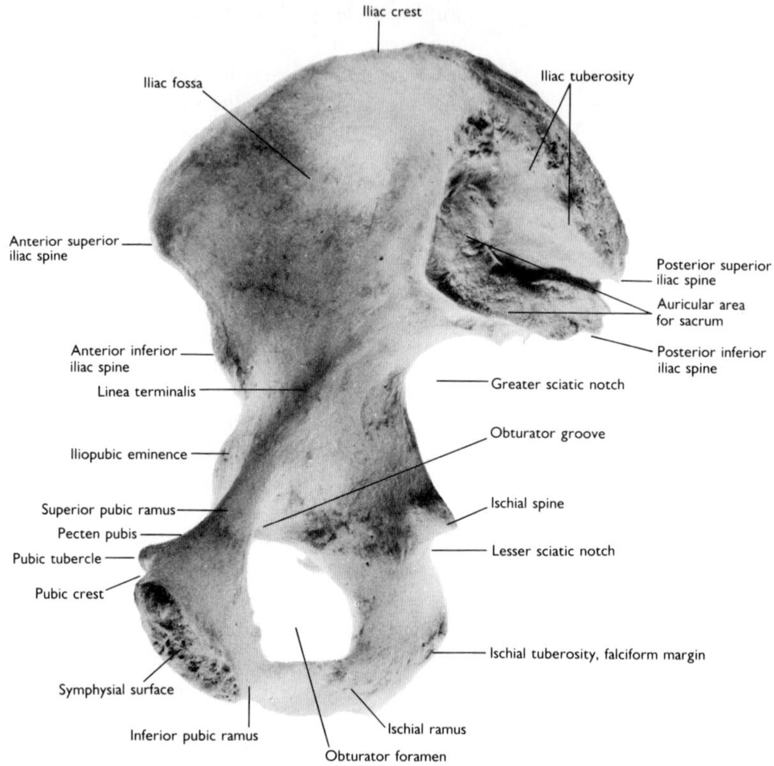

Fig. 100. Right hip bone seen from the medial side. Cf. Fig. 259.

The hip bone

This bone has the appearance of a propeller with a large blade (the ilium) directed upwards and a smaller blade, perforated by a large aperture (the **obturator foramen**) directed downwards. The two blades are almost at right angles to one another and meet at a narrow, thick hub where the head of the femur articulates in the **acetabulum**. The small blade consists of the **pubis** anteromedially and the **ischium** posterolaterally. These two fuse in the bar of bone inferior to the obturator foramen (**inferior ramus of the pubis** and **ramus of the ischium**) and at the hub where they meet in the acetabular notch.

The body of the pubis articulates with its fellow at the inferior extremity of the anterior abdominal wall (**pubic symphysis** [p. 215]). The anterosuperior margin of the body of the pubis (**pubic crest**) extends laterally from the symphysis to a small, blunt **pubic tubercle** 2.5 cm from the median plane. The crest and tubercle may be palpated, though the tubercle is covered in the male by the soft, cylindrical **spermatic cord**. Lateral to the tubercle, a resilient band is felt in the fold of the groin between abdomen and thigh. This is the **inguinal ligament** which extends from the tubercle to the anterior superior iliac spine. This ligament is the inrolled edge of the aponeurosis of the most superficial muscle of the anterior abdominal wall—the external oblique. On the bone, a sharp ridge (**pecten pubis** [Fig. 304]) extends laterally from the tubercle on the **superior ramus of the pubis**. Deep fibres of the inguinal ligament curve posteriorly (**lacunar ligament**) into the pecten and continue along it as the **pectineal ligament**. The pecten and ligament reach a blunt ridge (**iliopubic eminence**) on the anterior wall of the acetabulum. This marks the line of fusion of the superior ramus of the pubis with the ilium. A less well defined ridge on the posterior wall of the acetabulum marks the fusion of the ischium with the ilium.

The **inferior rami of the pubic bones** diverge at the subpubic angle to form the **pubic arch** with the rami of the ischia. The margins of this horizontal arch are palpable between the anterior part of the perineum (urogenital triangle) medially and the thighs laterally. The ramus of the ischium expands posteriorly into the **ischial tuberosity** which gives attachment to the hamstring muscles of the thigh and has a rough medial ridge for attachment of the sacrotuberous ligament. Superior to the tuberosity, the **ischial spine** [Fig.

304] projects posteromedially and separates the **lesser sciatic notch** of the ischium, inferiorly, from the **greater sciatic notch** on the posterior margin of the ilium, superiorly. When the hip bone and sacrum are articulated, the two notches form the anterolateral margin of a deep bay between the bones. The bay is converted into two foramina (greater and lesser sciatic) by the **sacrospinous** and **sacrotuberous ligaments** which pass from the sacrum to the ischial spine and tuberosity respectively. The **greater sciatic foramen** leads from the lesser pelvis into the gluteal region, the lesser from the gluteal region into the perineum [Figs. 211, 212].

The **ilium** is a fan-shaped plate of bone which extends superiorly from the acetabulum to the sinuous **iliac crest** at the lower margin of the waist. The position of the crest is marked by a groove where the abdominal and gluteal fasciae are attached to the crest. In yourself, follow the crest forwards and backwards. Anteriorly, it slopes downwards and slightly medially to the **anterior superior iliac spine** [Fig. 304]. Posteriorly, it turns backwards and downwards to the **posterior superior iliac spine** which lies in a dimple at the level of the second sacral spine. Anterior and posterior **inferior iliac spines** lie on the margins of the ilium inferior to the corresponding superior spines. The posterior inferior spine marks the posterior limit of the auricular surface and the upper posterior margin of the greater sciatic notch at the level of the third sacral spine.

The greater part of the medial aspect of the ilium forms the smooth, concave **iliac fossa**. Posterior to this lie the auricular surface and tuberosity of the ilium. The iliac fossa (bony wall of the greater pelvis) is separated from the part of the ilium medial to the acetabulum (superior part of the bony wall of the lesser pelvis) by a thick, curved ridge (**arcuate line of ilium**) which crosses the ilium from the antero-inferior part of the auricular surface to the lateral end of the pecten pubis. This strong part of the ilium transmits compression forces from the auricular surface, and hence from the vertebral column, to the acetabulum and lower limb. The pubic crest, pecten pubis, arcuate line of ilium, and the promontory of the sacrum together form the rim of the **superior aperture of the (lesser) pelvis**—the **linea terminalis** of the pelvis. The internal surfaces of the pubis and ischium also form part of the bony wall of the lesser pelvis. The obturator foramen is filled by the obturator membrane—a fibrous sheet attached to the sharp margin of the foramen except anterosuperiorly where it is notched by the **obturator sulcus**. The membrane bridges the sulcus and turns it into the **obturator canal** which transmits the obturator vessels and nerve.

It is important to understand the *position of the hip bone*. The symphysial surface of the pubic bone lies in the sagittal plane. The pubic tubercle and anterior superior iliac spine lie in the same coronal plane. The linea terminalis of the pelvis lies at an angle of approximately 70 degrees to the horizontal, entirely superior to the pubic symphysis, with the sacral promontory at the level of the anterior superior iliac spines. Hence the superior aperture of the pelvis faces the lower part of the anterior abdominal wall. The upper borders of the ischial tuberosities and of the pubic symphysis lie in the same horizontal plane as the tip of the coccyx. The **inferior aperture of the pelvis** is formed by the pubic arch, the ischial tuberosities, and the coccyx, the last two united by the sacrotuberous ligaments. It is approximately horizontal and is filled by the perineum. In the median plane, the pubic symphysis forms the short antero-inferior wall of the lesser pelvis; the curve of the sacrum and coccyx forms the long posterosuperior wall.

Surface anatomy of anterior abdominal wall

On each side the muscles of this wall end inferiorly at the inguinal ligament, though the fascia superficial to them extends to the fold of the groin before fusing with the deep fascia of the thigh (fascia lata). For the purposes of description, the anterior abdominal wall is divided into nine regions by two vertical and two horizontal planes [Fig. 101]. The right and left vertical planes pass through the **mid-inguinal points**; i.e. a point on each inguinal ligament midway between the anterior superior iliac spine and the pubic symphysis. The **transpyloric plane** lies horizontally midway between the jugular notch of the sternum and the pubic symphysis, i.e. approximately

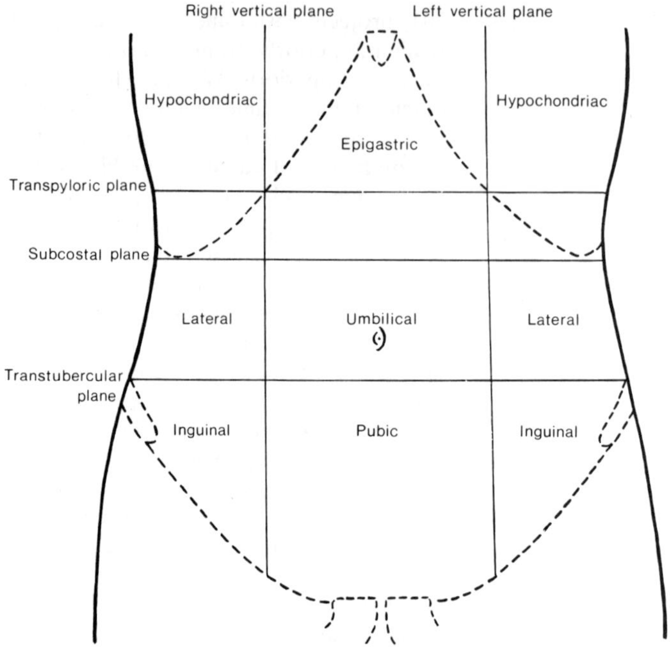

Fig. 101. Planes of subdivision of the abdomen proper, with the names of the nine abdominal regions.

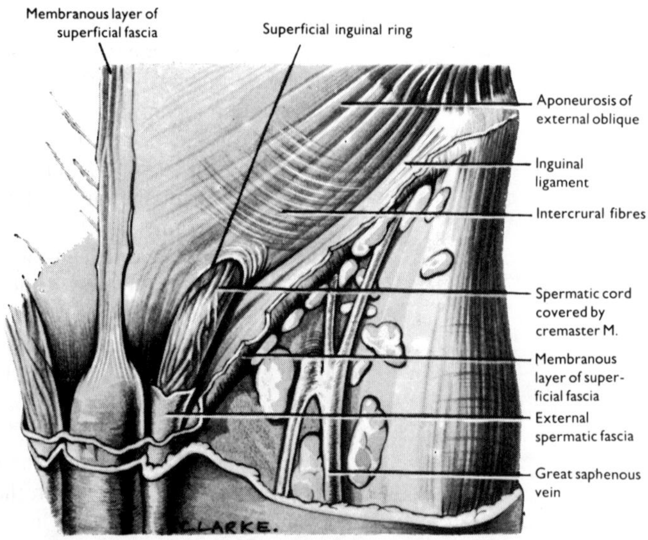

Fig. 102. A superficial dissection of the inguinal region.

midway between the xiphoid process and the umbilicus, at the level of the first lumbar vertebra. The **transtubercular plane** passes horizontally through the tubercles of the iliac crests at the level of the fifth lumbar vertebra.

The mid-inguinal point marks the position where, deep to the inguinal ligament, the external iliac artery escapes from the abdomen to become the femoral artery in the thigh. Feel the pulsations of your femoral artery at this point. Run your finger medially on the inguinal ligament to the pubic tubercle which is covered by the spermatic cord in the male. Immediately superolateral to the tubercle is the **superficial inguinal ring**—an aperture in the aponeurosis of the external oblique muscle of the abdomen. The **spermatic cord** descends in front of the pubis from this aperture to the scrotum [Fig. 102]. In the female, the **round ligament of the uterus** descends to the labium majus [Fig. 220]. The margins of the ring are easily felt in the male. Place the tip of your little finger on the loose skin of the upper part of the scrotum in front of the pubis and spermatic cord and invaginate the skin upwards along the line of the cord. Where the cord disappears through the ring, the sharp margins can be felt by pressing posteriorly. Pick up the spermatic cord between finger and thumb. Note the firm, cordlike **ductus deferens** buried in its posterior part. This is the duct of the testis. The ring is smaller in the female than the male and is more difficult to feel because of the amount of subcutaneous fat in the region.

There is a slight median groove on the anterior abdominal wall between the xiphoid process and the pubic symphysis. Deep to this is the **linea alba**—an extensive raphe formed by the interlocking of the aponeuroses of the three flat muscles on each side of the abdominal wall after they have ensheathed the **rectus abdominis** muscles which run longitudinally, one on each side of the midline [Figs. 107, 108]. The **umbilicus** lies in the linea alba, nearer the pubis than the xiphoid process. It is the scar formed from the remnants of the root of the umbilical cord through which the fetus *in utero* is attached to the placenta. The linea alba and umbilical scar are formed of relatively avascular, white fibrous tissue. Incisions into the abdominal cavity may be made through the linea alba without injury to nerves or blood vessels of any size, but the linea has poor healing qualities because of its avascularity and wounds are liable to break down because of the pull of the abdominal muscles on it.

The lateral edge of each rectus abdominis muscle is marked by a slight groove (**linea semilunaris**) which is visible in thin, muscular individuals. It is most obvious where the aponeuroses of the abdominal muscles split to enclose the rectus abdominis [Fig. 108] in the upper two-thirds of the abdomen. The linea semilunaris crosses the costal margin at the **ninth costal cartilage**, the position of the **fundus of the gall bladder** on the right. Three grooves may be seen crossing the rectus abdominis between the umbilicus and the xiphoid process. They are formed by tendinous intersections in the rectus abdominis muscles which fuse with the aponeuroses on the anterior surfaces of these muscles.

The anterior abdominal wall

Dissection

Make skin incisions 8 and 9 [Fig. 94]. Carry 8 round each side of the umbilicus and 9 posteriorly along the iliac crest. If the thorax has not been dissected, make incision 4 also. Carry it posteriorly at least to the midaxillary line. Reflect the flaps of skin leaving the superficial fascia on the anterior abdominal wall.

Superficial fascia

This contains a very variable amount of fat which is usually greatest over the inferior half of the abdomen. Here the fascia consists of superficial fatty and deep membranous layers. The **membranous layer** represents the elastic suspensory ligament of quadrupeds. On each side it is separated from the underlying muscle (external oblique) by a loose areolar layer which disappears superiorly and towards the median plane. Inferiorly [Fig. 103] the areolar layer disappears where the membranous layer fuses with the deep fascia of the thigh, medial part of the inguinal ligament, and pubic tubercle in the fold of each groin. From the pubic tubercle, on each side, the line of fusion extends downwards on the front of the body of the pubic bone and along the corresponding subcutaneous margin of the pubic arch. Thus a pocket-like extension of the areolar layer passes in front of the pubic bones into the anterior part of the perineum (**superficial perineal space**). The floor of this extension is formed by the membranous layer which closes it posteriorly by fusing, in front of the anus, with the posterior edge of the **urogenital diaphragm**—a musculofascial sheet which is stretched across the pubic arch at a higher level and forms the roof of the superficial perineal space.

In the male, the pocket contains the root of the penis and the spermatic cords passing to the testes in the scrotum. Both penis and scrotum, projecting from the pocket, receive a covering from the membranous layer. This forms the fascia and fundiform ligament of the penis and the smooth muscle, **dartos**, in the scrotal wall. If the penile urethra is ruptured within the superficial perineal space, urine escaping from the urethra fills the pocket and extends from it on to the anterior abdominal wall and into the scrotum deep to the fascia. The fundiform ligament usually prevents entry to the penis. It cannot extend into the thigh because of the attachments of the membranous

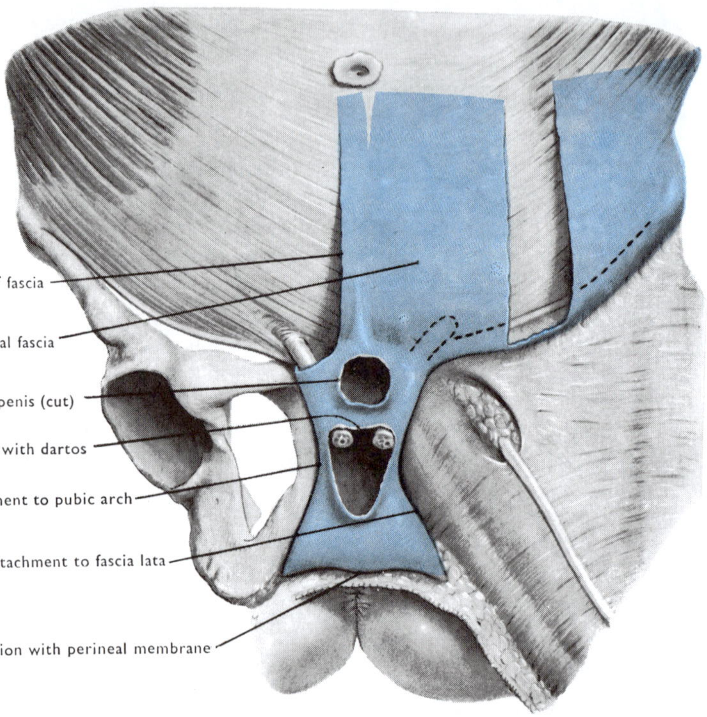

Fig. 103. A diagram to show the membranous layer of the superficial fascia of the abdomen and its extension into the perineum in the male. In the midline the fascia is fused with the external oblique aponeurosis to form the fundiform ligament of the penis. See also Fig. 221.

layer. Thus it produces a circumscribed swelling of the perineum, scrotum, and lower anterior abdominal wall.

In the female, the superficial perineal space is split in the median plane by the vulva. Thus a separate pocket extends into the base of each labium majus [Fig. 220] which corresponds to the scrotum.

Dissection

Make a transverse section through the entire thickness of the superficial fascia from the anterior superior iliac spine to the median plane. Raise the lower margin of the cut fascia and identify its fatty and membranous layers. Pass a finger deep to the membranous layer which separates easily from the aponeurosis of the external oblique muscle deep to it until a point is reached just inferior to the inguinal ligament where the membranous layer fuses with the fascia lata of the thigh. Medial to the pubic tubercle, a finger may be passed with the spermatic cord (or round ligament of the uterus), anterior to the body of the pubis, into the perineum. In this position movement of the finger laterally is limited by the attachment of the membranous layer of fascia to the pubic bone and arch.

Find the **superficial inguinal ring** immediately superolateral to the pubic tubercle. The ring is a triangular aperture in the aponeurosis of the external oblique muscle [Fig. 102] with the spermatic cord (or round ligament of the uterus) emerging through it. Note the anterior cutaneous branch of the **iliohypogastric nerve** piercing the aponeurosis of the external oblique muscle a short distance superior to the ring.

Cutaneous nerves

The muscles and skin of the abdominal wall are almost entirely supplied by the lower intercostal and subcostal nerves. Only the first of the lumbar nerves supplies the most inferior part through the **iliohypogastric** and **ilioinguinal nerves**. All these nerves are arranged on the same plan as the higher intercostal nerves [Fig. 17]. However, the ilioinguinal nerve lacks a lateral cutaneous branch and its anterior cutaneous branch passes through the superficial inguinal ring. This branch supplies skin on the medial side of the upper thigh and on the scrotum or labium majus.

Anterior cutaneous branches

These pierce the anterior wall of the sheath of the rectus muscle a short distance from the median plane. They are arranged in sequence with the corresponding branches of the upper intercostal nerves and supply a similar area. This branch of the tenth thoracic nerve emerges close to the umbilicus; the **first lumbar nerve** appears above the superficial inguinal ring (iliohypogastric nerve).

Dissection

Divide the superficial fascia vertically in the median plane, and in the line of the posterior axillary fold as far as the iliac crest. Reflect the fascia by blunt dissection from these two cuts and find the anterior and lateral cutaneous branches of the nerves emerging from the anterior and lateral parts of the abdominal wall.

Lateral cutaneous branches

These emerge through the external oblique muscle. The **subcostal** and **iliohypogastric branches** appear close to the iliac crest and descend over it to supply the skin in the upper anterior part of the gluteal region. The remainder give large anterior and small posterior branches. The anterior branches supply skin to the lateral margin of the rectus abdominis muscle.

Cutaneous vessels

The small arteries which accompany the lateral cutaneous branches of the nerves arise from the **posterior intercostal arteries**. Those with the anterior cutaneous branches arise from the superior and inferior **epigastric arteries** [p. 103] which anastomose within the sheath of the rectus abdominis muscle and so link the arteries of the upper and lower limbs.

Below the umbilicus, the skin and superficial fascia are supplied by three small branches from each femoral artery. The **superficial external pudendal** runs medially to supply scrotum (or labium majus) and penis. The **superficial epigastric** runs superomedially across the inguinal ligament as far as the umbilicus. The **superficial circumflex iliac** passes towards the anterior superior iliac spine supplying the adjacent abdominal and groin skin.

Superficial veins

Below the umbilicus these drain with the superficial arteries to the great saphenous vein in the groin, and thus eventually to the inferior vena cava. *Above the umbilicus* they pass to the axilla and so to the superior vena cava. Both groups anastomose freely with each other and with small veins which drain to the umbilicus from the liver alongside the obliterated umbilical vein. In obstruction of the superior or inferior vena cava, these veins may be distended as an alternative route for venous return. If the venous drainage through the liver is blocked, backflow may occur to the umbilicus from the liver. This is then drained in both directions on each side forming, in the later stages, a pattern of distended veins radiating from the umbilicus—'caput medusae'.

Muscles of anterior abdominal wall

These are in three layers each of which is muscular posterolaterally and aponeurotic anteromedially. As the three **aponeuroses** pass towards the median plane, they partially enclose the rectus abdominis muscle (see rectus sheath [p. 97]) and then fuse with each other and with the aponeuroses of the opposite side in the median **linea alba** from xiphoid process to pubis.

The outer two layers (external and internal oblique muscles) are approximately fan-shaped. The **external oblique** arises from the external surfaces of the lower eight ribs and radiates downwards and forwards. The **internal oblique** arises from the lumbar fascia, the iliac crest, and the lateral two-thirds of the inguinal ligament (q.v.) and radiates upwards and forwards. Thus the lower (posterior) fibres of the external oblique and the upper (posterior) fibres of the internal oblique are almost vertical and unite the iliac crest and rib cage. While the upper fibres of the external and the lower fibres of the internal are nearly horizontal, the middle fibres cross each other at right angles.

The innermost layer, **transversus abdominis**, is horizontally disposed. It runs from the internal surface of the rib cage, the lumbar fascia, the iliac crest, and the lateral third of the inguinal ligament to the linea alba. Thus its fibres lie at an angle to the intermediate fibres of both the other muscles, but are parallel to those of the external oblique, superiorly, and to the internal

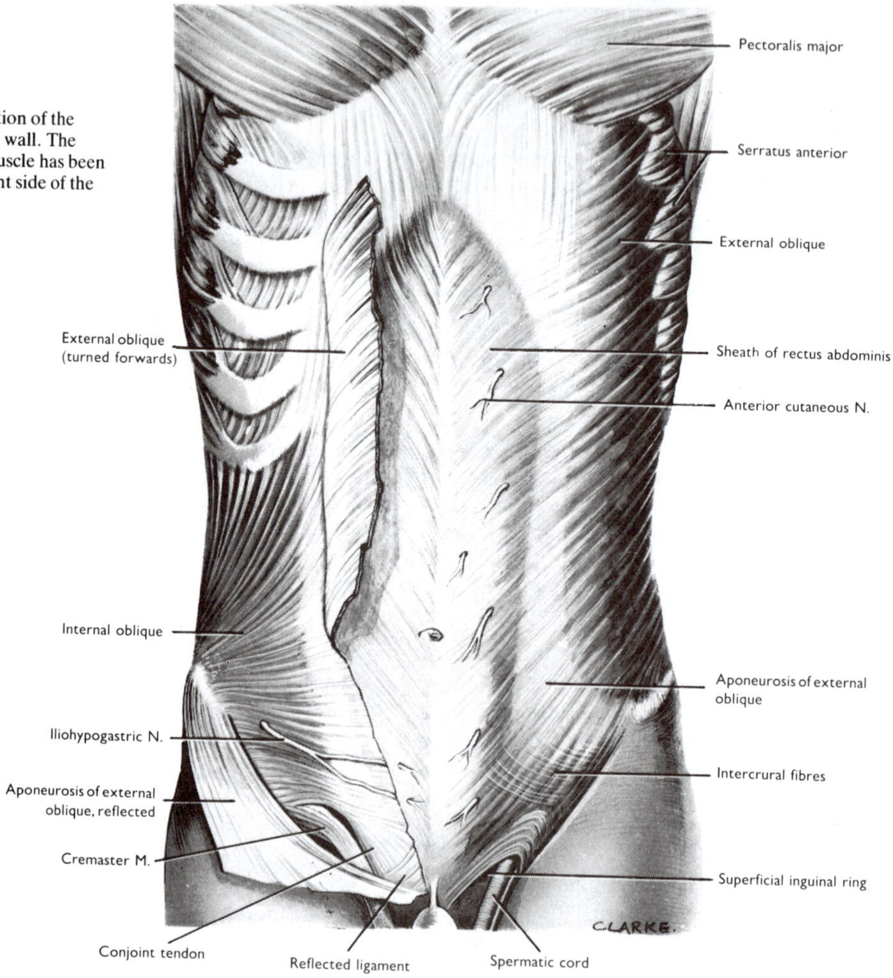

Fig. 104. A dissection of the anterior abdominal wall. The external oblique muscle has been reflected on the right side of the body.

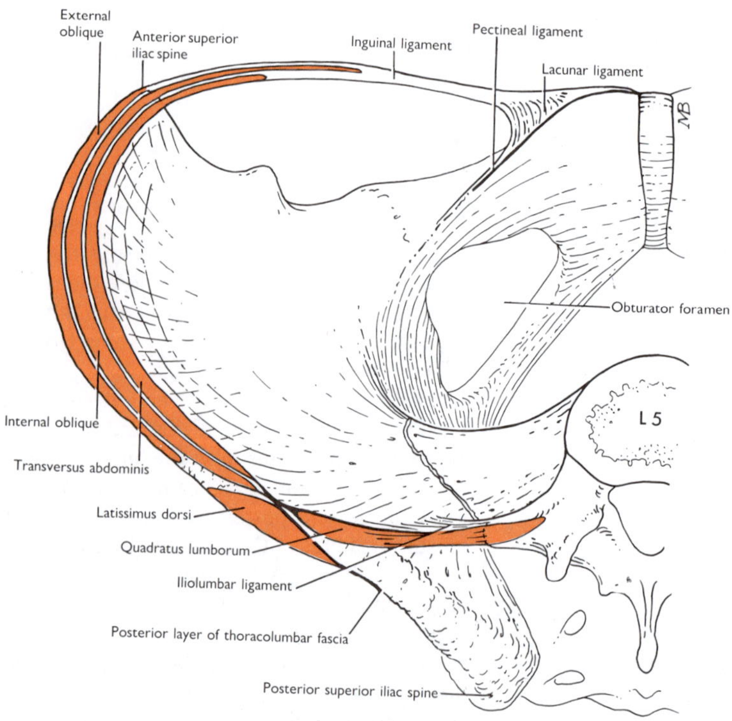

Fig. 105. The bony pelvis and fifth lumbar vertebra seen from above.

oblique, inferiorly. This arrangement gives maximum strength to the abdominal wall and helps to prevent the abdominal contents from bursting through the wall when the intra-abdominal pressure is raised by contraction of these muscles.

The lower, parallel fibres of the aponeuroses of the internal oblique and transversus abdominis do not reach the linea alba but fuse to form the **conjoint tendon** [Fig. 107] which turns downwards to be attached to the pubic crest and the pecten pubis [Fig. 206].

Transversalis fascia

The deep surface of the transversus abdominis is covered by a layer of transversalis fascia. This is a part of a continuous fascial lining of the abdominal and pelvic cavities. Each part of this fascia takes its name from the structures on which it lies. Thus there is also **diaphragmatic fascia** on the diaphragm, **iliac fascia** on the iliacus and psoas muscles, **renal fascia** surrounding the kidneys, and **pelvic fascia** in the pelvis. Internal to this layer is the serous lining of the abdomen (**peritoneum**) separated by a variable amount of extraperitoneal fat.

Actions of external oblique, internal oblique, and transversus abdominis muscles
[see also pp. 11, 102; Table 2, p. 265]

These muscles have a number of important actions many of which are concerned with compression of the abdominal contents. When the thoracic cage and diaphragm are relaxed, the three muscles produce forced expiration by pulling down the lower ribs (assisted by rectus abdominis) and by forcing the abdominal contents and diaphragm upwards. When such actions are violent, they produce the force for *coughing, sneezing*, and *vomiting*. When the ribs and diaphragm are fixed, the abdominal muscles raise the pressure in the abdomen and pelvis. This assists with *defecation, micturition*, and *childbirth* (parturition), but is also used to turn the trunk into a rigid pillar when the thoracic expiratory muscles also contract but the inspired air is prevented from leaving the lungs because the outflow tract is blocked by closure of the glottis and pharynx [see Vol. 3]. This action is used in any forced movement such as pushing or lifting heavy weights. In such actions, the *intra-abdominal pressure rises to very high levels*. This may cause discharge or urine through a weakened sphincter of the urinary bladder (stress incontinence) or abdominal contents may be forced through any weak points in the abdominal or pelvic walls—a condition known as *hernia*. This tends to occur where structures enter or leave the abdominal or pelvic cavities and the wall is intrinsically weak, or where the wall has been weakened by surgery. Hernia can also occur more easily when the abdominal wall is stretched by excessive accumulation of fat in the abdomen or following repeated pregnancies. In addition these muscles help to support the abdominal contents against gravity, and they also rotate the trunk—the internal oblique of one side acting with the external oblique of the other.

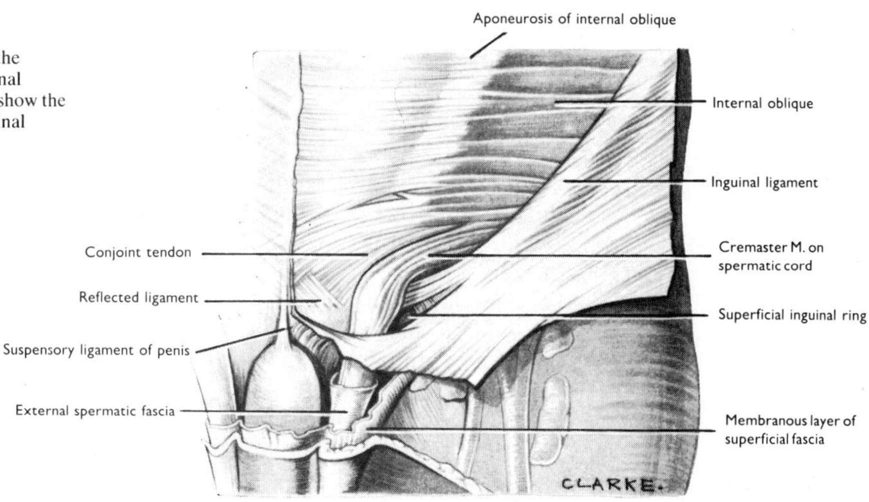

Fig. 106. A dissection of the inguinal region. The external oblique is turned down to show the spermatic cord in the inguinal canal.

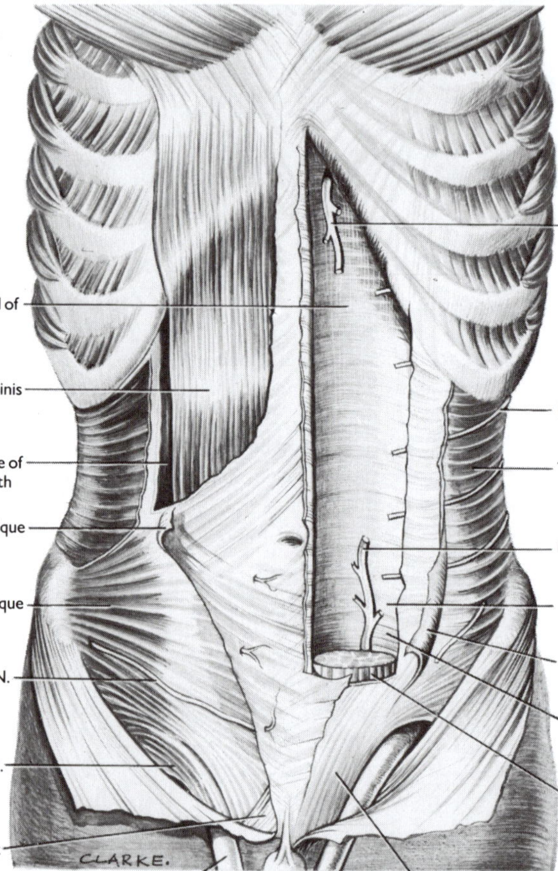

Fig. 107. A deep dissection of the anterior abdominal wall. On the left side of the body, the external and internal oblique muscles, the anterior wall of the rectus sheath, and the greater part of the rectus abdominis have been removed. On the right side of the body, the external oblique and upper parts of the internal oblique muscles and the upper part of the anterior wall of the rectus sheath have been removed.

Dissection

Remove any fascia from the surface of the external oblique muscle and its aponeurosis. Take special care superiorly where the aponeurosis is thin and easily removed, and also antero-inferiorly where the **superficial inguinal ring** forms a triangular deficiency in the aponeurosis immediately superolateral to the pubic tubercle. In the male, identify the **spermatic cord** emerging from this ring and note that it is attached to the margins of the ring by the layer of **external spermatic fascia**. In the female, the fatty, fibrous tissue emerging from the ring is the **round ligament of the uterus**. In either sex, define the margins of the ring by blunt dissection.

Identify the origin of the **external oblique** from the lower eight ribs. Here it interdigitates with serratus anterior and latissimus dorsi. Separate the upper six digitations from the ribs and cut vertically through the muscle to the iliac crest posterior to the sixth digitation. Separate the external oblique from the iliac crest in front of this, but avoid injury to the lateral cutaneous branches of the nerves which pierce it close to the crest.

Turn the superior part of the external oblique forwards and expose the **internal oblique** and its aponeurosis to the line of its fusion with the aponeurosis of the external oblique, anterior to rectus abdominis. Divide the external oblique aponeurosis vertically, lateral to this line of fusion, and turn the muscle and aponeurosis inferiorly as you do so. The cut should pass medial to the superficial inguinal ring as far as the pubis. This exposes the remainder of the internal oblique and the inrolled margin of the aponeurosis of the external oblique between its attachments to the anterior superior iliac spine and the pubic tubercle. This is the **inguinal ligament**. Note that this ligament gives origin to the internal oblique muscle from its lateral part and has the spermatic cord or the round ligament lying on its superior surface medially. Lift the cord or round ligament and identify the deep fibres of the inguinal ligament passing posteriorly to the pecten pubis. This is the **lacunar ligament** on which these structures also lie. Follow the lateral margin (**lateral crus**) of the **superficial inguinal ring** to the **pubic tubercle** and note the relationship of the crus and tubercle of the spermatic cord. The **medial crus** may be followed anterior to the pubis.

Remove the fascia from the surface of the internal oblique and its aponeurosis. Identify the part of the internal oblique which passes on to the spermatic cord. This **cremaster muscle** forms loops which extend down the cord and turn upwards towards the pubis. It is poorly developed in the aged but can usually be demonstrated. When it contracts, the testis is elevated in the scrotum towards the superficial inguinal ring. This movement can be produced in the living by stroking the medial side of the upper thigh (the **cremasteric reflex**). It tests the integrity of the first and second lumbar spinal nerves which supply the cremaster muscle (**genitofemoral nerve**) and the skin on the medial side of the proximal thigh (**ilio-inguinal nerve**).

Lift the internal oblique and cut carefully through its attachments to the inguinal ligament, iliac crest, and costal margin. Do not cut deeply or the nerves of the anterior abdominal wall which lie between internal oblique and transversus abdominis will be divided. Cut vertically through the internal oblique from the twelfth costal cartilage to the iliac crest and strip the muscle forwards from the transversus and the nerves. This is difficult superiorly because of the dense fascia between the muscles, and is impossible inferiorly where the aponeuroses of the two muscles fuse in the **conjoint tendon** [Fig. 107]. At the lateral edge of the rectus abdominis, the aponeurosis of the internal oblique splits to pass partly posterior and partly anterior to the rectus abdominis, the anterior layer fusing with the aponeurosis of the external oblique, the posterior layer with that of the transversus abdominis. This is the **rectus sheath**. Inferior to a horizontal line midway between the umbilicus and the symphysis pubis, the aponeuroses of all three muscles pass anterior to the rectus abdominis which then lies on the transversalis fascia posteriorly. The inferior edge of the posterior layer of the rectus sheath often forms a sharp margin, the **arcuate line**. This will be seen when the rectus sheath is opened.

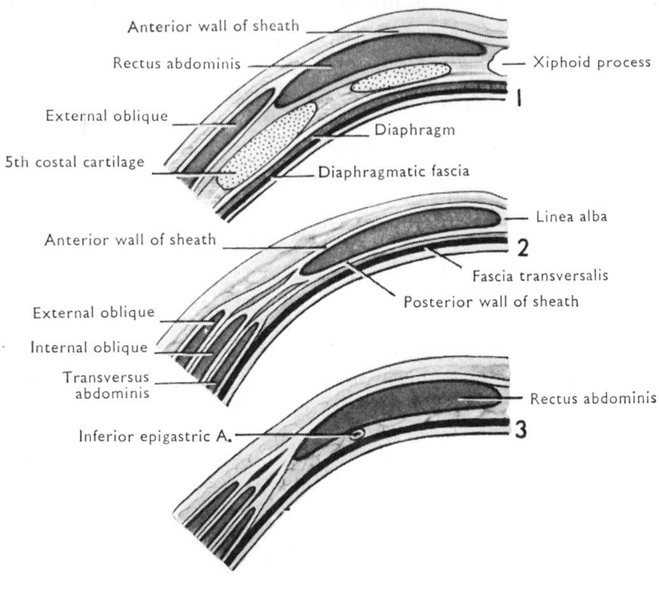

Fig. 108. Transverse sections of the anterior abdominal wall to show the varying formation of the rectus sheath.
1. Above the costal margin.
2. Upper three-quarters of the abdominal wall.
3. The lower quarter of the wall.

Remove the fascia from the surface of the transversus abdominis and from the nerves and vessels which lie on it. Confirm the continuity of the lateral cutaneous branches which have already been exposed with these nerves. Define the origins of the transversus and follow its aponeurosis to fuse with that of the internal oblique, posterior to the rectus abdominis above the arcuate line and anterior to the rectus below the line [Fig. 108]. Below the arcuate line, the aponeurosis of the external oblique is less firmly fused with that of the internal oblique than it is further superiorly [Fig. 112].

Open the rectus sheath by a vertical incision along the middle of the muscle. Reflect the anterior layer of the sheath medially and laterally, cutting its attachments to the **tendinous intersections** in the anterior part of the rectus muscle. Lift the rectus muscle and identify the intercostal and subcostal nerves entering the sheath and piercing the muscle. Confirm the method of formation of the rectus sheath.

On the lower part of the rectus, identify the **pyramidalis muscle** if present. This small triangular muscle arises from the upper surface of the pubis and pubic symphysis. It passes anterior to the rectus into the lowest part of the linea alba. It is supplied by a small branch of the subcostal nerve.

Divide the rectus abdominis transversely at its middle. Identify its attachments and expose the posterior wall of the rectus sheath by turning its parts superiorly and inferiorly, cutting the nerves as they enter it. Identify and follow the superior and inferior **epigastric arteries** passing longitudinally deep to the muscle within the rectus sheath [Fig. 107]. The tendinous intersections are only in the anterior part of rectus abdominis and so do not interfere with this longitudinal **anastomosis** between the subclavian (internal thoracic) and external iliac arteries. Try to define the **arcuate line** on the posterior wall of the rectus sheath. The inferior epigastric artery enters the sheath by passing anterior to this line.

Rectus abdominis

This muscle passes from the pubic crest posterior to the conjoint tendon to the anterior surfaces of the fifth, sixth, and seventh costal cartilages. Inferior to the arcuate line, the muscle lies between the transversalis fascia and the aponeuroses of the other muscles of the abdominal wall. Above the line, the **internal oblique aponeurosis** splits to enclose the rectus and fuses posteriorly with the transversus abdominis and anteriorly with the external oblique. Medially, all the aponeuroses fuse in the **linea alba**. This constitutes the **rectus sheath** [Fig. 108]. On the anterior surfaces of the costal cartilages, the posterior layer of the sheath is lost, transversus abdominis passing internal to the costal cartilages and internal oblique being attached to the costal margin, while the aponeurosis of the external oblique continues anterior to the muscle and gives attachment to the lowest fibres of pectoralis major.

Horizontal **tendinous intersections** in the anterior part of the rectus abdominis attach it to the anterior layer of the rectus sheath at the level of the umbilicus, at the tip of the xiphoid process, and midway between these. Occasionally a fourth is present between the umbilicus and the pubis.

Actions: the rectus abdominis is a powerful flexor of the vertebral column. It may be made to stand out when attempting to raise the head and shoulders (or lower limbs and pelvis) from the floor when lying on the back (supine position). When the extensors of the vertebral column (erector spinae) contract at the same time, the rectus muscles tighten the anterior abdominal wall against blows provided the ribs are fixed by inspiratory muscles. If the ribs are not fixed, the rectus is an expiratory muscle. It is not used in expulsive movements. **Nerve supply**: lower five or six intercostal and the subcostal nerves.

Dissection

Cut through the remaining ribs in the midaxillary line, and carefully turn down the sternum, costal cartilages, and the anterior parts of the ribs. Remove the pleura and fascia from the back of the sternum and the superior surface of the exposed part of the diaphragm and note the slips by which it arises from the xiphoid process and the costal cartilages. Identify the musculophrenic and superior epigastric branches of the **internal thoracic arteries**, the slips of origin of the transversus abdominis beside those of the diaphragm, and the continuity of the transversus abdominis with transversus thoracis superiorly.

Cut through the slips of origin of the diaphragm in front of the mid-axillary line and cut vertically through the transversus abdominis in that line to the iliac crest, avoiding injury to the peritoneum deep to the transversalis fascia. Turn down the remnants of the anterior abdominal wall with the sternum, costal cartilages, and ribs, attempting to strip the peritoneum from the transversalis fascia. Having identified the peritoneum, divide and reflect it with the anterior abdominal wall, cutting the fold of peritoneum which passes from the median part of the supra-umbilical anterior abdominal wall to the liver (**falciform ligament** [Fig. 141]). This fold contains the **ligamentum teres of the liver (obliterated umbilical vein** [Fig. 140]) in its free posterior border.

Examine the posterior surface of the reflected anterior abdominal wall. Identify five ill-defined peritoneal folds (two on each side and one median) which pass upwards towards the umbilicus. These are the lateral, medial, and median **umbilical folds**. They are formed respectively by the inferior epigastric vessels, the **lateral umbilicial ligaments (obliterated umbilical arteries**, which carry blood to the placenta in the fetus and ascend posterior to the conjoint tendons), and the **median umbilical ligament** (the remnant of the intra-abdominal part of the **allantois**—the **urachus** [Fig. 236]) which is attached inferiorly to the apex of the bladder. Strip the peritoneum from the posterior surface of the infra-umbilical abdominal wall to expose these structures and the attachments of transversus abdominis and the conjoint tendon. Before removing the transversalis fascia from the deep surface of the inguinal ligament, pull on the spermatic cord or round ligament of the uterus from the anterior surface to confirm the continuity of that fascia over these structures as the **internal spermatic fascia**.

The intrinsic weaknesses in the abdominal wall lie in the region of the groin (femoral and inguinal canals) and at the umbilical scar in the linea alba.

Femoral sheath and canal

At the groin, the anterior and posterior abdominal walls meet but only their fascial linings (transversalis and iliac fascia respectively) are continuous with each other. The muscles of the anterior abdominal wall end at the free, inrolled margin of the external oblique aponeurosis (**inguinal ligament**) which is fused to the deep fascia on the anterior surface of the thigh and is stretched

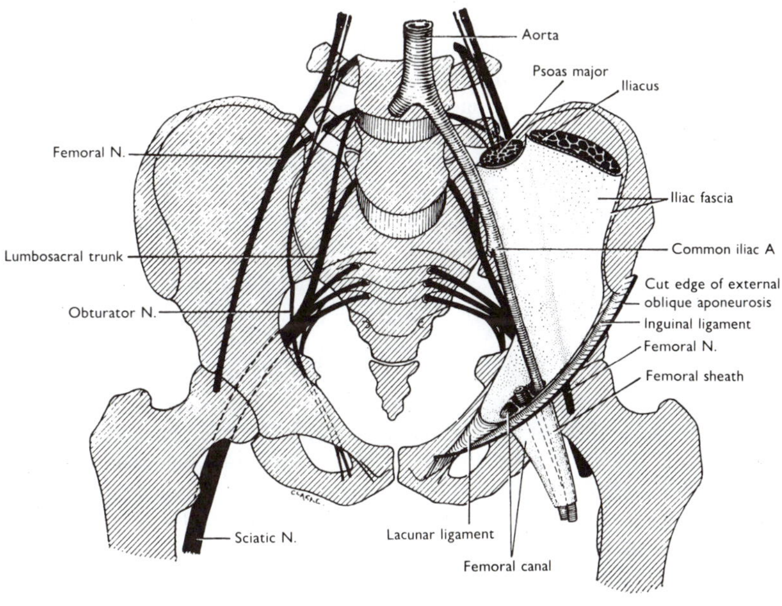

Fig. 109. A diagram to show the structures in the inguinal region and the nerves of the lower limb related to the pelvis.

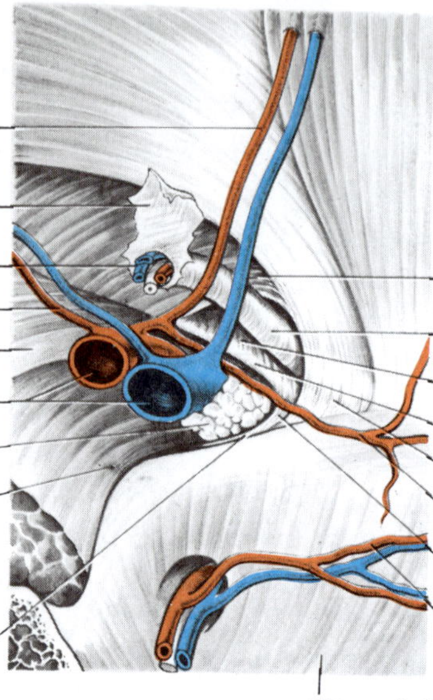

Fig. 110. A dissection of the posterior surface of the anterior abdominal wall in the inguinal region. Note the pubic branches of the obturator and inferior epigastric arteries which anastomose. They may replace the proximal part of the obturator artery (abnormal obturator artery).

between the anterior superior iliac spine and the pubic tubercle. This leaves a gap between the ligament and the hip bone through which structures of the posterior abdominal wall escape into the thigh [Figs. 105, 109, 113]. The **iliacus** and **psoas muscles**, the **femoral nerve**, and the **lateral cutaneous nerve of the thigh** lie behind the iliac fascia and descend posterior to the lateral half of the ligament which is fused with the transversalis and iliac fasciae. Medially these fasciae pass downwards behind the ligament to form a sheath (the **femoral sheath** [Fig. 109]) for the femoral vessels which, as the external iliac vessels, lie within the fascial lining of the abdomen. Not all the sheath is filled by the femoral vessels; its medial part (the **femoral canal**), which allows for distention of the femoral vein on exercise, is filled with fat, some lymph vessels, and an occasional lymph node.

Towards the pubic tubercle, the deep fibres of the inguinal ligament curve horizontally backwards (the **lacunar ligament**) to the medial part of the pecten pubis and continue along it to the iliopubic eminence (the **pectineal ligament**). The sharp lateral edge of the lacunar ligament lies hard against the femoral canal which is the site of production of a **femoral hernia**. In this condition, the peritoneum overlying the abdominal end of the femoral canal is forced through it into the proximal part of the thigh [p. 95]. This forms the hernial sac which may contain any mobile part of the abdominal contents. The deep fascia which overlies the canal in the proximal part of the thigh is the thin **cribriform fascia** pierced by the great saphenous vein [Fig. 113]. Thus any protrusion of the abdominal contents along the femoral canal bulges forwards distal to the inguinal ligament. Such a hernial sac passes through the constricting ring formed by the inguinal, lacunar, and pectineal ligaments. The pressure of this ring on the contents may be sufficient either to obstruct a loop of small intestine in the sac, or even to cut off its blood supply so that it becomes gangrenous, and rupturing. infects the sac. Both conditions are surgical emergencies. Relief of the obstruction is usually achieved by dividing the lacunar ligament, but this may injure an **abnormal obturator artery** [p. 103] and lead to severe haemorrhage unless care is taken. The possibility of femoral hernia is greater in women than in men because of the wider pelvis in the female and the greater space posterior to the inguinal ligament.

Inguinal canal

This is an intermuscular passage parallel with and immediately superior to the medial half of the inguinal ligament. It is the canal through which the **testis** descends from within the fascial lining of the abdomen to the scrotum. The canal therefore contains the duct (ductus deferens), the blood and lymph vessels, and the nerves of the testis. Together these constitute the **spermatic cord**.

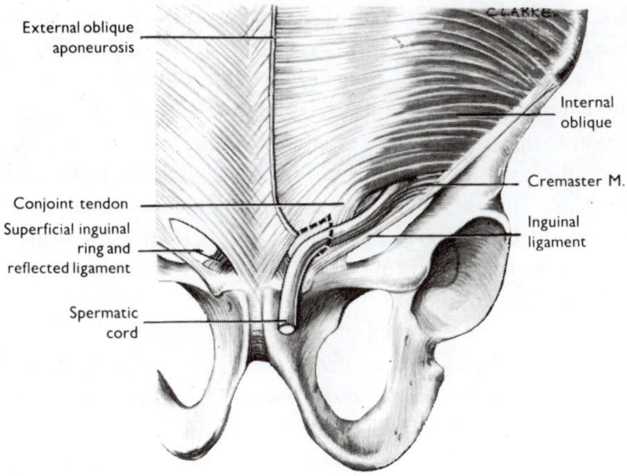

Fig. 111. A diagram of the inguinal canal to show the conjoint tendon and the internal oblique muscle. Note that the internal oblique muscle arches over the spermatic cord and sends fibres (cremaster muscle) on to it.

Fig. 112. A deep dissection of the inguinal region. Parts of the internal and external oblique muscles have been reflected. The spermatic cord and internal spermatic fascia are cut across.

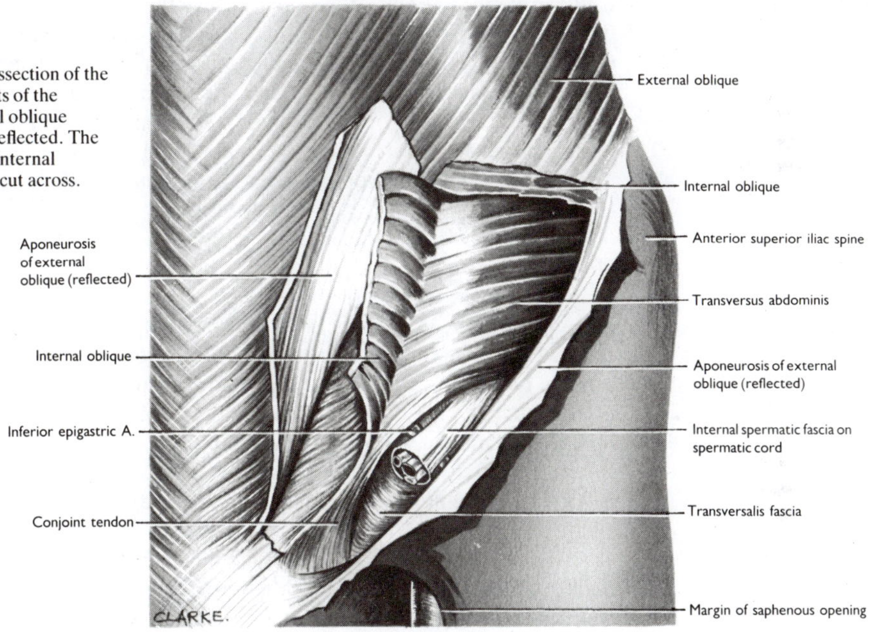

Fig. 113. A diagram of a sagittal section along the external iliac and femoral veins, to show the fasciae and muscles of the inguinal region.

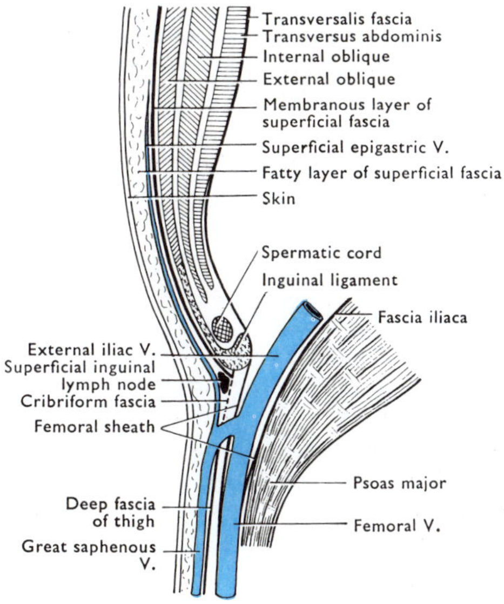

The inguinal canal begins at the **deep inguinal ring**, immediately superior to the inguinal ligament, at the mid-inguinal point [p. 89]. The ring is medial to the attachment of the transversus abdominis to the inguinal ligament and immediately lateral to the **inferior epigastric artery** [Figs. 110, 112; p. 103]. At this point, the descending testis carries the transversalis fascia and the most medial fibres of the internal oblique muscle before it [Fig. 106]. Respectively, these form the internal (**internal spermatic fascia**) and middle (**cremaster muscle** amd **cremasteric fascia**) coverings of the testis and spermatic cord. From the deep inguinal ring, the canal and spermatic cord turn inferomedially and run on the **inguinal** and **lacunar ligaments** (*floor of the canal*) deep to the aponeurosis of the external oblique and, for about 1 cm, deep to the internal oblique also (*anterior wall of the canal*) and superficial to the **transversalis fascia** (*lateral part of the posterior wall of the canal*). The lower margins of the transversus abdominis and internal oblique muscles arch over the deep inguinal ring (*roof of the canal*) and, becoming aponeurotic, fuse to form the **conjoint tendon**. This turns downwards between the transversalis fascia and the canal to be attached to the pubic crest and the pecten pubis at right angles to the lacunar ligament. Thus the conjoint tendon forms a strong *posterior wall for the medial part of the canal* where the anterior wall is weakened by the separation of the fibres of the external oblique to form the **superficial inguinal ring**, the superficial opening of the canal, immediately superolateral to the pubic tubercle [Figs. 104, 111]. The spermatic cord passes through this ring and receives its outer covering (**external spermatic fascia**) from the margins of the ring. Thus the spermatic cord comes to lie anterior to the pubis, deep to the membranous layer of the superficial fascia as it descends to the scrotum.

When the muscles of the anterior abdominal wall contract, the aponeurosis of the external oblique is pulled firmly against the taut conjoint tendon. The contraction of the fibres of the internal oblique and transversus which pass into the conjoint tendon pulls the arched roof of the canal downwards and narrows the deep ring and the canal. Thus the tendency to hernia through the canal is reduced as the intra-abdominal pressure rises.

In the female, the ovary remains intra-abdominal and the inguinal canal is small containing only the round ligament of the uterus, the homologue of the gubernaculum testis in the male [pp. 104, 260]. Hence inguinal hernia is much more common in the male than in the female (see also congenital inguinal hernia below).

The presence of the femoral and inguinal canals on each side at the lowest part of the abdomen means that there is continuous pressure on these canals from the weight of the abdominal contents. Thus the erect posture makes man particularly susceptible to inguinal and femoral hernia. It is obvious that weakness of the abdominal muscles, distention of the abdomen, the presence of a chronic cough, the lifting of heavy weights, or straining to pass urine through a partially obstructed urethra may cause or aggravate a hernia.

Inguinal hernia may be predisposed to by the persistence of the **processus vaginalis**. This is the tube of peritoneum which extends from the abdomen into the scrotum and along which the testis descends [p. 104]. Normally the processus obliterates shortly after birth leaving only that part of it which surrounds the testis (**tunica vaginalis**). When the processus persists, it forms a ready-made hernial sac along which a loop of intestine may pass. This is **congenital inguinal hernia** which traverses the inguinal canal and may enter the tunica vaginalis. It is one type of *oblique hernia*, so-called because it traverses the oblique inguinal canal. The other type arises as a secondary hernial sac passing along the inguinal canal from deep to superficial inguinal rings. *Direct inguinal hernia* usually arises from the weakening of the conjoint tendon with a hernial sac pushing directly through the tendon and distending the superficial inguinal ring. Thus direct inguinal hernias lie medial to the **inferior epigastric artery**, while oblique (indirect) inguinal hernias pass lateral to it.

Umbilical hernia usually occurs as a result of abdominal distention, e.g. by repeated pregnancies. The umbilical scar in the linea alba tends to stretch and thin. Unlike the muscular parts of the abdominal wall it does not return to its normal thickness and may subsequently bulge outwards forming a hernial sac. *In utero*, there is an extension of the peritoneal cavity into the root of the umbilical cord. If this persists, there may be a **congenital umbilical hernia** at birth—a condition which is almost normal in some races. The presence of a peritoneal dimple at the umbilicus, as at the deep inguinal ring, following obliteration of the peritoneal extension, may also facilitate hernia at these points.

Nerves of abdominal wall

These are the ventral rami of the lower six **thoracic nerves** and the **first lumbar nerve** (iliohypogastric and ilioinguinal).

The lower five intercostal nerves leave the intercostal spaces between the slips of transversus abdominis arising from the internal surfaces of the costal cartilages, and pass, either directly (eleventh) or deep to the upturned end of the costal cartilages, between the transversus and the internal oblique. Here they run antero-inferiorly into the rectus sheath. They supply and pierce rectus, and emerge through the anterior wall of the sheath as anterior cutaneous branches. These nerves, with the subcostal, iliohypogastric and ilioinguinal nerves supply the muscles of the abdominal wall. The last three pierce the transversus abdominis posteriorly to enter the same layer as the others, but differ from them in that: (1) The **lateral cutaneous branches** of the **subcostal** and **iliohypogastric nerves** pierce the oblique muscles close to the iliac crest and descend over it to the gluteal skin. (2) The iliohypogastric nerve pierces the internal oblique close to the anterior superior iliac spine [Fig. 107] and becomes cutaneous by piercing the external oblique 2–3 cm superior to the superficial inguinal ring. (3) The **ilioinguinal nerve** has no lateral cutaneous branch. It accompanies the spermatic cord or round ligament through the superficial inguinal ring to supply skin on the front of the thigh and the anterior parts of the external genitalia. Although these nerves run an oblique course, the lateral cutaneous branches descend to such an extent that the parts of each dermatome which they supply are much more horizontal than the ventral rami from which these branches arise.

Arteries of anterior abdominal wall

Most of the skin of the lower anterior abdominal wall is supplied by superficial branches of the femoral artery [p. 93].

From internal thoracic artery

1. The **superior epigastric artery** enters the rectus sheath deep to the seventh costal cartilage. It lies deep to rectus abdominis, supplies that muscle, and sends branches through it to the overlying skin. Small branches may enter the falciform ligament and anastomose with the hepatic artery, but its main anastomosis is with the inferior epigastric artery.

2. The **musculophrenic artery** runs along the upper surface of the costal origin of the diaphragm to the eighth intercostal space. It gives branches to the diaphragm and anterior abdominal wall.

From external iliac artery

1. The **inferior epigastric artery** arises immediately superior to the inguinal ligament at the mid-inguinal point. It ascends towards the umbilicus in the extraperitoneal tissue. At the lateral border of rectus abdominis it pierces the transversalis fascia and passes on the deep surface of the muscle to anastomose with the superior epigastric artery, supply the muscle, and send branches to the overlying skin.

Branches

(a) The **pubic branch** runs inferomedially on the inguinal ligament. It crosses the lacunar ligament and anastomoses with the **pubic branch** of the **obturator artery** on the posterosuperior surface of the body of the pubis [Fig. 110]. This small branch may replace the proximal part of the obturator artery (**abnormal obturator artery**). It is then greatly enlarged and may be damaged in surgical division of the lacunar ligament.

(b) As the inferior epigastric artery passes medial to the deep inguinal ring, it supplies the small **cremasteric artery** to the cremaster muscle. This may anastomose with the testicular artery near the testis. In the female there is a smaller artery of the round ligament.

2. The **deep circumflex iliac artery** arises close to the inferior epigastric

artery. It passes to the anterior superior iliac spine deep to the inguinal ligament, giving an ascending branch between the transversus and internal oblique muscles. Then coursing deep to the iliac crest, it pierces transversus abdominis about the middle of the crest, and branches in the abdominal wall deep to the internal oblique muscle.

The male external genital organs

These are the penis, the scrotum and its contents, and the spermatic cords. For development, see p. 263.

Scrotum

This pendulous sac of dark coloured, rugose skin contains the testes, their associated ducts, and the lower parts of the spermatic cords, all in their coverings. In the median plane there is a ridge or raphe which indicates the embryological line of fusion of the two halves of the scrotum.

The superficial fascia has no fat, is reddish in colour, and contains a layer of involuntary muscle (**dartos**) which decreases the surface area of the scrotum by its contraction. This helps to regulate the loss of heat through the thin, fat-free skin and so control the temperature of the testes—an essential prerequisite for normal spermatogenesis. The dartos layer also forms an incomplete **septum** between the testes, each of which is separately covered by external spermatic fascia, cremasteric fascia (and muscle), and internal spermatic fascia. Here these layers are fused together and difficult to differentiate except by the presence of loops of cremaster muscle. In addition each testis is invaginated into the posterior wall of a serous sac (**tunica vaginalis testis**). In the fetus, this is the distal end of a tubular extension of the peritoneal cavity (processus vaginalis [Fig. 115]) which passes through the inguinal canal into the corresponding half of the scrotum.

The precise mechanism of *descent of the testis* is unknown. However, a fibromuscular band (**gubernaculum testis**) extends from the caudal pole of each developing testis down the posterior abdominal wall immediately posterior to the peritoneum, and passes through the inguinal canal to the scrotum. As the gubernaculum shortens relative to the growing fetus, the peritoneum on its anterior aspect is drawn through the inguinal canal to the scrotum (**processus vaginalis**) and the testis descends on the posterior wall of the abdomen and processus. Subsequently the cavity of the part of the processus within the spermatic cord is obliterated, and the processus reduced to a fibrous thread or lost. Occasionally parts of the processus vaginalis may remain patent. Such isolated cavities can become swollen with fluid and form hydroceles of the spermatic cord [see also p. 108].

The descent of the testis may be arrested at any stage, e.g. in the abdomen, in the inguinal canal, or in the groin. Such undescended testes usually do not produce spermatozoa and are more commonly the site of cancers than the normally placed testis.

Dissection

Beginning at the superficial ring, make a longitudinal incision downwards through the skin of the anterolateral aspect of the scrotum. Carefully reflect the skin from the dartos which is attached to it. Reflect the dartos layer from the layer of loose areolar tissue (external spermatic fascia) deep to it. Towards the median plane, the dartos layer extends superiorly between the testes [Fig. 114]. Complete the separation through the layer of areolar tissue to the superficial inguinal ring. Lift the testis and spermatic cord from the scrotum.

Carefully lift the peritoneum away from the extraperitoneal tissue at the deep inguinal ring by blunt dissection. A fine thread, representing the remnants of the processus vaginalis, may be seen passing from the peritoneum into the beginning of the spermatic cord.

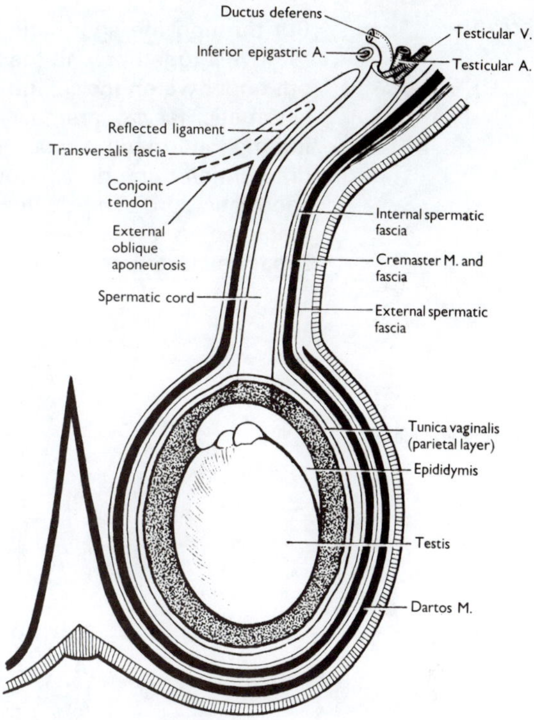

Fig. 114. A diagram of a coronal section through the spermatic cord and scrotum.

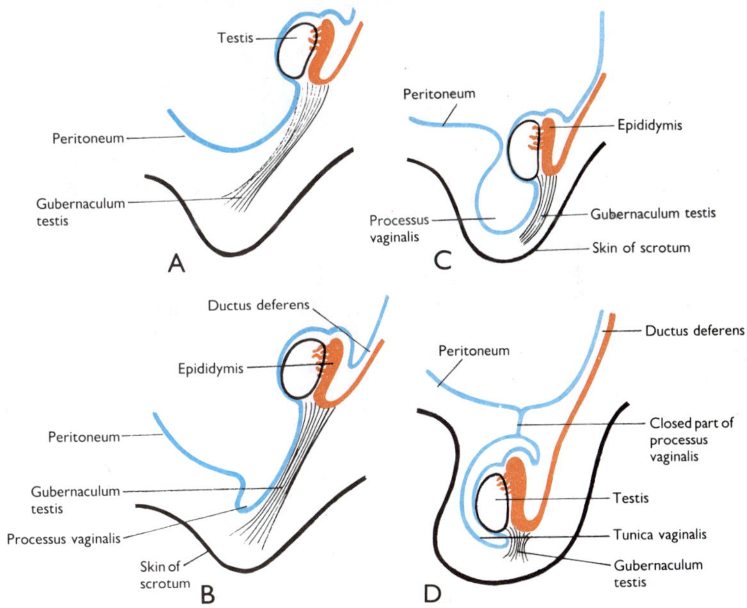

Fig. 115. Diagrams to illustrate the descent of the testis and the formation of the tunica vaginalis.

Spermatic cord

This bundle of structures passes to and from the testis. It is wrapped in three concentric layers of fascia derived from the layers of the anterior abdominal wall [p. 102]. It begins at the deep inguinal ring and ends at the superior pole of the testis [Figs. 290, 291].

Structures in spermatic cord

1. The ductus deferens, the duct of the testis.

2. Blood vessels
   - Arteries: of ductus deferens; Testicular
   - Veins: Pampiniform plexus

The cremasteric artery is in the sheath of the spermatic cord.

3. Lymph vessels which drain the testis and immediately associated structures, but *not the scrotal wall*.

4. Nerves. Sympathetic filaments on the arteries and pelvic autonomic fibres on the ductus deferens.

Dissection

Cut through the spermatic cord at the superficial inguinal ring and remove it together with the testis to a tray on which it may be pinned out under water. Incise and reflect the *coverings,* remains of external spermatic fascia, cremaster muscle and cremasteric fascia, and internal spermatic fascia. Begin superiorly for the layers cannot be differentiated inferiorly. Now separate the various structures in the spermatic cord. The ductus deferens and the blood vessels can be identified, but the nerves and lymph vessels are not visible as separate structures.

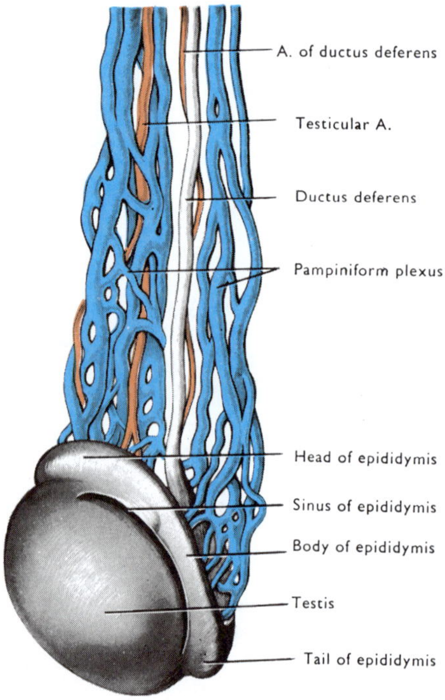

Fig. 116. A dissection of the left spermatic cord.

Ductus deferens

This is the thick-walled muscular part of the duct system of the testis. Spermatozoa are stored in and transported through it to the urethra. It is firm and readily palpable in the living. The thick muscular wall is responsible for the sudden discharge of mature spermatozoa from it. The first part of the ductus is convoluted and is continuous with the lower pole of the **epididymis** [Figs. 119, 120]. It ascends along the medial aspect of the epididymis, posterior to the testis, and runs in the posterior part of the spermatic cord to the deep inguinal ring. Here it hooks round the lateral side of the inferior epigastric artery, and leaving the other structures of the spermatic cord, arches inferomedially into the pelvis. It is accompanied by the **artery of the ductus deferens** [p. 222] which anastomoses with the testicular artery at the testis.

Testicular artery

This vessel arises on each side from the front of the abdominal aorta at the level of the second lumbar vertebra (level of origin of the testis). It descends on the posterior abdominal wall to the deep inguinal ring, enters the spermatic cord, and runs through it to the posterior border of the testis. Small branches enter the posterior border of the testis, while larger branches pass forwards on both sides of the testis and form a vascular layer deep to the dense layer of fibrous tissue (**tunica albuginea**) which encloses the testis [Fig. 117].

Veins

Numerous veins leave the posterior border of the testis to form the extensive **pampiniform plexus** [Fig. 119] which makes up a large part of the spermatic cord. At or near the deep inguinal ring, the plexus is replaced by the testicular vein. This ascends over the posterior abdominal wall to end either in the renal vein (left side) or in the inferior vena cava (right side) at the same level. The functions of the pampiniform plexus are not known. It probably

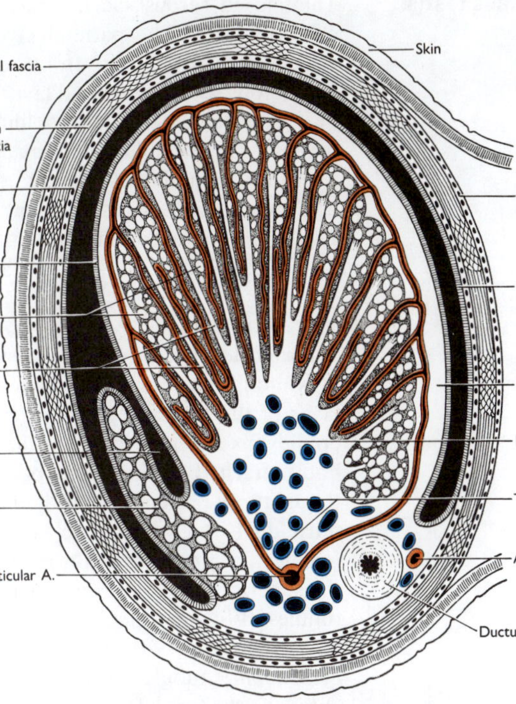

Fig. 117. A diagrammatic horizontal section through the left half of the scrotum and left testis. The cavity of the tunica vaginalis (black) is distended to make it obvious.

maintains the temperature of the ductus at a similar level to that of the testis and may cool the blood in the testicular artery. The venous channels of the plexus may be greatly distended to produce a varicocele of the spermatic cord.

Lymph vessels

The testicular lymph vessels, but *not those of the scrotum*, ascend through the spermatic cord. They pass over the posterior abdominal wall and enter the **lumbar lymph nodes** at the side of the aorta from its bifurcation to the level of the renal veins [Fig. 200].

Nerves

Sympathetic nerves run with the testicular artery from the renal or aortic plexuses. Small ganglia may be found along the artery. Sympathetic and parasympathetic nerve fibres run on the ductus deferens (deferential plexus) from the inferior hypogastric plexus in the pelvis.

Dissection

With a hypodermic syringe and needle or a blowpipe, force some air or water into the tunica vaginalis of the testis through the anterior wall. This demonstrates the extent of the cavity which extends upwards in front of the lower part of the spermatic cord [Fig. 118]. Open the cavity through its anterior wall.

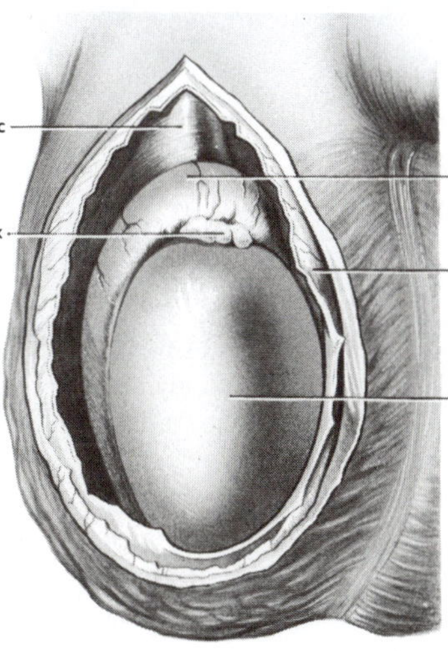

Fig. 118. The right testis and epididymis exposed by removal of the anterior wall of the scrotum and tunica vaginalis.

Tunica vaginalis testis

This closed serous sac has the testis and epididymis invaginated into its posterior wall. The parietal layer lines the internal spermatic fascia; the visceral layer covers the front and sides of the testis and epididymis and is continuous with the parietal layer near the posterior border of the testis [Fig. 117]. Normally there is only a film of fluid between the two layers. In certain pathological conditions the space may be distended with fluid to form a hydrocele. On the lateral side, the visceral layer is tucked between the epididymis and testis to form the slit-like **sinus of the epididymis** [Figs. 116, 117]. Rarely it is continuous with the peritoneal cavity through a persistent processus vaginalis in the spermatic cord.

Testis

This oval body is variable in size—approximately 4 cm long, 2.5 cm anteroposteriorly, and 2 cm transversely. It is enclosed in a thick, dense layer of white fibrous tissue, the **tunica albuginea**. This is covered by the visceral layer of the **tunica vaginalis** except where it is directly in contact with the epididymis superiorly and posteriorly. The **appendix testis** is a small, sessile body attached to the upper part of the anterior border of the testis. It is thought to be a remnant of the proximal end of the embryonic **paramesonephric duct** which forms the fimbriated extremity of the uterine tube in the female. The **appendix of the epididymis** is a small, pedunculated structure on the superior pole of the epididymis. It represents the degenerated remains of tubules of the mesonephros of the embryo cephalic to those which form the **efferent ductules of the testis** [Fig. 120]. Caudal to the efferent ductules, other mesonephric tubules may persist. These form small **aberrant ductules** which enter the ductus deferens at the tail of the epididymis.

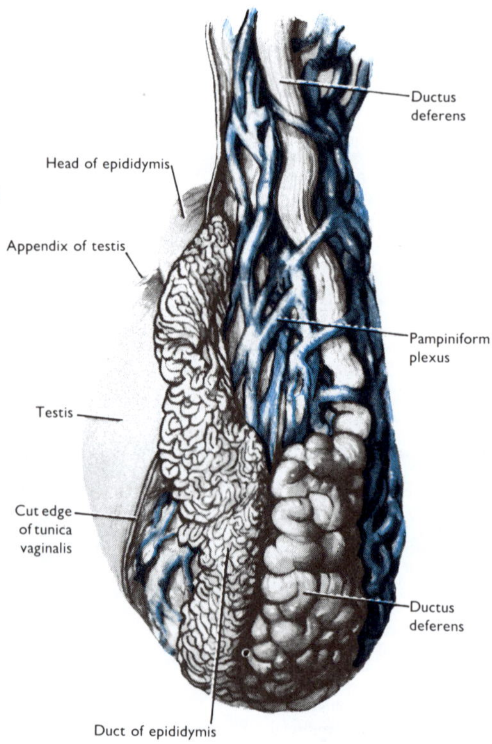

Fig. 119. The left testis, epididymis, and lower part of spermatic cord seen from behind

Epididymis

This comma-shaped structure overlies the superior and posterolateral surfaces of the testis. The superior and inferior extremities are the **head** and **tail** respectively. The intermediate part, partly separated from the testis by the sinus of the epididymis, is the **body**.

The epididymis consists almost entirely of the single, complexly convoluted **duct of the epididymis**. This duct is continuous with the ductus deferens at the tail of the epididymis [Fig. 120].

Structure of testis

The testis is enclosed in the thick, fibrous **tunica albuginea** which projects forwards into the posterior border of the testis forming a longitudinal thickened ridge (the **mediastinum testis** [Fig. 117]). The mediastinum is

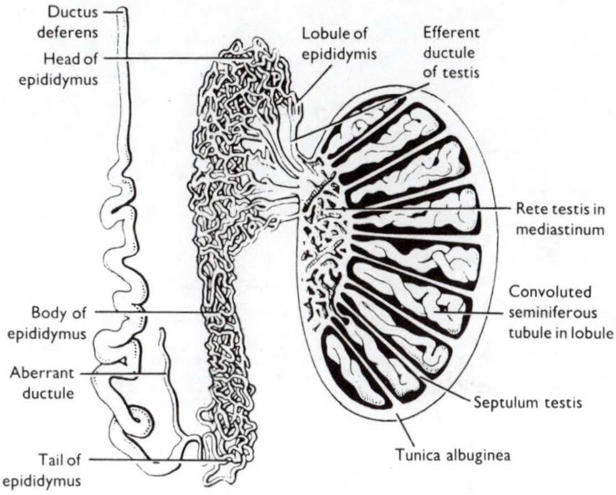

Fig. 120. A diagram of a sagittal section of the testis, epididymis, and ductus deferens.

transversed by the blood and lymph vessels of the testis and by a communicating network of seminal channels, the **rete testis**.

Fibrous strands pass radially from the mediastinum to the tunica albuginea. These are the incomplete **septula** which divide the testis into two or three hundred lobules. The lobules contain the **convoluted seminiferous tubules** which are lined with a thick, multi-layered germinal epithelium that produces immature spermatozoa. The convoluted tubules appear as fine, highly plicated, thread-like loops which join each other and become straighter as they pass towards the mediastinum. These **straight seminiferous tubules** do not produce spermatozoa, but discharge into the spaces of the rete testis which are lined by cubical epithelium. Each lobule contains two to four convoluted tubules. These measure approximately 60 cm in length. Thus the overall length of seminiferous tubules is approximately 500 m. Groups of **interstitial cells** which are responsible for secreting male sex hormones lie in delicate areolar tissue between the convoluted tubules.

Structure of epididymis

Fifteen to 20 delicate **efferent ductules** pass from the rete testis to the epididymis. In this structure they become spirally coiled to form the conical **lobules of the epididymis**. These unite in the head with the **duct of the epididymis** which is approximately 6–7 m long. This duct is lined by tall columnar epithelial cells which have long, non-motile processes (**stereocilia**). The spermatozoa go through the latter part of their maturation as they travel slowly along the duct.

Dissection

Trace the blood vessels into the testis, then free the tail and body of the epididymis from it. Make a transverse cut through the testis, and examine its structure with a hand lens. Attempt to unravel some of the tubules on the cut surface of the testis by drawing them out with a needle under water. Only a general idea of the arrangement can be obtained by this method. With the aid of a stream of water and gentle agitation with the needle, remove the tubules from part of the testis and uncover the fibrous septula.

At the superior pole of the testis, divide the tunica vaginalis which joins it to the head of the epididymis. Separate the testis and epididymis by gentle blunt dissection. This may demonstrate the efferent ductules passing from the rete testis to the head of the epididymis. Make an attempt to unravel at least part of the duct of the epididymis.

Penis

[Figs. 121–123; Vol. 1: Figs. 160, 161]

The penis is described as if erect. It consists of three parallel, cylindrical bodies. (1) The two dorsally placed **corpora cavernosa** which are fused together in the body of the penis, but diverge in the perineum to form the **crura** of the penis which are attached to the sides of the pubic arch. (2) The **corpus spongiosum** lies on the ventral (urethral) surface between the corpora cavernosa. It transmits the **urethra** and enlarges proximally to form the **bulb of the penis**. Here it is attached between the crura to the inferior surface of

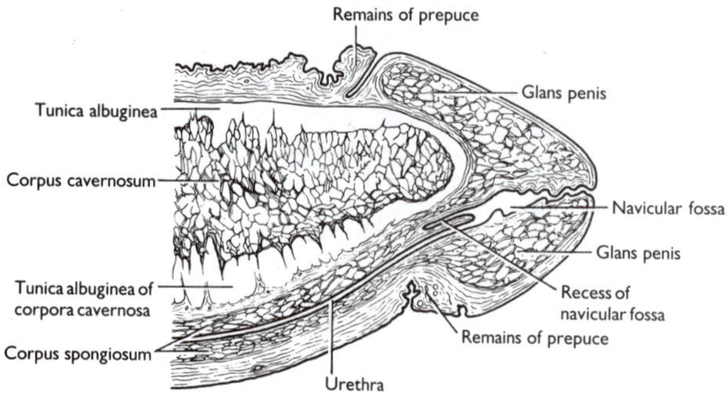

Fig. 121. A median section through the terminal part of a circumcised penis.

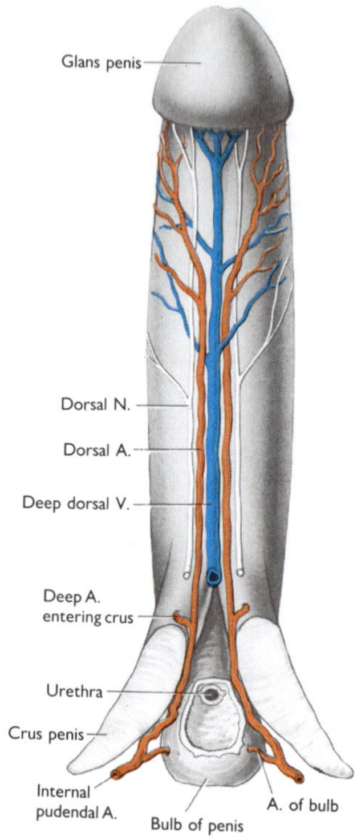

Fig. 122. A dissection of the dorsal surface of the penis.

the urogenital diaphragm (perineal membrane). Distally it expands to form the **glans penis** into which the tapered ends of the corpora cavernosa are inserted. The urethra traverses the glans and opens through its extremity as a vertical slit, the external urethral orifice. The glans penis is shaped like a helmet and is much more extensive on the dorsal and lateral surfaces than on the urethral surface. The projecting margin of its base is the **corona glandis**.

The skin of the penis is delicate, elastic, and hairless except at the base. It is freely movable over the surface of the penis, and distally forms a tubular fold (the **prepuce** [Figs. 121, 235]) which extends over the glans for a variable distance. The skin turns inwards at the distal end of the prepuce and lines its deep surface, becoming continuous, just proximal to the corona (**neck of the glans**) with the skin which encloses the glans and is firmly bound to its surface. In the midline, a narrow, free fold of skin (**frenulum of the prepuce**) passes from the urethral surface to the deep aspect of the prepuce. The greater part of the prepuce is removed in the operation of circumcision [Fig. 121].

The superficial fascia of the penis is composed of loose areolar tissue without fat. The deep fascia forms a close-fitting sheath around the corpora.

Dissection

Cut through and reflect the skin along the dorsum of the penis from the symphysis pubis to the end of the prepuce. Find the extension of the membranous layer of the superficial fascia of the abdominal wall on to the penis (**fundiform ligament**). The superficial dorsal vein of the penis lies in the superficial fascia. Trace it proximally towards the superficial veins of the thighs. Deep to this vein is the deep fascia and suspensory ligament of the penis. Divide the deep fascia in the same line as the skin incision. Reflect it to uncover the deep dorsal vein with the dorsal arteries and nerves on each side of it [Fig. 122].

The suspensory ligament is a fibro-elastic structure which spreads out from the anterior surface of the pubic symphysis to fuse with the deep fascia on the dorsum and sides of the penis. The dorsal vessels and nerves lie deep to it.

Dorsal vessels and nerves of penis

The superficial and deep dorsal veins are both median structures. The superficial vein lies in the superficial fascia and divides proximally into right and left branches which pass to the external pudendal veins of the corresponding thigh. The **deep dorsal vein** lies deep to the deep fascia. It drains to the prostatic plexus of veins by passing below the pubic symphysis into the pelvis. The vein has a thick muscular wall close to the pubis.

The two dorsal arteries and nerves are the terminal branches of the internal pudendal arteries and the pudendal nerves. The nerves are lateral to the arteries, and both supply skin and the glans of the penis.

Dissection

Make a transverse section through the body of the penis, but leave the two parts connected by the skin of the urethral surface. Examine the cut surface.

Structure of penis

The **corpora cavernosa** are a pair of cylindrical bodies each consisting of a mass of cavernous **erectile tissue** enclosed in a dense sheath of white fibrous tissue, the **tunica albuginea**. Medially the tunicae albugineae fuse to form an incomplete median **septum** through which the cavernous tissue of the two corpora is continuous. A **deep artery** of the penis lies near the centre of each corpus cavernosum. When these arteries are dilated, the cavernous spaces are inflated with blood under pressure turning the corpora cavernosa and the dense tunicae albugineae into a rigid structure.

The **corpus spongiosum** has a finer mesh of erectile tissue and a more delicate fibrous capsule (tunica albuginea). Thus it does not prevent distention of the urethra when the cavernous tissue is filled with blood. The **arteries of the bulb** [Fig. 122] traverse the corpus spongiosum inferior to the urethra. Thus each part of the penis has a separate blood supply.

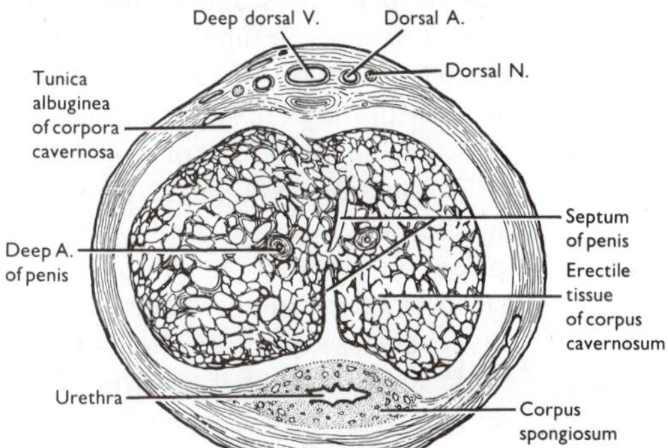

Fig. 123. A transverse section through the body of the penis.

The dissection of the loin

Dissection

With the body in the prone position, follow the inferior part of latissimus dorsi to the iliac crest and expose the free, posterior border of the external oblique muscle. Note the interval between these muscles (**lumbar triangle**) immediately superior to the iliac crest [Fig. 124: Fig. 28 Vol. 1]. Reflect the remains of latissimus dorsi inferiorly and those of the external oblique anteriorly. This exposes the posterior part of the internal oblique and the thoracolumbar fascia to which it is attached.

Thoracolumbar fascia

This fascia extends from the sacrum to the neck. It binds the long extensor muscle of the vertebral column (**erector spinae**) to the posterolateral surfaces of the vertebral bodies, and encloses the quadratus lumborum in the lumbar region.

In the *lumbar region*, the fascia is very strong. Laterally it gives origin to the internal oblique and transversus abdominis muscles [Fig. 124]. Medially it splits into three layers.

The **posterior layer** passes behind the erector spinae muscle and is attached to the tips of the spines of the lumbar vertebrae. It is this layer which extends superiorly into the thoracic and cervical regions and downwards into the

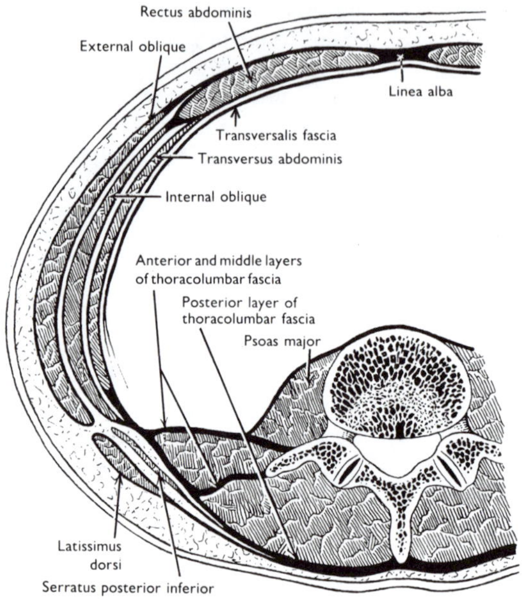

Fig. 124. A horizontal section through the abdominal walls at the level of the second lumbar vertebra, to show the thoracolumbar fascia.

sacral region. In the *thoracic region* it forms a thinner, transparent lamina attached to the spines of the thoracic vertebrae and the angles of the ribs. It lies deep to the scapular muscles (trapezius and rhomboids) and serratus posterior superior, and extends into the cervical region. In the *sacral region* it stretches from the sacral spines to the ilium and sacrotuberous ligaments, and fuses with the periosteum on the back of the sacrum and coccyx inferior to the attachment of erector spinae to the sacrum.

The **middle layer** passes medially between erector spinae and quadrat lumborum to the tips of the lumbar transverse processes. The **anterior layer** passes in front of quadratus lumborum and is attached to the anterior surfaces of the lumbar transverse processes. Thus the anterior and middle layers enclose **quadratus lumborum**. This muscle is attached to the anterior surfaces of the lumbar transverse processes and extends from the twelfth rib superiorly to the iliolumbar ligament and iliac crest [Fig. 105] inferiorly. Thus the middle and anterior layers end superiorly and inferiorly by being attached to the same structures as quadratus lumborum, respectively posterior and anterior to it.

The anterior layer is thin but strong. It has a thickened tendinous strip (**lateral arcuate ligament**) from which the fibres of the diaphragm, which are anterior to quadratus lumborum, arise. This ligament extends from the transverse process of the first lumbar vertebra to the twelfth rib lateral to the attachment of quadratus lumborum. The subcostal vessels and nerve pass from the thorax into the posterior abdominal wall posterior to the ligament.

Dissection

Remove the remains of latissimus dorsi and detach serratus posterior inferior from the posterior layer of the thoracolumbar fascia to expose the posterior layer. Cut vertically through this layer from the level of the last rib to the iliac crest and make transverse cuts through it at the upper and lower ends. Reflect the layer and expose erector spinae. Pull this muscle medially and follow the middle layer anterior to it. When the attachments of this layer have been defined, cut through it along its superior, medial, and inferior attachments and reflect it laterally.

Push quadratus lumborum medially and run your finger over the posterior surface of the anterior layer. This layer may also be divided to expose the lower part of the kidney and the subcostal, iliohypogastric, and ilioinguinal nerves passing posterior to it. It is better to leave the layer intact at this stage and see these structures from in front later in the dissection.

The abdominal cavity

The abdominal cavity is enclosed by the abdominal walls and is completely filled by the abdominal viscera. These are the stomach and intestines, their associated glands (liver and pancreas with their ducts), blood and lymph vessels, the spleen, kidneys, and suprarenal glands. The kidneys, their ducts (the ureters), and the suprarenal glands lie on the posterior abdominal wall enclosed in the fascial lining of the abdominal cavity [p. 95]. The other structures lie anterior to this and are surrounded to a greater or lesser extent by the peritoneal cavity.

The **peritoneum** is a tough layer of elastic areolar tissue lined with simple squamous epithelium. It forms the largest of the serous sacs of the body, but is similar to the pleura and pericardium in consisting of **parietal** and **visceral layers** which are separated from each other by a thin film of fluid in the peritoneal cavity. This fluid lubricates the smooth peritoneal surfaces and facilitates the movement of those parts of the abdominal viscera which are ensheathed by the visceral layer. The most mobile parts of the intra-abdominal gut tube are surrounded by visceral peritoneum except for a narrow strip where (like a cloth draped over a tube) it passes from the gut tube to the posterior abdominal wall as two parallel layers (suspensory folds of peritoneum, **mesentery**, or ligament). Between these layers is a variable amount of extraperitoneal fatty areolar tissue in which blood and lymph vessels and nerves run to and from the gut tube. Where the layers meet the fascial lining of the posterior abdominal wall, they become continuous with the parietal peritoneum, while the areolar tissue between them is continuous with the extraperitoneal tissue of the abdominal walls.

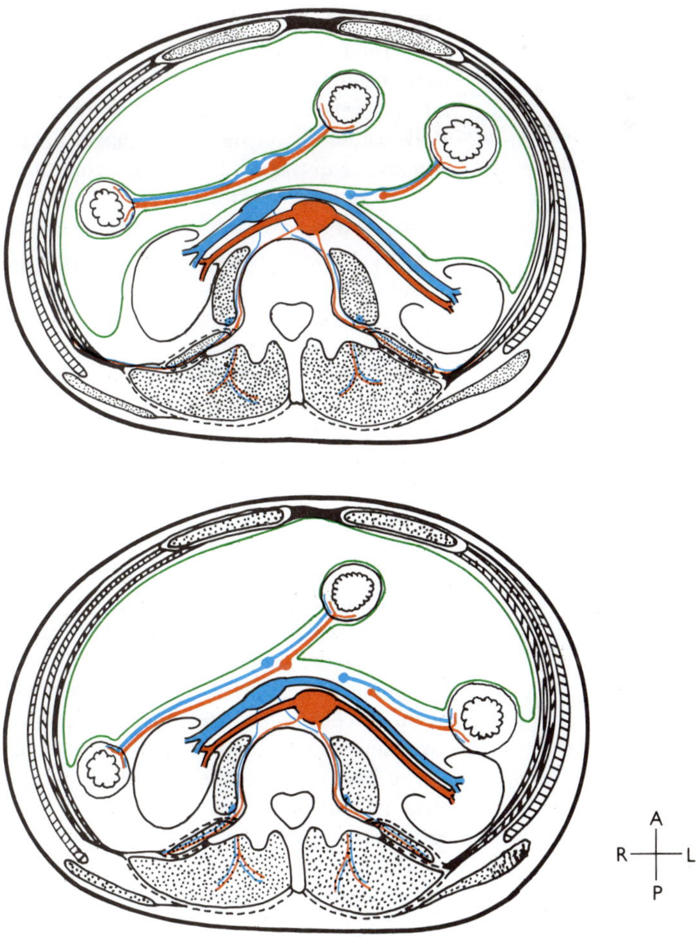

Fig. 125. A diagram to show the effects of adhesion of some mesenteries to the posterior abdominal wall during development. This results in the structures contained in these mesenteries being incorporated in the posterior abdominal wall anterior to those which form or lie on the posterior abdominal wall from the beginning. Thus there are three layers: (1) the posterior abdominal wall proper (muscles, bones, vessels, and nerves); (2) the urogenital apparatus (kidneys and ureters, gonadal vessels) and suprarenals; and (3) the mesenteric structures (vessels, nerves, and lymph nodes) of those organs (omental bursa, duodenum, and ascending and descending colon) which adhere secondarily to the abdominal wall. Within the middle layer, the gonadal vessels are anterior to the ureters [see p. 259]. Green, peritoneum.

Dissection

At this stage, it is important to avoid cutting any structure within the abdomen. Time should be taken to explore the peritoneal cavity without damage to the peritoneum or the structures which it covers.

The **parietal peritoneum** is a simple layer on the internal surface of the abdominal walls. The arrangement of the **visceral peritoneum** is complex. It forms mesenteries which surround the intricately folded and tightly packed gut tube, the liver, and the spleen. The **peritoneal cavity** is the slit-like interval between the parietal and visceral layers of the peritoneum and between the parts of the visceral peritoneum surrounding the separate structures packed together within the abdomen. Since these structures fill the abdomen, the peritoneal cavity has a very small volume, but it may be distended as far as the abdominal walls will allow by the introduction of fluid or air.

In the embryo, all parts of the gut tube have a mesentery. During development certain parts of this tube (duodenum, ascending and descending colon) and its glandular outgrowth, the pancreas, together with their mesenteries are applied to and fused with the peritoneum of the posterior abdominal wall so that the parietal peritoneum comes to run directly over their anterior surface [Fig. 125]. As a result, the blood and lymph vessels and the nerves which originally ran in these mesenteries now lie on the posterior abdominal wall anterior to the paired viscera (suprarenal glands, kidneys, and gonads) and their vessels which lie on the posterior abdominal wall behind the parietal peritoneum.

Thus there are *three distinct layers* of structures posterior to the peritoneal cavity, each with its own blood and lymph vessels and nerves. From behind forwards these are:

1. The **posterior abdominal wall** consisting of the vertebral column and the muscles attached to it [Fig. 124]. It contains the lumbar vessels and nerves.

2. The **kidneys** (and their ducts the **ureters**) and the **suprarenal glands** on each side of the vertebral column, and the great vessels (**abdominal aorta** and **inferior vena cava**) on the anterior surface of the vertebral column [Figs. 138, 199]. These lie on the abdominal wall, enclosed in its fascial lining. The gonads are displaced downwards from this layer, but their blood and lymph vessels and nerves still traverse it as do the paired suprarenal and renal vessels and nerves.

3. The unpaired viscera (**duodenum, pancreas, ascending** and **descending colon**) which are adherent to the posterior wall of the peritoneal cavity. This layer contains the branches of the unpaired vessels to these viscera.

The unpaired viscera which remain free—stomach, jejunum, ileum, transverse and sigmoid colon—do so by retaining the mesenteries which attach them to the posterior abdominal wall (**dorsal mesenteries**). They lie anterior to layer 3 and, like it, are supplied by unpaired visceral vessels.

In addition to the dorsal mesentery which all parts of the free gut tube have, the stomach and proximal 2–3 cm of the duodenum also have a **ventral mesentery** which attaches them to the anterior abdominal wall. The liver develops in this ventral mesentery and so divides it into a part which joins the stomach and proximal duodenum to the liver (**lesser omentum**) and a part which passes from the liver to the anterior abdominal wall (**falciform ligament**)—the only attachment of the abdominal viscera to the anterior abdominal wall. When the anterior abdominal wall is removed, the only parts of the viscera immediately visible are the liver, the free gut tube, and the ascending and descending parts of the colon.

The **cavity of the lesser pelvis** is a curved tube. It begins at the linea terminalis of the pelvis in continuity with the postero-inferior part of the abdominal cavity [Fig. 127]. The short antero-inferior wall consists of the pubic symphysis. The long roof and posterior wall are formed by the curved sacrum and coccyx. The floor is the diamond-shaped **perineum**, a fibromuscular diaphragm between the pubic symphysis and coccyx. This is pierced by the rectum and urethra and by the vagina in the female. The lateral walls are the hip bones covered by the obturator internus muscles. The peritoneal cavity extends into the superior part of the pelvis above the urinary bladder (and uterus in the female) and anterior to the rectum. *In the male* it is a closed sac. *In the female* the uterine tubes open into it and form direct channels to the exterior through the uterus and the vagina.

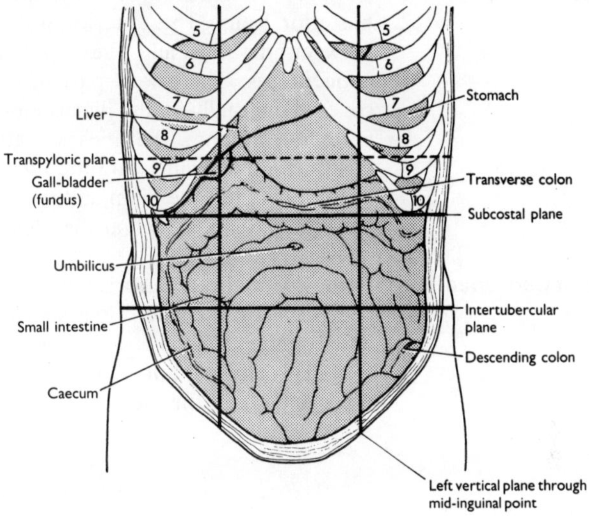

Fig. 126. The abdominal viscera after removal of the anterior abdominal wall and greater omentum. Note that the eighth costal cartilage reaches the sternum in this case.

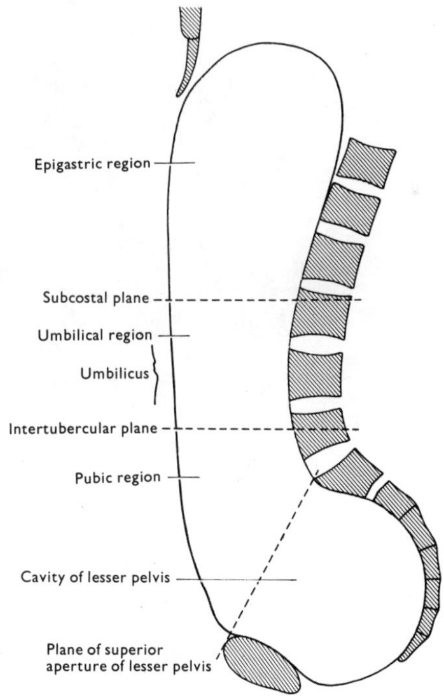

Fig. 127. An outline of the abdominal and pelvic cavities as seen in the median section.

Shape of abdominal cavity

[Figs. 127, 128, 130, 132, 137, 283–291]

In transverse section the abdominal cavity is kidney-shaped because the vertebral column protrudes into it in the midline posteriorly. Thus there is a deep paravertebral groove on each side which is separated from its thoracic counterpart by the diaphragm. Each groove lodges a kidney and a suprarenal gland and the ascending (right) or descending (left) part of the colon. Because of the curvatures of the vertebral column, the upper lumbar vertebrae lie further posteriorly than the lower. The anteroposterior extent of the abdominal cavity is therefore much greater in the superior than the inferior parts, though it is reduced in the uppermost part where the diaphragm arches forwards, anterior to the pleural cavity, above the first lumbar vertebra [Fig. 130]. Thus, in the supine position, the anterior abdominal wall may be less than 5 cm from the great vessels on the anterior surface of the lower lumbar vertebral column. Similarly, the **paravertebral grooves** slope posterosuperiorly from the anterior surface of the lateral part of the sacrum. Consequently, free fluid in the peritoneal cavity gravitates to the upper abdomen when a patient lies flat on his back—the reason for sitting patients up when there is infection in the lower peritoneal cavity, e.g. ruptured appendix.

Boundaries of abdominal cavity

The roof is the diaphragm which also forms the upper parts of the lateral and posterior walls. The anterior wall and a small part of each lateral wall between the ribs and the hip bone are formed by muscles and their aponeuroses. The lowest part of each lateral wall is formed by the ilium covered internally by the iliacus muscle. The posterior wall is formed by the vertebral column, the muscles attached to it (diaphragm, psoas, and quadratus lumborum), and the thoracolumbar fascia, and below this by the posterior part of the ilium and the iliacus muscle covering it which meet the anterior abdominal wall at the inguinal ligament.

Divisions of peritoneal cavity

Removal of the anterior abdominal wall exposes the greater part of the peritoneal cavity. There is a smaller extension of this cavity which passes between the stomach and the posterior abdominal wall [Figs. 128, 130, 136, 137]. This **omental bursa** arises as an extension of the peritoneal cavity into the right side of the mesentery of the stomach. It forms a sac in the dorsal

Fig. 128. A horizontal section through the abdomen at the level of the pylorus. Blue: peritoneal cavity. Red: omental bursa. See also Fig. 286A.

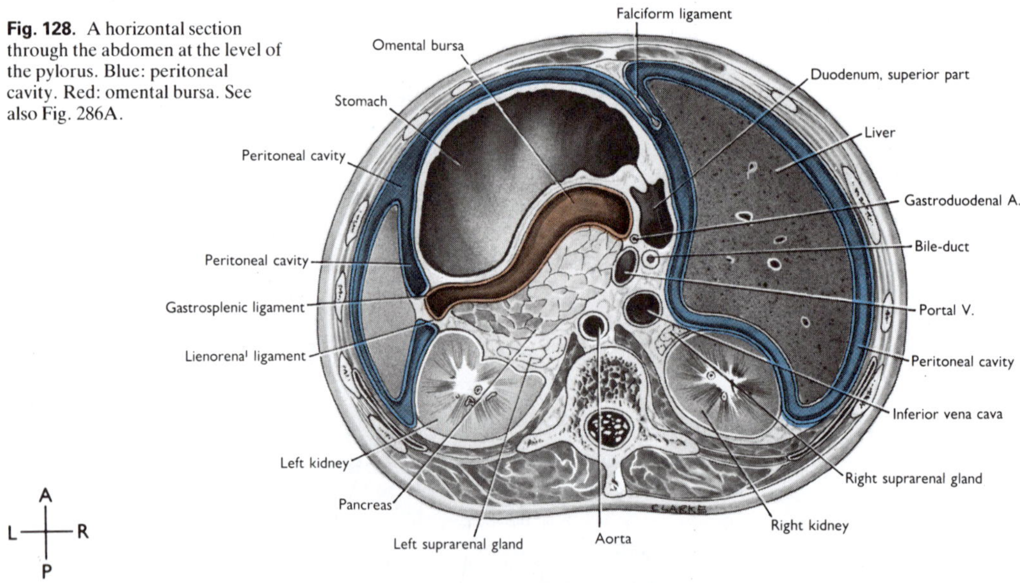

Fig. 129. A diagrammatic horizontal section through the abdomen at the level of the fourth lumbar vertebra. The peritoneal cavity is shown distended. Blue: peritoneal cavity. Red: omental bursa of peritoneal cavity. See also Fig. 288.

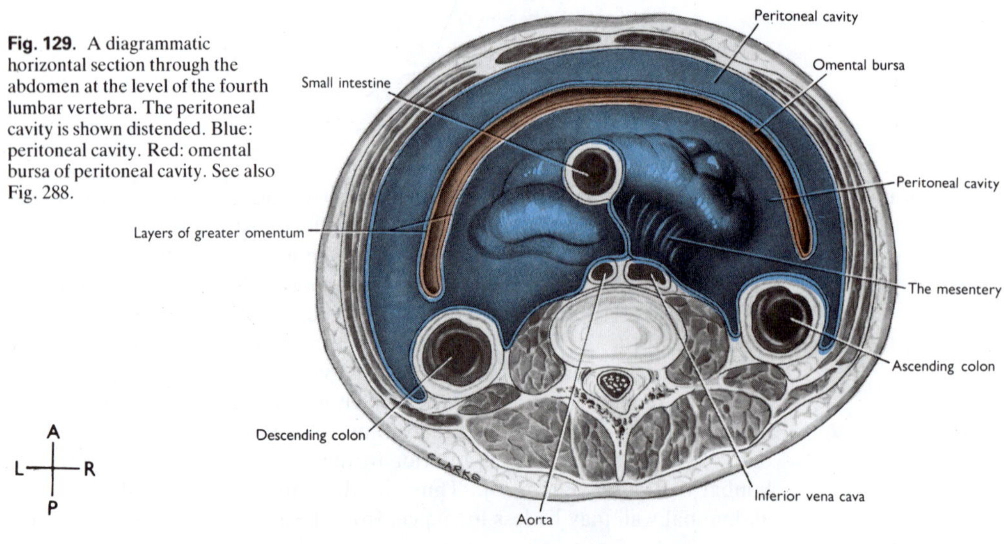

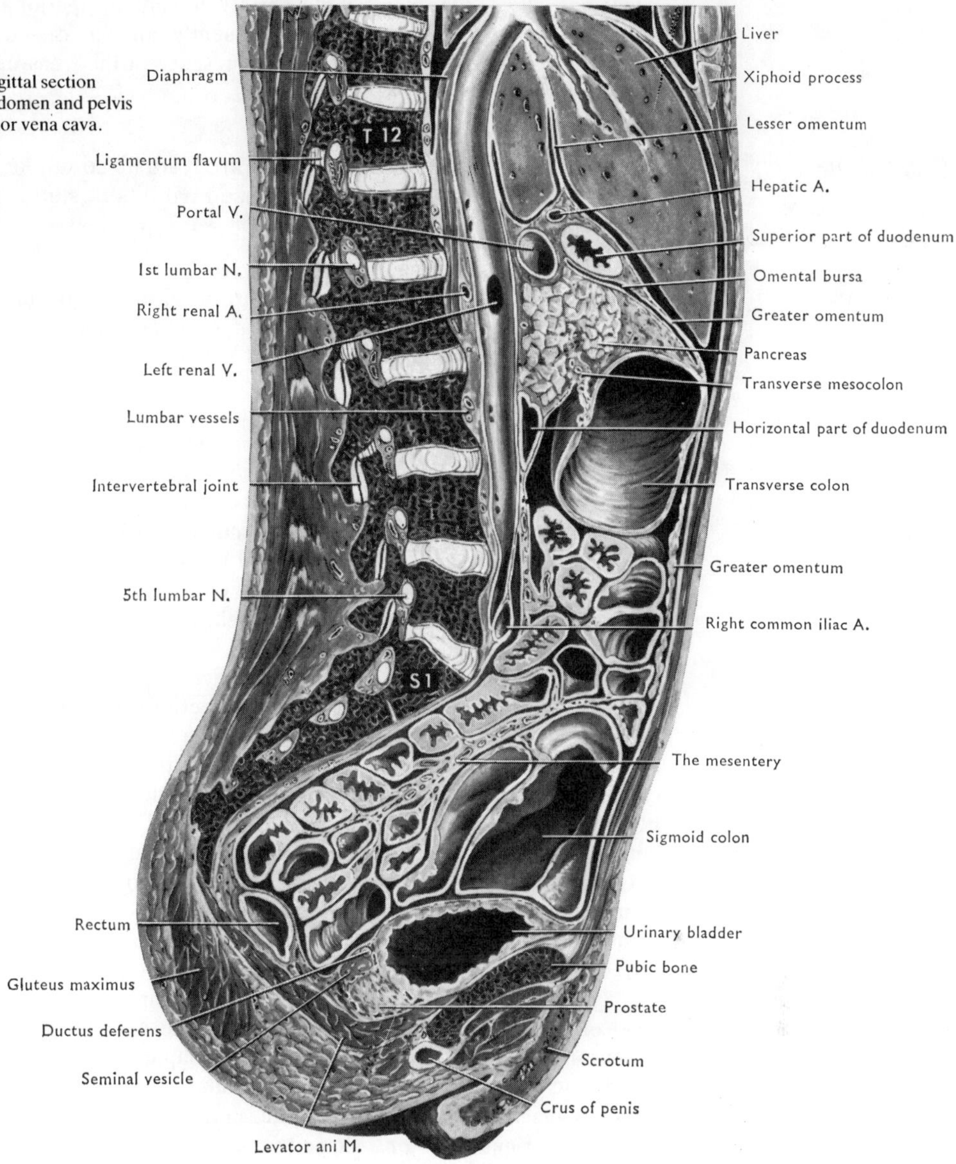

Fig. 130. A sagittal section through the abdomen and pelvis along the inferior vena cava.

mesentery which expands to the left and inferiorly ballooning the mesentery beyond the limits of the stomach [Fig. 135]. Superiorly the wall of the sac is carried to the left against the diaphragm, and the spleen develops as a projection on the left surface of this wall. Thus the spleen is held in position against the diaphragm by the left wall of the omental bursa, the anterior part of which passes from the stomach to the spleen (**gastrosplenic ligament**), while the posterior part passes from the spleen to the posterior abdominal wall in the region of the kidney (**lienorenal ligament** [Fig. 128]). These are simply parts of the dorsal mesentery of the stomach and are not specially strengthened in spite of their names. Superior to the spleen, the dorsal mesentery passes directly from the fundus (superior part) of the stomach to the diaphragm (**gastrophrenic ligament**).

The part of the dorsal mesentery of the stomach which is carried inferiorly by the expanding omental bursa forms a flattened bag of peritoneum (the **greater omentum**) between the parietal peritoneum on the anterior abdominal wall and the anterior surface of the abdominal viscera inferior to the stomach [Figs. 129, 136]. Initially the greater omentum contains part of the cavity of the omental bursa, but the walls fuse and convert it into a simple flap of peritoneum which often contains a considerable quantity of extraperitoneal tissue and fat. The greater omentum overlies the transverse part of the large intestine (**transverse colon**). This, together with its mesentery, fuses with the posterior surface of the greater omentum, thus forming a compound flap which partially divides the peritoneal cavity into anterosuperior and postero-inferior compartments. These are frequently known as supracolic and infracolic compartments because of the presence of the transverse colon in the flap [Fig. 137].

Dissection

Identify and lift up the greater omentum. Note its continuity with the stomach, and the transverse colon fused with its posterior surface a short distance inferior to the stomach.

The **supracolic compartment** of the peritoneal cavity surrounds the liver, stomach, spleen, and the superior part of the duodenum. It lies anterior to the pancreas, duodenum, kidneys, and suprarenal glands. The following brief description gives only the general arrangement of the abdominal viscera which may be examined without dissection. *It is important to confirm the various points on the specimen without damage to the structures which will be dissected later*. The positions given for the various structures are approximate because the abdominal viscera move with respiration, and alter their position with the age and bodily habitus of the individual. The relative position of organs is also changed by distention and movement of the hollow viscera, particularly those which are free to move on a mesentery.

The liver fills the greater part of the right hypochondrium, mainly under cover of the ribs and diaphragm. Most of the liver surface is covered with peritoneum, and it is divided into large right and small left **lobes** by the **falciform ligament** which is attached to its anterior surface to the right of the median plane. The sharp **inferior margin** of the right lobe lies approximately along the costal margin as far anteriorly as the tip of the ninth costal cartilage. Close to this, the rounded fundus of the **gall-bladder** protrudes below the inferior margin of the liver. The right lobe then appears from behind the costal cartilages and almost immediately joins the left lobe between the right and left costal margins. The inferior margin of the left lobe continues in the same direction to the eighth left costal cartilage. Here it turns more steeply upwards to meet the superior surface, posterior to the fifth costal cartilage, close to the fifth rib [Fig. 126]. The superior surface of the **right lobe** fits into the right dome of the diaphragm. Thus it reaches the level of the upper border of the fifth rib in the mid-clavicular line, while posteriorly it lies on the posterior part of the diaphragm, the right suprarenal gland, and the superior part of the right kidney [Fig. 139].

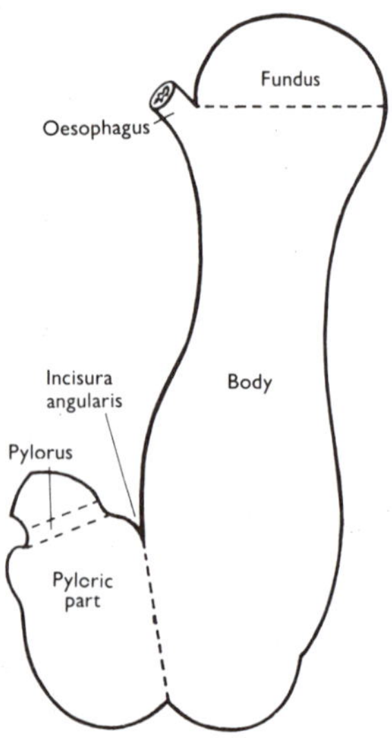

Fig. 131. A diagram of the anterior surface of the stomach to show its parts.

The stomach lies obliquely across the supracolic compartment from upper left to lower right in a J- or C-shaped curve. The greater part is hidden by the liver, diaphragm, and ribs, but part of its anterior surface is in contact with the anterior abdominal wall inferior to the left lobe of the liver. Pass a hand upwards over the anterior surface of the stomach and identify its superior, rounded **fundus** and the **oesophagus** entering the right border inferior to the fundus, immediately posterior to the liver. Lift up the inferior margin of the liver and trace the right, concave border of the stomach (**lesser curvature**) downwards from the entry of the oesophagus till a thickening (**pyloric sphincter**) is felt in the wall of the stomach where it meets the small intestine (superior part of the duodenum). Note a sharp angulation of the lesser curvature (**incisura angularis**) which marks the junction of the body of the stomach with the pyloric part [Fig. 131].

Identify the thin sheet of peritoneum (**lesser omentum**) that passes from the lesser curvature of the stomach to the liver. It is short where the abdominal part of the oesophagus abuts on the liver but lengthens towards the pylorus. The lesser omentum ends in a free edge on the superior part of the duodenum. This thick edge contains the **portal vein**, **proper hepatic artery**, and **bile-duct**, all of which run between the superior part of the duodenum and the small area on the liver (**porta hepatis**) to which the edge is attached superiorly.

Pass a finger to the left, posterior to the free edge of the lesser omentum. The finger passes through the **epiploic foramen** into the **omental bursa** posterior to the lesser omentum and stomach. If the finger is directed upwards as it passes through the foramen, it enters a narrow extension of the omental bursa (the **superior recess** [Fig. 138]) between the liver and the diaphragm. A finger in the thorax pushed inferiorly between the descending aorta and the diaphragm lies immediately posterior to the finger in the superior recess, but separated from it by the diaphragm.

Trace the left, convex border of the stomach from the fundus to the pylorus. The sheet of peritoneum which passes from this curvature is the **dorsal mesentery of the stomach**. Superiorly it passes to the diaphragm (**gastrophrenic ligament**). Inferior to this it extends first to the spleen (**gastrosplenic ligament**) and then forms the **greater omentum**. This ends where the superior part of the duodenum becomes adherent to the posterior abdominal wall.

Pull the upper part of the greater curvature to the right and expose the **spleen** deep in the left hypochondrium, posterior to the stomach and anterior to the upper part of the left kidney. Posterolaterally the spleen lies against the diaphragm which separates it from the pleural cavity [Figs. 283, 284]. Confirm this with a finger in the pleural cavity, and note that the long axis of the spleen lies parallel to the tenth rib, between the ninth and eleventh ribs, posterior to the mid-axillary line. The gastrosplenic and lienorenal ligaments are attached to a narrow strip (**hilus**) on the medial aspect of the spleen which is otherwise completely surrounded by peritoneum [Fig. 128].

Follow the **superior part of the duodenum** posterosuperiorly till it turns abruptly downwards. Continuing vertically as the **descending part**, it is adherent to the adjacent anterior surfaces of the right psoas muscle and kidney. It passes posterior to the attachment of the mesentery of the transverse colon [Fig. 138] and so connects the parts of the intestine in the supracolic and infracolic compartments. The head of the pancreas lies medial to this part of the duodenum.

Infracolic compartment

Turn the greater omentum upwards and find the **transverse colon** adherent to its posterior surface. The colon can be differentiated from the small intestine (1) by the sacculation of its wall between three thickened bands of

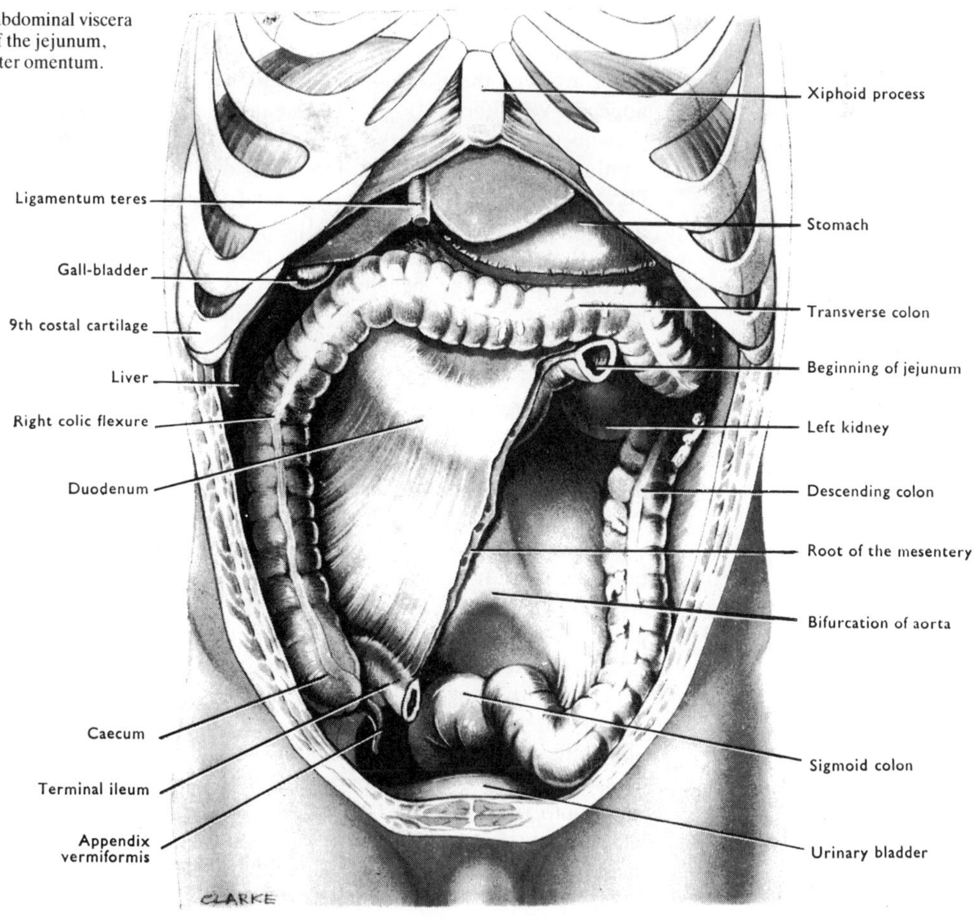

Fig. 132. The abdominal viscera after removal of the jejunum, ileum, and greater omentum.

longitudinal muscle—**taeniae coli** [Fig. 133], and (2) by the small projecting sacs of peritoneum filled with fat—**appendices epiploicae**. Trace the transverse colon and its mesentery in both directions. The **mesentery**, mainly fused with the greater omentum, is attached to the front of the pancreas and descending part of the duodenum [Fig. 138]. The transverse colon is continuous through the right and left **flexures** with the **ascending** and **descending parts of the colon** which are adherent to the posterior abdominal wall in the right and left paravertebral gutters respectively. The parts of these gutters lateral to the colon (**paracolic gutters**) form a route of communication between the infracolic and supracolic compartments [p. 118].

The **right colic flexure** lies anterior to the inferior part of the right kidney, close to the inferior margin of the liver. The **left colic flexure** lies at a much higher level [Fig. 164] in contact with the anterior (colic) surface of the spleen [Fig. 283].

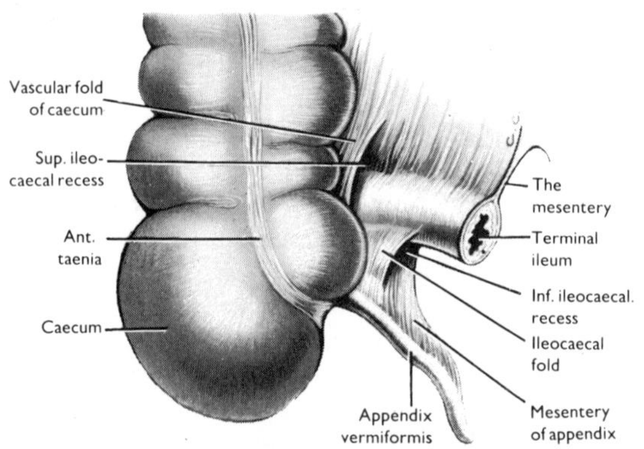

Fig. 133. The anterior surface of the ileocaecal region.

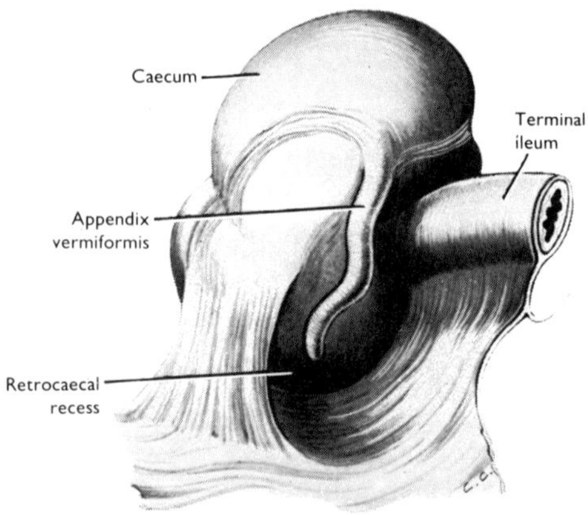

Fig. 134. The inferior surface of the ileocaecal region. The caecum has been turned forwards to open the retrocaecal recess in which the appendix vermiformis commonly lies.

The **caecum** is a blind-ended sac in the right iliac fossa. It is continuous superiorly with the ascending colon and medially with the terminal ileum and **appendix vermiformis** [Fig. 133]. The taeniae coli pass over the surface of the caecum and converge on the base of the appendix vermiformis. Here they are continuous with the uniform longitudinal muscle layer of the appendix. A blind extension of the peritoneal cavity (**retrocaecal recess**) extends upwards posterior to the caecum [Fig. 134].

At the superior aperture of the lesser pelvis, the descending colon is continuous with the **sigmoid colon**. This loops postero-inferiorly into the lesser pelvis to join the **rectum** on the pelvic surface of the third piece of the sacrum. Here the taeniae coli spread out into the more uniform longitudinal muscle layer of the rectum. The short **mesentery of the sigmoid colon** is attached across the margin of the superior aperture of the lesser pelvis [Fig. 138].

The inferior half of the duodenum, the jejunum, and the ileum form the infracolic part of the **small intestine**. This is centrally placed within a frame formed by the caecum and colon. Between the caecum and sigmoid colon, the frame is incomplete and coils of small intestine descend into the lesser pelvis. The infracolic part of the **duodenum** completes this C-shaped structure. It consists of the lower half of the descending part, the **horizontal part** which crosses the vertebral column immediately anterior to the inferior vena cava and aorta on the third lumbar vertebra, and the short **ascending part** which joins the jejunum on the left side of the second lumbar vertebra. The jejunum and ileum lie in the free edge of *the* **mesentery** which runs obliquely across the central region from the duodenojejunal junction to the ileocaecal junction. Thus it partly divides the infracolic part of the peritoneal cavity into right superior and left inferior regions, both of which are filled with coils of the small intestine. The appendix vermiformis lies at the right extremity of the left inferior region where it is directly continuous with the pelvic peritoneal cavity.

Pick up the mesentery. Note the short attachment to the posterior abdominal wall and the long, complexly folded free margin containing the jejunum and ileum. The **jejunum** and **ileum** cannot be differentiated from each other clearly. There is usually less fat in the mesentery of the thicker-walled jejunum so that the vessels and the spaces between them are more clearly visible than in the ileal mesentery. The jejunum is usually taken as two-fifths of the 6 m which this part of the intestine is said to measure. The length is very variable in life. Certain methods of measurement give readings as low as 2.5 m.

A number of variable **accessory peritoneal folds** are found in relation to the duodenum and caecum [Figs. 133, 134]. Each of these produces a peritoneal recess within which a loop of small intestine may become lodged and obstructed, thus forming an internal hernia. These folds and recesses should be noted as they are exposed.

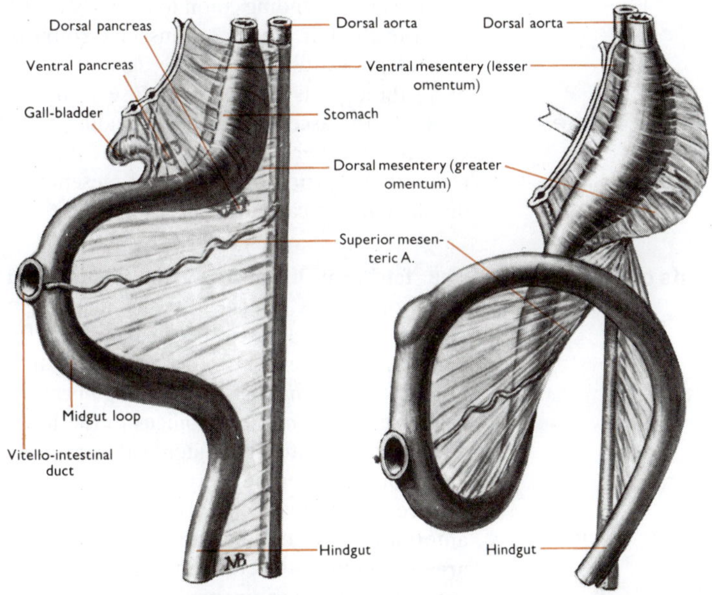

Fig. 135. A diagram to show two early stages in the development of the abdominal part of the gut tube and its mesenteries. Note the rotation of the midgut loop and the ballooning of the dorsal mesentery of the stomach to the left by the extension of the omental bursa (indicated by the arrow) into that mesentery.

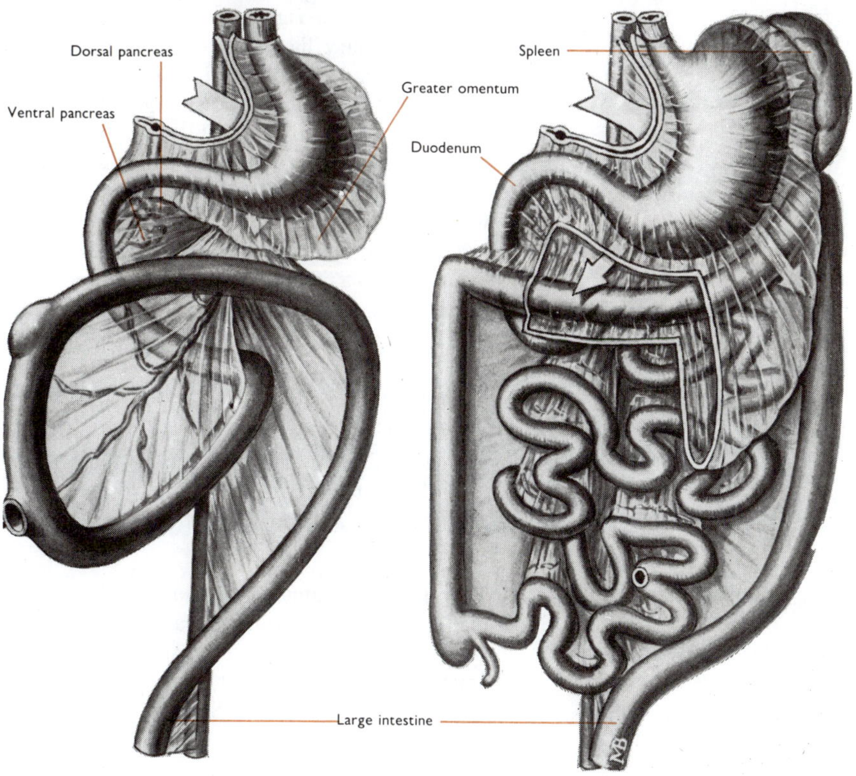

Fig. 136. A diagram of two later stages in the development of the abdominal part of the gut tube and its mesenteries. Note the changes in position of the various parts of the gut tube and the extension of the omental bursa with consequent formation of the greater omentum and the ligaments of the spleen from the dorsal mesentery of the stomach. The duodenum and the ascending and descending parts of the colon become fused to the posterior abdominal wall while the other parts of the gut tube retain their mesenteries. Cf. Fig. 135.

The apparently complex arrangement of the viscera described above is readily appreciated from its development [Figs. 135, 136]. The **midgut**, which extends from the descending part of the duodenum, is initially a simple loop protruding through the umbilical orifice. This loop rotates 180 degrees anticlockwise (as seen from the anterior surface) on itself. Thus the ends of the loop, the terminal part of the duodenum and the future left end of the transverse colon, take up reversed positions—the duodenal part inferior to the colonic part and to the right of the descending colon (hindgut) and its mesentery. The rotation also imparts to the duodenum its final C-shape. When the midgut loop returns to the abdomen from its original position in the root of the umbilical cord, the small intestine falls into the central region, while the caecum and other midgut parts of the colon lie across the abdomen (anterior to the descending part of the duodenum) superior and to the right of the small intestine. The centrally placed small intestine increases in length and displaces the surrounding parts of the large intestine outwards—the caecum and ascending colon to the right, the hindgut [Fig. 135] or descending colon to the left, and the transverse colon (which lies anterior to the small intestine) upwards and forwards against the greater omentum. The mesenteries of all three parts of the colon fuse with the peritoneum to which they are applied—the ascending and descending colon with the posterior abdominal wall, the transverse colon with the greater omentum. The ileum and jejunum retain their portion of the midgut mesentery between their fixed ends at the duodenum and caecum.

Ligaments of liver

The **falciform ligament** is the ventral part of the ventral mesentery. Anteriorly, it is attached to the diaphragm and supra-umbilical anterior abdominal wall close to the median plane [Fig. 138]. Posteriorly, the upper part passes to the right to be attached to the liver, the lower part has a free border which contains the **round ligament of the liver** (obliterated umbilical vein) passing from the umbilicus to the liver.

Trace the falciform ligament superiorly. Above the liver, its right and left layers of peritoneum diverge and are reflected separately from the superior surface of the liver on to the diaphragm [Fig. 138]. Thus they form the anterior margins of an area on the posterosuperior surface of the liver (**bare area of the liver**) where diaphragm and liver are directly in contact without any intervening peritoneum [Fig. 178]. The right layer is the superior layer of the **coronary ligament**. Followed to the right and posteriorly, it ends in a sharp margin (the **right triangular ligament**) where it meets the inferior layer of the coronary ligament. This layer may be felt by pressing the fingers upwards posterior to the right lobe of the liver and anterior to the right kidney. It forms the inferior margin of the bare area and will be seen when the liver is removed. The left layer of the falciform ligament passes to the left as the anterior layer of the **left triangular ligament**. This ends in a sharp, left margin where it becomes continuous with the posterior layer [Fig. 138], which can be traced to the lesser omentum.

The **round ligament of the liver** passes from the free edge of the falciform ligament into a fissure on the postero-inferior (visceral) surface of the liver. It passes in this fissure to the left extremity of the porta hepatis where it fuses with the left branch of the portal vein [Figs. 176, 286].

Dissection

Identify the arterial arcade (gastro-epiploic arteries) in the greater omentum, 2–3 cm from its junction with the greater curvature of the stomach. Cut through the anterior layers of the greater omentum 2–3 cm inferior to the arteries to open the lower part of the omental bursa sufficiently to admit a hand. Explore the bursa.

Omental bursa

The **epiploic foramen** opens into the right extremity of the omental bursa from the general peritoneal cavity. This foramen is posterior to the portal vein, proper hepatic artery, and bile-duct in the **free edge of the lesser omentum** and anterior to the inferior vena cava which lies on the right crus of the diaphragm [Fig. 139]. Superiorly the portal vein enters the liver and the inferior vena cava grooves it. Here a narrow strip of liver (caudate process

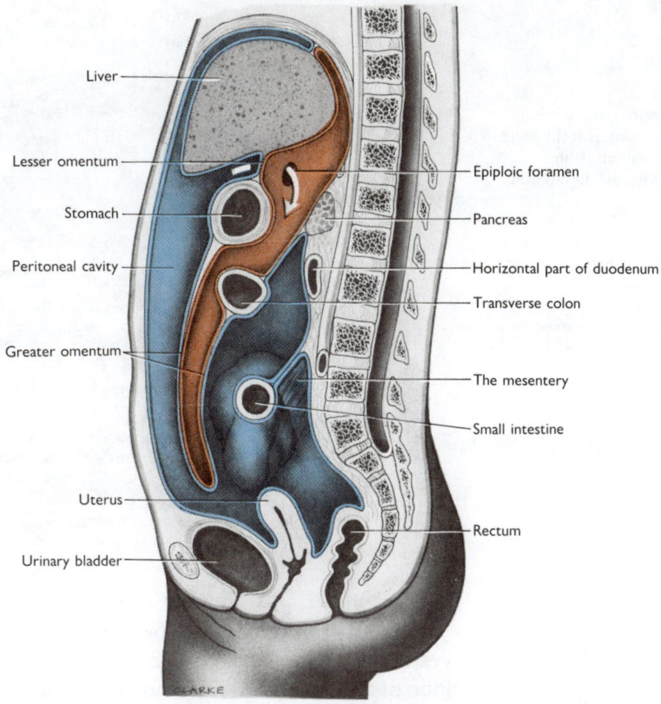

Fig. 137. A diagrammatic median section of the abdomen and pelvis to show the arrangement of the peritoneum. Normally the abdominal viscera completely fill the abdominal cavity and the peritoneal cavity is reduced to a slit. In the diagram the cavity has been distended to make it obvious. Blue: peritoneal cavity. Red: omental bursa of peritoneal cavity. The arrow traverses the epiploic foramen.

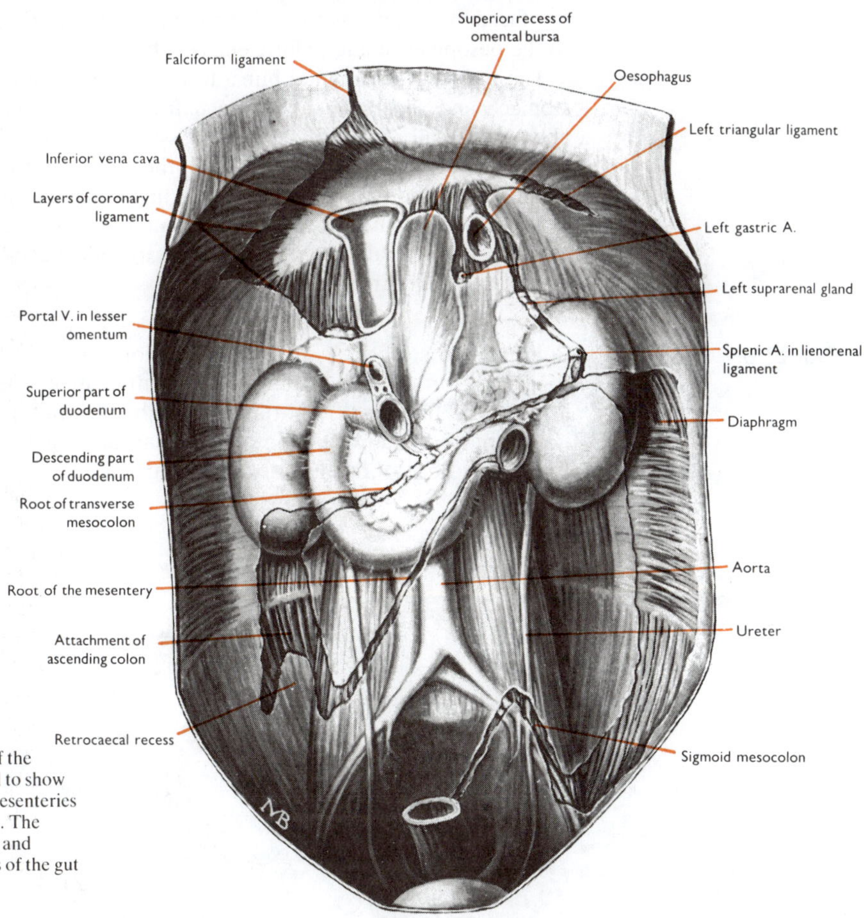

Fig. 138. A dissection of the posterior abdominal wall to show the attachments of the mesenteries and peritoneal ligaments. The oesophagus, duodenum, and rectum are the only parts of the gut tube left *in situ*.

[Fig. 176]) between them forms the superior limit of the foramen. The inferior boundary is formed by the portal vein and bile-duct passing posterior to the superior part of the duodenum. The epiploic foramen leads immediately into the vestibule of the bursa.

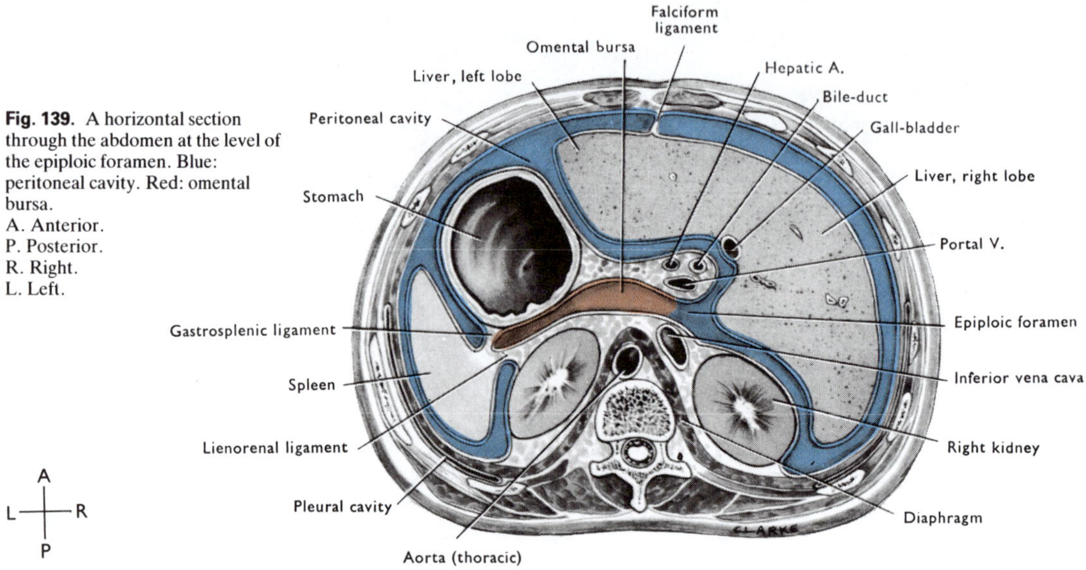

Fig. 139. A horizontal section through the abdomen at the level of the epiploic foramen. Blue: peritoneal cavity. Red: omental bursa.
A. Anterior.
P. Posterior.
R. Right.
L. Left.

The **superior recess** of the omental bursa passes superiorly from the vestibule, on the left of the inferior vena cava. It is posterior to the caudate lobe of the liver [Fig. 176] and is separated from the lower thoracic aorta by the diaphragm. To the left, the vestibule opens into the main body of the bursa between the **gastropancreatic folds**. These peritoneal folds are produced by the left gastric and common hepatic arteries passing respectively to the oesophageal and pyloric ends of the lesser curvature of the stomach.

The **body** of the omental bursa lies posterior to the lesser omentum and stomach and separates the stomach from the structures on the posterior abdominal wall (stomach bed). It passes for a variable distance into the greater omentum (**inferior recess**). On the left the bursa extends to the hilus of the spleen and the gastrosplenic and lienorenal ligaments (**splenic recess**).

The omental bursa gives added freedom of movement to the stomach, allowing it to expand after a meal and to slide freely on the surrounding tissues during contraction.

Dissection

Pull the liver superiorly and tilt its inferior margin anteriorly to expose the lesser omentum. If this gives insufficient exposure, remove the left lobe of the liver by cutting through it to the left of the falciform ligament, the fissure for the round ligament (ligamentum teres), and the attachment of the lesser omentum.

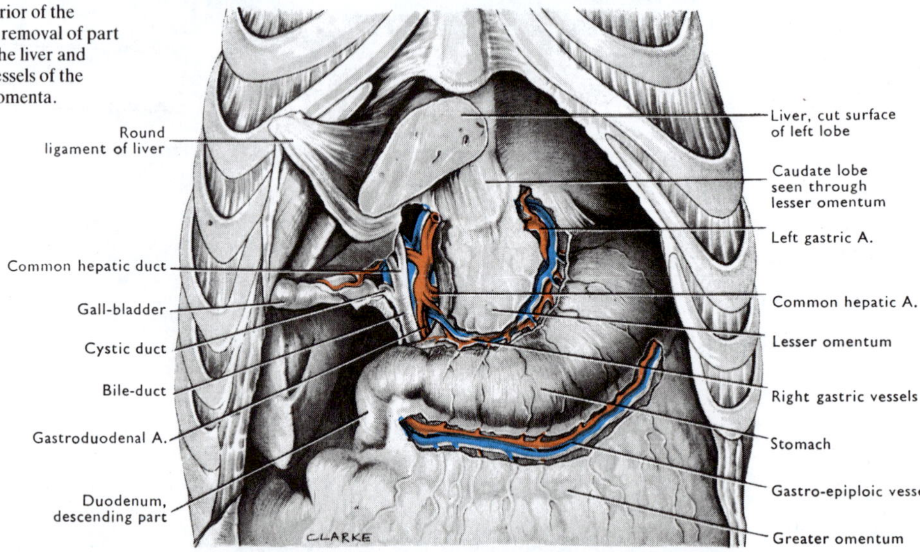

Fig. 140. The interior of the abdomen after the removal of part of the left lobe of the liver and dissection of the vessels of the lesser and greater omenta.

Lesser omentum

This double layer of peritoneum passes from the abdominal oesophagus, the lesser curvature of the stomach, and the first 2 cm of the duodenum to be attached to the liver in the depths of the fissure for the ligamentum venosum [Figs. 176, 283] and around the margin of the porta hepatis. Between the porta hepatis and the duodenum, the omentum ends in a *free edge*. Here the two layers meet around the **portal vein, proper hepatic artery**, and **bile-duct**. With these are (1) sympathetic **nerves** on the artery, (2) parasympathetic fibres from the anterior gastric nerves (vagus) to the gall-bladder, (3) **lymph vessels** and nodes which drain the liver and the adjacent part of the stomach. Elsewhere the layers of the omentum enclose only extraperitoneal tissue and the right and left **gastric vessels** close to the lesser curvature of the stomach. These vessels anastomose with each other, and the left gastric artery may send a branch in the omentum to supply part of the left lobe of the liver.

Dissection

Remove the anterior layer of peritoneum from the lesser omentum close to the lesser curvature of the stomach. Find and trace the left **gastric vessels** towards the oesophagus till they curve posteriorly round the superior surface of the omental bursa. Trace the **oesophageal branch** to the oesophagus. Find the anterior vagal trunk on the anterior surface of the oesophagus. Trace its branches on to the stomach.

Trace the right gastric artery to the proper hepatic artery, and the vein to the portal vein. Expose the proper hepatic artery and its branches to the porta hepatis. Trace the **cystic duct** from the neck of the gall-bladder to its junction with the common hepatic duct to form the bile-duct. Follow the **common hepatic duct** and its tributaries (right and left hepatic ducts) to the porta hepatis and the bile-duct till it passes posterior to the duodenum. Displace the artery and bile-duct and expose the portal vein posterior to them.

Remove the remainder of the lesser omentum, leaving the vessels intact, and examine the abdominal wall posterior to the omentum and omental bursa.

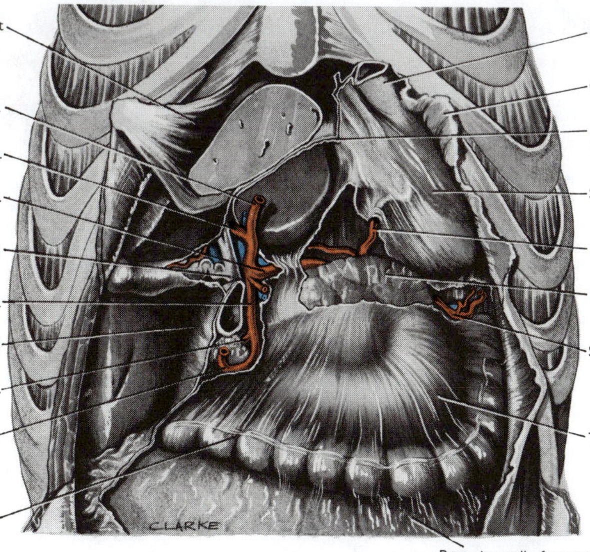

Fig. 141. The posterior wall of the omental bursa. The superior part of the duodenum and the greater part of the lesser omentum are divided and the stomach turned upwards with the anterior layers of the greater omentum.

The lesser omentum lies posterior to the left lobe of the liver, and posteriorly is separated from the pancreas, coeliac trunk (branch of aorta), and posterior diaphragm by the omental bursa. The free edge is continuous with that of the falciform ligament.

Lienorenal and gastrosplenic ligaments

Confirm the position of these [p. 117] by placing one hand between the diaphragm and the spleen and the other in the omental bursa. Posterior to the spleen, feel the thick lienorenal ligament which contains the **tail of the**

pancreas and the **splenic vessels**. Anterior to the spleen is the thin gastrosplenic ligament which contains branches of the splenic artery to the stomach (**short gastric** and **left gastro-epiploic arteries**) and the corresponding veins draining to the splenic vein. **Lymph vessels** and nodes are also present in both ligaments. They drain the territories supplied by the blood vessels.

Dissection

Identify and follow the vessels in the gastrosplenic ligament to the hilus of the spleen. Confirm the attachment of the ligament to the hilus, then follow the left gastro-epiploic artery through the greater omentum parallel to the greater curvature of the stomach.

Spleen

[Figs. 139, 142, 143, 149, 179, 283, 284]

This is the largest single mass of **lymph tissue** in the body. It does not receive afferent lymph vessels, and gives rise to few efferent lymph vessels in proportion to its size. It has a much richer blood supply than lymph nodes, but its thick **capsule** does not contain smooth muscle as it does in other animals where it serves as a blood store which can be emptied rapidly in response to blood loss.

The spleen lies deep in the left hypochondrium wedged obliquely between the diaphragm, stomach, and left kidney. The left colic flexure is applied to its **anterior extremity**. The spleen is covered by peritoneum except at the long, linear **hilus** on the medial part of its concave, anteromedial, **gastric surface**. Here the gastrosplenic and lienorenal ligaments are attached, the multiple branches of the splenic artery and the corresponding tributaries of the splenic vein pierce its surface, and the tip of the **tail of the pancreas** may reach it through the lienorenal ligament [Fig. 142].

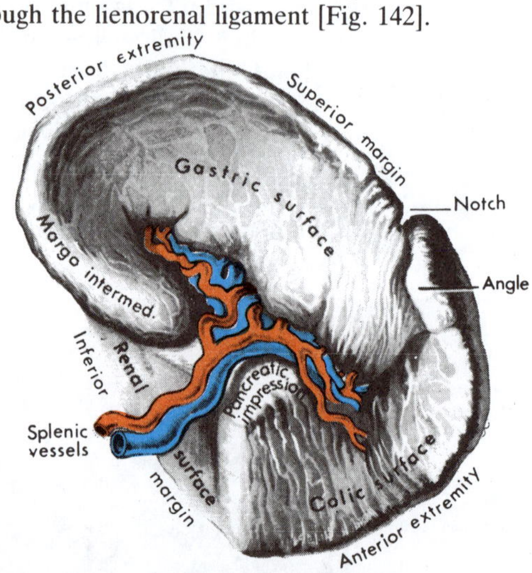

Fig. 142. The visceral surface of the spleen.

The convex, posterolateral, **diaphragmatic surface** lies on the diaphragm, parallel and deep to the posterior parts of the ninth to eleventh ribs, but separated by pleural cavity and lung. This surface meets the gastric surface at the relatively sharp **superior margin** which is notched towards its anterior end. The **notches** may be palpated through the anterior abdominal wall when a grossly enlarged spleen projects below the left costal margin at the ninth costal cartilage.

The **renal surface** is in contact with the lateral part of the upper half of the left kidney. It faces inferomedially and meets the diaphragmatic and gastric surfaces respectively at the blunt **inferior margin** and a low ridge (the intermediate margin) close to the hilus.

The spleen *develops* in the dorsal mesogastrium as a number of separate masses each with its own blood supply. These aggregate but retain their separate circulations. Thus blockage of a branch of the splenic artery leads to death (infarction) of a segment of the spleen. Accessory splenic nodules may be found in the gastrosplenic ligament.

Structure and function

The thick fibro-elastic capsule sends a network of **trabeculae** into the pulp of the spleen to join those which arise in the hilus around the entering blood vessels. There is red and white pulp. The **white pulp** consists of **lymph follicles** scattered throughout the spleen. These produce lymphocytes. The **red pulp** consists of many **sinusoids** separated by reticular fibres, phagocytes, and red and white blood cells some of which are being phagocytosed. The branches of the arteries which leave the trabeculae are ensheathed in lymphocytes, and pass to supply the lymph follicles. They then branch into contractile vessels (**ellipsoids**) which discharge into the sinusoids. These permit the passage of cells through their walls in both directions, and drain into the splenic venules.

The spleen is the major site of destruction of red and white blood cells and platelets. The products of their destruction are carried through the splenic and portal veins to the liver [p. 151]. In common with other lymph tissue masses, it plays a considerable role in the development of immunity; and though not essential to life, its removal tends to increase the susceptibility of the individual to infections.

Dissection

Complete the exposure of the gastro-epiploic vessels in the greater omentum. Follow them as far as possible in both directions. A plexus of sympathetic nerve fibres and an occasional lymph node may be found with them.

Cut through the stomach and the right gastric and gastro-epiploic vessels immediately to the left of the pylorus. Turn them to the left to expose the omental bursa. Remove the peritoneum from the left and posterior walls of the bursa as far inferiorly as the attachment of the greater omentum. Note the **lymph nodes (pancreaticosplenic)** on the superior border of the pancreas as it is uncovered.

Identify the coeliac trunk [Fig. 143] and remove the dense autonomic plexus from its branches. Expose the superior part of the left kidney and suprarenal gland, the numerous **suprarenal arteries** and single **vein,** and the **inferior phrenic artery** on the left crus of the diaphragm. Identify the **coeliac ganglia**, one on each side of the coeliac trunk, and trace the **splanchnic nerves** superiorly from them. Remove the peritoneum from the posterior surface of the stomach, tracing the posterior vagal trunk and its gastric branches.

Coeliac trunk

This large vessel is the most cephalic of the unpaired branches of the aorta to the gut tube. It passes forwards for approximately 1 cm from the uppermost part of the abdominal aorta and divides into common hepatic, splenic, and left gastric branches. These supply the gut tube from the lower oesophagus to the descending part of the duodenum and the liver, pancreas, and spleen. It is surrounded by a dense plexus of autonomic and sensory nerve fibres. These are distributed with its branches [Fig. 286].

Left gastric artery [Figs. 138, 143]

This small branch ascends on the posterior part of the diaphragm towards the oesophagus. It then arches forwards in the superior gastropancreatic fold, and runs inferiorly along the lesser curvature of the stomach to anastomose with the right gastric artery. Ascending **oesophageal branches** anastomose with oesophageal branches of the aorta in the thorax. **Gastric branches** pass to both surfaces of the stomach adjacent to the lesser curvature.

Fig. 143. The coeliac trunk and its branches.

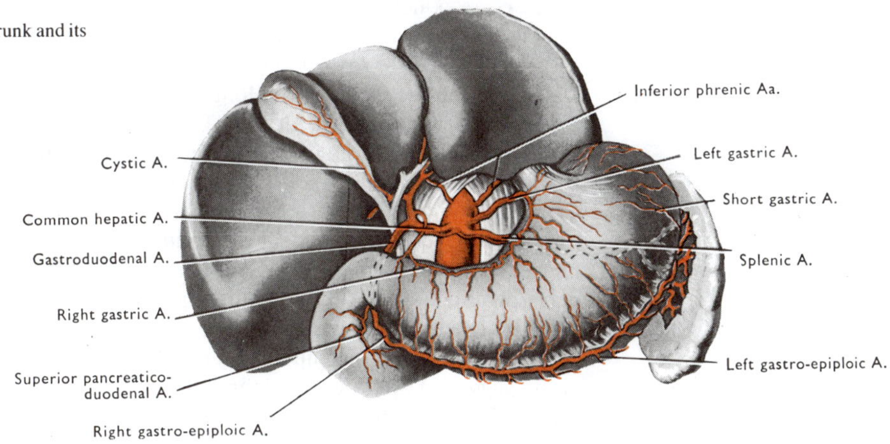

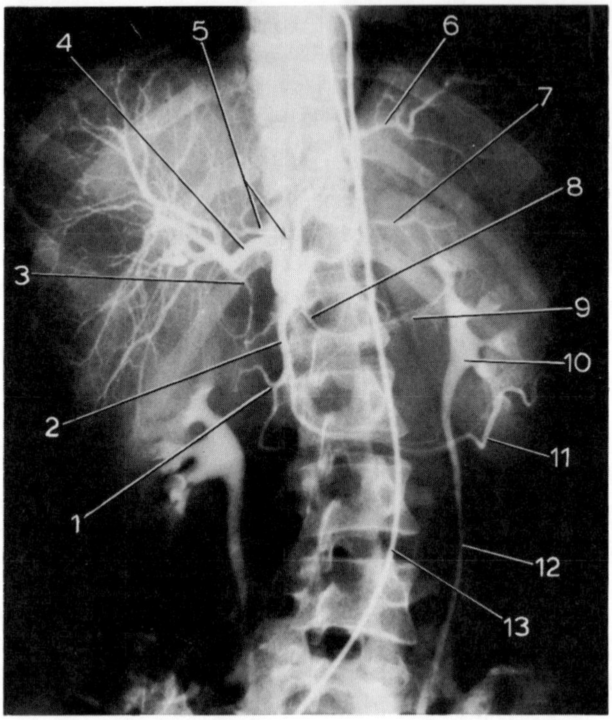

Fig. 144. An angiogram (a radiograph taken immediately after the injection of contrast material into an artery) of the coeliac trunk injected through a catheter passed into the aorta through the femoral artery, a test injection having been made to confirm entry into the coeliac trunk. This test injection has already been cleared by the kidneys and outlines their calyces, pelves, and ureters. In this case the splenic artery has not filled and there are some unusual features—a situation which is common in the arteries in this region. The main difference from normal is the origin of the left hepatic and left gastric arteries by a common stem and the presence of a middle hepatic artery where the left hepatic artery would be expected.

1. Superior pancreaticoduodenal artery [cf. Fig. 155].
2. Gastroduodenal artery.
3. Cystic artery.
4. Right hepatic artery.
5. Middle hepatic artery.
6. Left hepatic artery arising from a stem in common with 7.
7. Left gastric artery.
8. Right gastric artery.
9. Anastomosis of gastric arteries on lesser curvature.
10. Pelvis of left kidney.
11. Right gastro-epiploic artery.
12. Left ureter.
13. Catheter in aorta.

Such angiograms can show the presence of (1) abnormal masses by displacement of the arteries; (2) blockage of arteries or their narrowing by disease; (3) arteriovenous abnormalities or vascular tumours.

The **left gastric vein** runs along its artery to the coeliac trunk accompanied by branches of the vagal trunks to the coeliac ganglia. The vein then follows the common hepatic artery to the portal vein. The tributaries correspond to the branches of the artery. The most important are from the **oesophagus** for they anastomose with thoracic oesophageal veins which drain to the azygos system. This communication forms an alternative route for portal venous blood when its flow is obstructed in liver disease. Greatly distended submucous veins in the lower oesophagus may result, and these may be a source of severe haemorrhage [Fig. 170].

Splenic artery

[Figs. 142, 149, 284A, 285A]

This is the largest branch of the coeliac trunk. It runs a sinuous course to the left along the superior border of the pancreas, posterior to the omental bursa and anterior to the left kidney, to enter the lienorenal ligament.

Branches

(1) Small twigs pass to the body and tail of the **pancreas**. (2) Five or six branches enter the hilus of the **spleen**. (3) Five or six slender, **short gastric arteries** pass from the trunk and its splenic branches through the gastrosplenic ligament to the fundus of the stomach. (4) The **left gastro-epiploic artery** runs through the gastrosplenic ligament and greater omentum parallel to and a short distance from the greater curvature of the stomach. It anastomoses with the right gastro-epiploic artery, supplies both surfaces of the stomach adjacent to the greater curvature, and sends small twigs into the greater omentum.

The corresponding **veins** drain into the splenic vein. This lies inferior to the splenic artery, and runs to the right, posterior to the pancreas.

Common hepatic artery

[Figs. 141, 143, 286B]

This artery passes to the right along the superior border of the pancreas to the superior part of the duodenum. Here it divides into gastroduodenal and proper hepatic arteries. The **proper hepatic artery** turns forwards between the duodenum and epiploic foramen, gives off the right gastric artery, and ascends through the lesser omentum to the porta hepatis, lying anterior to the portal vein to the left of the bile-duct [Fig. 139]. Inferior to the porta hepatis it divides into right and left hepatic arteries which enter the corresponding lobes of the liver through the porta.

In the lesser omentum, the proper hepatic artery may give a descending duodenal branch to the superior part of the duodenum. The right hepatic artery sends the **cystic artery** along the cystic duct to supply the gall-bladder [Fig. 143]. The **cystic vein** enters the right branch of the portal vein.

Gastroduodenal artery

This descends posterior to the superior part of the duodenum, and divides into superior pancreaticoduodenal and right gastro-epiploic arteries [Figs. 141, 143].

The **superior pancreaticoduodenal arteries** form an arcade on or in the anterior and posterior surfaces of the head of the pancreas with the inferior pancreaticoduodenal branches of the superior mesenteric artery [Figs. 144, 155]. Each arcade sends branches to the duodenum and the pancreas. The corresponding veins drain to the portal and superior mesenteric veins.

The **right gastro-epiploic artery** runs to the left between the layers of the greater omentum. It anastomoses with the left gastro-epiploic artery and sends branches to the superior part of the duodenum, the right part of the stomach, and the greater omentum. The corresponding **vein** usually enters the superior mesenteric vein.

Right gastric artery

This branch passes to the left on the first centimetre of the duodenum, the pylorus, and the lesser curvature of the stomach. It supplies these and anastomoses with the left gastric artery. The corresponding **vein** enters the portal vein, and is united to the right gastro-epiploic vein by the **prepyloric vein**. This crosses the front of the pylorus and is a landmark for the surgeon.

Variations in the arrangements of the branches of the common hepatic artery are frequent. Occasionally the entire artery may arise from the superior mesenteric artery through enlargement of a pancreaticoduodenal arcade.

Abdominal part of oesophagus

The oesophagus pierces the muscular part of the diaphragm (right crus) posterior to the central tendon, 2–3 cm to the left of the median plane. It is accompanied by the vagal trunks, the oesophageal branches of the left gastric artery, and the corresponding veins. It grooves the left lobe of the liver, and almost immediately enters the stomach in line with the lesser curvature and at an acute angle (**cardiac notch**) to the fundus [Figs. 150, 152, 283].

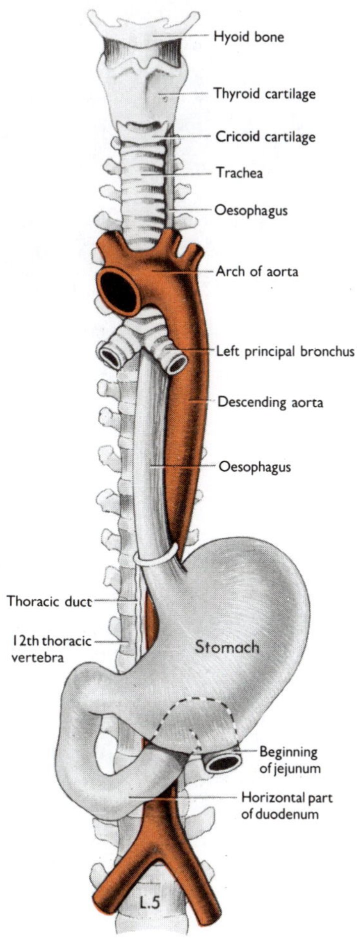

Fig. 145. The oesophagus, stomach, and duodenum.

Vagal trunks

On the lower thoracic oesophagus, the oesophageal plexus condenses into anterior and posterior vagal trunks. These pass through the diaphragm on the oesophagus and break up into anterior and posterior **gastric branches** respectively. Each vagal trunk contains fibres from both vagus nerves and sympathetic fibres from the greater splanchnic nerves [p. 28].

The **anterior gastric branches** supply the stomach and send nerve fibres to the duodenum and pancreas, and to the liver through the lesser omentum.

The **posterior vagal trunk** sends **posterior gastric branches** to the stomach. **Coeliac branches** of both trunks, especially the posterior, descend to the coeliac plexus with the left gastric vessels. These preganglionic parasympathetic nerve fibres are distributed with the sympathetic fibres which accompany visceral branches of the abdominal aorta, though pelvic parasympathetic and not vagal fibres run with the inferior mesenteric artery.

Replace the stomach and the left lobe of the liver if it has been removed. Review the shape and position of the stomach.

Stomach

[see also p. 118 and Figs. 131, 283–285]

The stomach is the most distensible organ of the body. It receives food mixed with and softened by saliva. The **body** of the stomach adds a considerable volume of fluid (containing hydrochloric acid, pepsin, rennin, and lipase) and churns the food to a semifluid mass (**chyme**) by its muscular action. It also adds mucus to the food, particularly in the pyloric part [Fig. 131] through which the chyme passes to be discharged slowly through the pylorus into the superior part of the duodenum. This mucus adsorbs a considerable quantity of hydrochloric acid, and helps to protect the gastric mucous membrane from digestion by the chyme.

The stomach passes downwards and to the right across the supracolic compartment of the peritoneal cavity. It tapers from the **fundus**, on the left of the median plane, to the narrow **pylorus** slightly to the right of the median plane. Together with the superior part of the duodenum it is bent across the prominent vertebral column—the fundus and superior part of the duodenum lying in the corresponding paravertebral gutters, the pyloric part anteriorly on the prevertebral structures [Fig. 146]. This **pyloric part** consists of a proximal dilated portion, the **pyloric antrum**, and a narrow, cylindrical portion (**pyloric canal**) 2–3 cm long, which is continuous distally with the pylorus. The **pylorus** is the portion of the stomach thickened by an increase in the amount of circular muscle to form the **pyloric sphincter** which controls

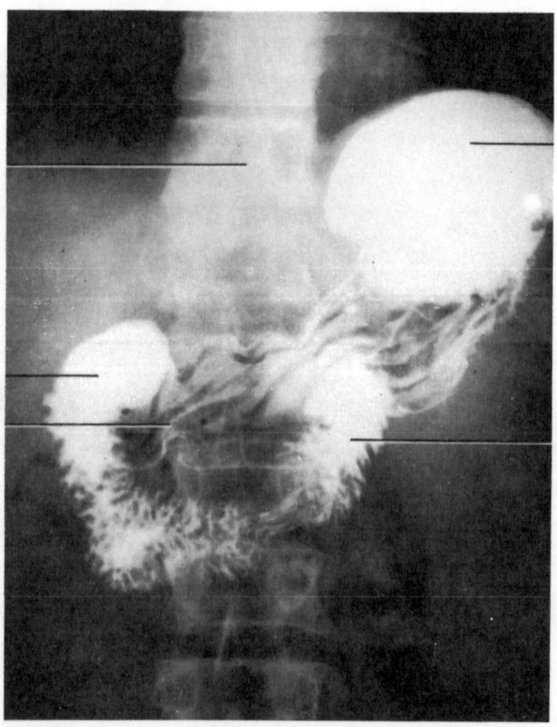

Fig. 146. A radiograph of the transverse type of the stomach taken in the recumbent position. Note that the gas bubble in the stomach lies in the part anterior to the vertebral column and outlines the folds of gastric mucosa. The heavy-contrast medium gravitates into the fundus and into the superior part of the duodenum which lie posteriorly in the paravertebral gutters. Cf. Figs. 140, 148, and 150.

the rate of discharge of stomach contents into the duodenum. It prevents too much hydrochloric acid passing at one time into the alkaline medium of the duodenum. The pylorus is highly mobile because the omenta are attached to it. It may lie anywhere between the first and third lumbar vertebrae. It is 2–3 cm to the right of the median plane, but is further displaced to the right when the stomach is full. In its higher positions the pylorus is posterior to the quadrate lobe of the liver and is separated from the pancreas by the omental bursa.

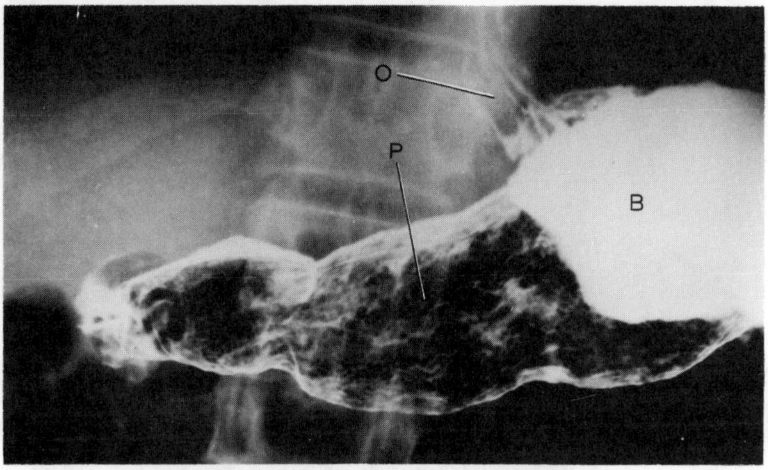

Fig. 147. A double contrast (X-ray-opaque medium and air) radiograph of the pyloric part of the stomach to show the mucosal pattern due to the opaque medium lying in the grooves between the mamillae [Fig. 151]. Such radiographs show early changes in the surface of the gastric mucosa, e.g. gastric ulcer or cancer, by comparison with the conventional silhouette radiographs of a hollow organ filled with opaque medium [Fig. 148] when the only surface visible is that directly at a tangent to the X-ray beam—a linear strip—and even then only gross changes are visible. This radiograph, like Fig. 146, was taken with the patient supine and the air in the prevertebral part of the stomach.
B. Body of stomach.
O. Oesophagus.
p. Pyloric part of stomach.

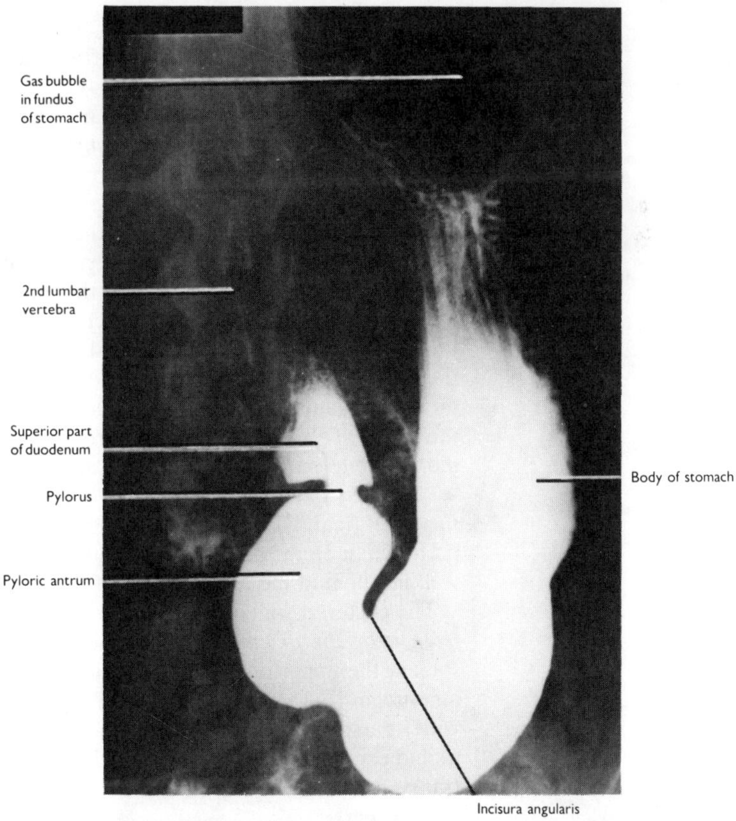

Fig. 148. A radiograph of J-shaped stomach taken in the erect posture. Note the level of the pylorus and compare this with Fig. 146.

The **fundus** abuts on the left dome of the diaphragm under cover of the rib cage, and reaches the level of the fifth rib in the midclavicular line anteriorly. Here it is inferior and slightly posterior to the apex of the heart. In the erect posture it is filled with a bubble of swallowed air [Fig. 148] which moves into the pyloric portion, anterior to the vertebral column, in the supine position [Fig. 146].

The **cardiac** (oesophageal) **orifice** lies approximately 10 cm posterior to the

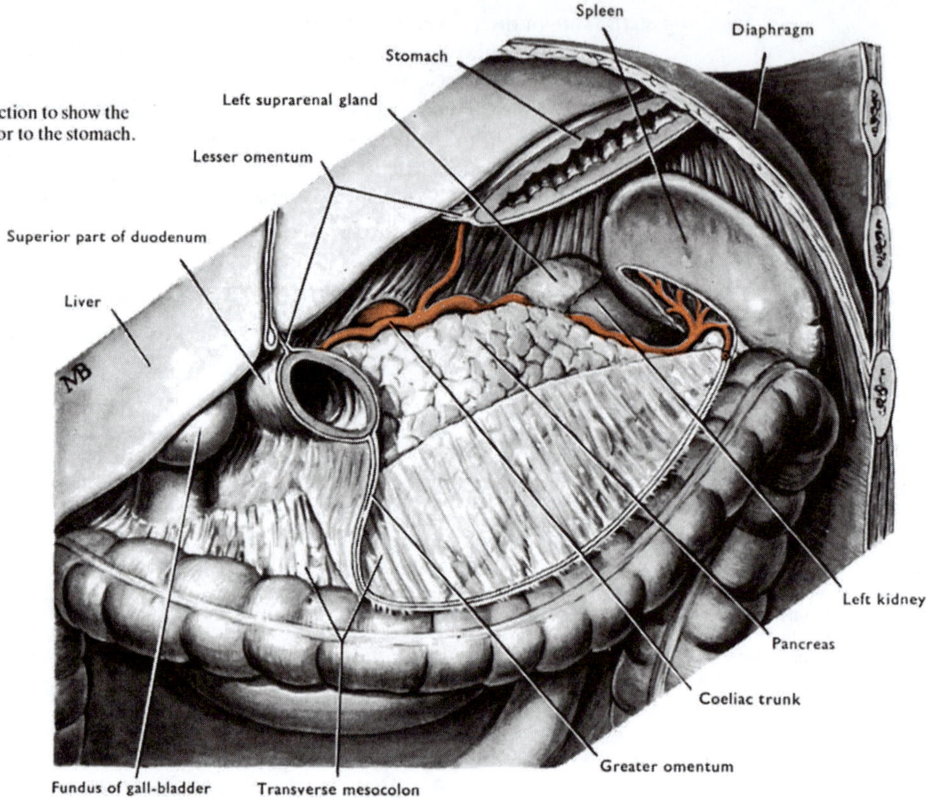

Fig. 149. A dissection to show the structures posterior to the stomach.

seventh left costal cartilage 2–3 cm from the median plane, between the liver and the diaphragm.

The cardiac orifice and fundus are relatively fixed and only move with respiratory excursions of the diaphragm. The shape and position of the remainder of the stomach varies considerably from individual to individual and in the same individual with age, degree of distention, position of the trunk, and state of contraction of the gastric muscle. These differences are partly due to the freedom of movement of the stomach imparted by the presence of the omental bursa and the loose omenta. However, in thick set individuals and children the stomach tends to lie almost transversely across the abdomen [Fig. 146], but in most people it is J-shaped. When J-shaped, the pyloric part lies horizontally or ascends to the superior part of the duodenum, and the lowest part of the greater curvature may even extend into the greater pelvis in the erect posture. Thus the structures in contact with the most mobile parts of the stomach are variable. Nevertheless, the anterior wall of the stomach adjacent to the lesser omentum is usually overlapped by the liver (mainly the left lobe) and inferior to this is in contact with the peritoneum on the rectus sheath. Further to the left, the superior part of this wall lies behind the anterior part of the diaphragm and rib cage.

The posterior wall of the stomach lies on the stomach bed, but is *separated from it by the omental bursa*. Superiorly the stomach bed consists of the spleen, the upper pole of the left kidney, the left suprarenal gland, and the diaphragm [Fig. 149]. Inferiorly is the upper part of the pancreas [Fig. 128] with its associated vessels and the mesentery of the transverse colon attached to and extending inferiorly from it. In the low type of J-shaped stomach, the transverse colon and even coils of small intestine may lie posterior to its inferior part.

Vessels and nerves

The rich arterial supply is derived from all three branches of the coeliac trunk. The right and left gastric arteries anastomose on the lesser curvature, while the right and left gastro-epiploic arteries unite near the inferior part of the greater curvature, the superior part of which is supplied by the short gastric arteries. Branches of all these arteries pass to both walls of the stomach at right angles to its long axis. The anastomoses are sufficient to permit the tying of one or more of the major arteries without ill effects. The **veins** drain with the corresponding arteries to reach the portal vein.

Lymph vessels run with the blood vessels to occasional small nodes lying beside them. The main **lymph nodes** (pancreaticosplenic and pyloric) lie on the posterior abdominal wall adjacent to the pancreas.

Parasympathetic nerve fibres reach the stomach through the anterior and posterior **vagal trunks** and their branches. The **sympathetic** nerve fibres reach the stomach through the **coeliac plexus** on the branches of the coeliac trunk.

Dissection

The stomach may be removed by cutting through the oesophagus and left gastric vessels close to the diaphragm, the gastrophrenic and gastrosplenic ligaments, and the anterior layers of the greater omentum. However, it is best left in position if sufficiently mobile. Strip the peritoneum from one wall of the stomach and attempt to dissect the muscle layers. Open the stomach along the greater curvature and examine the mucous membrane with a hand lens. Then strip the mucous membrane from one part and expose the internal muscle coat.

Mucous membrane

This is a thick, smooth-surfaced layer which is thrown into longitudinal folds when the stomach is contracted, but is flattened out as it distends. It consists of a layer of **tubular glands**. Groups of these open into **pits** [Fig. 151] formed

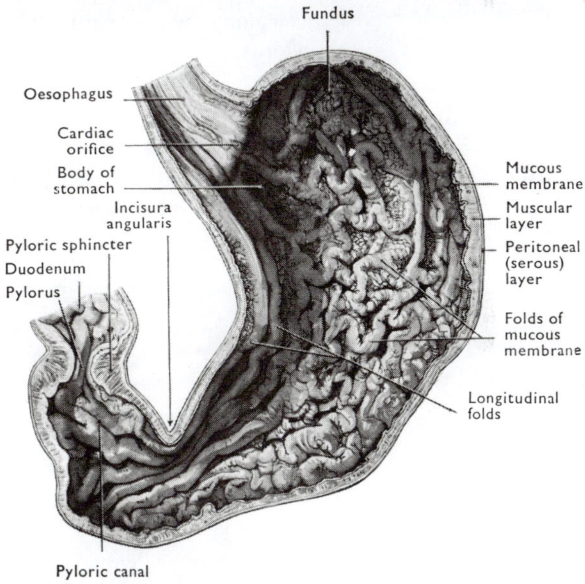

Fig. 150. The posterior wall of the empty, contracted stomach.

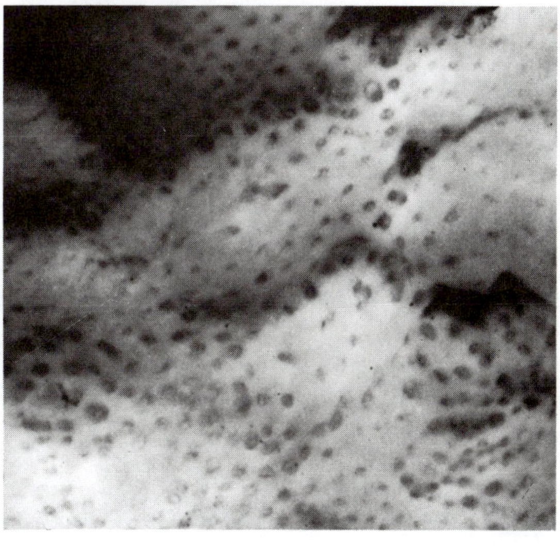

Fig. 151. A photograph of the surface of the human gastric mucosa. Note that it is not quite smooth but has a number of rounded protrusions (mamillae), and that the surface is covered with dark spots of variable size, the gastric pits. A number of simple tubular gastric glands open into the base of each pit.

by the tall columnar cells of the surface epithelium which produce a protective surface layer of mucus. In the **body** and **fundus** the pits are short and the glands are long, parallel, and tightly packed. They contain several different kinds of cells, including enzyme and acid-secreting types. In the **pyloric part** of the stomach the pits are deeper, and the glands are coiled, less tightly packed, and entirely of a mucus-secreting type. The deepest layer of the mucous membrane is the **muscularis mucosae**. This is thicker in the stomach than elsewhere, and may have three rather than two layers of muscle.

Muscle of stomach

There are three layers. The outer two are continuous with the muscle layers of the oesophagus and duodenum, the inner layer is peculiar to the stomach [Fig. 152].

The **outer layer** of longitudinal muscle is thickest at the curvatures, but is very thin or absent along the middle of each wall. Some of its fibres turn into the circular layer at the pyloric sphincter and may help to open the pylorus.

The **middle layer** is a complete circular layer. It gradually thickens in the pyloric canal and forms the pyloric sphincter. This thickening ceases abruptly at the duodenum [Fig. 153].

The **inner layer** consists of oblique fibres which loop over the cardiac notch. To the left the fibres fan out in the fundus and body of the stomach and a well-developed ridge passes towards the pylorus on each side of the lesser curvature. These fibres may approximate the ridges of mucous membrane which lie deep to them and thus cut off a tubular part of the stomach along the lesser curvature through which fluids may pass directly to the pylorus.

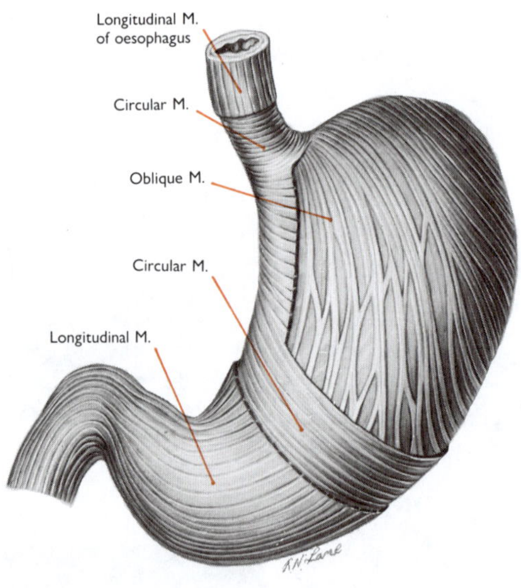

Fig. 152. A dissection of the muscle layers of the stomach.

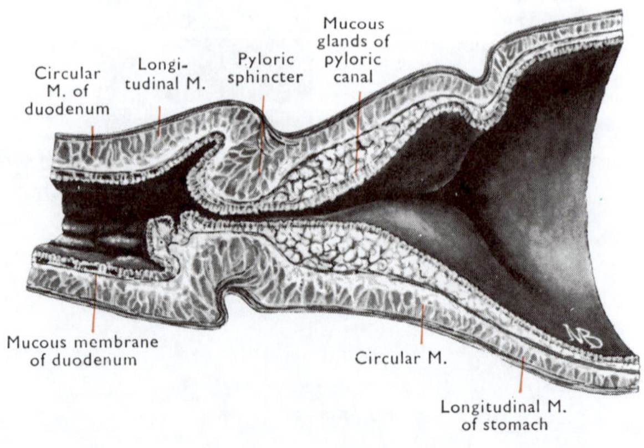

Fig. 153. A longitudinal section through the pyloroduodenal junction. Note the mass of mucous glands in the mucous membrane of the pyloric canal.

Dissection

Cut longitudinally through the wall of the superior part of the duodenum close to the pylorus and examine the duodenal aspect of the pylorus. Extend the cut through the pyloric wall to show the pyloric sphincter.

The **pyloric sphincter** bulges the mucous membrane into the pylorus and narrows the aperture so that it appears as a small opening in the centre of a rounded knob when viewed from the duodenal side.

Expose the mesentery of the small intestine in the infracolic compartment by turning the transverse colon and its mesentery upwards. Trace the oblique attachment of the mesentery of the small intestine on the posterior abdominal wall.

Turn the small intestine to the left, cut through the right layer of peritoneum of the mesentery along the line of its attachment to the posterior abdominal wall, and strip it from the mesentery. Remove the fat from the mesentery to expose the **superior mesenteric vessels** in its root and their branches and tributaries (jejunal and ileal) in the mesentery. Note the numerous lymph nodes and the complex mass of nerve fibres (**superior mesenteric plexus**) surrounding the vessels. Trace the superior mesenteric vessels proximally and distally and their branches to the caecum, ascending and transverse colon, and to the duodenum and pancreas.

The mesentery

This fold of peritoneum and extraperitoneal tissue attaches the whole length of the jejunum and ileum (up to 6 m) to an oblique line across the posterior abdominal wall from the duodenojejunal flexure towards the ileocaecal junction. The short (15 cm) **root** contains the superior mesenteric vessels and crosses the anterior surfaces of the horizontal part of the duodenum, the aorta, the inferior vena cava, and the testicular or ovarian vessels and ureter on the right psoas muscle [Figs. 132, 138]. *The* mesentery contains the jejunal and ileal blood vessels, large **lacteal lymph vessels** draining to the lymph nodes in and at the base of *the* mesentery, a considerable plexus of autonomic nerves, and extraperitoneal fatty tissue.

Superior mesenteric artery [Fig. 287]

This is the second median branch of the aorta supplying the gut tube. It arises at the level of the first lumbar vertebra, 0.5 cm inferior to the coeliac trunk, posterior to the body of the pancreas and the splenic vein. It descends anterior to the left renal vein, the uncinate process of the pancreas (q.v.), and the horizontal part of the duodenum, and runs in the root of *the* mesentery to the right iliac fossa. Here it ends by giving branches to the ileum and anastomosing with a branch of the ileocolic artery [Fig. 154].

Branches

The artery supplies the intestine from the descending part of the duodenum to the transverse colon. The branches anastomose freely with each other and with branches of the arteries supplying adjacent parts of the gut tube.

1. *From the right side of the artery*. The **middle colic artery** [Fig. 154] arises at the lower border of the pancreas. It turns forwards into the transverse mesocolon and divides into right and left branches. These either anastomose with each other close to the transverse colon or branch some distance from it, each branch then forming part of the **marginal artery**. This extends along the ascending, transverse, and descending parts of the colon and receives the branches of the other colic arteries. Branches pass from the marginal artery to the colon. Thus the middle colic normally supplies most of the transverse colon, but the anastomosis through the marginal artery is such that blocking of any one of the colic arteries would not imperil the blood supply of the colon.

The **inferior pancreaticoduodenal arteries** arise on the duodenum and pass upwards and to the right to form arcades with the superior pancreatico-duodenal arteries [Figs. 144, 155]. They supply duodenum and the head and uncinate process of the pancreas.

The **right colic artery** passes across the structures of the posterior

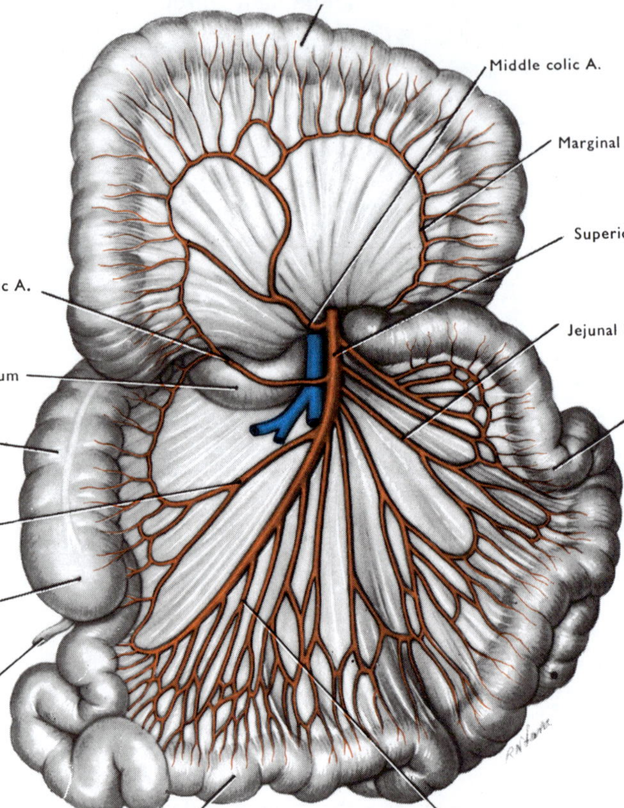

Fig. 154. The superior mesenteric artery and its branches.

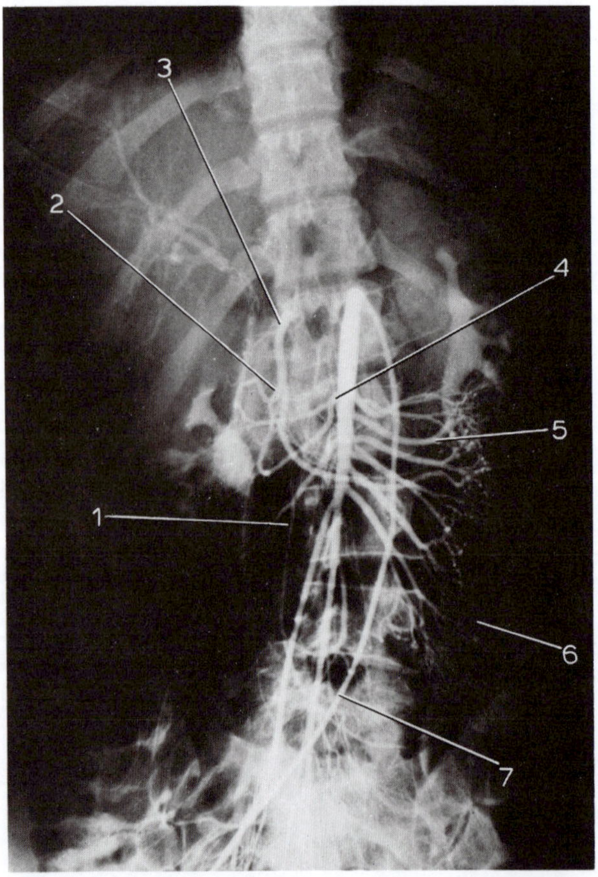

Fig. 155. Angiogram of the superior mesenteric artery in the same individual as that shown in Fig. 144 taken immediately after that angiogram. Hence some contrast medium is still in the branches of the coeliac trunk.
1. Right colic branch to marginal artery on transverse colon.
2. Superior pancreaticoduodenal artery.
3. Gastroduodenal artery.
4. Inferior pancreaticoduodenal artery.
5. Jejunal artery.
6. Marginal artery on transverse colon.
7. Catheter in aorta.

abdominal wall to join the marginal artery near the superior end of the ascending colon. It may be replaced by an enlarged ascending branch of the ileocolic artery.

The **ileocolic artery** may arise with the right colic artery. It passes downwards and to the right. An ascending branch is the beginning of the marginal artery. A descending branch supplies the colon, caecum, appendix vermiformis, and the terminal part of the ileum, and anastomoses with the last ileal branch of the superior mesenteric artery. The **appendicular artery** enters the lowest part of *the* mesentery, and passes posterior to the terminal part of the ileum into the mesentery of the appendix vermiformis [Fig. 160].

2. *From the left side of the artery*, the **jejunal** and **ileal branches** enter *the* mesentery. They branch and anastomose with each other to form a series of **arcades** from which further branches form a second, and in the lower part of *the* mesentery, a third and even a fourth tier of arcades. The last arcades send branches to each side of the small intestine and their branches anastomose in its wall.

Superior mesenteric vein

This large vein lies immediately to the right of the superior mesenteric artery. Superiorly it deviates to the right to join the splenic vein and form the portal vein posterior to the pancreas. It drains blood from the territory of the artery, but receives the right gastro-epiploic and pancreaticoduodenal veins and, occasionally, the inferior mesenteric vein.

Lymph nodes of the mesentery

These numerous nodes lie between the layers of *the* mesentery, and gradually increase in diameter towards its root.

The lymph vessels of the small intestine are known as **lacteals** because of the milky white emulsion of fat which they contain during life. They converge on and drain through a series of lymph nodes finally uniting at the root of the mesentery in the intestinal lymph trunk which passes to the cisterna chyli [Figs. 86, 200].

Dissection

Turn the small intestine and its mesentery to the right. Remove the peritoneum and fat on the posterior abdominal wall between *the* mesentery and the descending colon to expose the inferior mesenteric vessels and the autonomic nerves and lymph nodes associated with them [Fig. 163].

Inferior mesenteric artery

This is the third and last of the median branches of the aorta to the gut tube. It supplies the intestine from the left part of the transverse colon to the anal canal. The artery arises posterior to the horizontal part of the duodenum, and descends on the left of the aorta, posterior to the peritoneum, surrounded by the **inferior mesenteric plexus of nerves**. On the middle of the left common iliac artery it divides into sigmoid and superior rectal arteries.

Branches [Fig. 156]

These arteries cross the posterior abdominal wall anterior to the plane of the kidney, ureter, and gonadal vessels.

The **left colic artery** arises a short distance below the duodenum. It passes to the left and divides into ascending and descending branches which form part of the marginal artery. The ascending branch crosses the lower pole of the left kidney and unites with the middle colic part of the marginal artery, thus helping to supply the left flexure and left part of the transverse colon. The descending branch supplies the descending colon and anastomoses with the sigmoid arteries.

Two or more **sigmoid arteries** pass inferiorly and to the left. They anastomose with each other and continue the marginal artery to supply the descending colon in the left iliac fossa and the sigmoid colon. The lowest sigmoid artery anastomoses with the superior rectal artery by a small branch.

The **superior rectal artery** will be followed in the lesser pelvis.

Inferior mesenteric vein [Fig. 163]

This is the continuation of the superior rectal vein. It ascends lateral to the inferior mesenteric artery, and receives tributaries corresponding to the branches of that artery. The vein then passes lateral to the duodenojejunal

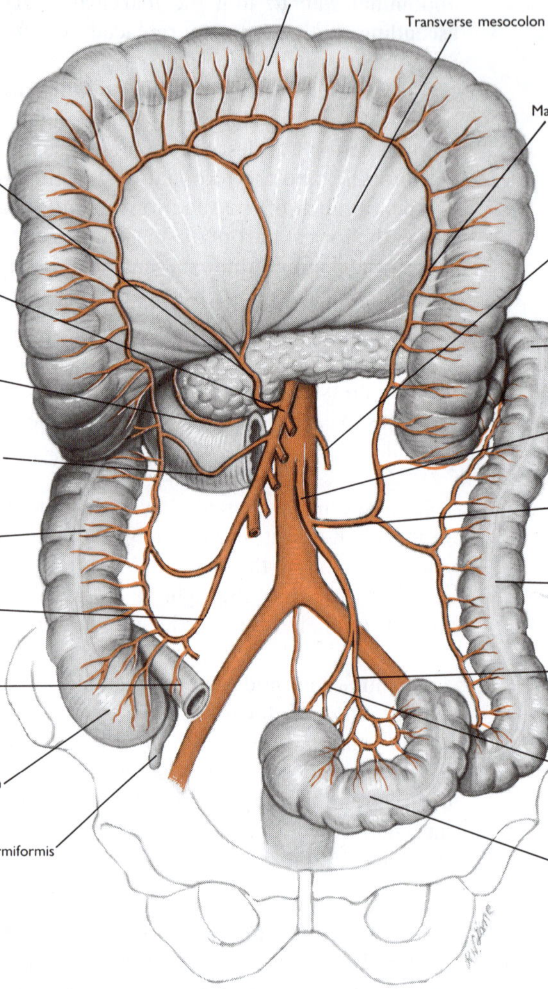

Fig. 156. The branches of the superior and inferior mesenteric arteries to the large intestine. Usually there is more than one sigmoid artery.

flexure and anterior to the left renal vein, to join the splenic vein posterior to the pancreas. It may deviate to the right and enter the superior mesenteric vein or its junction with the splenic vein.

Arterial anastomoses on gastrointestinal tract

The coeliac trunk, and the superior and inferior mesenteric are unpaired arteries that supply the gut tube, spleen, pancreas, and liver. They give branches which anastomose freely with each other and with the arteries supplying the adjacent parts of the gut tube. The **left gastric** (coeliac trunk) anastomoses with **oesophageal branches of the thoracic aorta**. The two **pancreaticoduodenal arteries** form a link between coeliac trunk and superior mesenteric artery [Figs. 144, 155]. Arcades unite the jejunal and ileal branches of the superior mesenteric artery and the marginal artery links its colic branches with each other and with the colic branches of the inferior mesenteric artery. Thus blockage of a single vessel or even of a group of vessels is not followed by degeneration of any part of the intestine. If a loop of intestine is compressed at the neck of a hernial sac or twisted upon itself (volvulus), none of the anastomoses can be effective, and death of the intestine with rupture of its wall will follow unless the condition is treated rapidly.

Abdominal aortic plexus

This consists of two or three intercommunicating strands of nerve fibres which descend over each side of the abdominal aorta. They arise in the coeliac and superior mesenteric plexuses (q.v.) and are reinforced by branches (**lumbar splanchnic nerves**) from each lumbar sympathetic trunk.

These descend obliquely at the sides of the aorta, and unite with the lowest part of the plexus. The plexus extends along the branches of the abdominal aorta below the superior mesenteric artery and continues, inferior to the bifurcation of the aorta, as the **superior hypogastric plexus** (presacral nerve) on the front of the fifth lumbar vertebra and the left common iliac vein. On the sacral promontory, this plexus divides into right and left **inferior hypogastric** (pelvic) **plexuses** [Fig. 202]. These surround the corresponding internal iliac arteries and are distributed with their branches to the pelvic viscera.

Structure of small intestine

The small intestine has the same four layers as the stomach. The outer, peritoneal or **serous layer** is tightly bound to the muscular layer by a thin but tough layer of extraperitoneal tissue.

The **muscular layer** consists of a complete outer, longitudinal layer, and an inner, thicker, circular layer of smooth muscle. It is sometimes stated that both these layers are spirally arranged, but this cannot be determined with certainty in a sheet of small, spindle-shaped muscle fibres. The layers are separated by a plexus of nerve cells and fibres, the **myenteric plexus**, in a little connective tissue. The plexus causes contraction of the muscle layers which together produce a peristaltic wave.

The **submucous layer** consists of areolar tissue containing blood and lymph vessels and the **submucous plexus** of the nerve cells and fibres.

The **mucous layer** is very different from that of the stomach. The functions of the small intestine are to complete digestion and to absorb from the fluid contents. The maximum area for absorption is achieved by three structural arrangements.

1. There are permanent **circular folds** of the whole thickness of the mucous membrane, including the muscularis mucosae [Figs. 157, 159].

2. The internal surface is covered with minute leaf-shaped or finger-shaped projections (**villi**, 0.5 mm or less in length). These are visible with a hand lens and give the mucous membrane a velvety appearance. Each villus contains a central lymph vessel (**lacteal**), a capillary loop, and some longitudinal smooth **muscle fibres** which allow it to contract and relax and may aid in the discharge of lymph from the lacteal [Fig. 158].

3. Each of the columnar cells which cover the villi as a single layer has a **brush border** of minute villous processes on its free surface. These microvilli are only clearly visible under the electron microscope, but greatly increase the surface area of the cells.

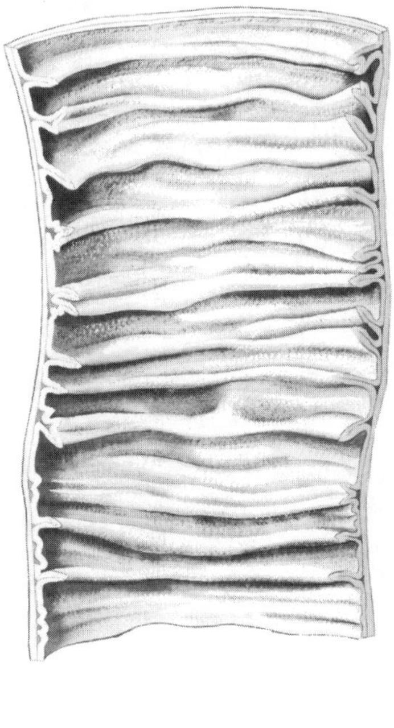

Fig. 157. A part of the interior of the jejunum to show the numerous circular folds of its lining. Cf. Fig. 146.

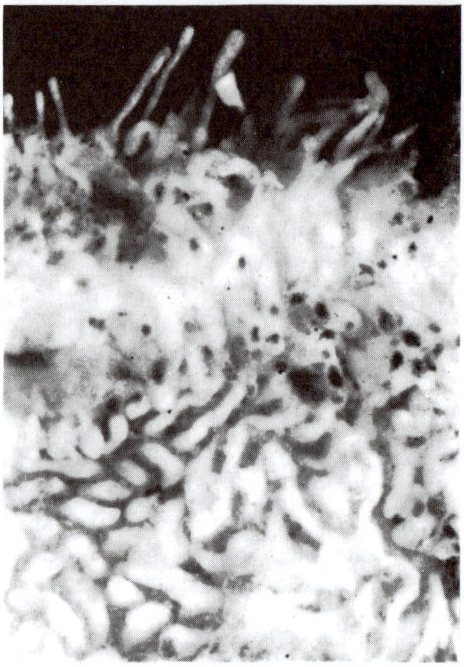

Fig. 158. A photograph of the surface of the mucous membrane of the human duodenum. Note the long villi which project from the entire surface, but which are only clearly seen at the edge.

Between the villi are **crypts**. These simple tubular glands dip into the mucous membrane. In the upper part of the duodenum there are complex **mucous glands** which extend from the crypts into the submucosa. Their alkaline mucus plays an important part in the neutralization of the acid in the stomach contents passed into the duodenum. Elsewhere the crypts are limited to the mucous membrane. The epithelial cells in the depths of the crypts show a high level of mitotic activity. Radioactive tracer techniques allow the cells formed here to be followed from the crypts, over the surfaces of the villi, to the tips of the villi where they are shed. In this way the entire epithelial lining of the small intestine is replaced every two to four days.

In addition to the absorptive cells, there are many **goblet cells** on the villi. These discharge their mucus content to protect the surface and reduce friction.

The mucous membrane also contains aggregations of lymph tissue. Many

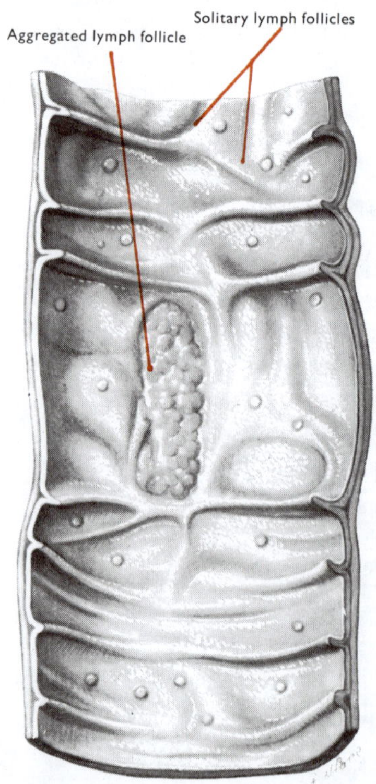

Fig. 159. The internal surface of part of the ileum for comparison with Fig. 157. Note the small, sparse, circular folds and the solitary and aggregated lymph follicles.

are **solitary lymph follicles** 1–2 mm in diameter, but large **aggregated lymph follicles** are occasionally found, especially on the antimesenteric wall of the ileum [Fig. 159].

Dissection

Examine the jejunum and ileum. Note the greater diameter and thickness of the jejunum, the smaller amount of fat in its mesentery, and the fact that the lumen is usually empty.

Tie a pair of ligatures round the jejunum close to the duodenojejunal flexure and another pair around the ileum close to the caecum. Cut through the small intestine between each pair of ligatures and remove it by dividing the mesentery close to the intestine. Wash out the piece of intestine with water. Remove a few inches of the jejunum and open it longitudinally. Pin this out flat and remove the peritoneal coat to expose the longitudinal muscle layer. On the mucosal surface, note the folds of mucous membrane which are not removed by stretching the intestinal wall. Identify the villi with a hand lens.

Strip the mucous membrane and submucosa from the wall of the intestine to expose the circular muscle layer.

Open the entire length of the remaining part of the intestine by a longitudinal cut and note the gradual change in structure of the mucous membrane along its length. The **circular folds** become progressively smaller and less numerous from the duodenum to the terminal ileum where they are missing. The **villi** are larger and more numerous in the jejunum than in the ileum, but the ileum contains aggregated lymph follicles. These are best seen in children and when viewed by transmitted light, but are difficult to demonstrate when atrophied in the aged.

The large intestine

[Figs. 132, 163, 164]

The large intestine extends from the caecum in the right iliac fossa to the anus in the perineum, and surrounds the centrally placed small intestine. It is much shorter (1.5 m) than the small intestine and decreases in diameter from the caecum to the descending colon. All parts of it are capable of considerable distention.

The large intestine consists of the caecum and appendix vermiformis; the ascending, transverse, and descending parts of the colon which meet at the right and left flexures; the sigmoid colon; the rectum; and the anal canal.

Caecum

This blind end of the large intestine is in the right iliac fossa. It is approximately 5–7 cm in length and width. Superiorly it joins the ascending colon and terminal ileum [Fig. 160]. It lies on the iliacus and psoas muscles and on the nerves (genitofemoral, femoral, and lateral cutaneous) and blood vessels (testicular or ovarian) anterior to them. It frequently overlaps the external iliac artery, and being relatively mobile, may lie in the lesser pelvis. The caecum is almost surrounded by peritoneum [Fig. 161], but is frequently

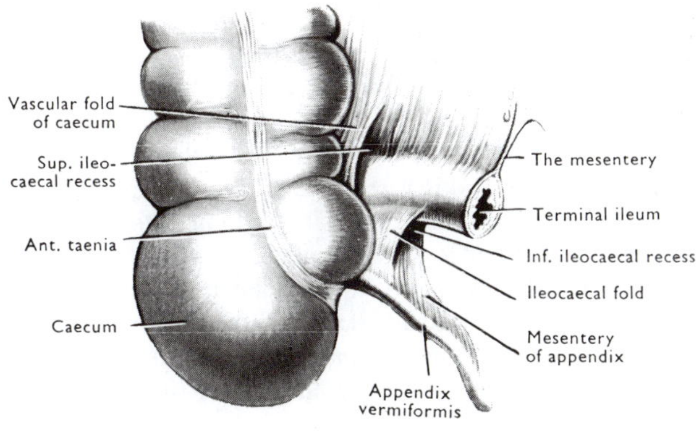

Fig. 160. The anterior surface of the ileocaecal region.

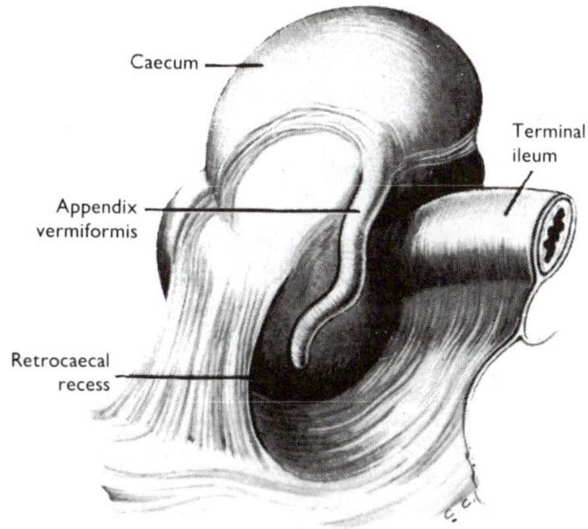

Fig. 161. The inferior surface of the ileocaecal region. The caecum has been pulled forwards to open the retrocaecal recess in which the appendix vermiformis commonly lies.

attached by it to the iliac fossa laterally and medially. This produces a wide, **retrocaecal peritoneal recess** which may ascend posterior to the inferior part of the ascending colon. The appendix vermiformis frequently lies in this recess. Rarely the caecum may lie at the level of the right colic flexure; the ascending colon is then absent.

Vermiform appendix

This is a narrow (approximately 5 mm) blind tube of very variable length (5–15 cm). It is suspended by a small extension of *the* mesentery which descends posterior to the terminal ileum. The base of the appendix is attached to the posteromedial surface of the caecum 2–3 cm inferolateral to the ileocaecal junction. The appendix is very variable in *position*. Frequently it lies in the retrocaecal recess, but may extend into the lesser pelvis to lie close to the ovary, uterine tube, and ureter [Fig. 236].

The appendix has the same peritoneal and muscle coats as the small intestine. At the base, the longitudinal muscle is continuous with the three **taeniae** of the caecum and colon [Fig. 162]. The mucous membrane consists mainly of **lymph follicles** partly separated by **crypts** of the columnar epithelial lining which contains many goblet cells. When swollen it readily blocks the lumen of the appendix.

Vessels and nerves

The caecum and appendix are supplied by the **ileocolic artery**. The appendicular artery passes in its mesentery posterior to the terminal ileum. **Lymph vessels** pass to nodes in the mesentery of the appendix and to others scattered along the ileocolic artery on which nerves from the **superior mesenteric plexus** reach caecum and appendix.

Dissection

Turn the caecum upwards and uncover the structures posterior to it. Trace the three taeniae on the external surface of the colon and caecum to the root of the appendix. Cut away the lateral wall of the caecum and examine the ileal and appendicular orifices.

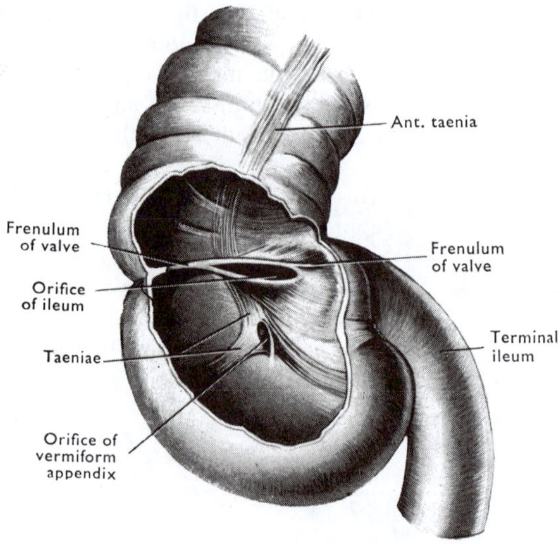

Fig. 162. A dried distended caecum opened to show the ileocaecal orifice and valve.

Ileocaecal orifice

This is very variable in appearance in the cadaver. Normally the ileum enters obliquely through a horizontal slit and is partly invaginated into the caecum to form folds (**ileocaecal valve**) above and below the opening. Medially and laterally these folds meet in single ridges, the **frenula of the valve** [Fig. 162]. The muscle in the valve is poorly developed and probably plays little part in preventing reflux of caecal contents into the ileum. Reflux is prevented by contraction of the circular muscle of the ileum and by the tightening of the frenula which draws the lips of the valve together when the caecum is distended.

Ascending colon

The ascending colon is 12–120 cm long. It begins in the right iliac fossa at the entry of the ileum. It ascends on iliacus, the iliac crest, and quadratus lumborum in the paravertebral gutter, crossing the **lateral cutaneous nerve of**

the thigh, and the **ilioinguinal** and **iliohypogastric nerves**. It ends in the right flexure which turns sharply to the left on the lower part of the right kidney, posterior to the liver [Fig. 191].

Peritoneum covers the front and sides of the ascending colon and binds it to the posterior abdominal wall, but sometimes there is a short mesentery. Anterior to the ascending colon is the anterior abdominal wall, but the greater omentum and small intestine may intervene.

Vessels and nerves

The ascending colon and right flexure are supplied by the **ileocolic** and **right colic arteries** which transmit nerves from the **superior mesenteric plexus. Lymph vessels** end in nodes on the medial side of the colon and along its vessels.

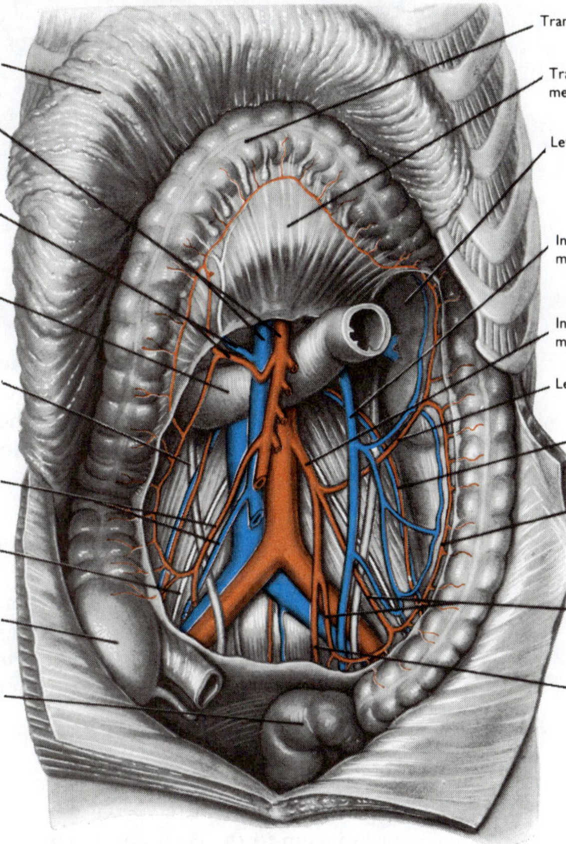

Fig. 163. Structures on the posterior wall of the infracolic compartment of the abdomen. The greater omentum and transverse colon are turned upwards, and the jejunum, ileum, *the* mesentery, and peritoneum covering the posterior wall are removed. See also Figs. 132, 166, and 199.

Transverse colon

This is usually the longest (40–50 cm) and most mobile part of the colon. It extends between the right and left flexures and forms a dependent loop between them. The lowest part may reach well below the umbilicus in the erect position, but is usually just superior to it in the recumbent position. If the intestines are distended, the transverse colon may be pushed superiorly. Occasionally it passes anterior to the stomach. If distended with gas, it may mask the dullness of the liver to percussion and mimic the presence of gas in the peritoneal cavity.

The transverse colon is suspended by the transverse mesocolon. This is fused to the posterior surface of the greater omentum [Fig. 137] except at the short extremities of the mesocolon [Figs. 138, 149]. The **transverse mesocolon** ascends from the colon to be attached to the descending part of the duodenum, the head and lower margin of the body of the pancreas, and the anterior surface of the left kidney [Fig. 138]. It contains the middle colic vessels and branches of the right and left colic vessels with their accompanying nerves and lymph vessels.

The transverse colon begins anterior to the descending part of the duodenum and the head of the pancreas, and posterior to the liver and the fundus of the gall-bladder. It then descends anterior to the coils of small intestine, and ascends on the left to the **left flexure**. Here it is anterior to the

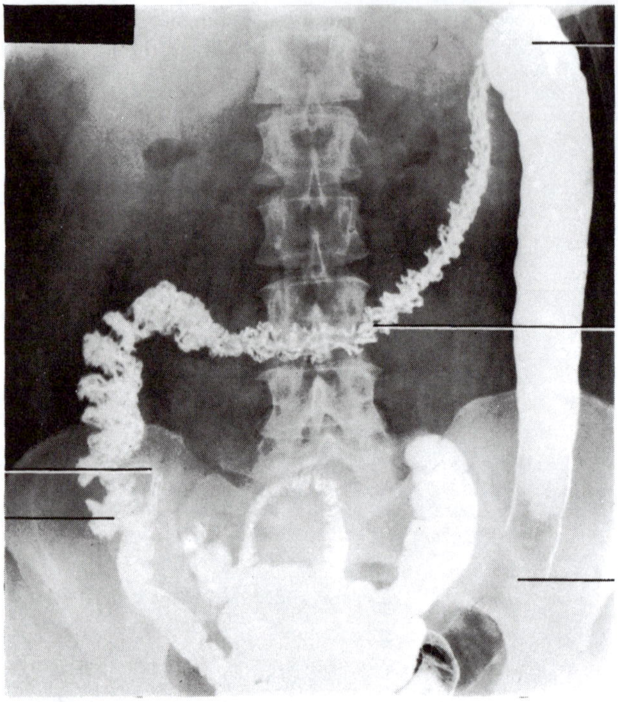

Fig. 164. A radiograph of the partly emptied colon outlined by barium introduced as an enema. The narrow, irregular parts of the lumen are produced by contraction of the muscles of the colon.

left margin of the **left kidney**, immediately inferior to the **spleen**, and posterior to the left margin of the greater omentum. This flexure lies at a higher level, is more acute, and further lateral than the right flexure. It is attached to the diaphragm by peritoneum (**phrenicocolic ligament**) and occasionally has a short mesentery.

Vessels and nerves

The transverse colon is mainly supplied by the **middle colic** vessels, but its extremities and the flexures also receive blood from the **right** or **left colic arteries**. Nerves accompany all these arteries. Those on the right and middle colic arteries (**superior mesenteric plexus**) transmit sympathetic and vagal nerve fibres; those on the left colic artery (**inferior mesenteric plexus**) carry sympathetic and pelvic parasympathetic nerve fibres. **Lymph vessels** and nodes lie on the arteries.

Descending colon

The descending colon passes from the left flexure to the margin of the superior aperture of the pelvis near the inguinal ligament. It is attached by peritoneum to the posterior abdominal wall in the left paravertebral gutter and iliac fossa. At first anterior to the lateral surface of the left kidney and medial to the diaphragm, it descends on transversus abdominis and quadratus lumborum to the iliac crest, anterior to the same nerves as the ascending colon [p. 143]. It continues in the left iliac fossa on iliacus to the anterior superior iliac spine. Here it turns medially, superior to the inguinal ligament, and lies on the femoral nerve, psoas, the testicular vessels, and the genitofemoral nerve, and joins the sigmoid colon anterior to the external iliac vessels [Fig. 163].

The pressure of the lowest part of the descending colon on the testicular and external iliac veins may be a factor in the greater frequency of varicose veins in the spermatic cord and lower limb on the left side.

Vessels and nerves

The blood supply is by the **left colic** and **upper sigmoid** branches of the inferior mesenteric vessels. These are accompanied by branches of the **inferior mesenteric plexus** and the corresponding lymph vessels and nodes [Figs. 199, 200].

Dissection

Divide the peritoneum along the lateral margin of the descending colon. Turn the colon medially to expose the structures posterior to it.

Sigmoid colon

This part of the colon varies in length from 15 to 80 cm. It extends from the end of the descending colon to the pelvic surface of the third piece of the sacrum where it joins the rectum. Usually it lies free in the lesser pelvis inferior to the small intestine; when long, it may extend into any part of the abdomen which the length of its mesentery (sigmoid mesocolon) permits.

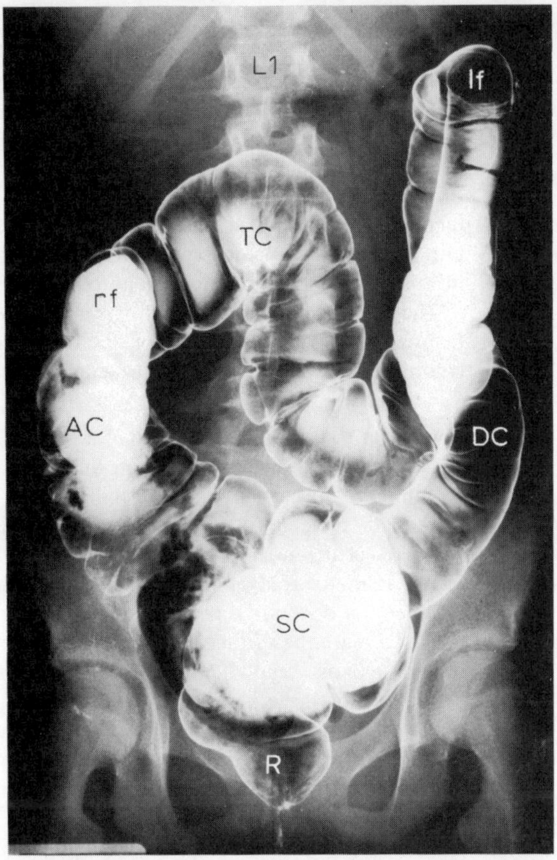

Fig. 165. Double-contrast (X-ray-opaque medium and air) radiograph of the distended large intestine. The caecum is partly hidden by the sigmoid colon [cf. Fig. 164]. This technique outlines the mucous membrane and allows changes, e.g. early cancers, to be seen anywhere on its surface.
AC, ascending colon.
DC, descending colon.
lf, left flexure of colon.
R, rectum.
rf, right flexure of colon.
SC, sigmoid colon.

The **sigmoid mesocolon** has a $\wedge$-shaped attachment. It begins at the end of the descending colon and ascends on the external iliac vessels to the middle of the common iliac artery. Here it turns sharply downwards and to the right across the lesser pelvis to the third piece of the sacrum [Fig. 138]. Just lateral to the apex of the $\wedge$, a pocket-like extension of the peritoneal cavity (**intersigmoid peritoneal recess**) passes upwards, posterior to the root of the mesocolon, in front of the left ureter. The **inferior mesenteric artery** divides near the apex of the $\wedge$, the superior rectal artery entering the right limb of the mesentery, the sigmoid arteries the left limb. Rarely the mesocolon begins at the iliac crest and runs directly to the third piece of the sacrum. In this case the sigmoid colon could be said to start at the iliac crest where the blood supply by the sigmoid arteries begins.

Taeniae coli

These three ribbon-like thickenings of the otherwise thin longitudinal muscle of the caecum and colon arise from the longitudinal muscle at the root of the appendix vermiformis, and end by spreading out in the terminal part of the sigmoid colon to become continuous with the longitudinal muscle of the rectum (q.v.). They are uniformly spaced around the circumference of the colon. Between them the wall of the colon and caecum bulges outwards forming three rows of puckered pouches (**sacculations**). In the ascending and descending parts of the colon the taeniae are anterior, posteromedial, and posterolateral. In the transverse colon, which is turned down, the corresponding positions are posterior, superior, and anterior.

Lymph nodes of large intestine

Small nodes lie near the marginal artery and along the arteries passing to it. The lymph draining through these nodes on the branches of the superior mesenteric artery passes to the **intestinal trunk** in the root of *the* **mesentery**. That draining with the inferior mesenteric artery enters the **lumbar lymph nodes** beside the aorta. Both reach the cisterna chyli [Fig. 200].

Dissection

Cut through the colon between ligatures at the junction of the descending and sigmoid parts. Remove the caecum and colon in one piece, dividing the peritoneum and blood vessels close to them.

Wash out the colon, examine its external surface, and open it longitudinally. Cut a transverse section through the appendix vermiformis, examine the cut surface with a hand lens.

Structure of large intestine

The same layers are present as in the stomach and small intestine.

The peritoneum, or **serous layer**, is firmly bound to the muscle but is an incomplete covering in the ascending and descending colon and the upper part of the **rectum** which are applied to the abdominal and pelvic walls. The inferior third of the rectum has no contact with the peritoneum.

The **appendices epiploicae** are small projecting pouches of peritoneum filled with fat. They are numerous on the sigmoid and transverse parts of the colon, but are absent from the caecum, appendix, and rectum.

Muscle layers

There is a thin, outer, longitudinal layer which is thickened in the taeniae. This layer is uniform and thick in the appendix and nearly uniform in the rectum and anal canal. The internal, circular layer is nearly uniform, but is thickened between the sacculations and especially where it forms the **internal sphincter of the anus**.

The **submucous layer** is similar to that in the ileum.

Mucosa

When not distended, the **mucous layer** forms a number of crescentic folds which increase the surface area for absorption. It consists of numerous simple tubular **glands** (crypts) united by very delicate connective tissue which is permeated by large numbers of cells of the lymphocyte series. They are so placed as to come into immediate contact with bacteria which may enter through abrasions of the epithelium. (The contents of the large intestine, unlike those of the upper parts of the small intestine, contain large numbers of bacteria.) Many small, **solitary lymph follicles** bulge the mucous membrane, but neither villi nor aggregated lymph follicles are present.

Vermiform appendix, see page 142.

Dissection

Expose the anterior surface of the pancreas and define the limits of the gland. Trace the duodenum from the pylorus to the duodeno-jejunal flexure.

Duodenum

This is the widest and most fixed part of the small intestine. It is approximately 25 cm long, bent in a C-shaped curve. The concavity faces upwards and to the left and is filled by the pancreas. It lies astride the vertebral column, and extends posteriorly on to the medial aspect of the right kidney in the paravertebral gutter [Figs. 138, 191]. The duodenum connects the supracolic and infracolic parts of the gut tube by passing posterior to the transverse mesocolon.

The **superior part** of the duodenum passes upwards, backwards, and to the right from the pylorus. Superior to the pancreas, it lies anterior to the portal vein (the gastroduodenal artery and bile-duct intervening) and the inferior vena cava, and then crosses their right sides. It lies posterior to the quadrate lobe of the liver, and ascends to the level of the neck of the gall-bladder. Here it turns sharply downwards to form the descending part. The superior part is approximately 5 cm long but appears much shorter (**duodenal cap**) in an anteroposterior radiograph because of its oblique direction [Fig. 148]. The first half has the greater and lesser omenta attached to it and is free to move with the stomach. The second half has no mesentery.

The **descending part** is 8 cm long and has no mesentery. It lies directly on the medial part of the right kidney and on psoas major (anterior to the renal vessels and ureter) down to the level of the third lumbar vertebra. At first posterior to the liver and **gall-bladder**, it passes posterior to the beginning of

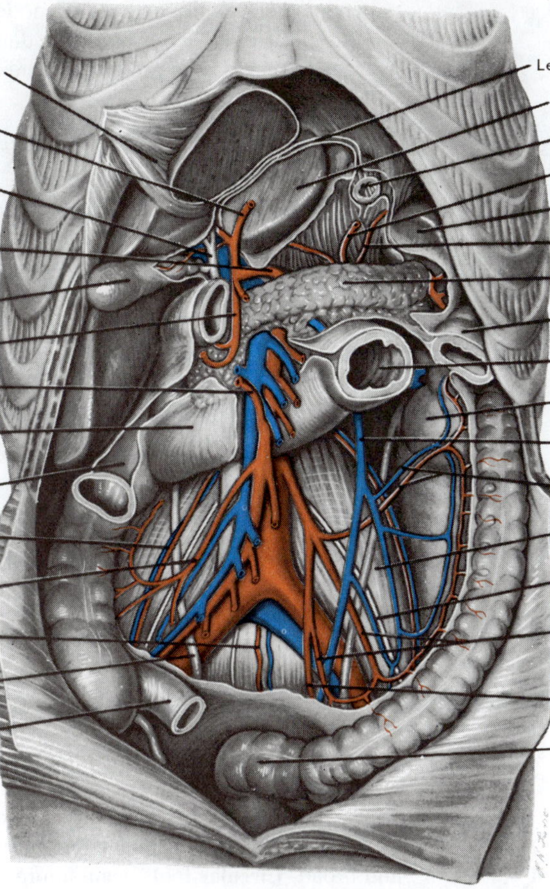

Fig. 166. Structures on the posterior abdominal wall.

the transverse colon to lie behind the jejunum in the infracolic compartment [Fig. 166]. Medially it is applied to the head of the pancreas, and two-thirds of the way along its length, the **bile** and **main pancreatic ducts** enter its posteromedial aspect together [Fig. 173].

The **horizontal part**, also adherent to the posterior abdominal wall, is nearly 10 cm long. It passes horizontally to the left, inferior to the pancreas and anterior to the right psoas muscle and vertebral column and the structures lying on them, i.e. the right ureter and testicular or ovarian artery, the inferior vena cava, and the aorta with the inferior mesenteric artery arising from it. The anterior and inferior surfaces are covered with peritoneum except where the root of *the* mesentery containing the superior mesenteric vessels crosses it anteriorly [Fig. 163].

The short **ascending part** passes upwards on the left psoas muscle to the left of the aorta and the head of the pancreas, lying anterior to the left sympathetic trunk and testicular or ovarian artery [Fig. 163]. It bends anteriorly (**duodenojejunal flexure**) 2–3 cm to the left of the median plane at the level of the second lumbar vertebra.

The position of the duodenum is variable. The first half of the superior part is very mobile. The horizontal part may pass to the duodenojejunal flexure without a recognizable ascending part, and the entire duodenum may lie at a higher or lower level.

Vessels and nerves

The superior part receives small branches from the **proper hepatic** (supraduodenal), **right gastric, right gastro-epiploic**, and **gastroduodenal** (retroduodenal) **arteries**. These anastomose poorly with each other and are said not to cross the pylorus to anastomose with the gastric vessels. The remainder of the duodenum is supplied by the superior and inferior **pancreaticoduodenal arteries**. These form arcades anterior and posterior to the head of the pancreas [pp. 129, 135]. Occasionally this anastomosis may replace the hepatic artery.

The **lymph vessels** drain to nodes that lie between the duodenum and pancreas. Thence drainage is to nodes on the coeliac trunk or superior mesenteric artery. Nerves reach the duodenum from the **coeliac** and **superior mesenteric plexuses** on the corresponding arteries.

Dissection

Divide the peritoneum along the right side of the descending part of the duodenum and turn it on to the anterior surface of the pancreas. Define the structures thus exposed. Replace the duodenum and remove the peritoneum and fat surrounding the ascending part. This exposes the **inferior mesenteric vein** lateral to the ascending part, the superior mesenteric vessels medial to it, and part of the left renal vein superior to it. A slender fibromuscular band may be seen passing from the superior surface of the duodenojejunal flexure to the right crus of the diaphragm. This is the **suspensory muscle of the duodenum.** It descends from the region of the oesophageal orifice, lying on the left crus and posterior to the pancreas and inferior mesenteric vein. It is large in the child, but difficult to define in the adult.

Open the entire length of the duodenum by cutting along its convex surface. Clean the interior to expose the mucosal surface.

Structure of duodenum

The duodenum has the same four layers as the other parts of the intestine.

The **serous**, peritoneal layer is incomplete except in the first 2–3 cm.

The **muscular layers** are the same as in the rest of the small intestine.

The **submucous layer** is thick and contains compound, mucous, **duodenal glands**, especially in the proximal third of the duodenum. The glands appear as reddish-grey bodies approximately 1 mm in diameter when the serous and muscle layers are carefully removed. They secrete an alkaline mucus through ducts which pierce the muscularis mucosae and enter the duodenal crypts.

The **mucous layer** is similar to that of the jejunum, but the **villi** are short and broad. **Circular folds** begin approximately 2 cm from the pylorus. They are small and irregular, but become large and numerous further distally. The **bile** and **pancreatic ducts** open by a common orifice on the **greater duodenal papilla**. This lies at the proximal end of a longitudinal fold on the posteromedial wall below the middle of the descending part, often covered by a circular fold [Fig. 167]. The papilla and longitudinal folds are variable in size and may be difficult to find. It is important to recognize the papilla because it can be catheterized under direct vision using a duodenal endoscope. The bile or pancreatic duct may then be filled with X-ray-opaque material. The position will be confirmed when the ducts are traced to the duodenum.

The **lesser duodenal papilla** is where the accessory pancreatic duct enters the descending part of the duodenum. The papilla is smaller and more difficult to find than the greater papilla, but lies superior and anterior to it.

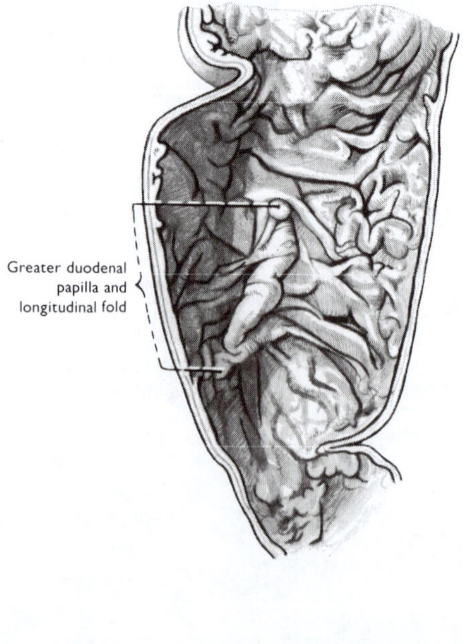

Fig. 167. The internal surface of the posterior wall of the descending part of the duodenum. The greater duodenal papilla lies at the upper end of the longitudinal fold, and is hooded by a circular fold.

Dissection

Lift the tail of the pancreas from the spleen, and ease the body from the posterior abdominal wall. Identify the **splenic vein** on the posterior surface of the pancreas, and follow it to its junction with the superior mesenteric vein to form the portal vein. Trace the **inferior mesenteric vein.** It usually enters the splenic vein, but may enter the beginning of the portal vein or the superior mesenteric vein. Follow the superior mesenteric vessels upwards, anterior to the uncinate process of the pancreas and posterior to the junction of its body and head. Follow the portal vein downwards to the junction of splenic and superior mesenteric veins.

Portal vein

[Figs. 168, 285, 286]

This vein drains the abdominal and pelvic parts of the alimentary canal (except the lowest part of the rectum and anal canal), the spleen, pancreas, and gall-bladder direct to the porta hepatis of the liver—hence its name. Here it branches to discharge into the sinusoids (large-diameter capillaries) of the liver. Such venous systems uniting two groups of capillaries elsewhere in the body are called **portal venous systems** after this the largest of them.

The portal vein begins posterior to the junction of the body and head of the pancreas by the union of the **splenic** and **superior mesenteric veins**. As it ascends posterior to the superior part of the duodenum, it receives a **pancreaticoduodenal vein** and then the right and left **gastric veins** as it enters the free edge of the lesser omentum. It ascends in this edge and divides into right and left branches which pass into the porta hepatis. The **right branch** receives the **cystic vein** from the gall-bladder and enters the right lobe of the liver. The **left branch** passes to the left end of the porta hepatis giving branches to the caudate and quadrate lobes and uniting with the **ligamentum teres** and **ligamentum venosum** before entering the left lobe of the liver. Some small, **para-umbilical veins** pass along the ligamentum teres from the left branch to the umbilicus.

The inferior vena cava lies posterior to the entire length of the portal vein, but is separated from it superiorly by the epiploic foramen. The **bile-duct** and first the gastroduodenal and then the **proper hepatic artery** are anterior to the portal vein from the superior part of the duodenum upwards.

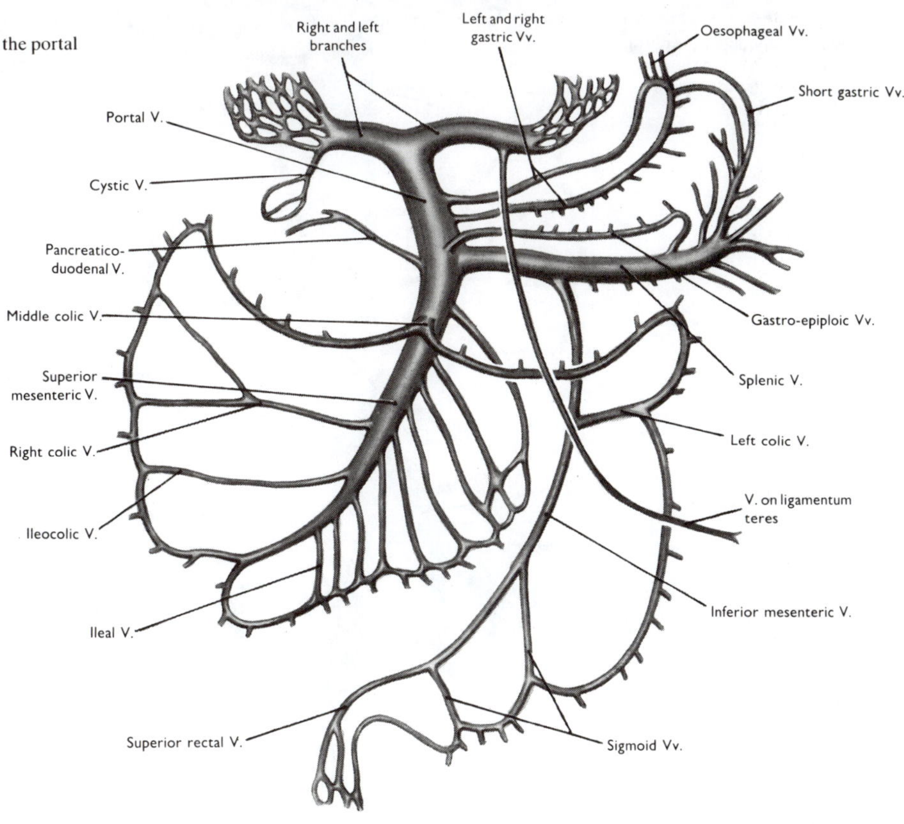

Fig. 168. A diagram of the portal venous system.

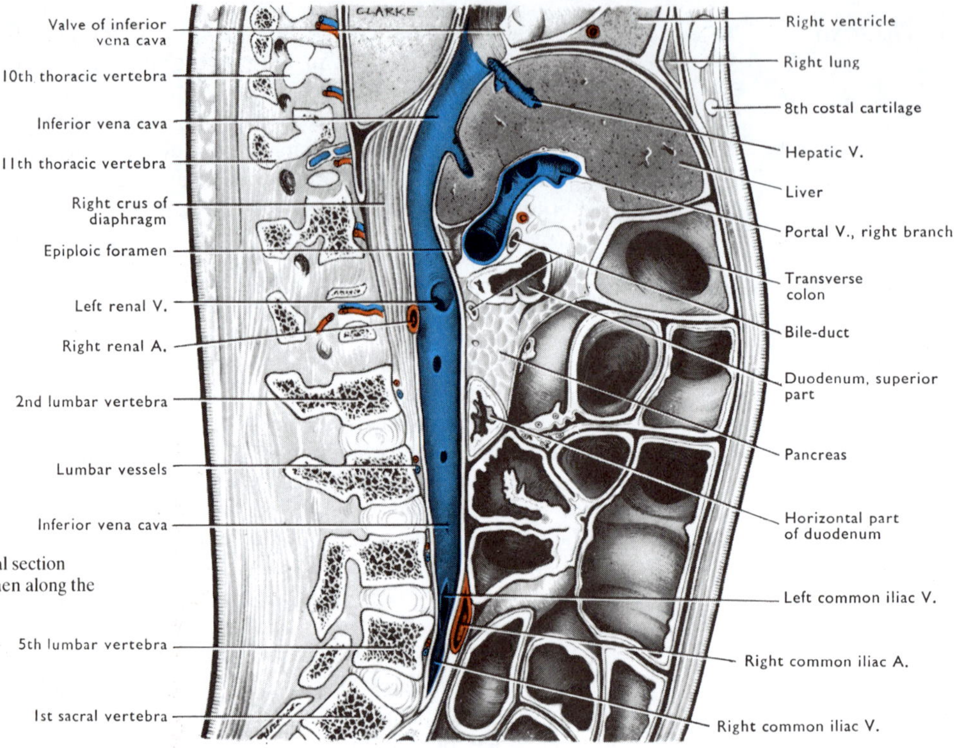

Fig. 169. A sagittal section through the abdomen along the inferior vena cava.

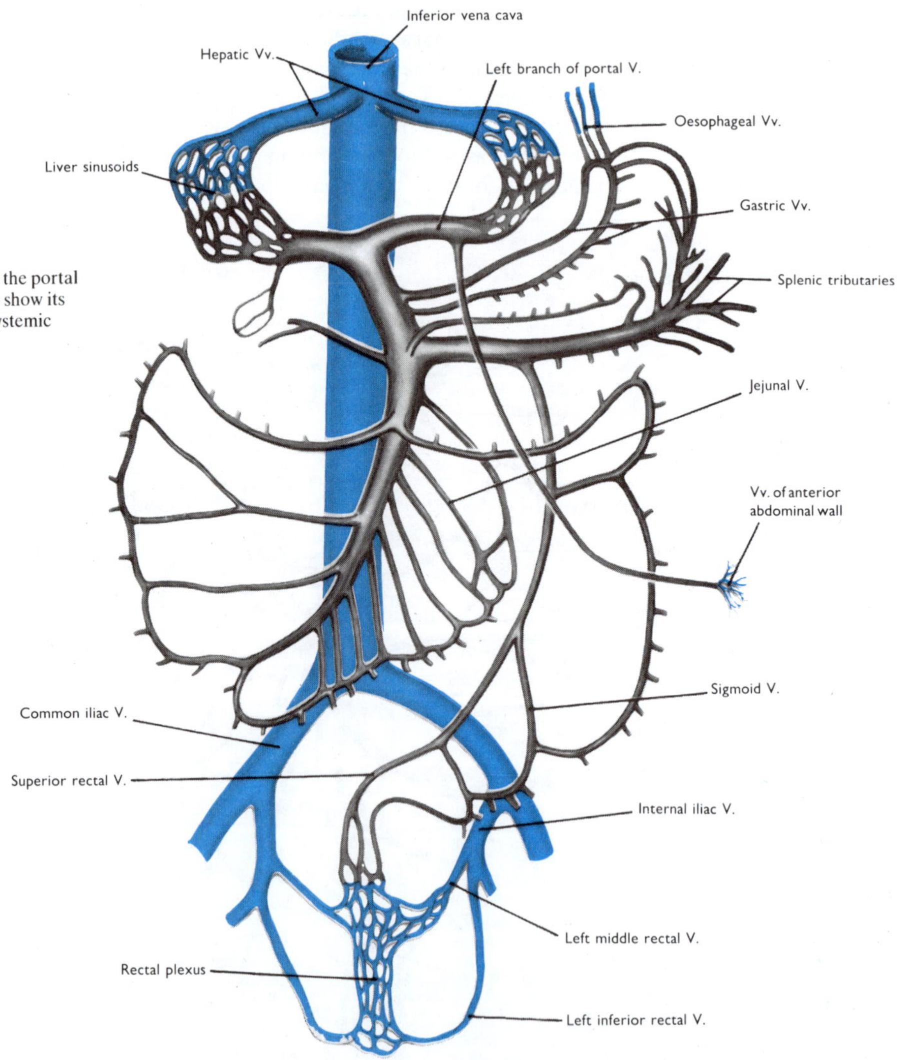

Fig. 170. A diagram of the portal venous system (grey) to show its anastomoses with the systemic venous system (blue).

The portal vein and the hepatic artery discharge their blood into the sinusoids of the liver. Here the blood is separated from the liver cells by a single layer of phagocytic, fenestrated endothelium and a perisinusoidal space [Fig. 171]. The portal vein transports the products of digestion of carbohydrates and proteins from the intestine and of red cell destruction (etc.) from the spleen to the liver. Fats are mostly transported through the lacteals to the thoracic duct.

The tributaries and branches of the portal vein contain up to one-third of the total volume of blood in the body.

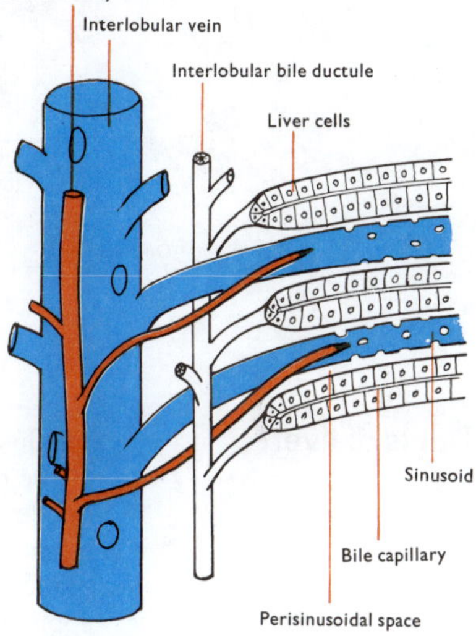

Fig. 171. A diagram to show the relationship of the interlobular branches of the hepatic artery, portal vein, and bile ductule to the liver cells and hepatic sinusoids.

Communications

The portal vein communicates with the systemic system [Fig. 170]: (1) at the gastro-oesophageal junction through the **oesophageal veins**; (2) at the umbilicus through the **para-umbilical veins**; and (3) in the rectum through the **superior rectal vein**. If the portal vein is obstructed, these communications may be greatly enlarged, and bleeding may occur from distended submucous venous plexuses in the lower oesophagus. The back pressure in the tributaries of the portal vein usually causes considerable enlargement of the spleen and may lead to accumulation of fluid in the peritoneal cavity (ascites).

Splenic vein

Five or six tributaries which emerge from the hilus of the spleen form the splenic vein. It passes to the right on the posterior surface of the pancreas, at first in the lienorenal ligament and then on the left kidney, left psoas muscle, left crus of the diaphragm, and the aorta between the origins of the coeliac trunk and superior mesenteric artery. It ends by forming the portal vein with the superior mesenteric vein, anterior to the inferior vena cava.

Tributaries

These correspond to the branches of the splenic artery [p. 125] with the addition of the inferior mesenteric vein which usually joins it near its termination.

Dissection

Free the horizontal part of the duodenum and the uncinate process of the pancreas from the posterior abdominal wall. Turn the descending part of the duodenum and the head of the pancreas to the left. Look for the posterior pancreaticoduodenal vessels and the bile-duct on the head of the pancreas. The **bile-duct** lies in a groove on the posterior surface of the head of the pancreas with the vein on its left side passing to the portal vein. Trace the bile-duct inferiorly from the lesser omentum, and find its union with the pancreatic duct close to the duodenum. Expose the structures posterior to the pancreas.

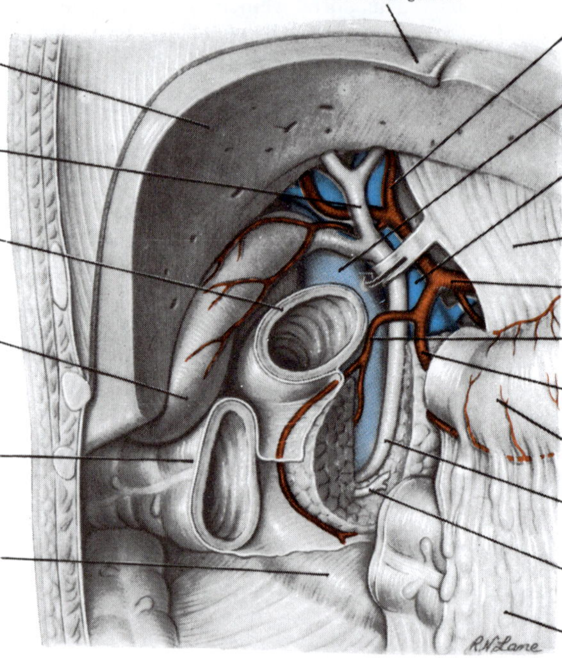

Fig. 172. A dissection to show the extrahepatic biliary system. The arrow indicates the epiploic foramen.

Ducts of liver

The liver is formed as a branching, hollow outgrowth of the epithelial lining of the duodenum. The lumen forms the system of bile-ducts leading to the duodenum. The terminal branches consist of a double row of cells with a minute extension of the lumen, the **bile canaliculus**, between them. These branches form the substance of the liver, and each has blood sinusoids applied to it through which portal venous and hepatic arterial blood passes [Fig. 171]. The bile canaliculi join to form **bile ductules** which, in their turn, form **interlobular ducts**. These unite and emerge from the porta hepatis as the right and left **hepatic ducts**, which join to form the **common hepatic duct** almost immediately. The common hepatic duct is directly continuous with the **bile-duct** where the **cystic duct** from the gall-bladder (a diverticulum of the biliary system) joins it.

Bile produced in the liver either flows directly to the duodenum or enters the gall-bladder when the sphincter on the bile-duct (q.v.) is closed. Bile is concentrated in the gall-bladder.

Bile-duct
[Figs. 181, 286, 287]

This duct is approximately 10 cm long and 0.5 cm wide. It begins by the union of the common hepatic and cystic ducts to the right of the proper hepatic artery, anterior to the portal vein. It descends first in the free edge of the lesser omentum, and then posterior to the superior part of the duodenum where it lies to the right of the gastroduodenal artery. It then deviates slightly to the right in a *groove on the posterior surface of the head of the pancreas*, and enters the posteromedial surface of the descending part of the duodenum a little inferior to its middle.

The duct passes obliquely through the duodenal wall, expanding to form the **ampulla** [Fig. 173] which bulges the mucous membrane of the duodenum inwards (**greater duodenal papilla**) where the duct pierces it. The **pancreatic duct** runs with the bile-duct for a short distance and joins it either before or during its passage through the duodenal wall. Here a **sphincter** of smooth muscle controls the discharge of bile and pancreatic secretions into the duodenum. The strongest part of the sphincter surrounds the bile-duct alone, and lies proximal to the ampulla and the junction with the pancreatic duct. When this contracts, bile passes along the cystic duct to the gall-bladder, but does not enter the pancreatic duct. The remainder of the bile-duct contains very little muscle.

The point of junction of the common hepatic and cystic ducts is very variable, but is usually close to the porta hepatis. The arrangement of the bile- and pancreatic ducts is also variable. Commonly (approx. 30 per cent) they do not join but open together on the greater duodenal papilla [Fig. 174].

Dissection

Turn the tail and body of the pancreas to the right stripping the splenic artery and vein from its posterior surface and identify the vessels passing to the gland from them. Ease the superior mesenteric vessels, portal vein, and gastroduodenal artery from the pancreas, identifying and then dividing their glandular branches or tributaries. Divide the bile-duct near the superior part of the duodenum, and remove the duodenum and pancreas in one piece.

On the posterior surface of the pancreas, make a cut into the gland parallel and close to the superior and inferior margins of the body. Pick away the lobules of the gland between the cuts to expose the greyish-white duct. Trace the duct in both directions [Fig. 173] taking care to expose the accessory duct and its tributaries in the head of the pancreas. Follow both ducts to the duodenum and identify their openings on the internal surface of the duodenum.

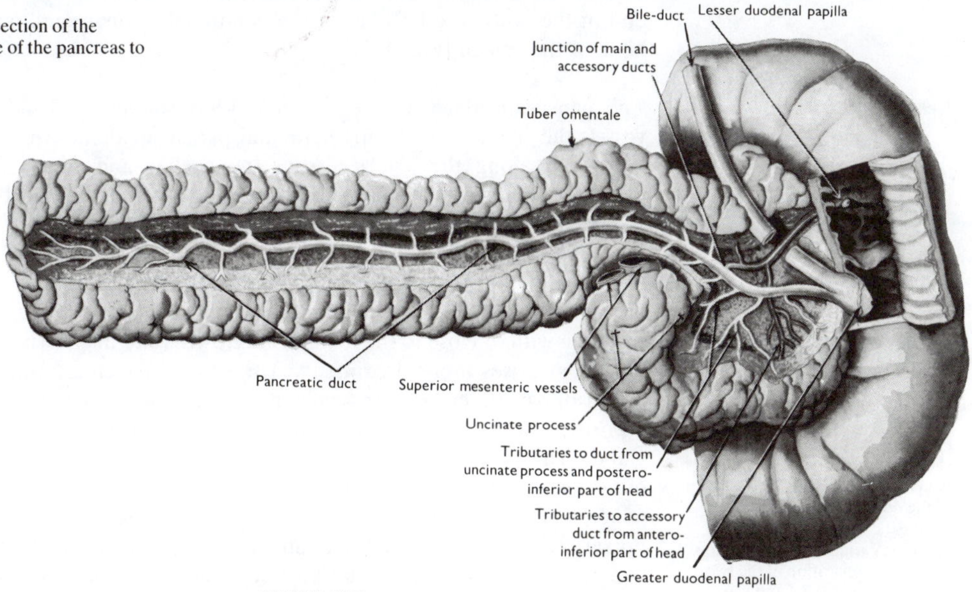

Fig. 173. A dissection of the posterior surface of the pancreas to show its ducts.

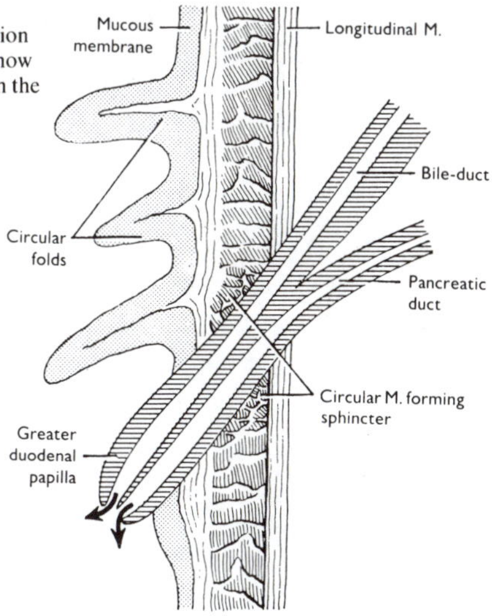

Fig. 174. A diagrammatic section through the duodenal wall to show one arrangement of the ducts in the greater duodenal papilla.

Pancreas

[Figs. 285–287]

This elongated gland lies across the upper part of the posterior abdominal wall from the duodenum to the spleen, at the junction of the supracolic and infracolic compartments of the peritoneal cavity. It is a compound gland whose *exocrine part* secretes a number of different enzymes that break down proteins, carbohydrates, and fats in the alkaline conditions of the duodenum. The *endocrine part* consists of minute islands (**islets**) of cells which are not connected with the duct system, but secrete insulin and glucagon directly into the blood stream for the control of blood sugar level, etc.

The gland consists of lobules of secretory tissue held loosely together with delicate areolar tissue, and is very pliable in life.

The expanded **head** lies in the concavity of the duodenum, overlapping the descending and horizontal parts. The head is anterior to the inferior vena cava [Fig. 169], to the bile-duct which grooves its superolateral part, and to the aorta where its inferomedial extension (**uncinate process**) passes posterior to the superior mesenteric vessels. The head is crossed anteriorly by the transverse colon or its mesentery, and superiorly by the first 2–3 cm of the duodenum, and joins the body, anterior to the formation of the portal vein.

The **body** passes to the left across the aorta (anterior to the superior mesenteric artery) the left crus of the diaphragm, psoas major, and the left renal vessels and kidney [Fig. 128]. It is posterior to the omental bursa and stomach, but its tuber omentale is in contact with the lesser omentum immediately inferior to the coeliac trunk, whence the **splenic artery** runs a sinuous course along its upper margin. The splenic vein lies on its posterior surface and is joined by the inferior and superior mesenteric veins. The blunt end of the body, the **tail**, lies in the lienorenal ligament and may touch the hilus of the spleen [Fig. 142].

Vessels and nerves

The **pancreaticoduodenal arteries** and **veins** supply the head, the **splenic vessels** the remainder. Sympathetic and parasympathetic **nerve fibres** reach the gland along the arteries from the coeliac and superior mesenteric plexuses. **Lymph nodes** lie along the superior border of the pancreas (pancreaticosplenic nodes) and on the pancreaticoduodenal arteries.

Ducts

Developmentally the pancreas arises as two separate, hollow, branching outgrowths from the duodenum. The smaller (ventral pancreas) arises in common with or close to the hepatic outgrowth (bile-duct). The other (dorsal pancreas) arises more proximally. The ventral pancreas, which forms the posterior part of the head and uncinate process, passes with the bile-duct into a position dorsal to the dorsal pancreas which forms the remainder of the gland. The two rudiments now fuse, and their ducts, the stems of the outgrowths, communicate in the gland so that the duct of the ventral pancreas forms the duodenal end of the main duct while the duct of the dorsal pancreas forms the remainder. The duodenal end of the dorsal pancreatic duct remains as the accessory duct which usually communicates with the main duct and opens into the duodenum 2–3 cm proximal to that duct [Fig. 175].

Fig. 175. (a, b, c, d) A diagram to show the formation of the adult pancreas and its ducts by the fusion of the dorsal and ventral pancreatic outgrowths in the embryo. Variations in the degree of fusion and separation of the two ducts account for the different arrangements of the main and accessory pancreatic ducts in the adult.

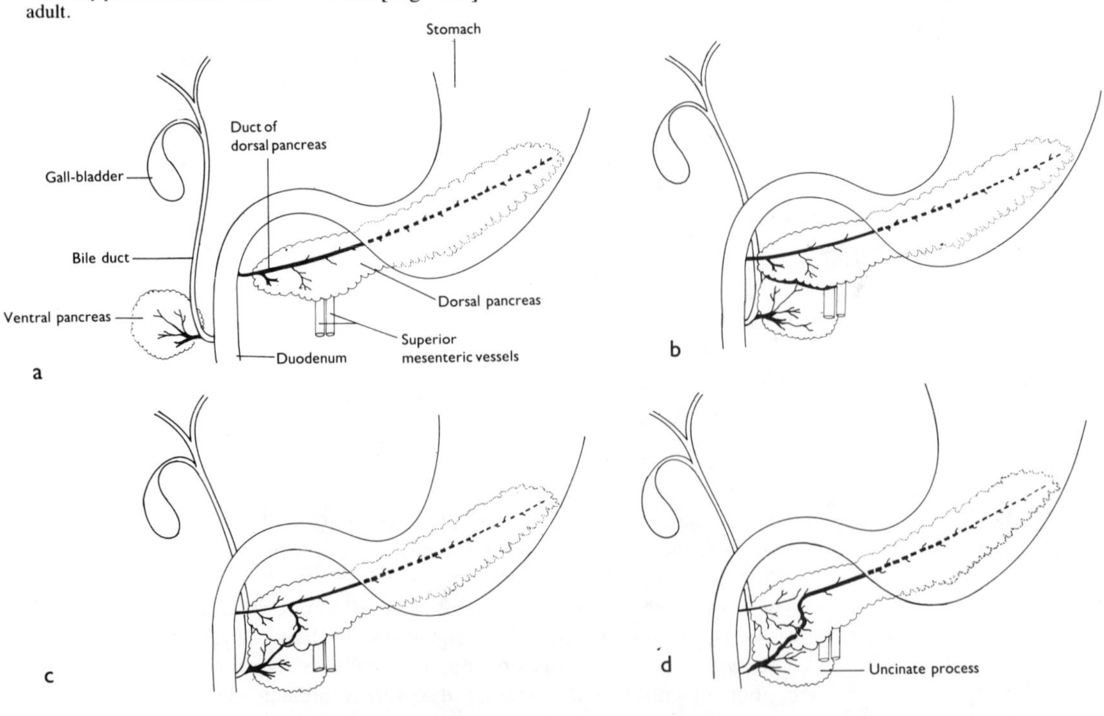

The **main duct** begins in the tail, runs through the body slightly superior to the centre, and receives small tributaries throughout. At the head it bends inferiorly, usually communicates with the accessory duct, and then drains the uncinate process and posterior part of the head of the pancreas. It then usually joins the bile-duct as it pierces the duodenal wall [Fig. 173].

The **accessory duct** passes through and receives tributaries from the upper part of the head and from its lower anterior part. Normally the accessory duct connects with the main duct, but it may be entirely separate or simply a tributary of the main duct without separate entry to the duodenum. This is a matter of some importance when the main duct is obstructed at the duodenum, as it may be by a gall-stone impacted in the **hepatopancreatic ampulla**, which is common to both ducts in approximately 50 per cent of individuals.

Where the pancreatic duct joins the bile-duct, weak **sphincters** are found in the pancreatic duct and on the combined channel. The pancreatic sphincter prevents the reflux of bile into the pancreatic duct if the common duct is closed. Sometimes the two ducts are entirely separate at the duodenum.

The liver

[Figs. 176–179, 283–287]

The liver is the largest gland in the body. It is responsible for: (1) metabolizing the products of digestion which reach it through the portal vein (principally degradation products of proteins and carbohydrates); (2) the storage and release of substances (principally glucose) so as to maintain a constant level in the blood; and (3) the synthesis, conjugation, and transformation of substances, e.g. formation of proteins, detoxication of poisonous substances, production of carbohydrates from proteins. All these are *endocrine functions* which alter the composition of the blood traversing the liver, but it also has an *exocrine or secretory function*, the formation of bile. Bile is an important agent in digestion, especially of fats. It is secreted into the bile canaliculi by the liver cells, and contains many substances, the most obvious of which are the bile pigments. These *pigments* are formed from the waste products of red cell destruction which reach the liver from the spleen through the portal vein. Such waste products accumulate in the blood stream (*jaundice*) when the liver cells are damaged by disease and can no longer process them, or are overwhelmed by the amount of them in excessive red cell destruction. Jaundice can also arise from blockage of the biliary tract which prevents excretion of the liver products.

The greater part of the liver lies under cover of the ribs and costal cartilages, and is in contact with the diaphragm which separates it from the pericardium and from the right pleural cavity and lung. With one hand in the pleural cavity and the other in the peritoneal cavity, examine the position of the liver. Note that the liver ascends to the level of the fifth rib in the right mid-clavicular line, filling this dome of the diaphragm and part of the left dome anterior to the stomach. The right lobe of the liver is separated from the costodiaphragmatic recess of the pleura by the diaphragm, but posteriorly the upper part of the right kidney and suprarenal gland intervene between the liver and diaphragm.

Dissection

Pull the liver downwards, and divide the anterior layers of the coronary and left triangular ligaments [p. 122], avoiding injury to the inferior vena cava. Identify the inferior vena cava between the liver and the diaphragm, and strip the liver downwards from it, finding and dividing the hepatic veins entering the inferior vena cava and the remaining peritoneal connections of the liver to the diaphragm. If the inferior vena cava is deeply buried in the liver, divide it and remove a segment with the liver.

The liver is a soft, dark brown, highly vascular organ which is readily torn in abdominal injuries and then causes severe intra-abdominal bleeding. It is approximately 2 per cent of the body weight in the adult, but is proportionately larger (5 per cent of body weight) in the new-born. This partly accounts for the protuberant abdomen in young children.

The shape of the liver is determined by the surrounding organs, but once fixed *in situ*, it retains the shape of a blunt wedge with its rounded base to the right. The liver has two surfaces. (1) The **diaphragmatic surface** is divisible into superior, anterior, right, and posterior parts, which together form the curved surface applied to the diaphragm. (2) The postero-inferior or visceral surface is indistinctly separated from the posterior part of the diaphragmatic surface, but slopes downwards, forwards, and to the right from it to meet its right and anterior parts at a sharp inferior margin.

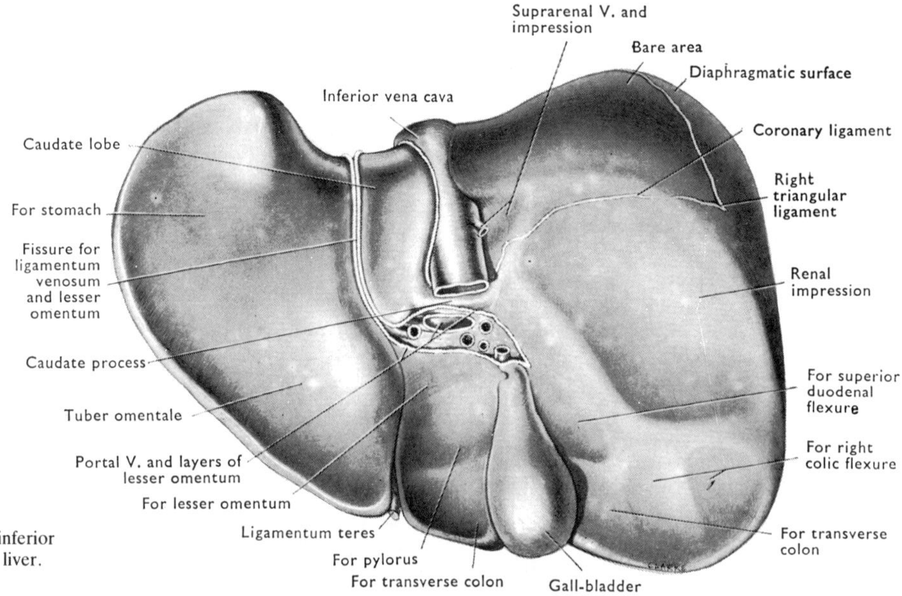

Fig. 176. The postero-inferior (visceral) surface of the liver.

Fissures of liver

A deep fissure extends almost vertically across the visceral surface and posterior part of the diaphragmatic surface. This fissure separates the left lobe of the liver from the **caudate lobe** [Fig. 176] superiorly, and the **quadrate lobe** [Fig. 178] inferiorly. Near its middle, the fissure is continuous with a short transverse fissure (**porta hepatis**) which extends to the right between the caudate and quadrate lobes. The inferior half of the vertical fissure contains the ligamentum teres of the liver (**fissure for ligamentum teres**); the superior half has the upper part of the lesser omentum attached in its depths where the ligamentum venosum lies (**fissure for the ligamentum venosum**). Superiorly, the layers of peritoneum of the **lesser omentum** pass from the fissure directly on to the oesophagus which grooves the liver at this point; inferiorly, they extend to the right to surround the porta hepatis and form the free edge of the lesser omentum at the neck of the gall-bladder [Fig. 176] and enclose the branches of the hepatic artery and portal vein and the hepatic and cystic ducts.

The right margins of the caudate and quadrate lobes are separated from the right lobe of the liver respectively by the **inferior vena cava** in its sulcus and the **gall-bladder** in its fossa. The inferior vena cava does not form a complete right margin for the caudate lobe. Inferiorly, a small strip of the lobe (**caudate process**) extends to the right between the inferior vena cava and the portal vein in the porta hepatis. This caudate process forms the upper wall of the **epiploic foramen** [Fig. 176] and unites the caudate and right lobes of the liver.

The ligamentum teres and the ligamentum venosum are fibrous remnants of the (left) umbilical vein and the ductus venosus of the fetus respectively. These are continuous with each other, and unite with the left branch of the portal vein at the porta hepatis. In the fetus, the ductus venosus is a bypass through which oxygenated umbilical venous blood passes directly to the inferior vena cava and the right atrium without traversing the liver. It curves to the right at the upper border of the caudate lobe to join the inferior vena cava. It is large in the early fetus, but becomes relatively smaller in the later stages when more umbilical blood traverses the liver.

Surfaces of liver

The right part of the **diaphragmatic surface** lies between the seventh and eleventh ribs in the mid-axillary line. The diaphragm separates it from the pleura down to the tenth rib, and from the lung down to the eighth rib in quiet respiration.

The anterior part of the diaphragmatic surface is triangular. A considerable part of it is in contact with the anterior abdominal wall between the right and left costal margins [Fig. 126], but a small part to the left and a large part to the right are in contact with the diaphragm. The **falciform ligament** is attached vertically to this surface [Fig. 177] and marks the division of the liver into right and left lobes anteriorly.

The superior part of the diaphragmatic surface is ovoid and convex. It rises almost to the level of the right nipple and to the level of the fifth intercostal space in the left mid-clavicular line. It is slightly flattened inferior to the pericardium (**cardiac impression**), and to the left meets the visceral surface at a sharp posterior edge [Fig. 178].

Fig. 177. The liver viewed from the front.

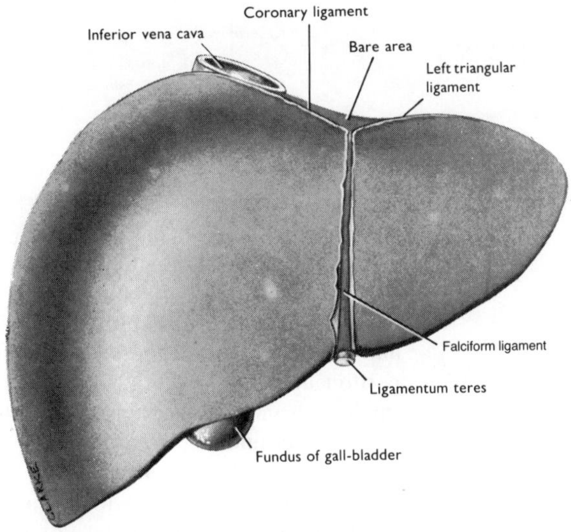

Fig. 178. The liver viewed from behind.

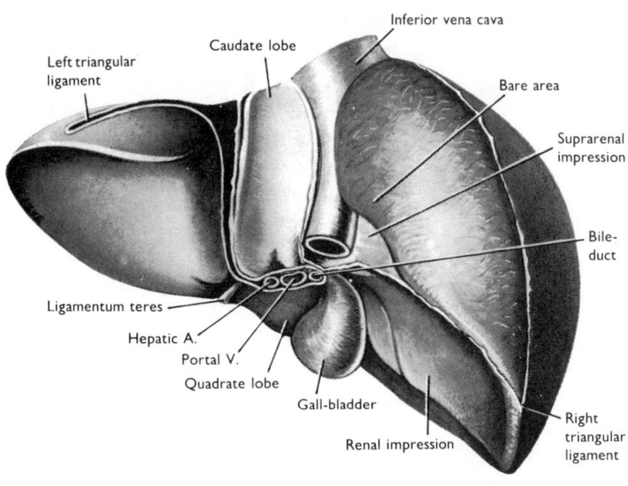

The posterior part of the diaphragmatic surface is narrow in the left lobe, but widens at the fissure for the ligamentum venosum to include the **caudate lobe**. This forms the anterior wall of the superior recess of the omental bursa. At its right margin, the peritoneum on the caudate lobe turns posteriorly on the inferior vena cava and extends to the left on the diaphragm, thus forming the right and posterior walls of the superior recess of the omental bursa.

The **inferior vena cava** lies in a deep groove (occasionally buried in the

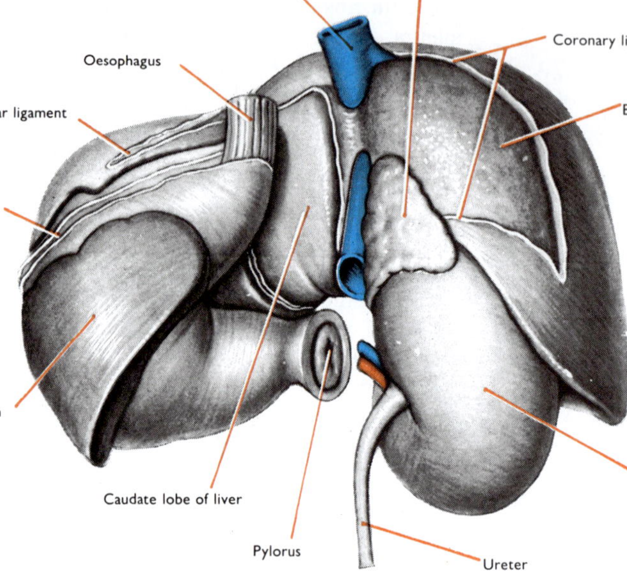

Fig. 179. The liver, right kidney, spleen, and stomach, as seen from behind.

liver) immediately to the right of the caudate lobe. The two main **hepatic veins** enter it at the upper end of the groove, some smaller veins at a lower level. To the right of the inferior vena cava, the posterior part of the diaphragmatic surface is broad and a large part of it (between the superior and inferior layers of the coronary ligament [Fig. 179]) is not covered by peritoneum (**bare area**). This permits the passage of the lymph vessels and small veins into the diaphragm. A slight depression immediately to the right of the lower end of the caval groove and partly in the bare area marks the position of the right suprarenal gland [Fig. 178]. The remainder of the bare area is directly in contact with the inferior vena cava.

The **visceral surface** [Fig. 176] is irregular in shape to fit the upper abdominal viscera which lie postero-inferior to it. In the left lobe, it lies on the stomach and oesophagus except for a small part (tuber omentale) which is in contact with the lesser omentum close to the porta hepatis.

The most obvious feature on the right lobe is the **gall-bladder**. It extends from the porta hepatis to a shallow notch on the inferior margin, and is anterior to the descending part of the duodenum and the transverse colon. To the left of the gall-bladder, the quadrate lobe overlies the lesser omentum, the pylorus and beginning of the duodenum, and the transverse colon. In addition the visceral surface is in contact with the junction of the superior and descending parts of the duodenum, the upper part of the right kidney, and the right flexure of the colon.

Peritoneum of liver

Peritoneum covers the surface of the liver, except the bare area (which includes the groove for the inferior vena cava) and the fossa for the gall-bladder. The peritoneal attachments of the liver are readily understood if it is realized that the liver develops in the ventral mesentery of the stomach and upper duodenum. As a result, the **ventral mesentery** is divided into a part which connects the liver to the anterior abdominal wall (**falciform ligament**), and a part which connects the liver to the stomach and duodenum (**gastrohepatic mesentery**). In addition, the thick gastrohepatic mesentery is split into right and left parts by the upward growth of the superior recess of the omental bursa to the right of the stomach; the right part,separated inferiorly from the remainder by the epiploic foramen, becomes the mesentery which transports the inferior vena cava to the liver. The left part remains attached to the stomach and cranial duodenum as the definitive lesser omentum. Hence two peritoneal folds, the lesser omentum and the

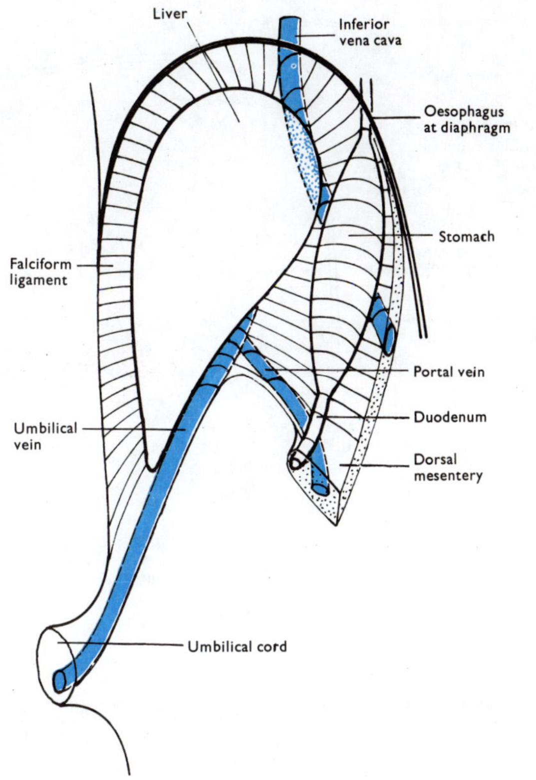

Fig. 180. (a) A theoretical diagram of the developing liver and stomach seen from the left side. This shows that the ventral mesogastrium (ventral mesentery of the stomach and upper duodenum) is divided by the liver into the gastrohepatic mesentery (containing the portal vein and inferior vena cava) and the falciform ligament (containing the umbilical vein). The liver has been drawn away from the diaphragm to show the continuity of the two parts of the mesentery superior to the liver.

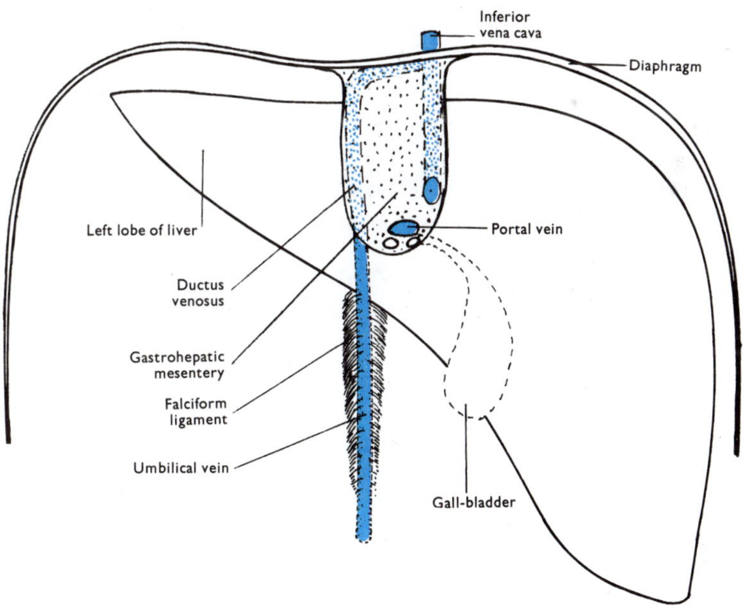

Fig. 180. (b) The posterior and visceral surfaces of the developing liver to show the thick gastrohepatic mesentery at its attachment to the liver.

mesentery of the inferior vena cava, pass to the visceral and posterior diaphragmatic surfaces of the liver and are separated at the liver by the caudate lobe—the anterior wall of the superior recess of the omental bursa [Fig. 180]. The mesentery of the inferior vena cava is further complicated by the posterior diaphragmatic surface of the liver abutting directly on the diaphragm and producing the bare area of the liver by displacing the right wall of this mesentery to the right as the coronary ligament [Fig. 179]. In spite of these complexities, the peritoneum of the coronary ligament and of the left wall of the lesser omentum can be traced into continuity with the two layers forming the falciform ligament; the left layer extending to the left as the left triangular ligament of the liver on the way [Figs. 177, 178].

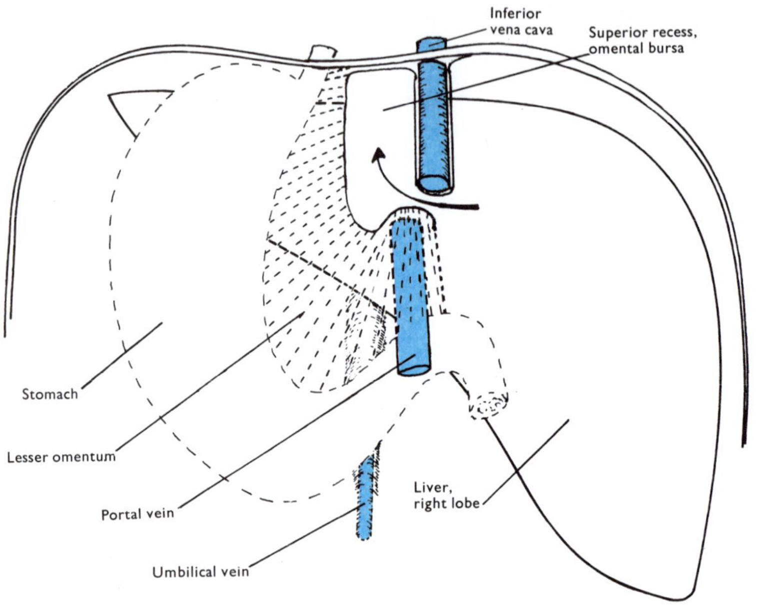

Fig. 180. (c) As in (b) but the superior recess of the omental bursa has extended into the gastrohepatic mesentery and split it into a part which surrounds the inferior vena cava (the caval mesentery) and a part (lesser omentum) which attaches the stomach and upper duodenum to the liver and contains the portal vein. The arrow passes through the epiploic foramen into the superior recess which forms the peritoneal surface on the caudate lobe of the liver.

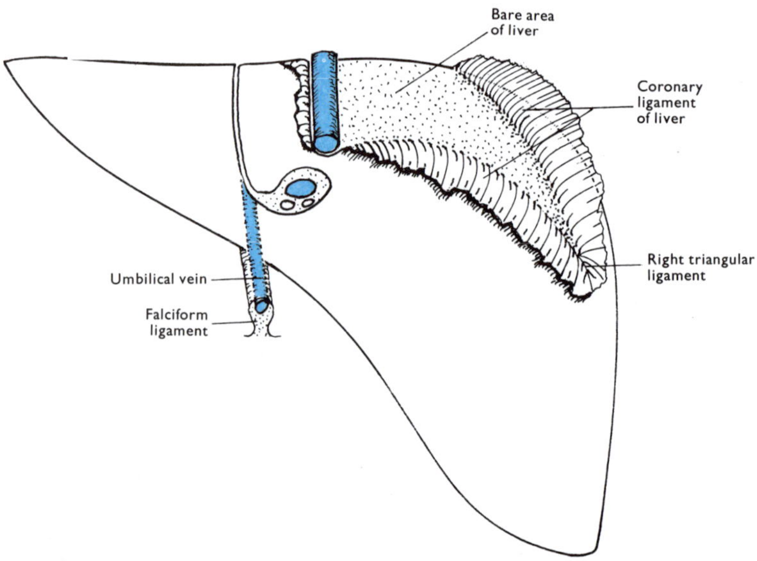

Fig. 180. (d) As in (c) but because the liver is directly applied to the diaphragm (bare area of the liver), the right and left surfaces of the part of the mesentery which attaches the liver to the diaphragm are spread apart to surround the bare area. The right surface forms the coronary and the right triangular ligaments. The left surface forms the left triangular ligament which is not seen because it is on the superior surface of the liver.

Vessels and nerves

The liver is supplied both by the **hepatic artery** and by the **portal vein**. When the mesenteric vessels are dilated, a large volume of blood traverses the liver. Venous blood drains from the liver to the inferior vena cava through right and left **hepatic veins** and by some smaller veins. Separate branches of the portal vein and hepatic artery, and tributaries of the hepatic veins and ducts serve the right and left **lobes of the liver**. All of the **quadrate lobe** and part of the **caudate lobe** are supplied and drained by the vessels of the left lobe.

The **left hepatic vein** usually emerges at the upper end of the fissure for the ligamentum venosum. It runs with the ligament along the upper margin of the caudate lobe to the inferior vena cava.

The **nerves** are derived from the coeliac plexus and from the gastric branches of the vagal trunks. Some sensory fibres in the right phrenic nerve appear to reach the gall-bladder and its ducts.

Lymph vessels emerge either through the porta hepatis to nodes in the lesser omentum, or pass from the bare area through the diaphragm to thoracic nodes. Hepatic lymph forms half of the lymph transmitted by the thoracic duct.

Gall-bladder

This piriform storage chamber of 30–60 ml capacity concentrates the bile (hence its tendency to form stones) and discharges it into the duodenum by muscular contraction. X-ray-opaque substances which are excreted

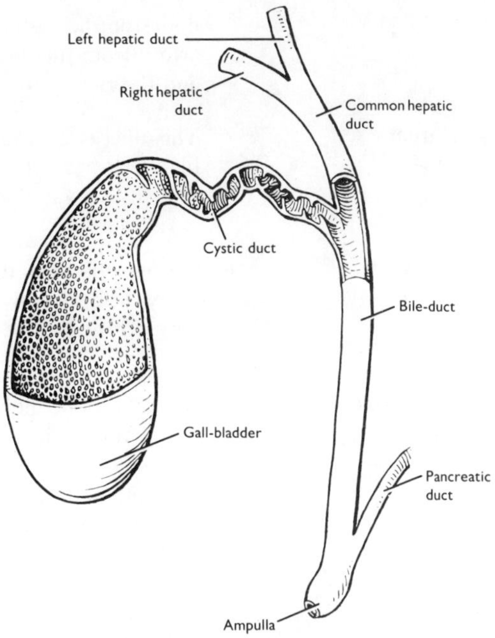

Fig. 181. A diagram of the extrahepatic parts of the biliary system.

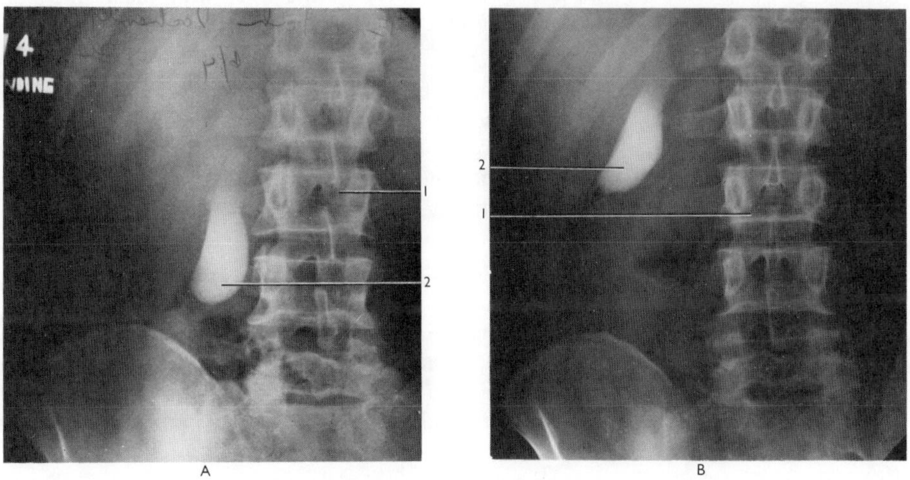

Fig. 182. Two radiographs to show the changing position of the gall-bladder in different positions of the body. The gall-bladder is filled with an X-ray-opaque material which is excreted by the liver in the bile. A is taken in the standing position, B is in the lying position.
1. 3rd lumbar vertebra.
2. Gall-bladder.

in the bile are also concentrated, and so are used to demonstrate the cavity of the gall-bladder and its ability to concentrate and to contract [Figs. 182, 286, 287].

The gall-bladder lies along the right edge of the quadrate lobe of the liver in a shallow fossa. Usually it is directly in contact with the liver substance and has venous communications with it, but it may be suspended from the liver by a short mesentery, or partly buried in it.

Antero-inferiorly, the rounded **fundus** protrudes below the inferior margin of the liver, and touches the anterior abdominal wall approximately where the right linea semilunaris meets the ninth costal cartilage. The fundus is continuous through the **body** of the gall-bladder with the narrow **neck** which is close to the right extremity of the porta hepatis. These parts of the gall-bladder lie respectively on the transverse colon, the descending, and superior parts of the duodenum [Figs. 172, 176].

Vessels and nerves

The gall-bladder is supplied by the **cystic artery** (branch of the right hepatic artery [Fig. 144]) and **vein** (tributary of portal vein). Its **lymph vessels** pass to nodes on the cystic duct and in the porta hepatis. Nerves reach it along the artery from the coeliac plexus (sympathetic), the vagus (parasympathetic), and the right phrenic nerve (sensory).

Cystic duct
[Fig. 181]

This duct is 2 cm or more in length. It descends from the neck of the gall-bladder to run in the lesser omentum with the common hepatic duct, and joins it at a variable point to form the bile-duct.

Dissection

Expose the structures in the porta hepatis, and follow them to their entry into the liver. Their arrangement is variable and may not correspond to the following description.

Structures in porta hepatis

Near the porta hepatis, the common hepatic duct, hepatic artery, and the portal vein divide into right and left branches. These pass together into the corresponding lobes of the liver with the hepatic ducts anterior to the arteries and both in front of the veins. The right branch of the portal vein receives the cystic vein and enters the right lobe of the liver almost immediately. The left branch passes between the caudate and quadrate lobes, and supplying both, sinks into the left lobe after uniting with the ligamentum venosum and ligamentum teres.

As these structures enter the liver they carry an extension of the fibrous capsule of the surface of the liver with them—the perivascular fibrous capsule. This extends around their branches and tributaries within the liver.

Dissection

Trace a branch of the portal vein with the corresponding artery and duct for some distance into the liver. Note their simultaneous branches to the liver tissue. Trace one of the hepatic veins from the inferior vena cava into the liver, and inspect the cut surface of a slice of liver with a hand lens.

Structure of liver

Within the liver, the branches of the vessels in the porta hepatis communicate with the smallest tributaries of the hepatic veins, between strands of liver cells which pass radially from the tributaries of the hepatic ducts (**interlobular ducts**) towards the surrounding tributaries of the hepatic veins (**central venules**). Each of the strands contains the ultimate tributary of a hepatic duct—a bile canaliculus. Between the strands of liver cells are the blood-

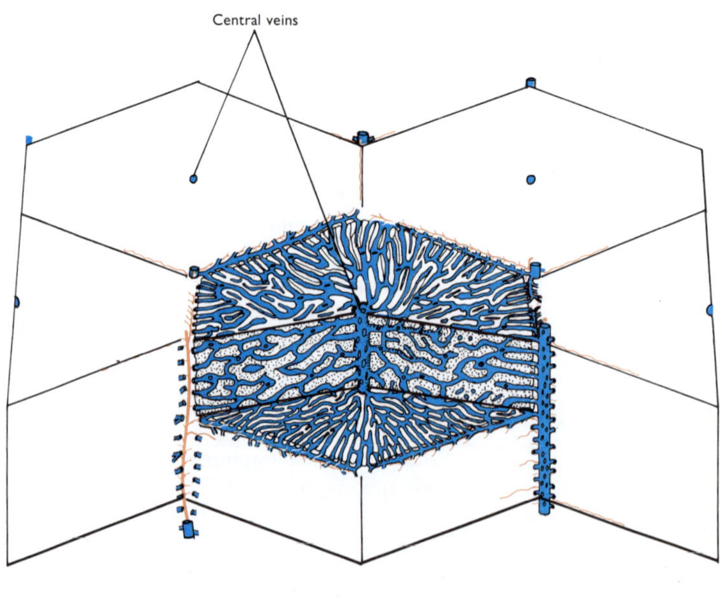

Fig. 183. A diagram to indicate the structure and vascular connexions of a hepatic lobule based on a central vein. The biliary passages are not shown.

filled **sinusoids**. These have a simple wall of phagocytic, fenestrated endothelial cells, and connect the terminal branches of the hepatic artery and portal vein to the central venules [Figs. 183, 184].

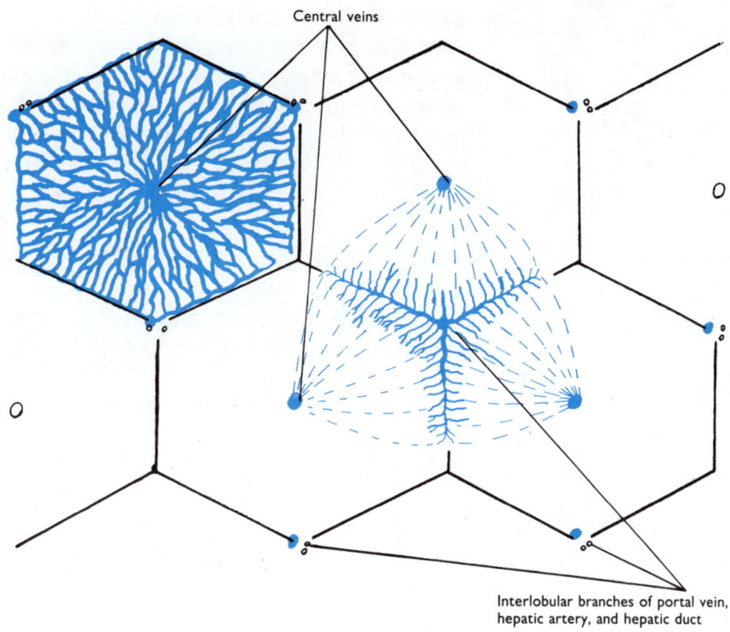

Fig. 184. A diagram of the two types of liver lobule described in the text. That on the right shows the lobule centred on the interlobular branch of the portal vein. That on the left shows the lobule centred on the central vein.

Various **lobules** have been described in the liver. These may be centred either on a central venule or on a **portal tract** (the terminal branch of the perivascular fibrous capsule and its contained structures). In most animals no clear-cut lobular pattern exists, though in the pig, sheets of the perivascular fibrous capsule join the various portal tracts and so outline lobules, each with a centrally placed venule. From the point of view of the biliary system, the lobule is the volume of liver that drains into a single interlobular ductule. Such a lobule has several central venules arranged around it, each of which drains parts of several hepatic lobules. Since the hepatic arterioles lie in the portal tracts, the oxygen tension is highest close to the tracts and lowest in the liver tissue adjacent to the central venules. Thus anything that slows the rate of hepatic circulation will affect the cells around the central venules, while poisons entering the liver through the portal vein or hepatic artery tend to damage the cells immediately round the portal tracts [Fig. 184].

Dissection

Make a longitudinal incision through the wall of the gall-bladder and cystic duct. Wash out the interior with a jet of water and examine the lining.

Structure of gall-bladder and cystic duct

The gall-bladder is lined with columnar epithelial cells which are of the absorptive type with numerous microvilli on their internal surfaces. They also secrete mucus. The mucous membrane is complexly folded to increase the surface area and has a honeycomb appearance to the unaided eye. There is no muscularis mucosae. The mucous membrane lies directly on a thin layer of smooth muscle with interlacing bundles running in many directions. This arrangement is found in many hollow organs which contract uniformly to force their contents through a single aperture.

From the neck of the gall-bladder a prominent fold of mucous membrane runs spirally along the cystic duct, the **spiral fold**. It may help to maintain the patency of the cystic duct [Fig. 181].

Abdominal structures in contact with diaphragm
[Figs. 282–286]

Posteriorly, each half of the diaphragm is in contact with the upper part of the corresponding kidney and suprarenal gland. Anterior to this, the right lobe of the liver fills the right dome of the diaphragm, while the spleen, stomach, and left lobe of the liver occupy the left dome. Where these organs are in contact with the diaphragm they are separated by it from the pleura, except those parts of the right and left lobes of the liver which lie inferior to the pericardium. To a lesser extent the liver, stomach, and spleen are separated by the diaphragm from parts of the pleural cavities which normally contain the lungs, though the parts of the 'diaphragmatic' surface of the liver which are in contact with the anterior abdominal wall and the anterior surface of the right kidney are related neither to pleura nor lungs.

Replace the upper abdominal organs that have been removed, and confirm their positions relative to the pleural cavities.

Dissection

Find a **coeliac ganglion** on each side of the coeliac trunk. They lie in the plexus of nerves on the aorta anterior to the corresponding crus of the diaphragm. Trace branches of the ganglia to the suprarenal glands, to the coeliac trunk, and inferiorly along the aorta to form plexuses on the superior and inferior mesenteric arteries. The aortic plexus receives the lumbar splanchnic nerves [p. 138].

The autonomic nervous system

The general arrangement of this system has been described already [p. 27]. This system consists of motor (or inhibitory) nerve cells whose cell bodies are situated in peripheral **ganglia**. These cells sends axons (**postganglionic fibres**) to innervate various organs in the body, especially smooth muscle and glands. The activity of these cells is controlled by axons of nerve cells in the central nervous system. These axons (**preganglionic fibres**) leave the central nervous system through the thoracic and upper two or three lumbar nerves (**sympathetic** preganglionic fibres), and also through certain cranial nerves (including the vagus) and the third and fourth sacral nerves (**parasympathetic** preganglionic fibres). They end on different groups of ganglion cells, the sympathetic usually at some distance from the organs they supply and commonly associated with the arteries; the parasympathetic in or near all parts of the gut tube and the structures developed on or from it, the eye, and the urogenital system.

Sympathetic nervous system

This part of the autonomic nervous system consists mainly of (1) the sympathetic trunks and their branches, and (2) the sympathetic plexuses.

A **sympathetic trunk** extends on the anterolateral surface of each side of the vertebral column from the upper cervical region to the coccyx. Each trunk consists of a series of ganglia united by nerve fibres. The cells in the ganglia send their **postganglionic fibres** principally to the spinal nerves (**grey rami communicantes**) for the supply of the body wall. Bundles of **preganglionic fibres** which enter each trunk through the **white rami communicantes**, extend along it and end on the cells of the ganglia at various levels. They also pass directly through the trunk and *descend* in front of it, as **splanchnic nerves**, to the **visceral plexuses** and **ganglia** on the aorta and its branches *at much lower levels*. Thus most of the **thoracic splanchnic nerves** pierce the crura of the diaphragm and reach the coeliac (greater and lesser splanchnic nerves) and renal plexuses (lowest splanchnic nerve). The **lumbar splanchnic nerves** [Fig. 202] join the inferior part of the abdominal aortic plexus. They pass mainly to the **inferior hypogastric plexuses** in the pelvis. Here they are joined by the small sacral splanchnic nerves and by the pelvic splanchnic nerves which are preganglionic parasympathetic fibres which arise from the third and fourth sacral ventral rami and pass through the hypogastric plexuses to ganglia on the pelvic organs and the descending colon.

The **abdominal** and **pelvic sympathetic plexuses** are extensions of the aortic plexus. They are the coeliac, renal, gonadal, superior and inferior mesenteric, and the superior and inferior hypogastric. All of these also transmit preganglionic parasympathetic fibres derived either from the vagus nerve or the pelvic splanchnic nerves.

Coeliac plexus

This plexus lies on the aorta and the crura of the diaphragm around the coeliac trunk. It is posterior to the omental bursa and partly overlapped by the pancreas and by the inferior vena cava on the right.

The large, nodular **coeliac ganglia** lie on each side of the coeliac trunk. They give rise to most of the postganglionic sympathetic nerve fibres in the plexus on the coeliac trunk. Preganglionic fibres also pass directly through the ganglia to the **suprarenal glands** and to the ganglia on the coeliac trunk and the superior mesenteric artery. The coeliac plexus is joined by **preganglionic parasympathetic fibres** from the vagal trunks and by *phrenic fibres* (sensory). These reach it along the left gastric and inferior phrenic arteries respectively. Both are distributed with the sympathetic fibres of the coeliac plexus. Vagal fibres also descend in the aortic plexus to join the **superior mesenteric plexus**.

The coeliac plexus is continuous with the abdominal aortic plexus (of which it is really a part), and through it with the **superior** and **inferior mesenteric plexuses** on the corresponding arteries. Inferior to the bifurcation of the aorta, the abdominal aortic plexus is continued as the **superior hypogastric plexus** (presacral nerve) between the two common iliac arteries. It then divides into right and left **inferior hypogastric plexuses** which surround the corresponding internal iliac arteries and their branches in the pelvis [Fig. 202].

The plexuses on the renal arteries (**renal plexuses**) form subsidiary plexuses along the gonadal arteries and the ureter. Small ganglia are scattered through all these plexuses and even in the walls of the viscera.

Dissection

Remove the fat and fascia from the anterior surface of the left kidney and suprarenal gland. Find the left suprarenal vein and the left testicular or ovarian vein, and trace both to the left renal vein. Follow this vein from the inferior vena cava to the left kidney, and note its tributaries. Displace the vein and expose the left renal artery, following its branches to the left suprarenal gland and ureter. Follow the ureter in the abdomen.

Turn the left kidney medially to expose its posterior surface and that of its vessels and the ureter, and the muscles, vessels, and nerves which are posterior to them. Carry out the same dissection on the right side, but note that the testicular (or ovarian) and suprarenal veins drain directly to the inferior vena cava.

Suprarenal glands

Each of these important endocrine glands consists of two parts—the **cortex** (developed from the mesodermal lining of the peritoneal cavity) and the **medulla** (developed from the neural crest and equivalent to a group of sympathetic ganglion cells).

The cortex secretes a considerable number of steroid hormones which are responsible for: (1) the control of electrolyte and water balance; (2) the maintenance of blood sugar concentration and of liver and muscle glycogen stores; (3) the control of inflammatory reactions and of connective tissues in general.

The medulla secretes **adrenaline** and noradrenaline into the blood stream. These sympathetic catecholamines are similar to those released by the postganglionic sympathetic nerve fibres, and they are stored in quantity in

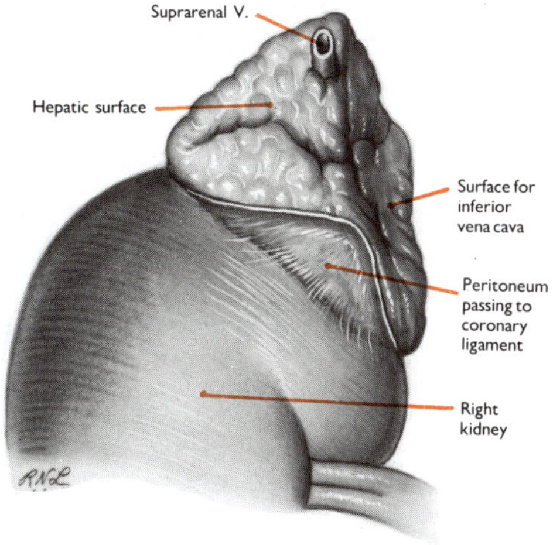

Fig. 185. The anterior surface of the right suprarenal gland.

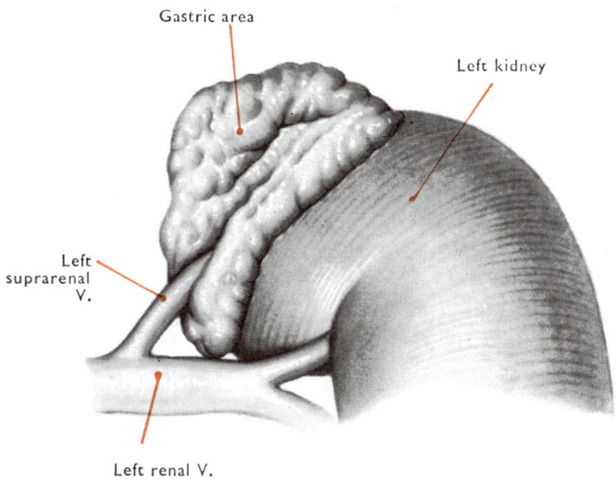

Fig. 186. The anterior surface of the left suprarenal gland.

the medulla. They are readily oxidized to a dark brown colour by potassium bichromate—a feature which makes the medulla part of the so-called **chromaffin tissue** of the body.

Position
[Figs. 149, 191, 199, 284A, 285, 286]

Each gland lies against the superomedial surface of the corresponding kidney, enclosed in the same fascial sheath (renal fascia [p. 168]). A little fatty connective tissue separates it from the kidney.

The pyramidal **right gland** is wedged between the diaphragm posteromedially, the inferior vena cava anteromedially, the liver anteriorly, and the kidney inferolaterally. Superiorly it lies on the bare area of the liver, but peritoneum intervenes inferiorly [Fig. 185].

The crescentic **left gland** lies between the diaphragm posteromedially, the stomach anteriorly (with the omental bursa and the pancreas and splenic artery intervening), and the kidney inferolaterally.

Vessels

The large blood supply is obtained through a considerable number of small **arteries** which enter the surface of the gland (cortex). They arise from the renal arteries, the aorta, and the inferior phrenic arteries, supply the cortex, and piercing it, enter the medulla. The **veins** run inwards from the cortex to the medulla, whence they emerge as a single vein, the right entering the inferior vena cava directly while the left joins the left renal vein.

Dissection

Make a series of sections through the right gland. Follow the left suprarenal vein into the gland, removing the anterior surface of the gland to expose the extent of the medulla. Examine the cut surfaces with a hand lens.

Structure

The cortex consists of three layers. (1) The outer, **zona glomerulosa** is composed of nests or clumps of cells. (2) The **zona fasciculata** is formed of parallel columns of cells. (3) The **zona reticularis** is a mesh of interlacing cords of cells. Each layer may have a different function, but new cells are formed at the junction of the outer two layers, and the cortex may be regenerated from this region. *In the fetus* the cortex is relatively very large and thick but its function is unknown. After birth the fetal cortex disappears and is replaced by the remaining outermost layer. The medulla consists of strands or clumps of chromaffin cells interspersed with sympathetic ganglion cells.

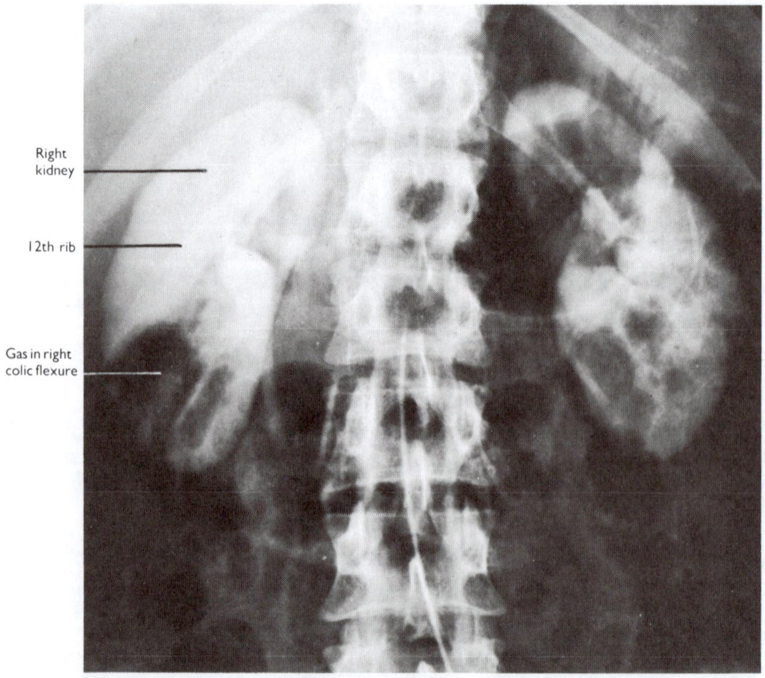

Fig. 187. An anteroposterior radiograph of the upper abdomen shortly after the injection of contrast material into the aorta, at the level of the renal arteries. The kidneys are outlined by the contrast material in their capillaries.

The kidneys

These organs are responsible for removing excess water, salts, and waste products from the blood, and for maintaining its pH. To achieve this the blood flow through the wide renal vessels is approximately one-quarter of the resting cardiac output, i.e. 1.2–1.4 litres per minute.

The kidneys are reddish-brown in colour and approximately 10 cm long, 5 cm wide, and 2.5 cm thick. They are ovoid in outline, but the medial margin is deeply indented and concave at its middle. Here a wide, vertical cleft (the **hilus**) transmits the structures entering and leaving the kidney, and leads to a space within the kidney, the **sinus** of the kidney. The hilus lies approximately at the level of the first lumbar vertebra.

The kidneys lie in the upper parts of the paravertebral gutters, posterior to the peritoneum, tilted against the structures on the sides of the lowest two thoracic and upper three lumbar vertebrae, so that the anterior and posterior surfaces face anterolaterally and posteromedially respectively, and the superior extremities are medial to the inferior extremities. In addition, the superior extremity of the right kidney lies at a lower level (eleventh intercostal space) than the left (eleventh rib) because of the presence of the liver [Figs. 190, 195].

The upper end of the ureter expands to form the **pelvis of the kidney** [Fig. 192]. This passes through the hilus into the sinus of the kidney. Here it is continuous with some short, funnel-like tubes (**calyces**) which unite it to the kidney tissue. The amount of the pelvis enclosed in the sinus is variable. The renal vessels lie anterior to the pelvis of the kidney, but some of their branches and tributaries pass posterior to it. Lymph vessels and autonomic and sensory nerve fibres also pass through the hilus into the sinus.

Each kidney is enclosed in a dense fibrous **capsule** which is readily stripped from its surface. The capsule passes through the hilus to line the sinus and become continuous with the walls of the calyces where they are attached to

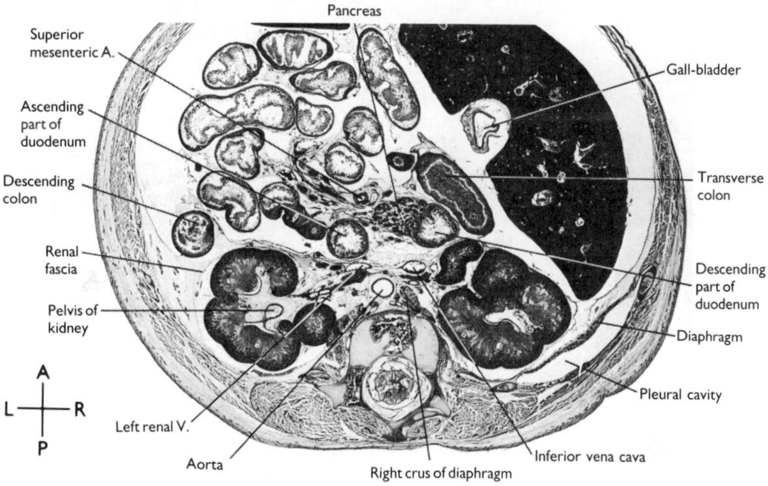

Fig. 188. A horizontal section through the abdomen of a seven-month human fetus. The levels of the various structures are not identical with those in the adult, but the absence of dense connective tissue makes the structures more obvious.

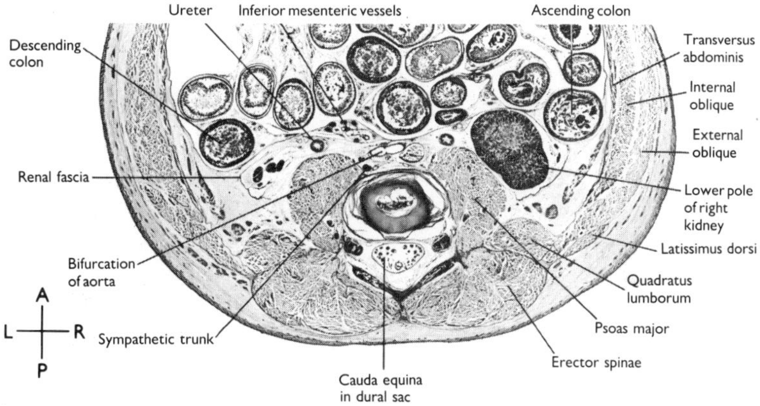

Fig. 189. A horizontal section through the abdomen of a seven-month human fetus at the level of the bifurcation of the aorta.

the kidney. The fibrous capsule is surrounded by a fatty capsule (**perirenal fat**) which fills the space inside the loosely fitting sheath of **renal fascia** enclosing the kidney and suprarenal. The renal fascia is continuous laterally with the transversalis fascia, superiorly with the diaphragmatic fascia, and medially with the fascia around the renal vessels. Inferiorly the walls of this sheath are only loosely united, and may be separated for some distance below the kidney [Figs. 188, 189]. Because of this, the kidney may descend to an unusually low level if the fatty capsule is absorbed; the renal vessels are then its only support, and kinking of the ureter may obstruct the flow of urine along it.

The *developing kidney* is first formed in the pelvis, and subsequently ascends to its final position. This ascent may stop at any point. During the ascent, the kidney receives its blood supply from successive sources. Thus an accessory renal artery from the aorta may be found entering the lower pole of a normally placed kidney. When first formed, the rudiments of the two kidneys are close together and may fuse to form a **horseshoe kidney** anterior to the aorta. The ascent of such a combined kidney is blocked by the inferior mesenteric artery so that the fused part always lies inferior to that vessel [p. 259].

There may be a considerable accumulation of extraperitoneal fat (**pararenal fat**) between the peritoneum and the renal fascia. Air injected into the loose extraperitoneal tissue anterior to the sacrum ascends to the level of the kidneys in this layer, and surrounding them, makes their outlines readily visible on X-ray examination.

Structures in contact with kidney
[Figs. 138, 188–191, 285–288]

Posteriorly, on both sides are the diaphragm (superiorly), psoas major (medially), and quadratus lumborum and transversus abdominis (laterally). The **subcostal** vessels and nerve and the **iliohypogastric** and **ilioinguinal nerves** lie between the kidney and the anterior layer of the thoracolumbar fascia which covers the anterior surface of quadratus lumborum [Fig. 201].

The **diaphragm** separates the upper part of each kidney from the pleura and twelfth rib. Occasionally there is a defect in the diaphragm between its costal origin and that from the lateral arcuate ligament [Fig. 198]. Then the kidney may be directly in contact with the pleura and last rib.

The upper part of the **right kidney** is wedged between the posterior abdominal wall and the visceral surface of the liver [Fig. 188]. Here it is separated from the liver by the suprarenal gland and the peritoneum of the

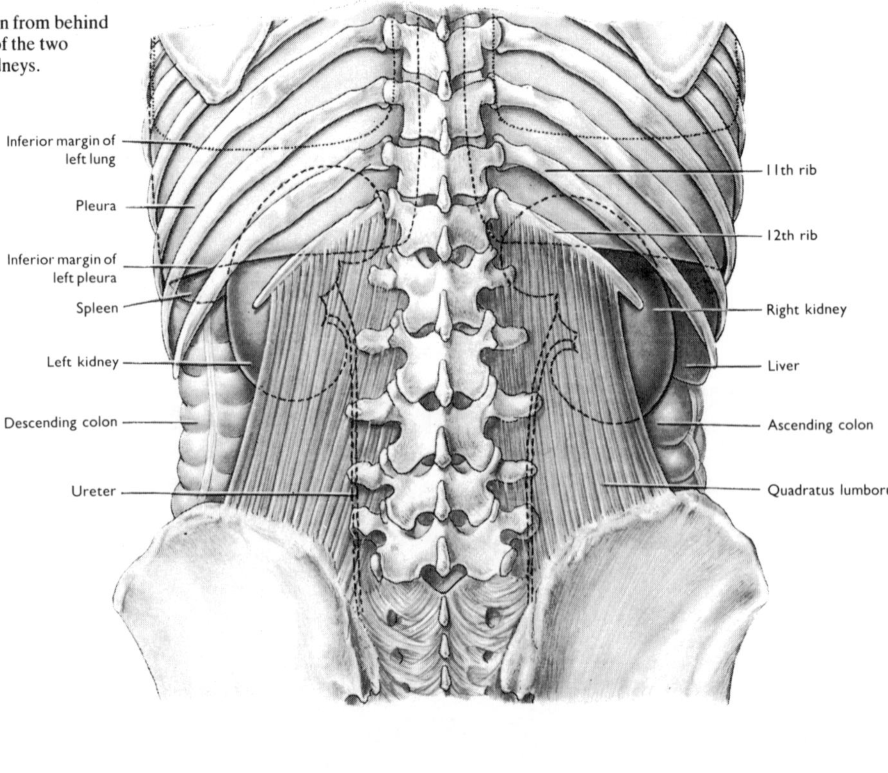

Fig. 190. A dissection from behind to show the relation of the two pleural sacs to the kidneys.

hepatorenal recess. Inferiorly, the kidney is separated from the liver and from the gall-bladder by the descending part of the duodenum medially, and the right flexure of the colon inferolaterally. The lower extremity lies in the infracolic compartment.

The upper part of the **left kidney** is posterior to the suprarenal gland, the omental bursa (with the stomach in its anterior wall), the attachment of the lienorenal ligament, and lateral to that, the spleen. At the renal hilus, the body of the pancreas [Fig. 138] with the splenic vessels and the attachment of the greater omentum and transverse mesocolon are anterior. Inferior to this, the left kidney lies in the infracolic compartment with the descending colon along its lateral margin, the jejunum anterior, and the duodenojejunal flexure medial to it. The descending colon, pancreas with splenic vessels, and the suprarenal gland are not separated from the kidney by peritoneum.

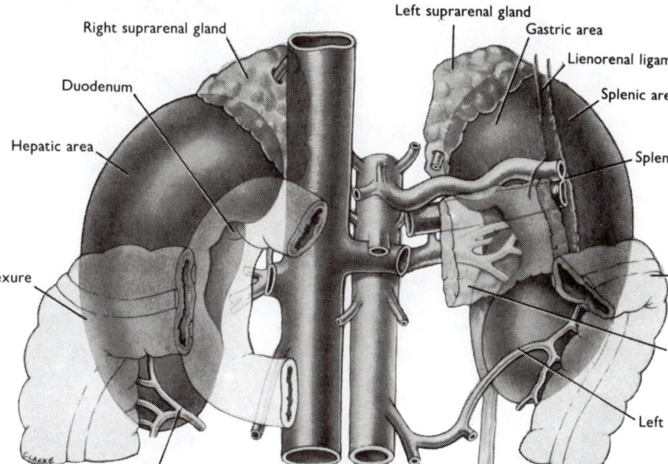

Fig. 191. A diagram to show the structures in contact with the anterior surfaces of the kidneys. The pancreas, colon, suprarenal glands, and duodenum are shown as though transparent.

Dissection

Remove the anterior wall of the renal sinus piecemeal, beginning at the hilus. Divide the vessels entering this wall of the sinus, and define and separate the calyces that are attached to it. Expose the contents of the sinus, and then remove the anterior part of the kidney by making a clean coronal slice from the lateral margin through the sinus.

The **sinus of the kidney** is a considerable space which takes up a large part of the interior of the kidney. It contains the greater part of the pelvis of the kidney, the calyces, blood and lymph vessels, and nerves of the kidney.

Structure of kidney [Fig. 192]

On the cut surface of the kidney, note the paler **cortex** adjacent to the capsule and the darker conical **pyramids** of the **medulla**. The pyramids are radially striated and are covered with cortex which extends inwards between them (**renal columns**). The apex of each pyramid extends into the sinus as a small, conical projection (**renal papilla**) covered by the extremity of a lesser calyx which is attached around the base of the papilla. Here the fibromuscular wall of calyx becomes continuous with the fibrous capsule lining the sinus, while the epithelial lining is continued over the surface of the papilla. **Collecting tubules** from a lobe of the kidney (one pyramid and its covering of cortical tissue) discharge urine into the calyx through apertures (**foramina papillaria**) on the papilla. The collecting tubules pass radially through the pyramid into the cortex. Here they take part in the formation of radial striations (the medullary rays) with other renal tubules, and receive urine from the excretory units of the kidney, the nephrons.

Each **nephron** consists of a filter or **renal corpuscle**. This is a tuft of capillaries with fenestrated endothelial walls (glomerulus) invaginated into the blind, expanded end (glomerular capsule) of a long tubule which leaves the renal corpuscle to form a **proximal convoluted tubule** in the cortex. In this tubule certain substances are reabsorbed (glucose, salt, etc.) and some are excreted by the epithelial lining. The proximal convoluted tubule leads into

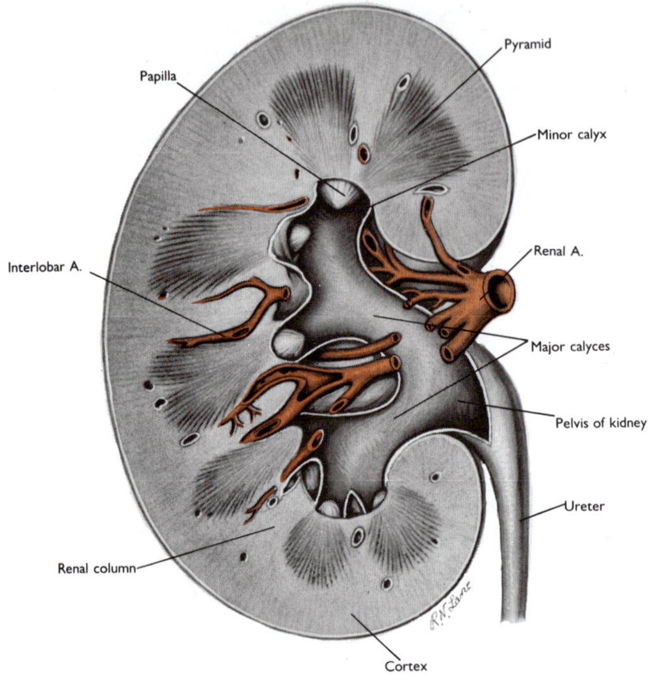

Fig. 192. A coronal section of the kidney. Note the papillae projecting into the minor calyces.

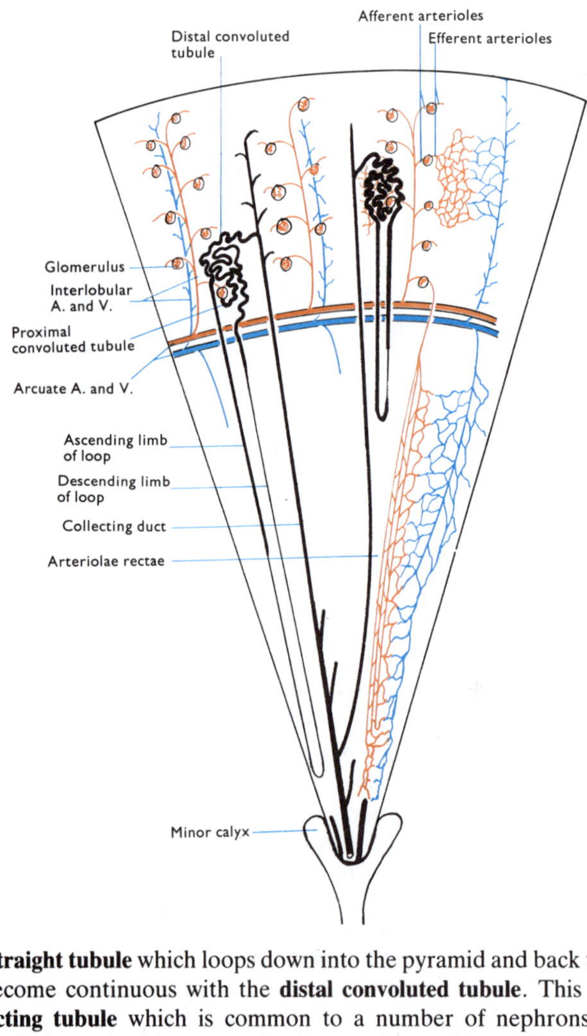

Fig. 193. A diagram to show the arrangement of the blood vessels, nephrons, and collecting ducts of a renal pyramid, and the minor calyx into which the collecting ducts drain. Only two nephrons and one collecting duct are shown out of the many that are present.

the **straight tubule** which loops down into the pyramid and back to the cortex, to become continuous with the **distal convoluted tubule**. This opens into a **collecting tubule** which is common to a number of nephrons, and passes through the pyramid to enter the lesser calyx at the papilla. In these parts, the urine is concentrated and other substances are added or removed by the epithelium.

The distal convoluted tubule comes into close association with the afferent glomerular arteriole and the cells of both are modified to form the **juxtaglomerular apparatus**. This is thought to be responsible for the release of substances which raise the blood pressure and thereby maintain the renal blood flow.

Vessels of kidney

The renal artery divides into four or five **segmental arteries** close to the hilus. The majority pass anterior to the pelvis of the kidney, but one or two pass posterior to it. They give twigs to the structures in the sinus and a **lobar artery** towards each papilla. These divide into **interlobar arteries** which enter the kidney substance near the papilla, and ascend at the sides of the pyramid. They give rise to **arcuate arteries** which run parallel to the surface of the kidney between the pyramid and its cortical cap. They do not anastomose with adjacent arcuate arteries, but send branches (**interlobular arteries**) towards the surface of the kidney. **Afferent arterioles** pass from these to the glomeruli. From the glomeruli, **efferent arterioles** either pass to further capillaries around the convoluted tubules, or form **straight arterioles** which run into the medulla from the glomeruli close to it. The capillaries drain into **interlobular veins** and thence to the **arcuate** and **interlobar veins**. These begin as **stellate veins** deep to the renal capsule, and pass through the kidney tissue to the sinus.

Pelvis of kidney and calyces
[Figs. 192–195]

The calyces are short, funnel-like tubes. They are the remnants of the main branches of the **ureteric bud** of the embryo, which forms the ureter, pelvis of the kidney, calyces, and collecting tubules. There are two orders of calyces, greater and lesser. The end of each lesser calyx (approximately ten in number) forms a cup-shaped expansion which surrounds one or two renal papillae and receives the urine from the collecting tubules piercing it. The lesser calyces are branches of two or three greater calyces which arise from the renal pelvis. The volume of the pelvis and calyces does not exceed 8 ml. If more than this volume of X-ray-opaque material is injected through the ureter to outline these cavities, the pressure may tear the epithelial junction of the minor calyces with the papillae, and allow the material to enter the adjacent renal veins.

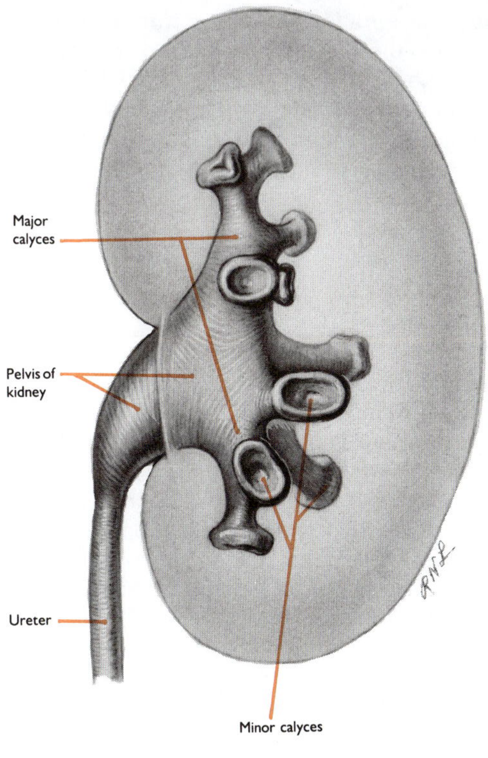

Fig. 194. The pelvis and calyces of the kidney, from a cast. The cupped appearance of the lesser calyces is due to each having a renal papilla inserted into it.

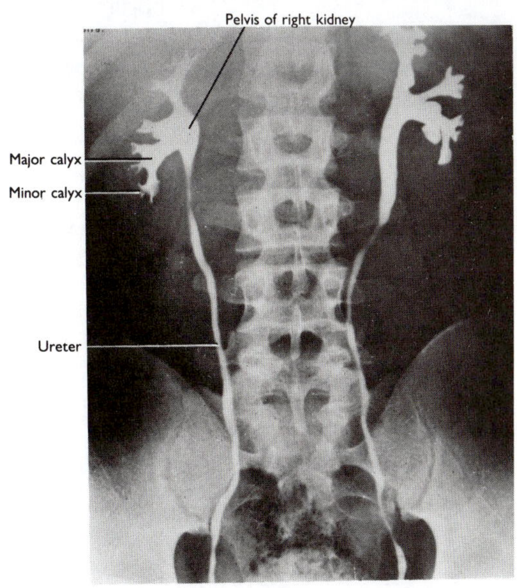

Fig. 195. A pyelogram. This radiograph shows the ureters, pelvis, and calyces of the kidneys outlined by a contrast medium filing their lumina.

The renal pelvis and calyces are surrounded by fat, vessels, and nerves in the renal sinus. The pelvis emerges through the lower part of the hilus and, tapering downwards on psoas major, joins the ureter near the inferior extremity of the kidney. The extrarenal part of the right pelvis is covered by the descending part of the duodenum and the renal vessels, while the renal vessels and pancreas partially cover it on the left [Fig. 191].

Abdominal part of ureter

This expansile, muscular tube is 25 cm long and 5 mm wide. From a slight constriction at its junction with the pelvis of the kidney, it descends almost vertically along the line of the tips of the lumbar transverse processes to its midpoint which lies on the origin of the external iliac artery. Here the ureter enters the lesser pelvis [Fig. 199].

Dissection

Remove a small part of the ureter, slit it open, and pinning it out under water, dissect its walls layer by layer.

Structure

The outer layer consists of connective tissue. The subjacent smooth muscle is arranged in bundles forming inner longitudinal and outer circular layers. In the inferior part of the ureter, a further longitudinal layer appears externally, and the circular layer disappears as the ureter reaches the bladder. In the pelvis of the kidney and the calyces, the muscle is mainly circular. The mucous membrane contains much **elastic tissue** and is lined by **transitional epithelium** (also elastic in character) which extends into the pelvis of the kidney, the calyces, and the urinary bladder.

Blood supply

Small branches pass to the ureter from the renal, testicular or ovarian, aorta, common and internal iliac, and vesical or uterine arteries. These form longitudinal anastomoses on it so that some of the branches may be divided without inferfering with its arterial supply. **Lymph vessels** drain to lumbar, common and internal iliac nodes. The **nerves** are derived from the renal plexus.

Dissection

Strip the peritoneum from the **diaphragm**, and expose its crura on the anterior surfaces of the upper two or three lumbar vertebrae. Find the **arcuate ligaments**. These are fibrous arches from which the diaphragm arises anterior to the aorta, psoas, and quadratus lumborum [Fig. 197]. Expose the slips of the diaphragm arising from the internal surfaces of the remaining costal cartilages, and identify the intercostal vessels and nerves entering the abdominal wall between them. Review the anterior attachments of the diaphragm.

The diaphragm [Figs. 197, 198, 282–286]

This thin, fibromuscular partition between the thoracic and abdominal cavities is an important muscle of respiration. When it contracts, it increases the vertical extent of the thoracic cavity by partially flattening its dome and displacing the abdominal contents downwards [see also p. 265]. The fibrous, central part of the diaphragm (**central tendon**) is slightly depressed by the heart, and thus it has right and left **domes**. The right dome, supported by the liver, lies at a slightly higher level (a little inferior to the nipple in the male) than the left. On full expiration, it may rise to the level of the fourth rib, superior to the nipple. For development see p. 255.

Attachments

The muscle fibres arise from the margins of the inferior aperture of the thorax, and pass upwards and inwards to the edges of the flat, C-shaped central tendon. The anterior fibres are nearly horizontal. The posterior fibres pass almost vertically upwards leaving a deep recess between the thoracic wall and the diaphragm—the **costodiaphragmatic recesses**—and the lowest part of the posterior mediastinum.

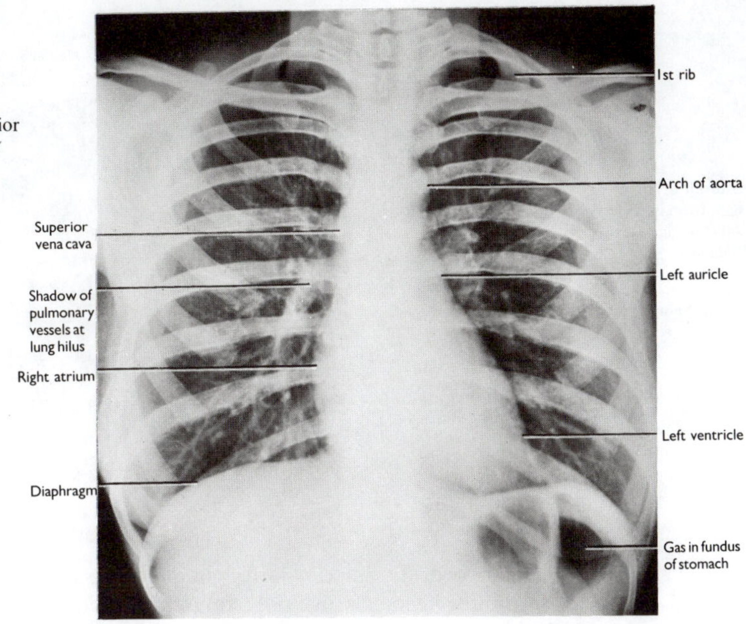

Fig. 196. An anteroposterior radiograph of the thorax in inspiration. Cf. Fig. 1.

Sternal part

Two small slips pass backwards from the xiphoid process.

The **costal part** arises by wide slips from each of the lower six costal cartilages, with slips of transversus abdominis fitted between them.

The **vertebral part** arises by the crura and by the arcuate ligaments.

Crura

These thick, fleshy bundles are attached on each side of the aorta to the anterior surfaces of the upper two (left) or three (right) lumbar vertebral bodies and the intervening discs, and from tendinous slips that bridge the lumbar vessels on the vertebral bodies. As the fibres of the right crus ascend towards the central tendon they deviate to the left and surround the oesophageal hiatus.

Arcuate ligaments

The medial sides of the two crura are united superiorly by a tendinous band (the **median arcuate ligament**) over the anterior surface of the aorta [Fig. 198]. The lateral side of each crus is connected to the transverse process of the first (or second) lumbar vertebra by a tendinous thickening of the fascia over psoas major, the **medial arcuate ligament**.

The **lateral arcuate ligament** is a linear thickening of the anterior layer of the thoracolumbar fascia [Fig. 201]. It passes from the medial arcuate

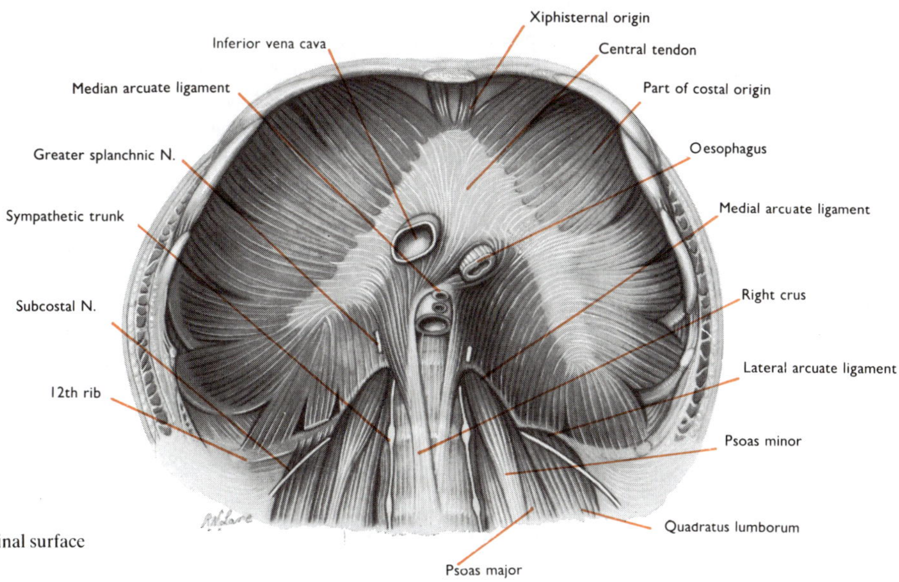

Fig. 197. The abdominal surface of the diaphragm.

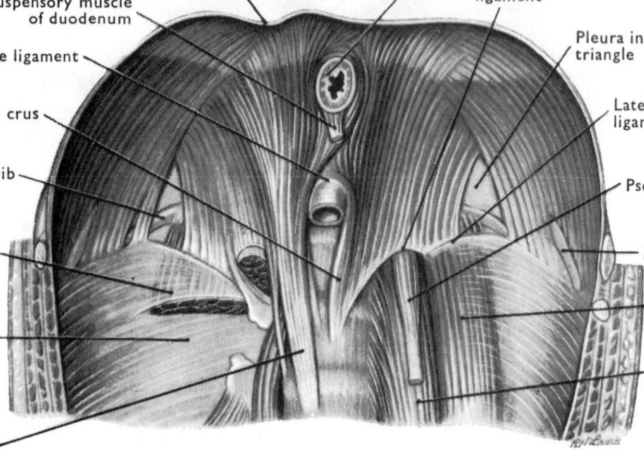

Fig. 198. The posterior origin of the diaphragm, seen from in front. The vertebrocostal triangles are particularly well marked.

ligament over the anterior surface of quadratus lumborum to the twelfth rib.

All three ligaments give rise to muscle fibres of the diaphragm. Those from the lateral part of the lateral ligament may be missing (**vertebrocostal triangle** [Fig. 198]). This leaves the pleura almost directly in contact with the kidney, and makes a potential site for herniation of abdominal contents into the thorax. This deficiency is thought to represent an incomplete closure of the embryonic **pleuroperitoneal canal** between the parts of the diaphragm derived from the dorsal mesentery and the pleuroperitoneal membrane [p. 255].

All the muscle fibres of the diaphragm converge on the strong, interlacing tendinous bundles of the C-shaped **central tendon**. This tendon has right and left horns which curve posteriorly into the corresponding halves of the diaphragm, while the larger, median part expands anteriorly towards the xiphoid process.

Foramina in diaphragm

The **inferior vena cava** pierces and fuses with the central tendon of the diaphragm 2–3 cm to the right of the median plane, approximately at the level of the eighth thoracic vertebra. When the diaphragm contracts, it compresses the abdominal viscera, lowers the intrathoracic pressure, and pulls the inferior vena cava open, thus facilitating the flow of blood from the abdomen into the thorax. Slender branches of the **right phrenic nerve** and some lymph vessels from the liver also traverse the foramen with the inferior vena cava [Fig. 60].

The **oesophagus** passes obliquely through an oval hiatus in the muscular (right crus) part of the diaphragm, posterior to the central tendon, 2–3 cm to the left of the median plane, approximately at the level of the tenth thoracic vertebra. With the oesophagus are the anterior and posterior **vagal trunks**, oesophageal branches of the left gastric artery, and communications between the veins of the stomach and thoracic oesophagus. When the portal vein is obstructed, these veins are distended as an alternative route for the drainage of portal venous blood.

The **aortic hiatus** lies posterior to the median arcuate ligament of the diaphragm and anterior to the twelfth thoracic vertebra. The hiatus also transmits the **thoracic duct**, the **azygos vein**, and lymph vessels which descend to the cisterna chyli (the saccular origin of the thoracic duct) from the thorax.

In addition to these three apertures, a number of smaller structures pass from the thorax to the abdomen through, or around, the diaphragm.

1. The **phrenic nerves**, the right lateral to the inferior vena cava, the left lateral to the pericardium.

2. The **superior epigastric vessels** between the sternal and costal attachments.

3. The **musculophrenic vessels**, between the slips from the seventh and eighth costal cartilages.

4. The lower five intercostal nerves, between the slips from the last six costal cartilages.

5. The **subcostal vessels** and **nerves**, posterior to the lateral arcuate ligaments.

6. The **sympathetic trunks**, posterior to the medial arcuate ligaments.

7. The **splanchnic nerves** pierce the crura, and the hemiazygos vein pierces the left crus.

Nerves and vessels

The motor supply to the diaphragm is from the **phrenic nerves**. These arise from the third to fifth cervical ventral rami (mainly the fourth), and ramify on the inferior surface of the diaphragm. The sensory supply is via the phrenic and lower intercostal nerves. The high level of origin of the phrenic nerves is due to the caudal movement of the diaphragm and viscera relative to the vertebral column during development. The oblique course of the splanchnic nerves and their cervical counterparts, the cervical cardiac branches of the sympathetic (and vagus), is similarly produced.

The principal vessels are the **inferior phrenic** from the abdominal aorta, the **musculophrenic** from the internal thoracic, and the **pericardiacophrenic** which accompany the phrenic nerves through the thorax.

The posterior abdominal wall

Vessels

Dissection

Expose the abdominal aorta and the inferior vena cava. Identify the lymph nodes which lie adjacent to them and the sympathetic trunks which lie on each side of the aorta on the anterior margins of the psoas muscles—the right posterior to the inferior vena cava. Trace the branches of the sympathetic trunks, and clean the proximal parts of the lumbar arteries. Between the right crus of the diaphragm and the aorta, expose the cisterna chyli and the azygos vein. Trace the cisterna chyli upwards to the thoracic duct and the azygos vein inferiorly to the posterior surface of the inferior vena cava at the level of the renal veins. Follow the testicular or ovarian vessels. For the layers of structures on the posterior abdominal wall see Fig. 125.

The abdominal aorta

This median vessel descends on the vertebral column from the aortic hiatus in the diaphragm (T. 12) to its bifurcation into the common iliac vessels on the fourth lumbar vertebra. It is partially surrounded by sympathetic plexuses and lymph vessels and nodes.

The aorta lies on the anterior longitudinal ligament and on the left lumbar veins which pass transversely to the inferior vena cava on its right side. Superiorly, it lies between the crura of the diaphragm; inferiorly it is between the sympathetic trunks with the ascending part of the duodenum and coils of the jejunum on its left side.

Anterior to the aorta, from above downwards, are (1) the pancreas and splenic vein, partly separated from the aorta by the superior mesenteric artery; (2) the left renal vein between the aorta and the superior mesenteric artery; (3) the horizontal part of the duodenum; (4) the root of the mesentery; (5) the peritoneum separating it from coils of small intestine.

In a slim person the inferior part of the abdominal aorta is very close to the anterior abdominal wall, and may readily be compressed against the convexity of the lumbar vertebral column by firm pressure on the anterior abdominal wall just above the umbilicus.

Branches

There are three sets of branches. (1) The unpaired ventral branches have been seen already. (2) Paired lateral branches to the structures derived from

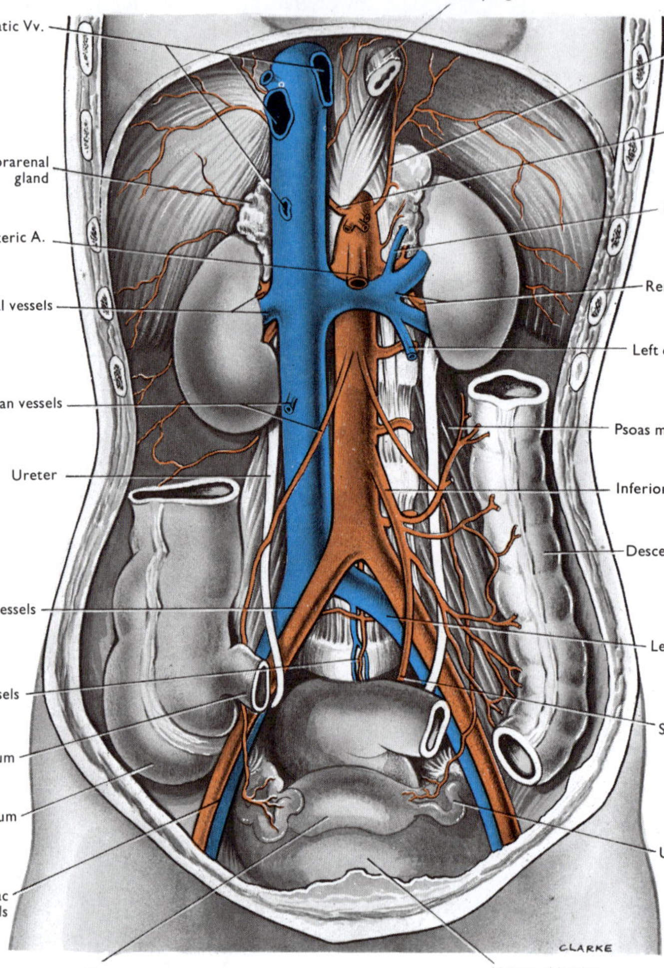

Fig. 199. The inferior vena cava and the abdominal aorta.

the intermediate mesoderm of the embryo (the suprarenal glands, the kidneys, and the ovaries or testes). (3) Paired posterolateral branches (lumbar arteries) to the abdominal wall [p. 184].

The *unpaired branches* are the coeliac trunk, the superior and inferior mesenteric arteries, and the median sacral artery. The last continues downwards into the lesser pelvis from the posterior surface of the aorta at its bifurcation.

Paired branches
[Fig. 199]

The **inferior phrenic arteries** pass superolaterally over the crura of the diaphragm near the superior margins of the suprarenal glands. They send many small **superior suprarenal arteries**, and then ramify on the inferior surface of the diaphragm. The diaphragmatic veins enter the inferior vena cava, though the left may pass with the left suprarenal vein to the left renal vein.

Small **middle suprarenal arteries** arise near the origin of the superior mesenteric artery. They pass laterally to the suprarenal glands, the right posterior to the inferior vena cava.

The **suprarenal veins**, one on each side, drain respectively into the left renal vein and the inferior vena cava. Occasionally the left vein passes across the anterior surface of the aorta to the inferior vena cava.

Renal arteries

These large arteries arise at the level of the upper part of the second lumbar vertebra, and cross the corresponding crus of the diaphragm and psoas muscle to the kidneys. Here each branches to supply the kidney [p. 171] and sends small arteries to the ureter and suprarenal gland (**inferior suprarenal artery**). The right renal artery passes posterior to the inferior vena cava and the right renal vein; the left is posterior to its vein [Fig. 191].

An **accessory renal artery** is not uncommon. It usually arises from the lower part of the aorta, passes anterior to the ureter (and inferior vena cava if right-sided), and enters the antero-inferior part of the kidney.

Renal veins

These enter the inferior vena cava on the right side of the median plane. Thus the right renal vein is much shorter than the left. Both veins lie anterior to the corresponding artery. The right vein passes posterior to the descending part of the duodenum, and may be overlapped by the right margin of the head of the pancreas. The long left vein is joined by the left suprarenal and testicular or ovarian veins, and usually by the hemiazygos vein close to the kidney. The left renal vein passes to the right, posterior to the inferior border of the pancreas and to the inferior mesenteric vein as it ascends to the splenic vein, and crosses the median plane in the angle between the aorta and the superior mesenteric artery [Fig. 199].

Testicular and ovarian vessels

Each testicular artery is a long slender vessel that arises from the front of the aorta a short distance inferior to the renal arteries. It runs inferolaterally between the ureter lying on the posterior abdominal wall and the intestines and mesenteric vessels, to reach the corresponding deep inguinal ring and enter the inguinal canal. Thus the **right testicular artery** lies anterior to the inferior vena cava, psoas, ureter, and external iliac artery, but is posterior to the horizontal part of the duodenum, the right colic, ileocolic, and superior mesenteric vessels, and the caecum. The **left testicular artery** has the same structures posterior to it (other than the inferior vena cava). It is posterior to the duodenum, the inferior mesenteric vein, the left colic and sigmoid arteries, and the inferior part of the descending colon [Figs. 125, 163].

The **ovarian arteries** are exactly similar to the testicular arteries except that they enter the lesser pelvis by crossing the external iliac arteries 2–3 cm inferior to their origins [Fig. 199]. Thus the left is posterior to the sigmoid colon and mesocolon, not the descending colon, and the right to the terminal ileum, not the caecum.

Each **testicular** or **ovarian vein** is formed by coalescence of a **pampiniform plexus**: the testicular at the deep inguinal ring, the ovarian at the margin of the superior aperture of the pelvis. The veins accompany the corresponding arteries. The **left** enters the left renal vein, the **right** enters the inferior vena cava inferior to the renal vein. This *apparent asymmetry* of the gonadal and suprarenal veins arises because that part of the left renal vein which these vessels enter is all that remains of a **left inferior vena cava**. This usually disappears early in development, but may persist between the left common iliac and left renal veins.

Lumbar arteries

Four pairs of these arteries arise from the posterior surface of the abdominal aorta in series with the posterior intercostal arteries. They pass laterally on the surfaces of the lumbar vertebral bodies, and then backwards deep to the psoas muscle with the corresponding lumbar veins and the rami communicantes of the lumbar nerves [p. 183].

The inferior vena cava [Figs. 282–288]

This is the widest vein of the body. It drains venous blood from the lower limbs, most of the abdominal wall, the urogenital apparatus, and the suprarenal glands. The venous blood from the remaining abdominal viscera drains to the liver in the portal vein, and reaches the inferior vena cava only after it has traversed the liver.

The inferior vena cava begins by the union of the two **common iliac veins** on the front of the fifth lumbar vertebra, posterior to the right common iliac artery [Figs. 199, 289]. It ascends to the right of the median plane, at first between the aorta and the right ureter, and anterior to the vertebral column, and the right psoas, sympathetic trunk, and lumbar arteries. It then arches forwards on the right crus of the diaphragm, anterior to the right renal artery, the right coeliac ganglion, and middle suprarenal artery, to reach a deep groove in the liver between the right and caudate lobes [Fig. 178]. Here it is anterior to the medial part of the right suprarenal gland and the posterior part of the diaphragm [Fig. 130].

Anterior to the inferior vena cava as it ascends are: (1) the superior mesenteric vessels in the root of the mesentery; (2) the ileocolic and right colic vessels; (3) the horizontal part of the duodenum and the right testicular or ovarian artery; (4) the head of the pancreas and the bile-duct; (5) the portal vein, at first posterior to the superior part of the duodenum, and then in the lesser omentum anterior to the epiploic foramen; (6) the liver tissue between the right and caudate lobes. Here it receives the **hepatic veins**, then pierces the central tendon of the diaphragm and the pericardium, and enters the postero-inferior part of the right atrium.

Tributaries

(1) Common iliac veins. (2) Third and fourth lumbar veins. (3) Right testicular or ovarian vein. (4) Renal veins. (5) Azygos vein. (6) Right suprarenal vein. (7) Inferior phrenic veins. (8) Hepatic veins.

Common iliac arteries
[Figs. 199, 233]

These terminal branches of the abdominal aorta arise on the anterior surface of the fourth lumbar vertebra, and are accompanied by extensions of the aortic sympathetic and lymph plexuses. Each passes inferolaterally to the superior surface of the sacro-iliac joint, where it divides into internal and external iliac arteries. *Both* common iliac arteries are anterior to the corresponding sympathetic trunk and are crossed by its branches and those of the aortic plexus passing to the hypogastric plexuses. The superior rectal vessels and some sigmoid arteries lie anterior to the *left* common iliac artery, while the *right* artery lies directly on the beginning of the inferior vena cava and the right common iliac vein.

Common iliac veins
[Fig. 199]

These veins begin on the medial surface of the psoas muscle by the union of the internal and external iliac veins. They end by uniting in the inferior vena cava 2 cm to the right of the median plane on the fifth lumbar vertebra. Each receives an iliolumbar vein, and the median sacral vein joins the left common iliac vein.

The right vein is posterior to the corresponding artery. The left is inferomedial to its artery and runs a longer course to reach the inferior vena cava.

External iliac arteries

They begin immediately anterior to the sacro-iliac joints as the direct continuation of the common iliac arteries. They pass inferolaterally along the margins of the superior aperture of the lesser pelvis, at first medial and then anterior to the psoas. Each gives off a **deep circumflex iliac artery** and an **inferior epigastric artery** immediately superior to the inguinal ligament at the mid-inguinal point, and then becomes the femoral artery by passing posterior to the ligament.

Each artery is at first anterior and then lateral to its vein, and is crossed proximally by the ureter and distally by the ductus deferens (or round ligament of the uterus) and the deep circumflex iliac vein. The genital branch of the genitofemoral nerve runs on the distal part of the artery, and the ovarian vessels cross it 2–3 cm inferior to its origin [Fig. 199]. On the right, the caecum and appendix may overlie it; on the left, the end of the descending colon is directly anterior to its distal part.

External iliac veins

Each ascends with its artery, passing from its medial to its posterior surface, and being crossed by the same structures. Each vein receives an inferior epigastric and a deep circumflex iliac vein, and passing lateral to the internal iliac artery, unites with the internal iliac vein.

The lymph nodes of the posterior abdominal wall
[Figs. 200, 255]

These are scattered along the iliac vessels, the aorta, and the inferior vena cava.

The **external iliac nodes** lie on the corresponding vessels. Inferiorly the medial nodes receive lymph from the lower limb and pelvic viscera, while the lateral nodes drain the territories of the inferior epigastric and deep circumflex iliac vessels. All this lymph ascends through other external iliac nodes to the **common iliac nodes** which lie along the common iliac vessels (lateral group) and in the angle between them (medial group). The lateral group receive lymph from the lower limb and pelvis through the external and internal iliac nodes. The medial group drains the pelvic viscera directly and

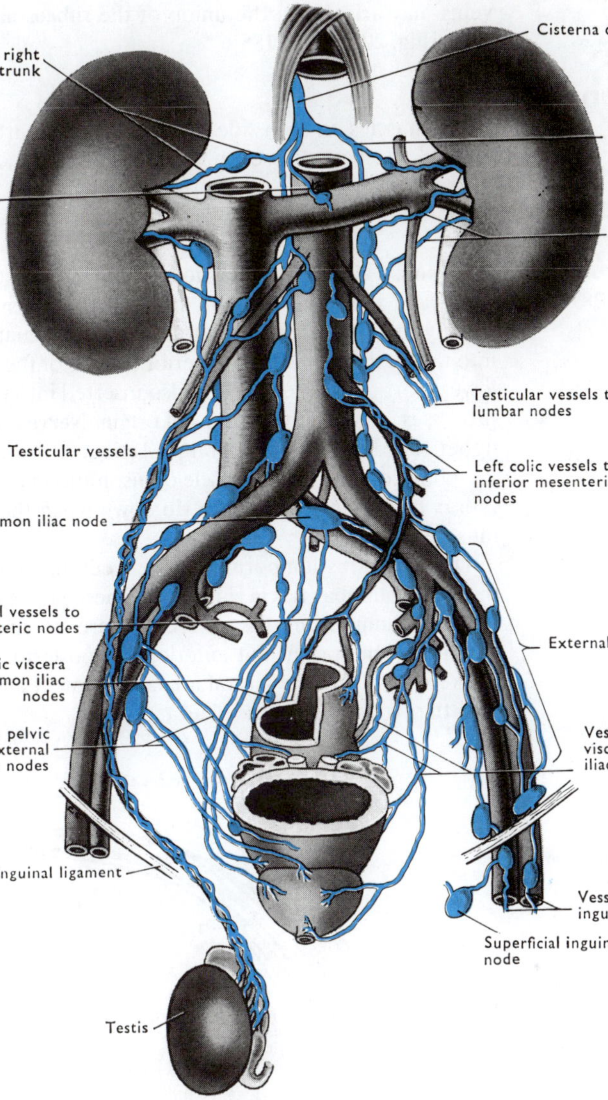

Fig. 200. A diagram to show the lymph vessels and nodes of the male pelvis and abdomen.

through the internal iliac and sacral nodes. The efferents of the common iliac nodes pass to the lumbar nodes.

The **lumbar nodes** are scattered along the aorta and the inferior vena cava. They receive lymph *directly* from adjacent structures, i.e. posterior abdominal wall, kidneys, and ureters, and from the **testes** or from the **ovaries, uterine tubes, uterus**, and the remainder of the abdominal contents (except the liver, stomach, and small intestine. They also receive lymph from the descending colon, pelvis, and lower limbs through inferior mesenteric and common iliac nodes. The efferent vessels from the lumbar nodes form the right and left **lumbar lymph trunks**, which drain to the cisterna chyli.

Cisterna chyli

This long (5 cm), white lymph sac, approximately 4 mm wide in the cadaver, is often tortuous and branched. It lies on the upper two lumbar vertebrae between the aorta and the azygos vein, hidden by the right crus of the diaphragm. It receives the **lumbar lymph trunks** inferiorly, the **intestinal lymph trunk** (which drains the liver, stomach, and small intestine) about the middle, and lymph vessels from the lower intercostal nodes superiorly. Above it continues through the aortic hiatus as the **thoracic duct** [Fig. 86]. A similar, distended lymph sac may be present on the left of the aorta.

The azygos and hemiazygos veins

Both these veins usually begin in the abdomen; the hemiazygos from the posterior surface of the left renal vein, the azygos from the inferior vena cava at the same level. They ascend into the thorax through the aortic hiatus (azygos) and the left crus (hemiazygos) of the diaphragm. Either or both veins may arise from the union of the **subcostal** with the **ascending lumbar veins** [Fig. 205 and p. 185].

The muscles and fasciae of the posterior abdominal wall

Three muscles on each side form the greater part of the posterior abdominal wall, and each is enclosed in fascia.

Quadratus lumborum [Figs. 105, 190, 197, 287, 288]

This muscle arises from the iliolumbar ligament, the adjacent part of the iliac crest, and the lower two to four lumbar transverse processes. Narrowing slightly, it ascends posterior to the lateral arcuate ligament, and is inserted into the medial part of the anterior surface of the twelfth rib, posterior to the lowest part of the pleura. It is also inserted into the upper lumbar transverse processes, posterior to its slips of origin. **Nerve supply:** direct branches of the upper four lumbar ventral rami. **Action:** it is a lateral flexor of the lumbar vertebral column, and a muscle of inspiration because it helps to elongate the thorax by holding the twelfth rib down when the diaphragm and intercostal muscles contract.

The quadratus lumborum lies between the anterior and middle layers of the **thoracolumbar fascia** [Fig. 201]. These layers fuse at the lateral margin of quadratus lumborum. Elsewhere they are attached to the same structures as quadratus lumborum, but anterior and posterior to it. The anterior layer is thickened to form the lateral arcuate ligament and continues upwards to the twelfth rib posterior to the pleura.

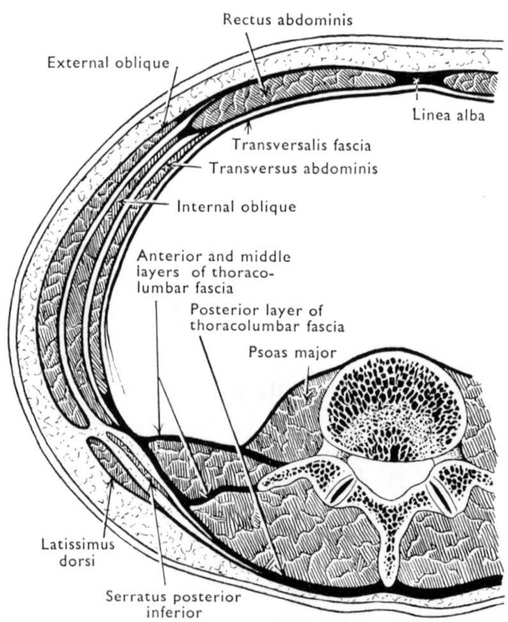

Fig. 201. A horizontal section through the abdominal walls at the level of the second lumbar vertebra, to show the thoracolumbar fascia.

Psoas major [Figs. 197, 201, 287–291]

This long muscle arises from the anterior surfaces of the upper four lumbar transverse processes, medial to quadratus lumborum; from sides of the last thoracic and upper four lumbar intervertebral discs and the adjacent margins of the vertebral bodies; from the tendinous arches which unite these margins lateral to the lumbar arteries.

The muscle continues along the margin of the superior aperture of the lesser pelvis, and enters the thigh posterior to the inguinal ligament. Here its tendon passes postero-inferiorly to the lesser trochanter of the femur [Fig. 204]. **Nerve supply:** direct branches from the second to fourth lumbar ventral rami and from the femoral nerve. **Action:** see under iliacus.

Psoas minor [Fig. 197]

This small muscle is present in only 60 per cent of cadavers. It arises with the uppermost fibres of psoas major, descends on the anterior surface of that muscle, and forming a slender tendon, is inserted into the thickened lower part of the fascia covering psoas and iliacus. Through this it is inserted medially to the arcuate line of the ilium [Figs. 207, 259] and laterally with the iliac fascia to the inguinal ligament. **Nerve supply:** first lumbar ventral ramus. **Action:** see under iliacus.

Iliacus
[Figs. 204, 259, 289–291]

This muscle arises from the upper part of the floor of the iliac fossa. It converges on and fuses with the lower part of psoas major which it accompanies to the lesser trochanter of the femur and an area immediately inferior to the trochanter. **Nerve supply:** the femoral nerve.

Actions of psoas and iliacus

They are flexors of the hip joint. Inserted lateral to the axis of rotation which passes through the head of the femur, they rotate the thigh medially, e.g. the flexed medially rotated thigh in psoas spasm of acute appendicitis. When the neck of the femur is broken, the axis becomes the shaft of the bone so they rotate the limb laterally and the toes characteristically point in this direction. The psoas muscles are lateral flexors of the lumbar vertebral column.

Fascia of psoas and iliacus

Psoas is enclosed in a sheath of fascia which fuses above with the periosteum of the vertebral column and the anterior layer of the thoracolumbar fascia and is thickened to form the **medial arcuate ligament** where the diaphragm is attached to it. Below it fuses with the arcuate line of the pelvis and the fascia covering iliacus (iliac fascia). This long tubular sheath forms a route along which infected material may travel from the thoracic vertebral column to the groin.

Iliac fascia is attached to the internal lip of the iliac crest, to the inguinal ligament and transversalis fascia [Fig. 109] and forms the posterior wall of the femoral sheath anteromedially [Fig. 113]. It is often thickened by the insertion of psoas minor into it.

Dissection

Expose the muscles of the posterior abdominal wall by removing their fascial coverings. Avoid injury to the vessels and nerves related to the muscles (the main vessels lie anterior to the fascia while the nerves are posterior to it). The vessels on iliacus are branches of the iliolumbar artery.

Push the inferior vena cava laterally and expose the right sympathetic trunk. Trace both trunks superiorly to the medial arcuate ligaments, and inferiorly into the pelvis, posterior to the common iliac vessels. Find and trace the branches of both trunks to the superior hypogastric plexus [p. 139]. Detach psoas major from the intervertebral discs and vertebral bodies, and trace the **lumbar vessels** and the rami communicantes posteriorly deep to the tendinous arches from which psoas arises.

The nerves of the posterior abdominal wall

Sympathetic trunk
[Fig. 197]

The thoracic part of each sympathetic trunk is continuous with the lumbar part posterior to the medial arcuate ligament. In the abdomen, the trunk lies in the groove between the anterior border of psoas major and the vertebral bodies, anterior to the lumbar vessels. It enters the pelvis by passing posterior to the common iliac vessels [Fig. 289B].

Branches

The **rami communicantes** [p. 28] are long. They run with the lumbar vessels to the ventral rami of the lumbar nerves buried in the posterior part of psoas. White and grey rami communicantes unite the trunk to the first two or three lumbar ventral rami, but only a grey ramus unites it to each of the remaining lumbar and to the sacral ventral rami.

Visceral branches (**lumbar splanchnic nerves**) arise irregularly from the trunk. They pass to the pelvis through the aortic and hypogastric plexuses.

Subcostal nerve

This is the ventral ramus of the last thoracic nerve. It sends a branch to the ventral ramus of the first lumbar nerve, and then passes inferolaterally on the

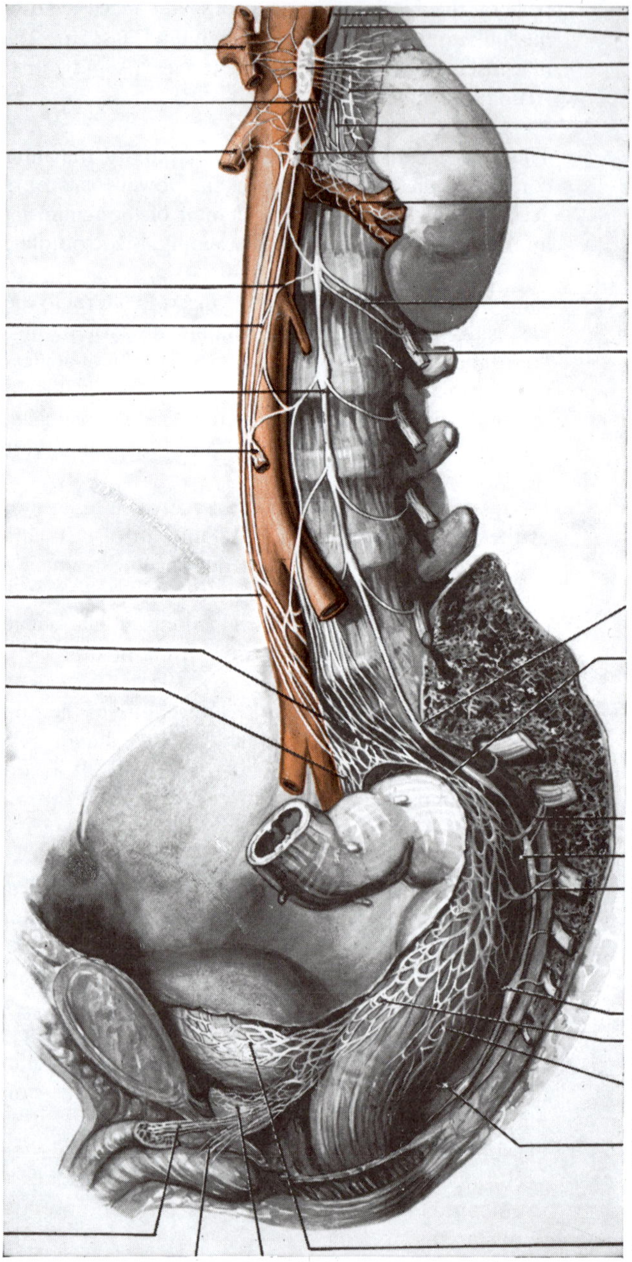

Fig. 202. Plexuses of autonomic system in abdomen and pelvis.

anterior surface of quadratus lumborum to enter the abdomen posterior to the lateral arcuate ligament. At the lateral border of quadratus lumborum, it pierces transversus abdominis to run in the abdominal wall between that muscle and the internal oblique [p. 103].

Dissection

Find the genitofemoral nerve on the anterior surface of psoas [Fig. 204] and trace it through that muscle to the lumbar nerves. Carefully complete the removal of psoas from the transverse processes of the lumbar vertebrae, disentangling the ventral rami of the lumbar nerves from its substance. Expose these nerves and their branches.

Lumbar nerves

The five lumbar nerves emerge through the intervertebral foramina below the corresponding vertebrae, and their ventral rami pass into the posterior part of psoas major. Here they are connected to the sympathetic trunk by rami communicantes, and give branches to supply the intertransverse muscles, psoas, and quadratus lumborum. The ventral rami then divide. The upper branch of the **fourth lumbar ventral ramus** joins with the branches of the first to third to form the lumbar plexus, while its lower branch joins the fifth lumbar ventral ramus to form the **lumbosacral trunk** which descends to the sacral plexus. Because it divides to send nerve fibres to both plexuses, the fourth lumbar ventral ramus is sometimes called the nervus furcalis.

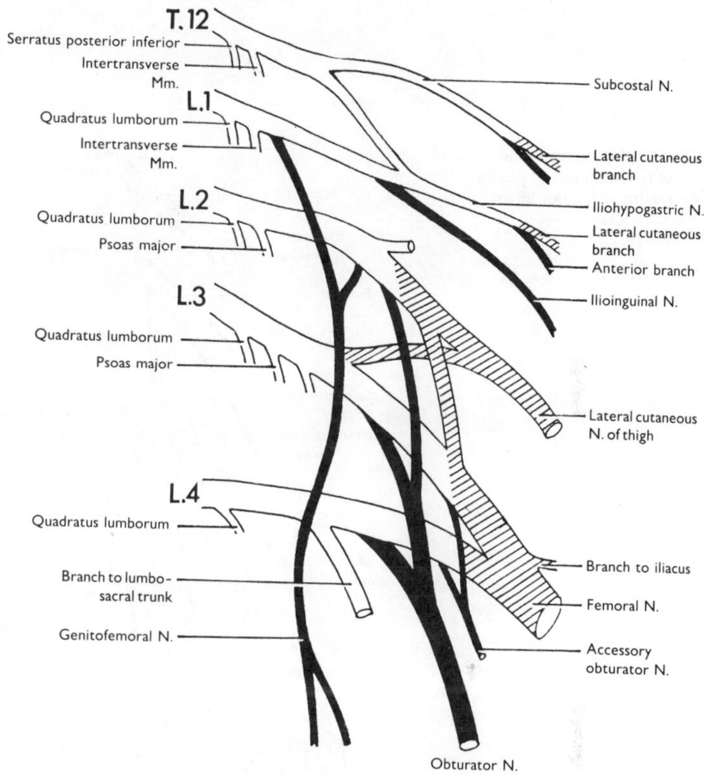

Fig. 203. A diagram of the lumbar plexus. Ventral divisions of the ventral rami, black; dorsal divisions, cross-hatched. See also Fig. 256.

Lumbar plexus
[Fig. 288]

This plexus is formed in the substance of the psoas major by the ventral rami of the first three lumbar nerves with part of the fourth, and a contribution from the subcostal nerve. These do not form dorsal and ventral divisions as in the brachial plexus, but the major nerves arising from the lumbar plexus can be recognized as belonging to one or other division [Fig. 203].

The **iliohypogastric nerve** (L. 1, T. 12) emerges from psoas, and passes inferolaterally between quadratus lumborum and the kidney. It pierces transversus abdominis a short distance superior to the iliac crest, and runs in the abdominal wall [p. 103].

The **ilioinguinal nerve** (L. 1) takes the same course as the iliohypogastric but at a slightly lower level. It has no lateral cutaneous branch.

The **genitofemoral nerve** (L. 1, 2; ventral divisions) passes forwards through psoas, and runs inferiorly on that muscle dividing into femoral and genital branches. The **femoral branch** follows the lateral side of the external iliac artery into the femoral sheath. It pierces the anterior wall of the sheath and the fascia lata to supply skin over the femoral triangle. The **genital branch** pierces the psoas sheath, and runs to the deep inguinal ring. It traverses the inguinal canal supplying the **cremaster muscle** and skin of the scrotum in the male, or sensory fibres to the round ligament of the uterus and the skin of the labium majus in the female.

The **lateral cutaneous nerve of the thigh** (L. 2, 3; dorsal divisions) emerges from psoas above the iliac crest. It passes obliquely across iliacus towards the anterior superior iliac spine, and enters the thigh posterior to the lateral end of the inguinal ligament.

The **femoral nerve** (L. 2, 3, 4; dorsal divisions) emerges from psoas below the iliac crest. It descends in the groove between psoas and iliacus (posterior to the iliac fascia and the caecum or descending colon) and enters the thigh lateral to the femoral sheath. In the abdomen, it supplies psoas and iliacus.

The **obturator nerve** (L. 2, 3, 4; ventral divisions) leaves the medial border of psoas on the base of the sacrum, and enters the lesser pelvis [p. 237].

An **accessory obturator nerve** may arise from the obturator nerve or from the third and fourth lumbar nerves. It runs to the thigh along the medial side of psoas, gives branches to the hip joint and sometimes to pectineus, and joins the obturator nerve.

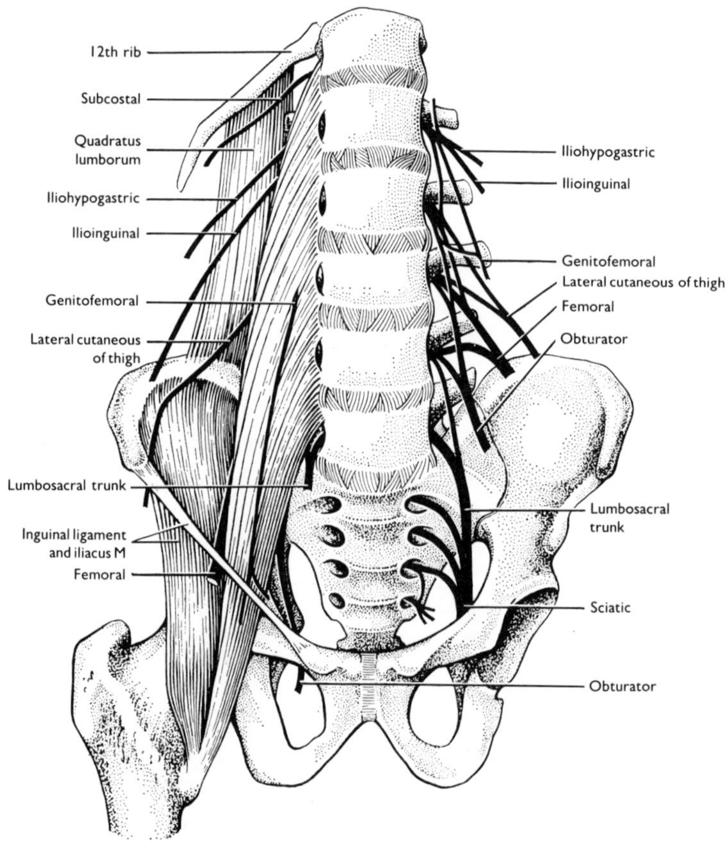

Fig. 204. A semidiagrammatic drawing of the lumbosacral plexus and the quadratus lumborum and iliopsoas muscles.

Lumbosacral trunk

The inferior branch of the fourth lumbar ventral ramus descends through psoas on the medial part of the fifth lumbar transverse process. It forms the trunk by uniting with the ventral ramus of the fifth lumbar nerve, and enters the lesser pelvis on the base of the sacrum, posterior to the common iliac vessels and psoas.

The roots of the obturator and femoral nerves and the contribution from the fourth lumbar ventral ramus to the lumbosacral trunk all run anterior to the **fifth lumbar transverse process**. Any or all of them may be damaged in injuries of this process.

Subcostal and lumbar vessels

The **subcostal artery** is the last parietal branch of the thoracic aorta. It passes with the subcostal nerve into the abdominal wall. The **subcostal vein** lies superior to the artery and enters the azygos (right) or hemiazygos (left) vein, sometimes forming that vein with the ascending lumbar vein.

Lumbar arteries

The upper four pairs arise from the posterior surface of the abdominal aorta on the lumbar vertebral bodies. They curve over the vertebral bodies passing deep to the sympathetic trunk (and to the cisterna chyli and inferior vena cava on the right) and the fibrous arches of origin of the psoas. The upper one or two are also deep to the azygos or hemiazygos veins and the crura of the diaphragm. At the root of the transverse process, each artery gives off a posterior branch, then passes posterior to quadratus lumborum to end as a number of small branches between transversus abdominis and the internal oblique muscles.

The **posterior branch** accompanies the dorsal ramus of the spinal nerve. It sends a **spinal branch** through the intervertebral foramen to the contents of the vertebral canal, and ends in the erector spinae muscle and the overlying skin.

A small **fifth** pair of lumbar **arteries** arise from the median sacral artery or from the iliolumbar arteries.

Lumbar veins

These accompany the lumbar arteries. The first and second join the ascending lumbar vein on the lumbar transverse processes. The third and fourth enter the inferior vena cava, the left vessels passing posterior to the aorta. The fifth enters the iliolumbar vein.

The **ascending lumbar vein** unites the lateral sacral, iliolumbar, and upper four lumbar veins to the subcostal vein. It ascends in psoas major anterior to the lumbar transverse processes. The major tributaries are the communications through the intervertebral foramina with the **internal vertebral venous plexuses** [Fig. 205].

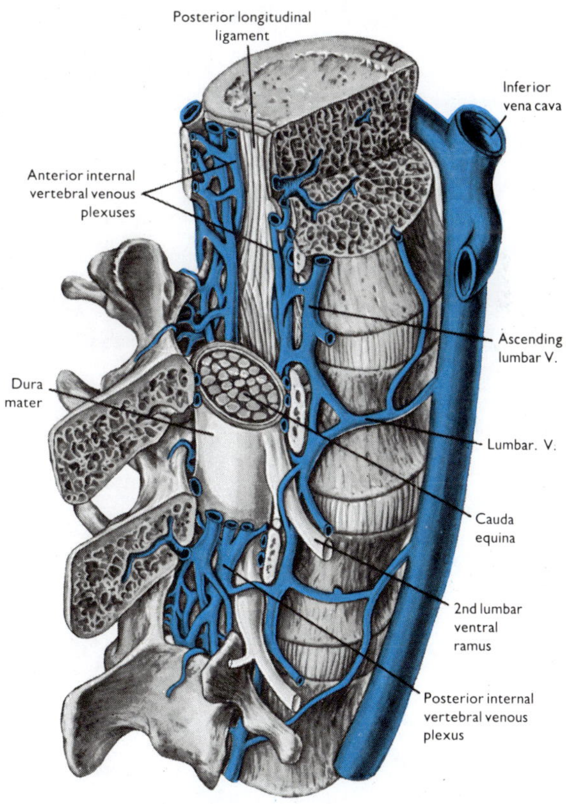

Fig. 205. Dissection of the upper four lumbar vertebrae to show the internal vertebral venous plexuses and their communications with the inferior vena cava.

Dissection

It is an advantage to remove the pelvis and lower limb from the trunk at this stage, but this can only be done without damage if the erector spinae muscle and the lumbar vertebral canal have been dissected. If this has not been done by the dissectors of the head and neck, then the appropriate pages of Volume 3 of this Manual should be read and the dissections carried out on the lumbar and sacral regions only.

Then cut through the intervertebral disc between the third and fourth lumbar vertebrae and all the other soft structures on each side

of the vertebral column at this level. Identify the joints between the articular processes, and divide the ligaments uniting them. This separates the pelvis and lower limbs from the remainder of the trunk.

Intervertebral joints

Examine the joints between the lumbar vertebrae [Figs. 95, 96], and compare them with those in the cervical and thoracic regions [p. 81]. Review the structure of the intervertebral disc [p. 79] and the arrangement of the ligaments uniting the vertebrae.

If the dissectors of the abdomen and pelvis are to dissect the lower limb later, *there is considerable advantage in dissecting the thigh and gluteal region before continuing with the pelvis.* If this is possible, then pages 125–60 of Volume 1 of this Manual should now be followed.

The pelvis and perineum

The bones of the pelvis consist of the two hip bones, the sacrum, and the coccyx. They are united by four joints; two synovial sacro-iliac joints posterosuperiorly, and two fibrocartilaginous joints—the pubic symphysis antero-inferiorly and the sacrococcygeal joint posteriorly.

In the erect position, the pelvis lies with the upper margin of the pubic symphysis and the anterior superior iliac spines in the same coronal plane. This is the position taken up by an articulated pelvis placed with these three points touching a vertical surface.

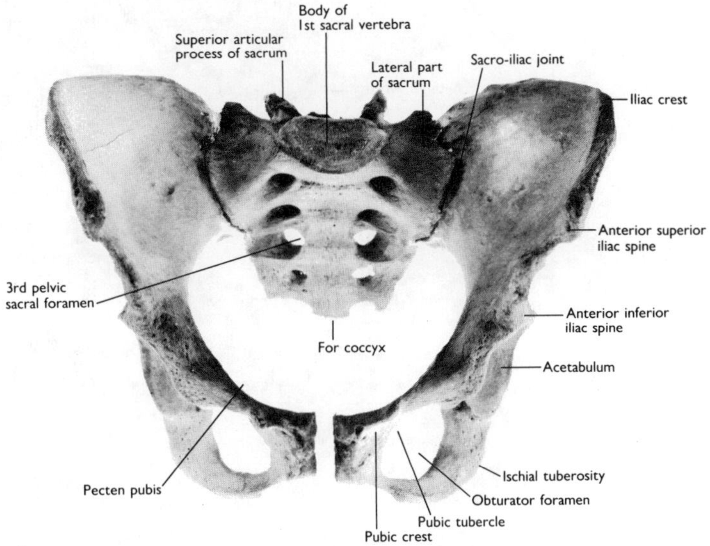

Fig. 206. The female pelvis seen from in front.

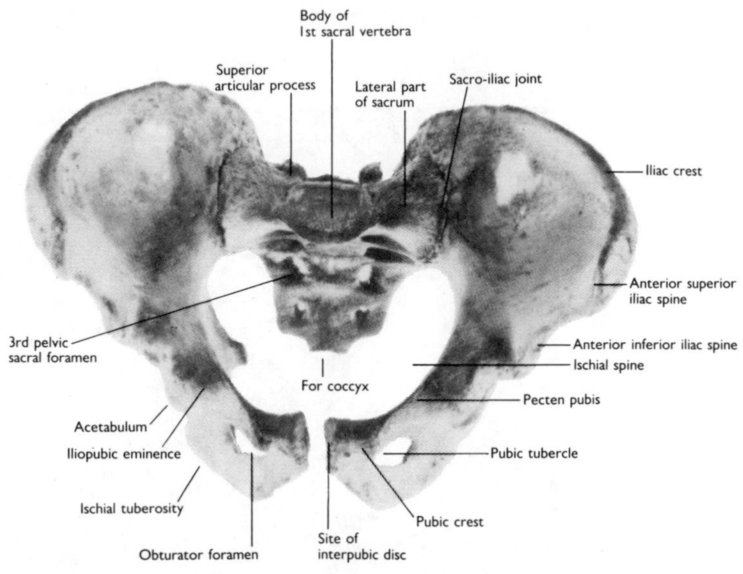

Fig. 207. The male pelvis seen from in front without coccyx.

The pelvis consists of two parts which are separated by the plane of the superior aperture of the lesser pelvis. This is an oblique plane passing from the sacral promontory to the upper surface of the pubic symphysis. The part anterosuperior to the plane, the greater pelvis, is formed by the iliac fossae and is part of the wall of the abdomen. The part postero-inferior to the plane is the lesser pelvis, to which the term pelvis is frequently applied.

The lesser pelvis

Begin by reviewing the bony walls of the lesser pelvis [pp. 85–9]. In the sagittal plane, the cavity of the lesser pelvis is C-shaped [Fig. 236] with a long, curved *posterosuperior wall* formed by the sacrum and coccyx, and a short *antero-inferior wall* which lies below the level of the coccyx and is formed by the bodies of the pubic bones and the pubic symphysis. The *anterolateral wall*

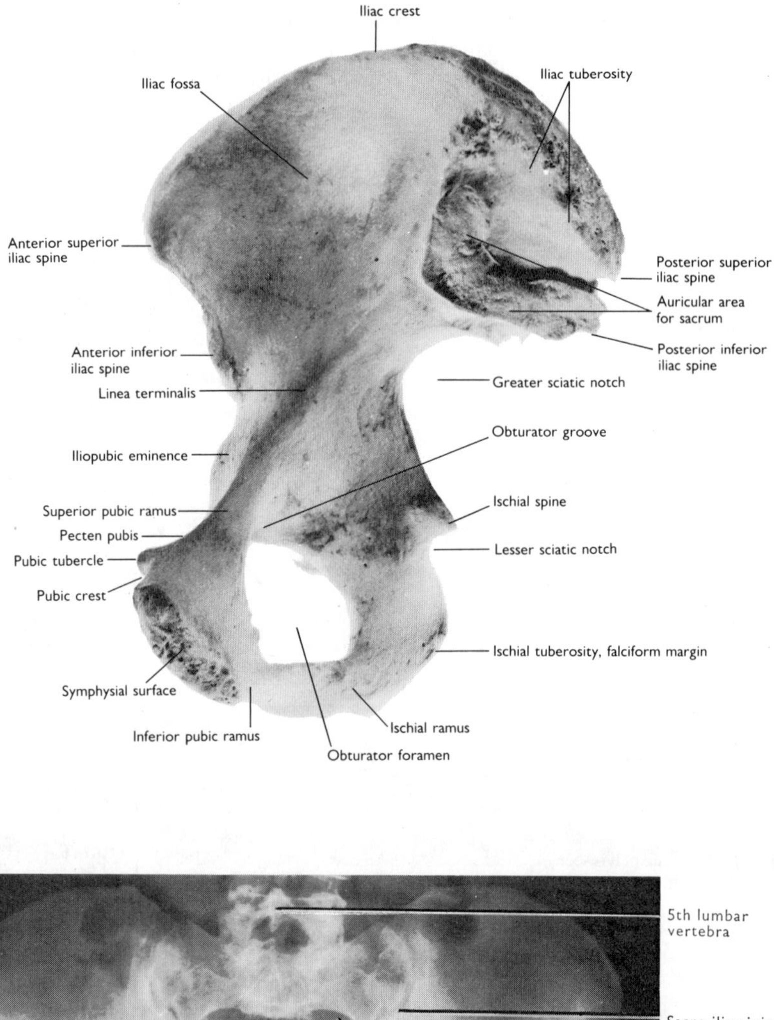

Fig. 208. The right hip bone seen from the medial side. Cf. Fig. 259.

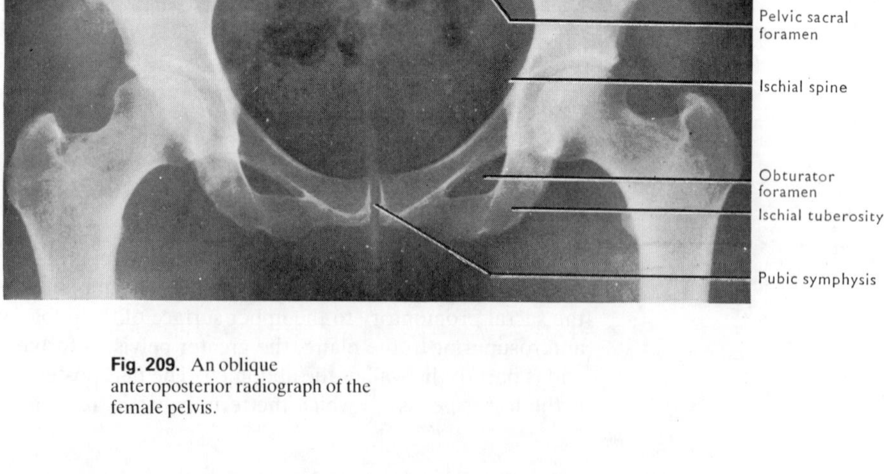

Fig. 209. An oblique anteroposterior radiograph of the female pelvis.

is formed inferiorly by the **rami of the pubis** and by the **ischium** which together surround the **obturator foramen**. Superiorly this wall is completed by the medial wall of the acetabulum (where pubis, ischium, and ilium unite) and above this by a small part of the ilium [Fig. 208]. Posteriorly, this part of the ilium curves medially to meet the sacrum at the **sacro-iliac joint**. Inferior to this joint, the *posterolateral wall* of the lesser pelvis is the gap between the hip bone and the sacrum and coccyx. This gap is partly filled by the **sacrotuberous** and **sacrospinous ligaments** which divide it into greater and lesser **sciatic foramina** [Figs. 211, 212]. The gap in the anterolateral wall (obturator foramen) is filled by the **obturator membrane** except anteriorly where the obturator vessels and nerve leave the lesser pelvis in the **obturator canal**.

The walls of the lesser pelvis end anterosuperiorly at the margin of the superior aperture—the **linea terminalis** of the pelvis. This consists of the anterior margin of the base of the sacrum, and on each side the **arcuate line** of the ilium, the **pecten pubis**, the **pubic crest**, and the **pubic symphysis**. Inferiorly the walls end in the boundaries of the **inferior aperture of the pelvis**. This is a diamond-shaped aperture with the pubic symphysis, the coccyx, and the ischial tuberosities at the angles. The anterolateral margins are the ischial and inferior pubic rami; the posterolateral margins are the sacrotuberous ligaments [Figs. 218, 219]. These are *boundaries of the perineum*.

The inferior aperture transmits the urethra, the vagina in the female, and the anal canal. Elsewhere it is closed, the anterior half by the **urogenital diaphragm**, the posterior half by the **levator ani muscles**. The walls of the lesser pelvis are lined by muscles—**piriformis** on the sacrum [Fig. 257], **coccygeus** on the sacrospinous ligament, and **obturator internus** on the anterolateral wall [Fig. 259]. All these are covered internally by a layer of **pelvic fascia**.

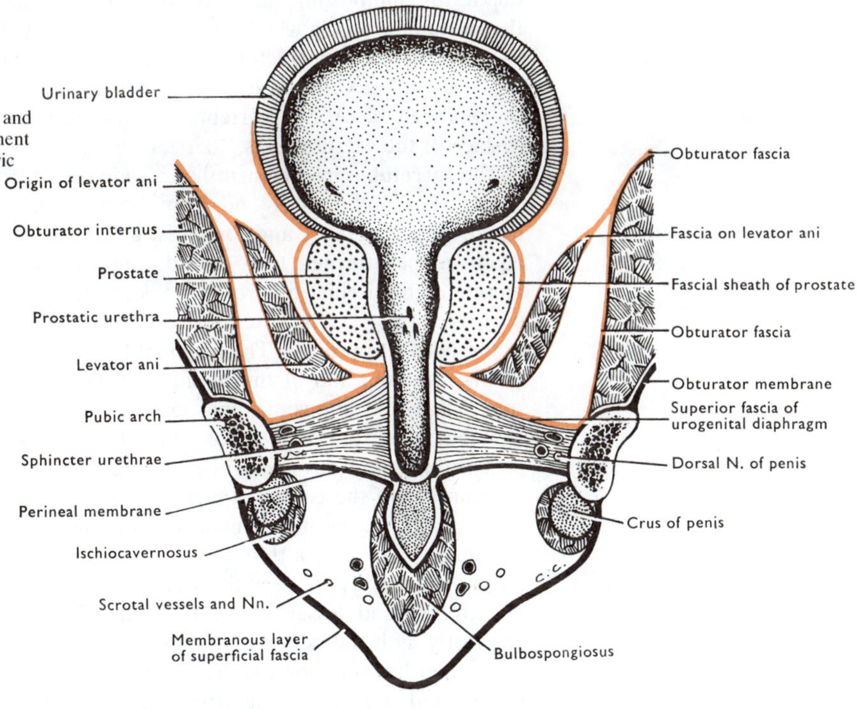

Fig. 210. A schematic coronal section through the male pelvis and perineum to show the arrangement of the parietal and visceral pelvic fascia (red).

The **levator ani muscles** run postero-inferiorly from the anterolateral walls of the lesser pelvis to meet one another in the median plane from the posterior margin of the urogenital diaphragm to the coccyx. Thus they divide the cavity of the lesser pelvis into an upper part containing the pelvic viscera (the **pelvic cavity**, for which they form a V-shaped floor—**pelvic diaphragm**), and a lower part consisting of an **ischiorectal fossa** on each side roofed by the levator ani muscles [Fig. 225].

The **parietal pelvic fascia** lines the walls of the pelvic cavity and covers the superior surfaces of the levator ani muscles. This part of the fascial envelope of the abdomen is continuous with the loose fascial layer (visceral pelvic fascia [Figs. 210, 222]) that surrounds the pelvic viscera where these structures lie on, or pierce, levator ani.

The **pelvic peritoneum** passes over the superior surfaces of the pelvic viscera and dips between them to form pouches. Elsewhere they are separated from the parietal pelvic fascia by fatty extraperitoneal tissue which contains their blood vessels and autonomic (hypogastric) nerve plexuses. The main nerves of the **sacral plexuses** lie external to the parietal pelvic fascia [Fig. 217].

Dissection

Assuming that the gluteal region has been dissected, expose the iliolumbar ligaments and the ligaments on the posterior surface of the sacro-iliac joints by removing the overlying erector spinae muscles and the posterior layer of the thoracolumbar fascia. Expose the dorsal sacral foramina [Fig. 98] and the dorsal rami of the sacral nerves passing through them together with small blood vessels. Define the attachments of the sacrotuberous ligament, then cut across the ligament at its middle, and separate it from the underlying sacrospinous ligament, noting any small nerves between them. Define the sacrospinous ligament and the spine of the ischium, and find the pudendal nerve, the internal pudendal vessels, and the nerve to obturator internus curving over the ligament and the adjacent part of the spine.

Vertebropelvic ligaments

[Figs. 211, 212, 218]

A strong, triangular **iliolumbar ligament** unites each thick transverse process of the fifth lumbar vertebra to the inner lip of the iliac crest posteriorly. Its lower fibres descend to the lateral part of the sacrum as the **lateral lumbosacral ligament**. The horizontal part gives origin to part of the quadratus lumborum, and to the anterior and middle layers of the **thoracolumbar fascia** which enclose it. Anteriorly the ligament is covered by psoas, posteriorly by erector spinae. It plays an important part in maintaining the fifth lumbar vertebra in position, resisting the tendency of the weight of the body to force that vertebra antero-inferiorly on the sloping superior surface of the sacrum [Figs. 105, 236].

The **sacrotuberous ligament** has a wide origin from the dorsal surfaces of the sacrum and coccyx and from both posterior iliac spines. It passes downwards, laterally, and forwards, at first narrowing and then expanding again, to be attached to a curved, sharp ridge of bone along the medial margin of the ischial tuberosity. It is partly continuous with the tendon of biceps femoris, and its anterior margin curves forwards on the ischial ramus as the **falciform process**. The ligament forms parts of the boundaries of both sciatic foramina and of the perineum [Figs. 211, 218, 291]. It gives origin superficially to gluteus maximus, and it crosses piriformis, the sacrospinous ligament, and the tendon of obturator internus. It is pierced by the **perforating cutaneous nerve**, the coccygeal and fifth sacral ventral rami, and by branches of the **coccygeal plexus.**

The **sacrospinous ligament** is the fibrous dorsal part of the **coccygeus muscle**. It extends as a thin, triangular sheet from the lateral margins of the coccyx and the last piece of the sacrum to the ischial spine. Thus it separates the greater and lesser sciatic foramina. These foramina are continuous anteriorly with the pelvic cavity and the ischiorectal fossa respectively, for the greater lies superior and the lesser inferior to the pelvic diaphragm. Thus vessels and nerves passing from the pelvis to the ischiorectal fossa and perineum emerge through the greater foramen and enter the lesser, hooking over the sacrospinous ligament (pudendal nerve) or the ischial spine (internal pudendal vessels and nerve to obturator internus). The medial part of the ligament is covered by the sacrotuberous ligament with the **perineal branch of the fourth sacral** and **perforating cutaneous nerves** between them.

The sacrotuberous and sacrospinous ligaments bind the sacrum to the ischium, and holding down the posterior part of the sacrum, prevent the weight of the body depressing its anterior part around the sacro-iliac joints.

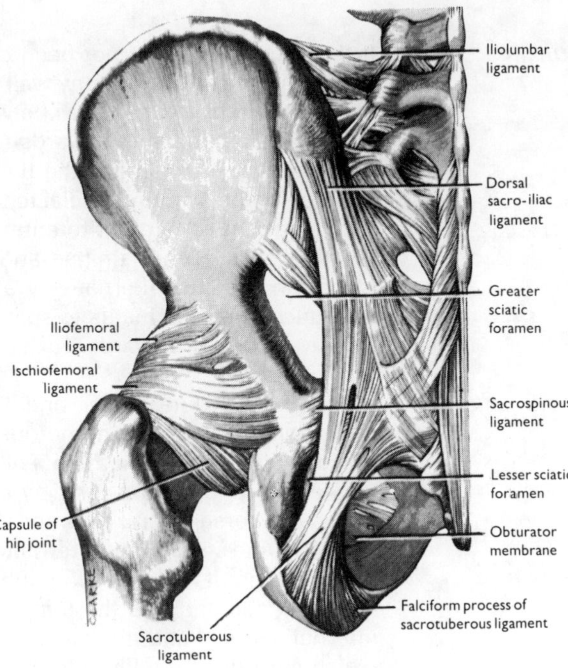

Fig. 211. Dorsal view of the pelvic ligaments and the hip joint.

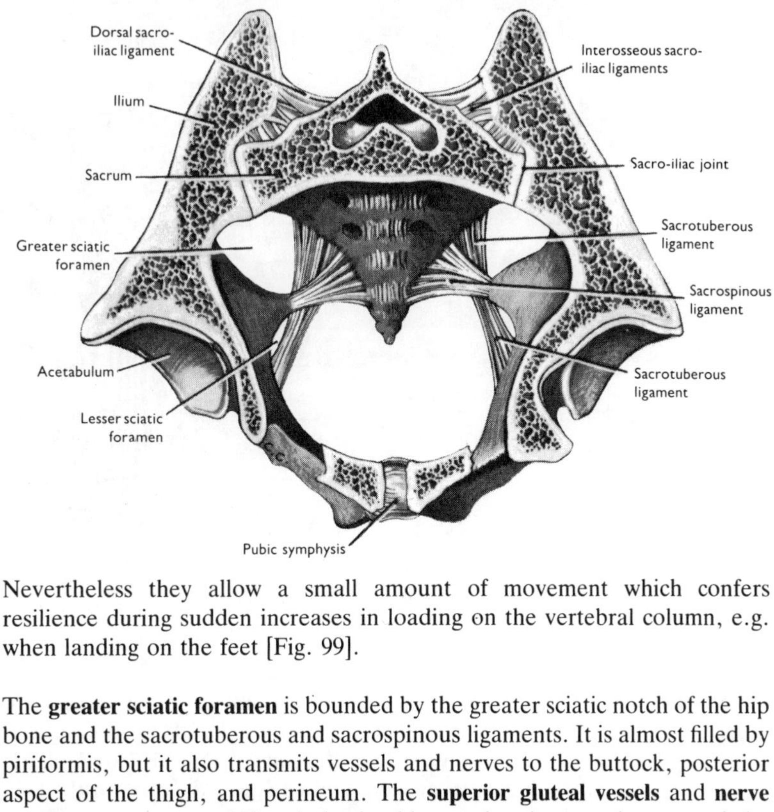

Fig. 212. An oblique section through the lesser pelvis to show the ligaments and sacro-iliac joints.

Nevertheless they allow a small amount of movement which confers resilience during sudden increases in loading on the vertebral column, e.g. when landing on the feet [Fig. 99].

Sciatic foramina

[Figs. 211, 212]

The **greater sciatic foramen** is bounded by the greater sciatic notch of the hip bone and the sacrotuberous and sacrospinous ligaments. It is almost filled by piriformis, but it also transmits vessels and nerves to the buttock, posterior aspect of the thigh, and perineum. The **superior gluteal vessels** and **nerve** emerge superior to piriformis by hooking under the superior part of the notch. *Inferior to piriformis*, the large sciatic nerve crosses the posterior wall of the acetabulum with the **nerve to quadratus femoris** between them. The **inferior gluteal vessels** and **nerve** and the **posterior cutaneous nerve of the thigh** emerge close to the medial side of the sciatic nerve. The vessels and nerves passing to the perineum have been seen already.

The **lesser sciatic foramen** is formed by the lesser sciatic notch and the two ligaments. The **tendon of obturator internus** emerges through it into the gluteal region, then turns laterally under cover of the gemelli. The nerve to obturator internus, the internal pudendal vessels, and the pudendal nerve pass through the foramen.

Dissection

If the sacral canal has not been opened already, proceed to identify the gap in the posterior bony wall of the canal—the **sacral hiatus.** This varies in extent from a notch between the sacral cornua [Fig. 98] to a large hiatus extending upwards to the second sacral spine. Remove the membrane which fills the hiatus and cut through the remaining laminae of the sacrum, medial to the intermediate crest. If this is done with a saw, take care not to enter the canal, but cut through most of the thickness of the laminae and then lever them up with a chisel placed in the cut. Alternatively a fine pair of bone forceps may be introduced into the hiatus to split the laminae, one at a time on each side, from below upwards. Take care not to catch the sacral nerves in the forceps.

Expose the dura mater and the nerves in the sacral canal by removing the fat and numerous veins (**internal vertebral venous plexus**) which surround them. Follow each **sacral nerve** to its division into dorsal and ventral rami by extending the opening of the canal into each dorsal sacral foramen. Find the end of the dural sac, and trace the fine strand (**filum terminale**) from its caudal extremity to the coccyx where it is close to the fifth sacral and coccygeal nerves. Open the dural sac and find the thin, transparent **arachnoid** applied to its internal surface, and the leash of nerve roots (**cauda equina** [Vol. 3]) which surrounds the filum terminale inside the arachnoid.

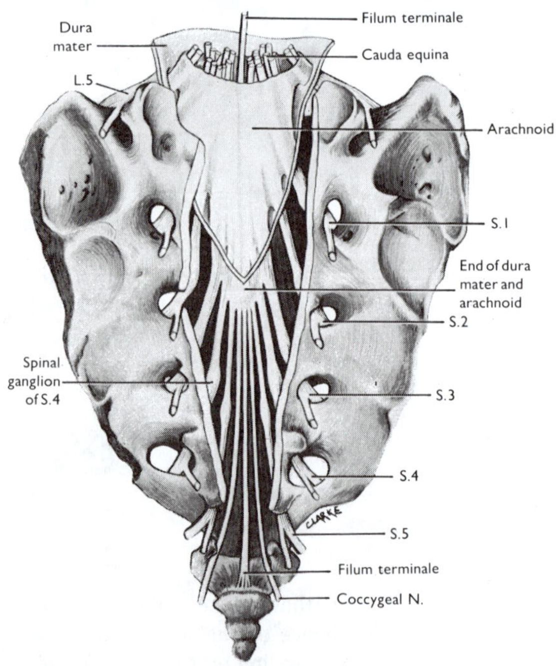

Fig. 213. A dissection to expose the sacral nerves and meninges within the sacral canal.

The sacral canal

Contents

1. The tubes of **dura mater** and **arachnoid** which surround the spinal medulla extend down to the level of the second sacral vertebra. Here they close down on the filum terminale [Fig. 213 and Vol. 3] which receives a thin covering from them and passes to the back of the coccyx.

2. The roots of five pairs of **sacral nerves** and one pair of **coccygeal nerves** pierce the arachnoid and dura and receive a sheath from each of them. The **roots** of the upper four sacral nerves unite at their spinal ganglia in the lateral part of the sacral canal, and divide almost at once into dorsal and ventral rami. The small **dorsal rami** pass through the dorsal sacral foramina. They supply the erector spinae and skin on the dorsum of the sacrum and adjacent gluteal region. The large **ventral rami** enter the pelvis through the pelvic sacral foramina to form the greater part of the sacral plexus.

The roots of each **fifth sacral nerve** unite in the lower part of the sacral canal, and their rami escape through its inferior end. The roots of the **coccygeal nerves** unite within the dural sac, pierce it, and leave with the fifth sacral nerve. The dorsal rami of these two nerves unite to supply the overlying skin. Their ventral rami run forwards through the sacrotuberous and sacrospinous ligaments, and enter the pelvis to form the coccygeal plexus.

The **internal vertebral venous plexus** surrounds the dural sac and nerves. It communicates with the pelvic veins through the pelvic sacral foramina and is directly continuous with the same plexus in the lumbar region [Fig. 205].

The position of the pelvic viscera

It is important that every student should study the pelvis of both sexes, and though the two have to be dissected separately, the corresponding features of each will be dealt with together.

In both sexes the **sigmoid colon** may be lifted out of the pelvis, but its inferior part is attached to the superior wall by the medial limb of the sigmoid mesocolon, and is continuous with the rectum on the third piece of the sacrum. The **rectum** follows the concavity of the sacrum, coccyx, and the posterior part of levator ani. Inferiorly it turns sharply downwards and backwards as the **anal canal**.

The **urinary bladder** lies in the antero-inferior part of the cavity, posterosuperior to the pubic bones and symphysis. Between the bladder and the rectum is a transverse septum of connective tissue (*genital septum*) which thickens as it passes towards the lateral wall of the pelvis. The ureters pass antero-inferiorly through this septum to the bladder. *In the male*, the septum is small and contains on each side only a **ductus deferens**, a **seminal vesicle**, and a **ureter**. Each ductus deferens sweeps postero-inferiorly from the deep inguinal ring across the anterolateral part of the pelvis, immediately inferior to the peritoneum. Then, hooking over the ureter, it runs medially in the septum on the posterior surface (base) of the bladder, superior to the seminal vesicle. Near the median plane, it turns downwards close to its fellow [Fig. 242], and ends by uniting with the duct of the seminal vesicle to form the **ejaculatory duct**, posterior to the junction of the bladder and **prostate**. The ejaculatory duct pierces the prostate to enter the urethra as it traverses that gland (prostatic part) from the neck of the bladder to the urogenital diaphragm.

In the female, the septum is large and extends upwards into the lesser pelvis covered with peritoneum. The superior part (the **broad ligament of the uterus** and its contents) is bent forwards and thus overhangs the posterior part of the urinary bladder, and has superior and inferior rather than posterior and anterior surfaces. This part of the septum contains the **uterus** in the midline and the **uterine tube** in the free margin on each side, with an **ovary** close to its lateral extremity [Fig. 215]. The **vagina** is in the inferior part of the septum which slopes antero-inferiorly posterior to the bladder and urethra, and

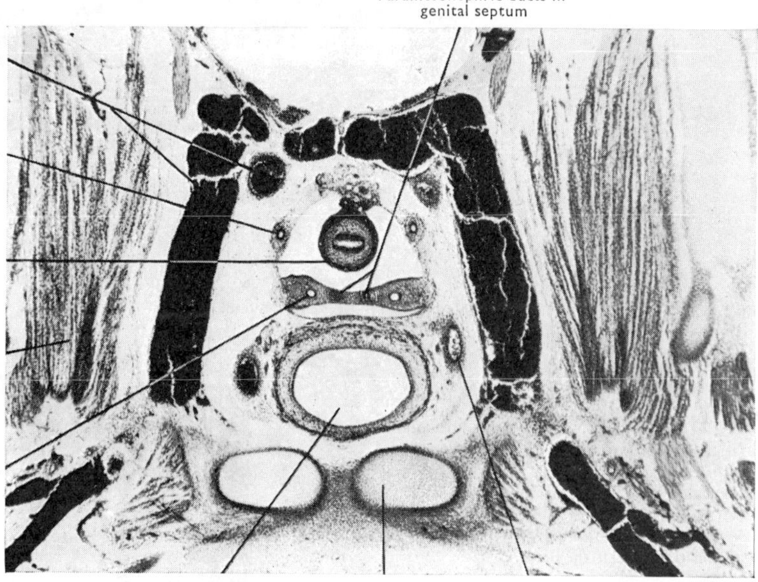

Fig. 214. A horizontal section through the lesser pelvis of an eight-week-old human fetus to show the subdivision of the pelvic cavity by the genital septum.

anterior to the rectum. It opens between them on the surface of the perineum.

The rounded, free end (fundus) of the **uterus**, in the margin of the septum, is continuous through the adjoining two-thirds (**body of the uterus**) with the narrower postero-inferior third, the **cervix** or neck of the uterus. This is partly inserted into the anterior wall of the vagina.

Each **uterine tube** extends laterally from the junction of the fundus and body of the uterus [Fig. 216] towards the lateral wall of the pelvis, and expanding (**ampulla**), recurves upon itself to end as the funnel-shaped **infundibulum** which is directed medially towards the ovary. *The infundibulum opens into the peritoneal cavity*, and is surrounded by finger-like extensions of its margin (**fimbriae** of the tube), one or more of which is attached to the ovary (ovarian fimbria).

Attached to the tubo-uterine junction are two ligaments. (1) The **round ligament of the uterus**, attached inferior to the tube, curves anterolaterally to the deep inguinal ring in a position similar to that occupied by the ductus deferens in the male. (2) The **ligament of the ovary**, attached superior to the tube, passes in the septum to the medial extremity of the ovary. In addition, a ridge of the pelvic fibrous tissue curves posterosuperiorly from the cervix of the uterus towards the lateral part of the sacrum. This forms the **uterosacral ligament** [p. 196] enclosed in the **recto-uterine peritoneal fold** [Fig. 215].

The ureter in the female follows the same course as in the male, but passes postero-inferior to the ovary and lateral to the uppermost part of the vagina, deep in the genital septum.

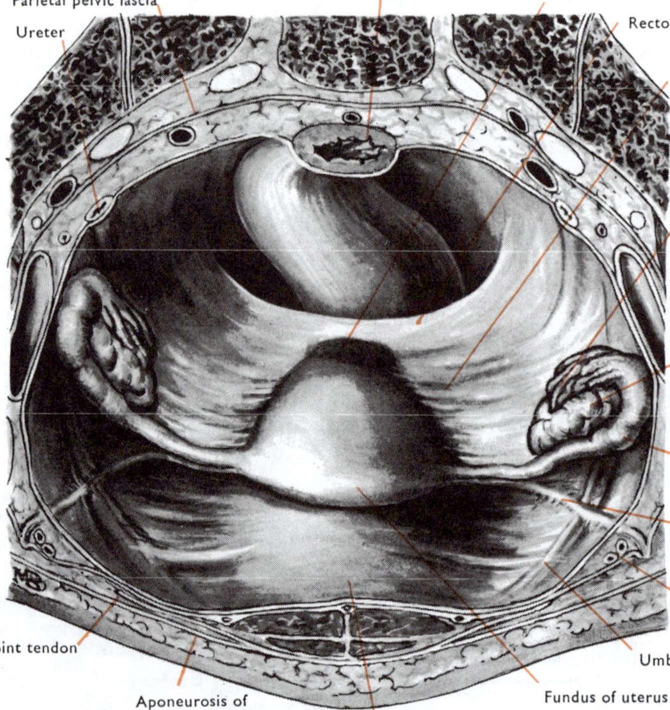

Fig. 215. The peritoneum of the lesser pelvis in the female.

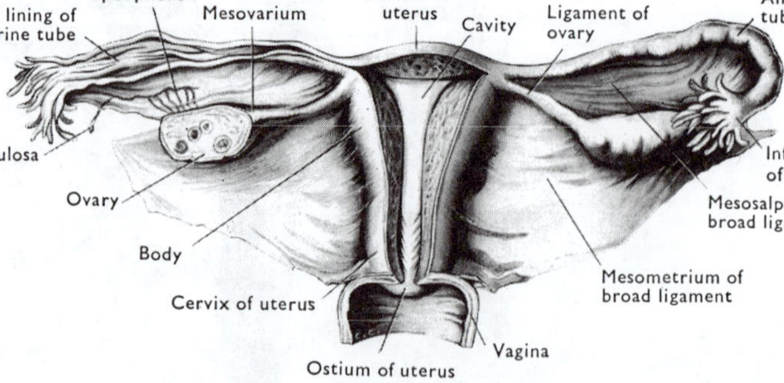

Fig. 216. The posterosuperior surface of the broad ligament and associated structures. The vagina, uterus, and left uterine tube have been opened, and the left ovary is sectioned parallel to the broad ligament.

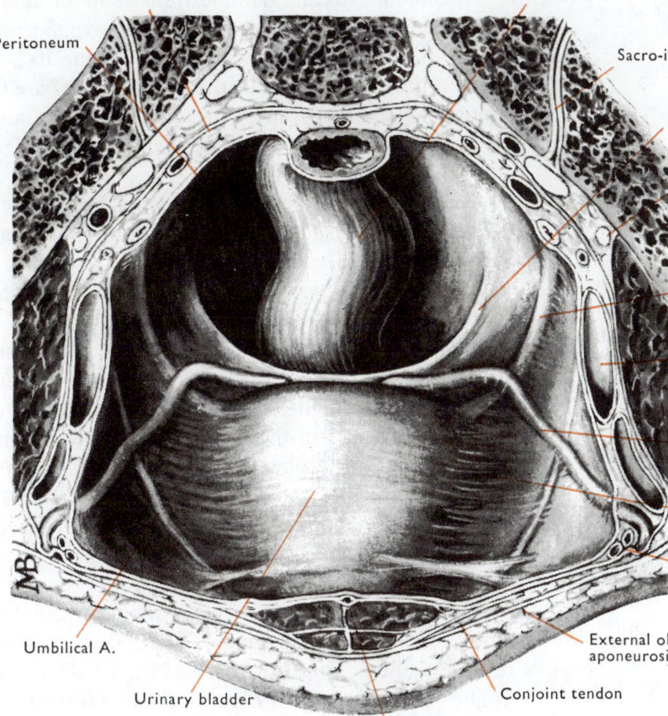

Fig. 217. The peritoneum of the lesser pelvis in the male, viewed from above and in front.

Pelvic peritoneum
[Figs. 215, 217]

The parietal abdominal peritoneum passes directly into the lesser pelvis over the margins of the superior aperture. It covers the superior surfaces of the pelvic organs, and dipping between them, produces peritoneal pouches and fossae. Anteriorly and posteriorly the arrangement of this peritoneum is virtually identical in the two sexes, but it differs in the intermediate region because of the presence of the large genital septum and its contained structures in the female.

The posterosuperior surface of the lesser pelvis is covered with peritoneum down to the second piece of the sacrum, except where the medial limb of the sigmoid mesocolon is attached [Fig. 138]. Inferior to this the rectum intervenes between the sacrum and the peritoneum. The peritoneum covers the front and sides of the upper part of the **rectum**, but leaves it by turning forwards from the anterior surface of its middle third to run upwards over the genital septum. Thus the peritoneum forms the **recto-uterine** (female) or **rectovesical** (male) **pouch** between the rectum and the contents of the genital septum. *In the female*, the peritoneum in the median plane passes from the recto-uterine pouch on to the superior part of the posterior vaginal wall; then covers the superior surfaces of the cervix and body of the uterus, and turns over the fundus to cover the inferior surface of the body of the uterus [Fig. 236]. On this surface, at the junction of the body and cervix, the peritoneum bends forwards over the superior surface of the bladder, thus forming the **uterovesical pouch** of peritoneum. It continues forwards on the bladder and passes directly on to the posterior surface of the anterior abdominal wall.

Lateral to the uterus, the peritoneum passes: (1) from the cervix as the **recto-uterine fold** on the uterosacral ligament; (2) from the body of the uterus as a double layer (superior and inferior) enclosing the connective tissue of the septum (**parametrium**), the round ligament of the uterus, the ligament of the ovary, and the uterine tube in its free, anterior margin. This **broad ligament of the uterus** is thickened laterally where the uterosacral ligament passes posteriorly and the round ligament of the uterus curves anteriorly. Its superior layer of peritoneum covers the ovary close to the attachment of the ligament to the lateral pelvic wall. The part of the broad ligament lateral to the ovary is the **suspensory ligament of the ovary**, the part between the ovary and the uterine tube is the **mesosalpinx** (mesentery of the tube), while the remainder is the **mesometrium** (mesentery of the uterus) [Fig. 216].

Thus the uterus and parametrium lie in a transverse peritoneal fold with a free anterior margin. This allows it to expand upwards into the abdominal cavity during pregnancy without disturbing its supporting structures which are composed of the connective tissue in the base of the broad ligament. This holds the cervix to the wall of the pelvis, and is especially thickened (**transverse ligaments of the cervix**) around the uterine arteries and as the **uterosacral ligaments**.

Anterior to the broad ligaments, and lateral to the bladder, the peritoneum passes forwards as the floor of a shallow **paravesical fossa** on each side [Fig. 217]. This is limited laterally by the ridge produced by the round ligament curving forwards to the deep inguinal ring, and has the obliterated umbilical artery passing forwards in its floor.

In the male, the peritoneum from the rectovesical fossa passes on to the superior part of the posterior surface of the bladder between the two deferent ducts. Occasionally it covers the superior surfaces of the seminal vesicles and the adjacent parts of the deferent ducts, which then raise a peritoneal fold which sweeps posterolaterally from the ducts towards the sacrum in the same position as the recto-uterine fold, the **rectovesical fold** [Fig. 217]. Anterior to this, the peritoneum covers the entire superior surface of the bladder, but laterally arches over the **ureter** which sweeps antero-inferiorly from the beginning of the external iliac artery to the superolateral angle of the base of the contracted bladder. The ureter forms the posterior limit of the paravesical fossa in the male. Here it is crossed by the ductus deferens turning medially on to the base of the bladder.

The greater part of the intra-abdominal **ductus deferens** lies immediately inferior to the peritoneum. Anteriorly it is in the same position as the round ligament of the uterus, but it extends further posteriorly to reach the base of the bladder [Figs. 215, 217].

The perineum

The perineum consists of the structures that fill the inferior aperture of the pelvis. This diamond-shaped aperture lies between the upper parts of the thighs and the lower parts of the buttocks, and is almost completely hidden by them in the erect posture.

The perineum extends from the inferior margin of the pubic symphysis to the coccyx. Its lateral *boundaries* are the inferior rami of the pubic bones, the rami and tuberosities of the ischia, and the sacrotuberous ligaments [Fig. 218, 219]. The perineum is considerably wider in the female than the male. In both it is divided into an anterior, urogenital region and posterior, anal region by a transverse line passing through the ischial tuberosities immediately anterior to the anus.

The **urogenital region** contains: *in the male*, the urethra enclosed in the root of the penis, partly hidden by the scrotum; *in the female*, the urethral and vaginal orifices, and the clitoris surrounded by the labia minora and majora. The anal region transmits the terminal 3–4 cm of the large intestine, the anal canal.

In the male, a median cutaneous ridge, the **raphe of the perineum**, extends from the anus over the inferior surface of the scrotum and the ventral surface of the penis. The raphe marks the line of fusion in the male of the structures that form the separate labia in the female—the floor of the urethra by fusion of the labia minora, the scrotum by fusion of the labia majora.

Female external genital organs

The pudendum femininum or **vulva** consists of the following structures [Fig. 220].

1. The **mons pubis** is a protrusion of hairy skin by subcutaneous fat anterior to the pubic bones. The hairs cease abruptly at a horizontal line where the mons meets the anterior abdominal wall. In the male, the corresponding pubic hairs extend upwards towards the umbilicus.

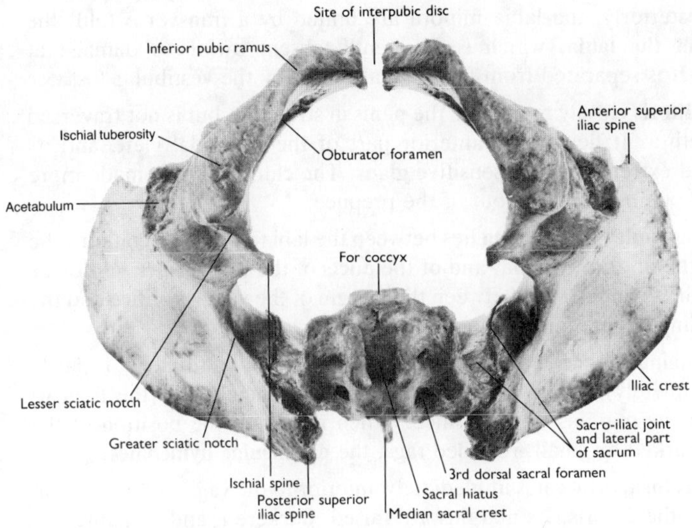

Fig. 218. The inferior aperture of the male pelvis without coccyx.

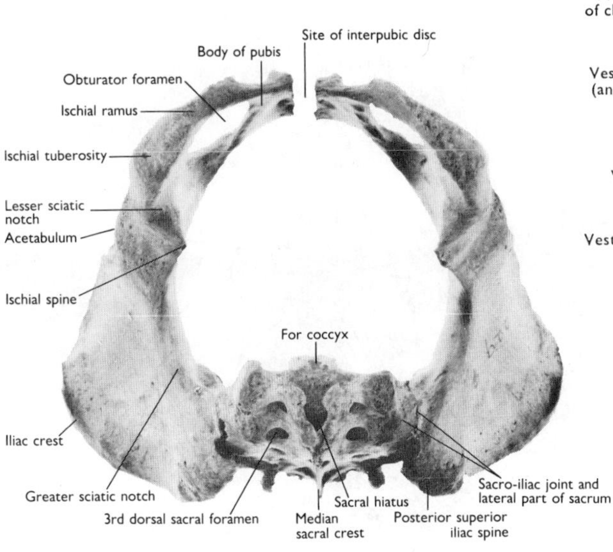

Fig. 219. The inferior aperture of the female pelvis without coccyx.

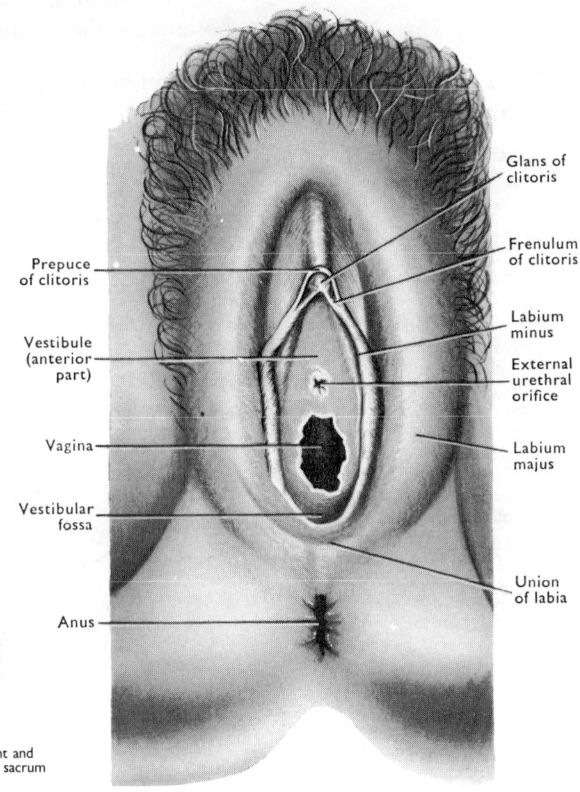

Fig. 220. The female external genital organs.

2. The labia majora are a pair of rounded folds covered with skin which extend postero-inferiorly from the mons to surround the **pudendal cleft**. They decrease in size posteriorly, and meet across the midline anterior to the anus. They carry hairs on their lateral parts, but their medial surfaces are smooth and lubricated by sebaceous glands. The remaining structures lie in the pudendal cleft.

3. The **labia minora** are a pair of smooth, pink folds, covered with stratified squamous epithelium [Fig. 220]. Anteriorly each splits into two as it approaches the clitoris. The smaller, posterior folds fuse and are attached to the inferior surface of the clitoris as the **frenulum of the clitoris**. The anterior

pair unite to form a hood over the tip of the clitoris, the **prepuce of the clitoris**. Posteriorly, the labia minora are united by a transverse fold, the **frenulum of the labia**, which is frequently absent owing to damage at childbirth. It is separated from the vaginal orifice by the vestibular fossa.

4. The **clitoris** closely resembles the penis in structure, but is not traversed by the urethra. It lies in the anterior part of the pudendal cleft, and its downturned extremity is the sensitive **glans**. The clitoris can be made more obvious by pulling the glans out of the prepuce.

5. The **vestibule of the vagina** lies between the labia minora. It contains the orifices of the urethra, vagina, and of the **ducts** of the two **greater vestibular glands**, each of which opens between the margin of the vaginal orifice and the corresponding labium minus.

6. The vaginal orifice lies in the posterior part of the vestibule. It is partly (rarely completely) closed in the virgin by a thin membrane (the **hymen**) attached to the margins of the orifice. When ruptured, the position of the hymen is marked by small, rounded tags, the **carunculae hymenales**.

7. The **urethral orifice** lies immediately anterior to the vaginal orifice, 2 cm posterior to the clitoris. Its margins are raised, puckered, and palpable.

The general arrangement of the perineum

The **urogenital region** has three layers of fascia separated by the superficial and deep **perineal spaces** filled by two layers of muscles and other structures. The fascial layers are most obvious in the male. They consist of a superficial

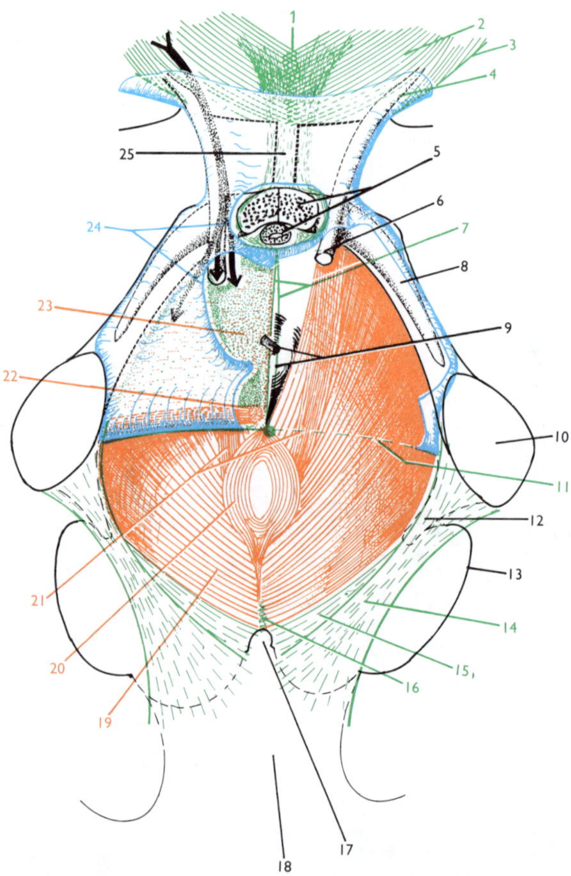

Fig. 221. A diagram to show the layers of the perineum. The lower anterior abdominal wall has been folded downwards so that it can be seen in this inferior view. The greater part of the extension of the membranous layer of the superficial fascia of the anterior abdominal wall (blue) into the perineum has been removed on the reader's right together with that half of the urogenital diaphragm (green) in order to expose most of levator ani (red) on that side. The extensions of the membranous layer of fascia over the scrotum (where it forms dartos) and the penis have been cut through together with the spermatic cords and the root of the penis all of which are shown in section. The bulb of the penis has been removed from the inferior surface of the urogenital diaphragm (inferior fascia or perineal membrane) and the membranous urethra sectioned longitudinally in the urogenital diaphragm to the point at which it emerges from the prostate. Blue, membranous layer of the superficial fascia of the anterior abdominal wall. Red, muscle. Green, fasciae of urogenital diaphragm, ligaments, and aponeuroses.

1. Linea alba.
2. External oblique aponeurosis.
3. Inguinal ligament.
4. Superficial inguinal ring.
5. Corpora cavernosum and spongiosum in root of penis.
6. Spermatic cord.
7. Cut edge of urogenital diaphragm (superior and inferior fasciae).
8. Crus of penis.
9. Membranous urethra and apex of prostate.
10. Ischial tuberosity.
11. Broken line indicating posterior edge of removed part of urogenital diaphragm and its line of fusion with the membranous layer of fascia.
12. Ischial spine.
13. Edge of greater sciatic notch.
14. Sacrotuberous ligament.
15. Sacrospinous ligament edge to edge with levator ani.
16. Anococcygeal raphe (ligament).
17. Coccyx.
18. Sacrum.
19. Posterior part of levator ani (ischiococcygeus).
20. External anal sphincter.
21. Puborectalis part of levator ani.
22. Superficial transverse perineal muscle.
23. Sphincter urethrae.
24. Cut edges of penile and scrotal extensions of membranous layer of fascia.
25. Pubic symphysis deep to the fundiform ligament of the penis which is fused to the membranous layer of the fascia superficial to it. The arrow shows the routes of communication between the zone of loose connective tissue deep to the membranous layer of the superficial fascia on the lower abdominal wall and similar zones in the perineum (superficial perineal space) around the spermatic cord, and into the scrotum. Cf. Fig. 103.

membranous layer which is attached laterally to the ischial tuberosities and to the lateral margins of the ischial and inferior pubic rami with the deep fascia of the thighs. Anteriorly, this layer continues its lateral attachments across the front of the bodies of the pubic bones towards the pubic tubercles, and is continuous with the membranous layer of the superficial fascia of the anterior abdominal wall [Fig. 103]. Between these attachments it forms the fascial sheath and fundiform ligament of the penis [p. 91] and the **dartos** layer in the scrotum. Anterior to the anal orifice, this membranous layer turns superiorly to fuse with the posterior border of the thick middle fascial layer (the **inferior fascia of the urogenital diaphragm** or **perineal membrane**) which is also attached laterally to the pubic arch [Fig. 223]. The superficial perineal space which lies between the two layers of fascia is closed posteriorly by their fusion. In the middle of the line of fusion, between the anus and the vagina (female) or the bulb of the penis (male), is the **central perineal tendon**, a fibrous mass to which a number of perineal muscles are attached.

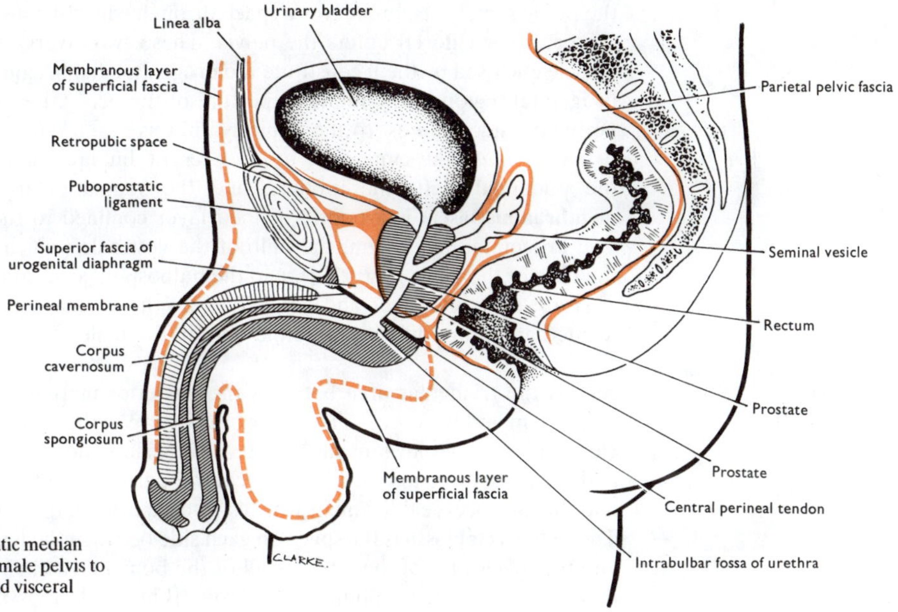

Fig. 222. A schematic median section through the male pelvis to show the parietal and visceral pelvic fascia (red).

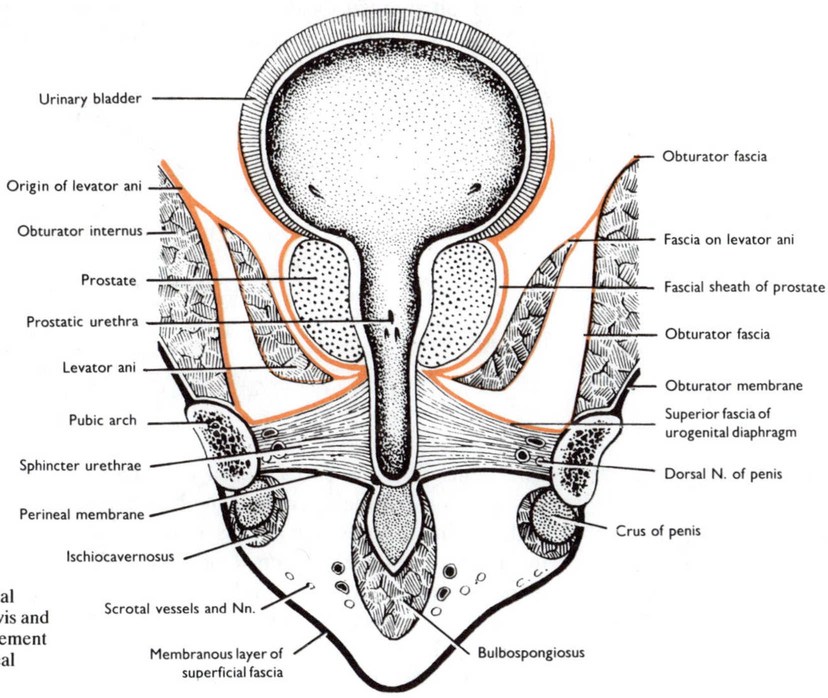

Fig. 223. A schematic coronal section through the male pelvis and perineum to show the arrangement of the pelvic (red) and perineal (black) fasciae.

In the male, the **superficial perineal space** [Fig. 226] contains a number of nerves and blood vessels, and the root of the **penis** separated into its three elements [Fig. 228]. (1) The two **crura** attached to the everted surfaces of the ischiopubic rami, each covered by an ischiocavernosus muscle. (2) The median **bulb of the penis**, covered by the bulbospongiosus muscles, is attached to the inferior surface of the perineal membrane through which the urethra passes to enter the bulb. The **superficial transverse perineal muscles** lie transversely across the posterior margin of the space from the tuberosities of the ischium to the central perineal tendon.

Superior to the perineal membrane is a thin layer of muscle which stretches across the pubic arch [Figs. 223, 230]. The main part surrounds the urethra (the voluntary **sphincter urethrae**), but the posterior fibres pass transversely as the **deep transverse perineal muscles**. This layer of muscle fills the **deep perineal space**, which is limited superiorly by the third layer of fascia (**superior fascia of the urogenital diaphragm**). This is attached laterally to the pubic arch and fuses anteriorly and posteriorly with the perineal membrane, thus closing the deep perineal space. Anteriorly, this fusion does not reach the pubic symphysis, but leaves a space through which the **deep dorsal vein of the penis** (or **clitoris**) enters the pelvis. These two layers of fascia and the muscle enclosed by them constitute the **urogenital diaphragm**. This closes the urogenital region of the inferior aperture of the pelvis, i.e. from the central perineal tendon almost to the pubic symphysis.

In the female, the same elements are present, but are split in the midline by the pudendal cleft, the urethra, and the vagina. Thus the superficial **membranous fascia** is a poorly defined layer confined to the labia majora. The urogenital diaphragm, the bulb of the vestibule (which corresponds to the bulb of the penis [Fig. 229]), and the bulbospongiosus muscles [Figs. 226, 227] are split into right and left halves by the vagina. They are less well formed and more difficult to define than in the male.

Anal region
[Figs. 226, 227]

This is the triangular area between the posterior margin of the urogenital diaphragm and the coccyx. The inferior aperture of the pelvis in this region is closed by the two **levator ani muscles**. They slope downwards, backwards, and medially to be inserted into the central perineal tendon, the anal canal, and the anococcygeal ligament which stretches from that canal to the coccyx. The **ischiorectal fossa** is the space on each side between the levator ani muscle and the lower part of the lateral wall of the bony pelvis, below the origin of that muscle, lined by obturator internus [Fig. 225]. It is filled with fatty superficial fascia which permits distention of the median **anal canal**. This canal is surrounded by the voluntary **sphincter ani externus** which extends forwards to the central perineal tendon and backwards to the coccyx [Fig. 226].

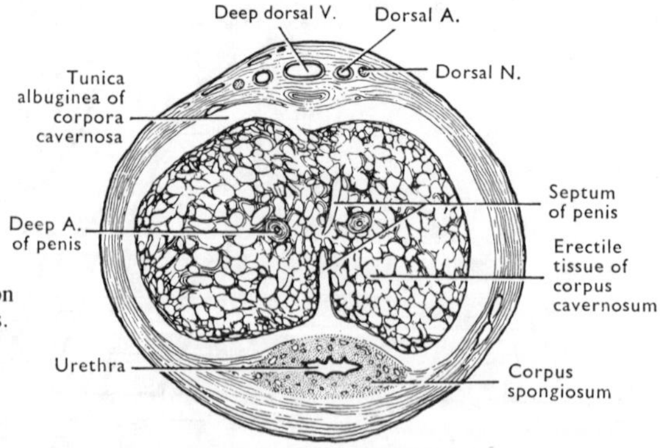

Fig. 224. A transverse section through the body of the penis.

Penis and urethra

The penis contains two **corpora cavernosa**. These are thick cylinders of spongy, fibro-elastic, erectile tissue bound together side by side [Fig. 224] by a thick sheath of tough fibrous tissue (**tunica albuginea**) which forms an incomplete septum between them. Their distal ends are embedded in the **glans penis**, the enlarged end of the third longitudinal body, the corpus spongiosum. Proximally the corpora cavernosa separate, and each, tapering to a point, is attached along the everted inferomedial surface of the ischiopubic ramus.

The **corpus spongiosum** lies between and inferior to the corpora cavernosa in the body of the penis. It consists of delicate erectile tissue and a thin **tunica albuginea**, and expands proximally to form the **bulb of the penis** [Fig. 228]. It transmits the spongy part of the urethra.

The **urethra** *in the male* is approximately 20 cm long. It extends from the most inferior part of the urinary bladder (neck) to the tip of the glans penis [Figs. 222, 235]. First it traverses the prostate (**prostatic part**, 3 cm long) from the base to a point anterior to the apex of the prostate [Fig. 222]. Then it pierces the urogenital diaphragm where it is surrounded by the sphincter urethrae (**membranous part**, 1 cm long). It then turns abruptly forwards, and sinking into the corpus spongiosum, dilates posteriorly to form the **intrabulbar fossa** [Fig. 222], and passes through the corpus spongiosum (**spongy part**) to expand in the glans (**navicular fossa**) and open on its apex.

Dissection

In the male, pass a greased bougie or blunt metal rod gently along the spongy part of the **urethra** in a plane parallel to the perineum. Direct the point towards the inferior surface of the penis to avoid recesses in the superior wall of the urethra, and palpate the point through the corpus spongiosum following its progress until it is arrested in the intrabulbar fossa, midway between the root of the scrotum and the anus. Now withdraw the point of the bougie slightly and carry the handle in the median plane towards the thighs, while applying slight pressure on the point with a finger on the perineum. The point should now enter the membranous part of the urethra without force and slip into the bladder. If this does not occur easily, do not attempt to force a passage or the tissues will be damaged.

With the bougie in position, note that it is easily palpated in the spongy part of the urethra. It can also be felt in the membranous part by a finger in the rectum, but is not palpable in the prostate from the rectum in the fixed body.

In the female, identify the urethral orifice, and pass a bougie along the **urethra** to the bladder. Note that the bougie is readily palpable through the anterior vaginal wall. If possible, introduce a speculum into the vagina and examine the **cervix** of the uterus projecting through the anterior wall of its uppermost part, with a sulcus separating it from the vaginal walls—the **fornices of the vagina**. The aperture of the cervix (**os uteri**) faces postero-inferiorly. It is small and is elongated transversely between the rounded lips of the cervix. In parous women, the os is often enlarged with lips that are cleft and scarred.

Make a transverse cut through the skin between the ischial tuberosities, immediately anterior to the anus. In the male, make a median incision in the skin from the coccyx to the scrotum, encircling the anus. *In the female*, make the same incision, but also encircle the pudendal cleft. Reflect the flaps of skin, and note the radiating strands of involuntary muscle passing outwards from the anus—**corrugator cutis ani**. These are the terminal fibres of the longitudinal muscle of the intestine.

Superficial fascia

In the **anal region** there is much lobulated fat which extends upwards into the ischiorectal fossa.

In the **urogenital region** the membranous fascial layer forms the floor of the superficial perineal space [Fig. 221]. *In the male*, a fibrous septum extends superiorly from the membranous layer to the raphe between the bulbo-spongiosus muscles [Fig. 226]. This septum is incomplete anteriorly where the fatty layer is progressively lost, and both fatty and membranous layers are replaced by smooth muscle (**dartos**) of the scrotum. *In the female*, both fatty and membranous layers are split by the pudendal cleft. The fatty layer is absent from the labium minus. The membranous layer is present in the labia majora and continues forwards, deep to the fat of the mons pubis into the anterior abdominal wall, as in the male.

Dissection

If the superficial perineal space has not already been entered from the anterior abdominal wall by passing a finger downwards and backwards deep to the membranous layer of the superficial fascia of the anterior abdominal wall, this should now be done. *In the female*, remove the fat from the labium majus and expose the membranous layer. Incise it and explore the posterior part of this space. Note the posterior limit where the membranous layer passes superiorly to fuse with the perineal membrane [p. 199]. *In the male*, expose the membranous layer in the perineum and explore one side of the superficial perineal space by pushing a finger into it through an incision in the membranous layer. Note the incomplete septum between the two sides, and the continuity of the space with the anterior abdominal wall. If the spongy part of the urethra is ruptured into the space, the urine will track forwards deep to the membranous layer into the anterior abdominal wall.

Divide the membranous layer in the median plane posterior to the scrotum or the frenulum of the labia, and carry the incision posterolaterally to each ischial tuberosity from the central perineal tendon. Reflect the fascia taking care not to damage the scrotal (labial) nerves and vessels which lie immediately deep to it. Confirm the attachments of the fascia.

The anal region

Anal canal

This canal extends postero-inferiorly from the lower extremity of the rectum to the anus. It is 4 cm long and its superior part lies in the pelvic cavity surrounded by the thickened inferior part of the circular muscle layer of the intestine (the involuntary **internal anal sphincter**) with the lower parts of the levator ani muscles on each side of it. The inferior part of the anal canal lies in the perineum surrounded by the voluntary **external anal sphincter**.

Anococcygeal ligament

This is a poorly defined, fibro-fatty raphe permeated with muscle fibres from the levator ani and external anal sphincter muscles. It extends from the anus to the tip of the coccyx, and helps to support the lower part of the rectum which lies on it.

Dissection

Remove the fascia from the external anal sphincter, the anococcygeal ligament, the margins of the anus, and the central perineal tendon, and find the inferior rectal vessesls and nerve in the ischiorectal fossa [Fig. 226]. Trace the perineal branch of the fourth sacral nerve over the surface of levator ani from the side of the coccyx to supply the external anal sphincter and the overlying skin.

Sphincter ani externus

This muscle has three parts which are indistinctly separated from each other. (1) The **subcutaneous part** surrounds the anal orifice. It has no bony attachments, but its fibres decussate anterior and posterior to the anus [Figs. 226, 227]. (2) The **superficial part** is oval in shape. Its fibres arise from the coccyx and anococcygeal ligament, and pass anteriorly around the anus to the central perineal tendon. (3) The **deep part** arises from the central perineal tendon. It encircles the lower half of the anal canal, and is fused with the puborectalis part of levator ani which reinforces its action [Fig. 221].

Nerve supply: the perineal branch of the fourth sacral nerve and the inferior rectal nerves. **Action:** the subcutaneous and superficial parts close the anus. The deep part, assisted by puborectalis, also draws the anal canal forwards, thus increasing the angle between it and the rectum [Fig. 235]. All parts of this sphincter are formed of striated muscle fibres, and it is under voluntary control.

Ischiorectal fossa

This wedge-shaped space lateral to the anus and levator ani is filled with fat. The *edge* lies superiorly where levator ani arises from the fascia covering obturator internus [Fig. 225]. The *base* is the perineal skin. The lateral and superomedial *walls* are formed by the fascia covering the perineal surfaces of obturator internus and levator ani respectively. Posteriorly, the fossa is

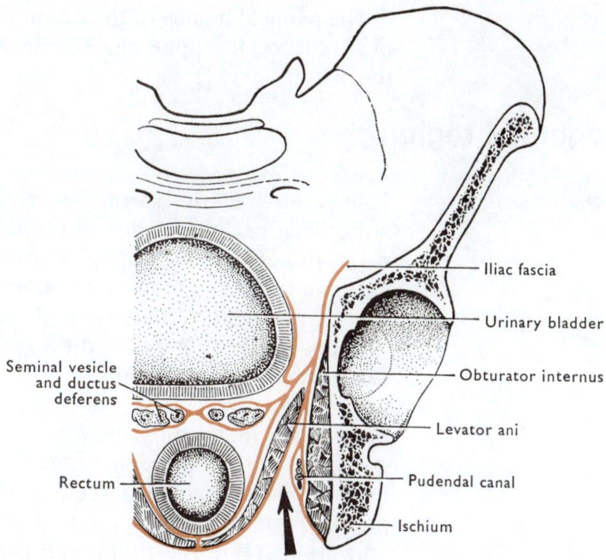

Fig. 225. A diagrammatic coronal section through the male pelvis to show the pelvic and perineal fasciae and levator ani.

continuous with the **lesser sciatic foramen** above the sacrotuberous ligament. Anteriorly, it is continuous with a narrow space, filled with loose areolar tissue, which extends forwards between levator ani and obturator internus superior to the urogenital diaphragm [Fig. 223].

The fossa is widest and deepest posteriorly, but becomes narrower and shallower anteriorly. Infections in the fat of the ischiorectal fossa are not uncommon either as a result of small tears of the anal mucous membrane or from disease of the perineal skin. If an abscess forms, it may either burst medially into the anal canal, or through the perineal skin, or both. In the last case a track may lead from the skin to the anal canal, a *fistula in ano*.

The ischiorectal fossa contains the branches of the vessels and nerves that enter it through the lesser sciatic foramen and run in the pudendal canal in its lateral fascial wall (pudendal nerve, internal pudendal vessels, and the nerve to obturator internus) and the perineal branch of the fourth sacral nerve.

Dissection

If the gluteal region has not been dissected, expose the lower border of gluteus maximus by incising the superficial fascia from a point 2 cm superior to the tip of the coccyx to the lateral side of the ischial tuberosity. Small gluteal branches of the **posterior cutaneous nerve of the thigh** may be seen curving round the inferior border of the muscle lateral to the ischial tuberosity. Identify the sacrotuberous ligament deep to the inferior border of gluteus maximus. Expose the posterior scrotal (labial) vessels and nerves near the lateral part of the posterior margin of the perineal membrane [Fig. 226] and follow them into the superficial perineal space. Complete the exposure of the **inferior rectal vessels** and **nerve,** following them to the lateral wall of the ischiorectal fossa. Remove the fat from the ischiorectal fossa. Find and follow the pudendal nerve and vessels in the fascial **pudendal canal** on the lateral wall [Figs. 225, 290, 291].

Pudendal nerve and internal pudendal vessels

These give off the inferior rectal branches immediately on entering the pudendal canal (the **inferior rectal nerve** may arise directly from the third and fourth sacral nerves in the pelvis). They pierce the medial wall of the canal, pass through the fat of the ischiorectal fossa, and supply levator ani, the external anal sphincter, the overlying skin, and the wall of the anal canal. The nerve communicates with the other cutaneous nerves of the perineum (*vide infra*). The **artery** sends branches over the margin of gluteus maximus into the buttock, and anastomoses with the other rectal arteries in the anorectal wall. The **pudendal nerve** divides into the **perineal nerve** and the **dorsal nerve of the penis** or **clitoris**. These continue through the canal with the internal pudendal vessels.

The perineal branch of the fourth sacral nerve enters the fossa at the side of the coccyx. It supplies the external anal sphincter and the skin posterior to the anus.

The urogenital region

Dissection

Follow the posterior scrotal (or labial) vessels and nerves through the superficial perineal space to the scrotum (or labium majus). Identify the **perineal branch** of the **posterior cutaneous nerve of the thigh** 2–3 cm anterior to the ischial tuberosity. Follow its branches to the scrotum or labium majus.

Expose the structures in the superficial perineal space [Fig. 226]. (1) An **ischiocavernosus muscle** covers the inferior surface of each crus of the penis or clitoris along the margin of the pubic arch. (2) The **bulbospongiosus muscles** *in the male* pass anterosuperiorly round each side of the bulb of the penis from a median, ventral raphe which begins posteriorly in the central perineal tendon. They pass to the perineal membrane or meet dorsal to the corpus spongiosum or corpora cavernosa. *In the female*, the muscles are smaller and surround the sides of the vestibule from the central perineal tendon to the crura of the clitoris [Fig. 227]. (3) The **superficial transverse perineal muscles** pass between the posterior ends of the other two muscles in both sexes. Part of the perineal membrane can be seen in the interval between these three muscles.

Nerves and vessels of superficial perineal space

Two **posterior scrotal** or **labial nerves** (lateral and medial, S. 3, 4) and arteries arise from each perineal nerve and internal pudendal artery in the anterior part of the pudendal canal. They cross the anterior part of the ischiorectal fossa, enter the superficial perineal space by piercing the membranous fascial layer, and supply the skin of the urogenital region, including the scrotum or labium majus. One of the arteries may give rise to a small **perineal artery** which runs on the superficial transverse perineal muscle to the central tendon of the perineum.

The **perineal branch of the posterior cutaneous nerve of the thigh** (S. 3) pierces the deep fascia anterolateral to the ischial tuberosity. It runs anteromedially across the pubic arch, and supplies the lateral and anterior parts of the scrotum or labium majus.

Dissection

Place a finger in the ischiorectal fossa and push it gently forwards. It will pass easily above the urogenital diaphragm, lateral to levator ani. The **urogenital diaphragm** can now be felt easily between finger and thumb. Note that it is a tough, rigid structure in both male and female, though it is difficult to define by dissection.

Divide the posterior scrotal or labial vessels and nerves and turn them aside. Separate the superficial perineal muscles and expose part of the perineal membrane between them. Cut the transverse perineal muscles from the central perineal tendon. Turn them aside, and expose the deep branches of the perineal nerve [p. 210]. *In the male*, separate the two bulbospongiosus muscles along the raphe. Turn them away from the corpus spongiosum, and follow the fibres to their terminations. *In the female*, lift the bulbospongisus muscles [Fig. 227] from the underlying masses of erectile tissue on each side of the vaginal orifice, the bulbs of the vestibule. In both sexes, strip the ischiocavernosus muscles from the crura of the penis or clitoris. Trace them to their termination.

Superficial perineal muscles

Each **superficial transverse perineal muscle** is a small strip that arises from the medial side of the ischial tuberosity and joins its fellow in the central perineal tendon. In the female, it is small, pale in colour, and difficult to define.

The **bulbospongiosus muscles** are different in the two sexes. *In the male* [Fig. 226], they arise from the central perineal tendon and from the median raphe, and curve anterosuperiorly round the bulb and posterior part of the

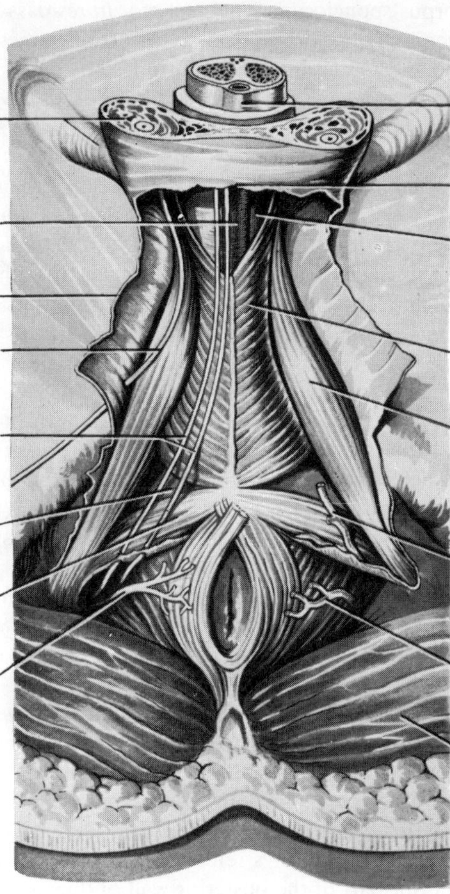

Fig. 226. A dissection of the male perineum. The penis and scrotum have been cut across and removed.

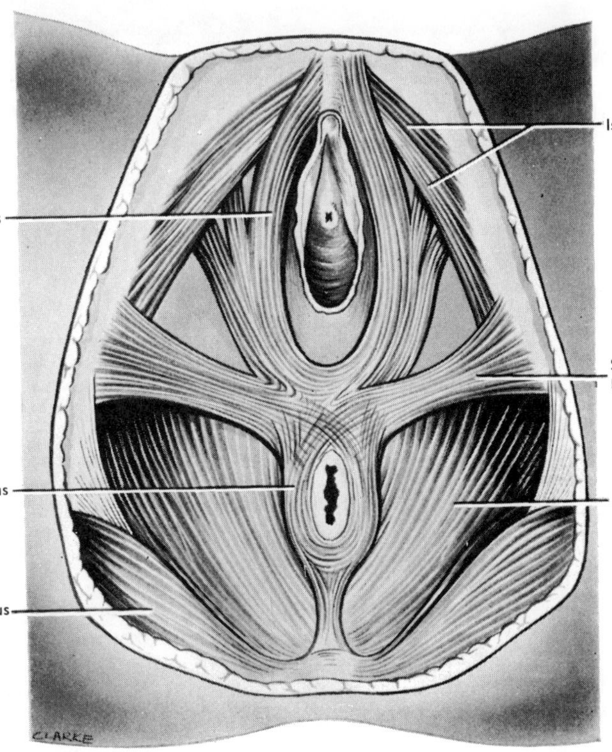

Fig. 227. The muscles of the female perineum.

corpus spongiosum. The *posterior fibres* pass round the bulb to the perineal membrane. The *middle fibres* (the largest part) encircle the corpus spongiosum and unite dorsal to it. The *anterior fibres* pass round the corpus spongiosum and the corresponding corpus cavernosum to join with its fellow dorsal to the penis (**bulbocavernosus**). *In the female* [Fig. 227], the fibres also arise from the central perineal tendon, but sweep round the sides of the vestibule inferior to the greater vestibular glands [Fig. 229] and the bulbs of the vestibule (the female equivalent of the corpus spongiosum), to be inserted into the sides and dorsum of the clitoris.

The **ischiocavernosus muscles** arise from the corresponding ramus of the ischium close to the tuberosity. Each runs forwards on the crus and is inserted into the inferior and lateral surfaces of its anterior part.

Nerve supply: the perineal nerve supplies all three muscles. **Actions:** the transverse perineal muscles help to fix the central perineal tendon and hence the posterior part of the perineal membrane and the structures superior to it, i.e. the prostate or vagina. The ischiocavernosus may assist with erection (which is due to the cavernous spaces of the penis or clitoris filling with blood) by compressing the deep vein leaving the crus. The bulbospongiosus *in the male* compresses the bulb and corpus spongiosum, thus emptying the urethra of any residual urine or semen. Its anterior fibres can assist with erection by compressing the deep dorsal vein of the penis, and impeding venous drainage from the cavernous tissue. *In the female*, it is a sphincter of the vagina, and is assisted by the underlying erectile tissue of the bulbs.

Central tendon of perineum

This indefinite mass of fibrous tissue lies between the anal canal and the bulb of the penis or the vagina. It gives attachment to the transverse perineal muscles, the bulbospongiosus, the superficial and deep parts of the external anal sphincter, the longitudinal muscle of the rectum, and some of the anterior fibres of levator ani. The tendon is an important structure in the female. Tearing or stretching of it in childbirth removes support from the inferior part of the posterior wall of the vagina. This facilitates the prolapse of a displaced uterus through the vaginal orifice.

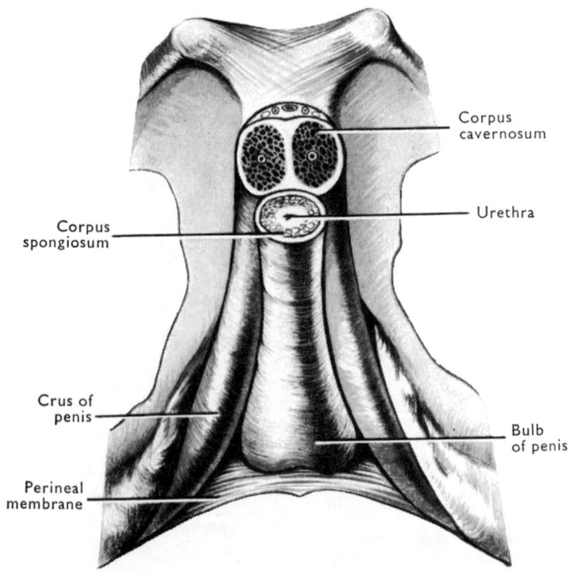

Fig. 228. The root of the penis. The corpora are shown in transverse section.

Crura of penis and clitoris

These divergent, posterior parts of the corpora cavernosa are attached to the everted, medial surfaces of the pubic arch and the adjacent parts of the perineal membrane. Each is covered by, and gives attachment to the corresponding ischiocavernosus muscle. The deep artery and vein enter and leave its superior surface. At their distal ends the corpora cavernosa are inserted into the glans of the penis or clitoris; the former is the expanded end of the corpus spongiosum, the latter is nearly a separate structure, but is united to the bulbs of the vestibule by connective tissue and a narrow strip of erectile tissue.

Bulb of penis
[Figs. 222, 228]

This expanded proximal part of the corpus spongiosum is attached to the inferior surface of the perineal membrane by fibrous tissue, by the bulbospongiosus muscles, and by the urethra which pierces the membrane to enter the corpus spongiosum in front of its posterior end. The urethra is accompanied by the **ducts of the bulbo-urethral glands** and by the arteries of the bulb, both of which arise in the deep perineal space.

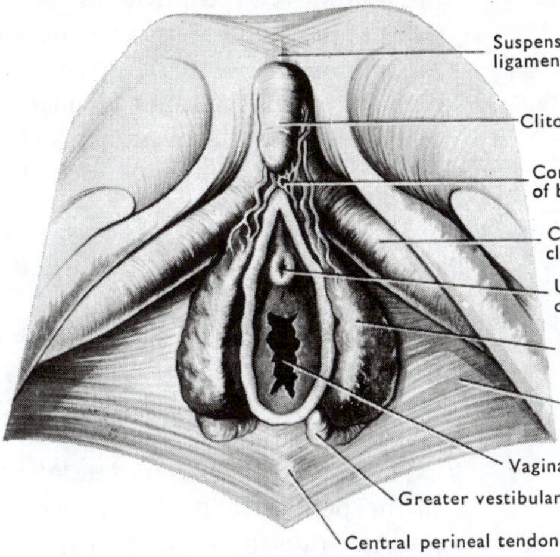

Fig. 229. A dissection of the superficial perineal space in the female.

Bulbs of vestibule

These oval masses of erectile tissue lie one on each side of the vaginal orifice. Each, covered by a fibrous sheath and a bulbospongiosus muscle, is attached to the perineal membrane and overlaps the corresponding greater vestibular gland posteriorly [Fig. 229]. The bulbs narrow anteriorly, and are united by a plexus of veins (the **commissure of the bulbs**) between the urethra and the clitoris. The commissure is attached to the glans of the clitoris by a thin strip of erectile tissue. This strip, the glans, the commissure, and the bulbs together correspond to the corpus spongiosum and glans penis.

Greater vestibular glands
[Fig. 229]

These glands lie beside the orifice of the vagina between the perineal membrane and the bulbs of the vestibule. Each has a long duct that opens at the side of the vaginal orifice, between the hymen and the labium minus.

Dissection

Remove the superficial perineal muscles, and detach one crus of the penis carefully from the ischiopubic ramus. Turn it forwards to expose the deep artery and vein on its superior surface. Find and trace the dorsal artery and nerve of the penis or clitoris. They lie close to the deep artery [Fig. 230] and pass into a position lateral to the **deep dorsal vein.** Trace this vein proximally till it disappears into the pelvis between the pubic symphysis and the anterior margin of the perineal membrane.

In the male, detach the bulb of the penis from the central perineal tendon. Turn it forwards to expose the **urethra** and the **artery of the bulb** piercing the perineal membrane to enter the bulb. The ducts of the bulbo-urethral glands lie at the sides of the urethra but are difficult to identify. Expose as much of the perineal membrane as possible without damage to these structures.

In the female, raise the posterior end of the bulb of the vestibule to expose the greater vestibular gland. Follow it forwards to its duct, and find the artery of the bulb. Divide this artery, and turn the bulb forwards to expose as much of the perineal membrane as possible.

Perineal membrane (inferior fascia of urogenital diaphragm)

This is a triangular fibrous sheet. Its base passes transversely through the central perineal tendon; its truncated apex almost reaches the pubic symphysis. Laterally, it is attached to the pubic arch. Posteriorly, it fuses with the membranous layer of the superficial perineal fascia and with the superior fascia of the urogenital diaphragm, thus closing both **perineal spaces** posteriorly [Fig. 222]. Anteriorly, it fuses with the superior fascia of the urogenital diaphragm closing the deep perineal space and thickening to form the **transverse perineal ligament** which is separated from the pubic symphysis by the **deep dorsal vein of the penis** or **clitoris**.

In the anatomical position, the perineal membrane lies horizontally between the superficial and deep perineal spaces and their contents. The **urethra** and **vagina** pierce the membrane in the median plane. *In the male*, the urethra is 2.5 cm from the pubic symphysis and is accompanied by the ducts of the bulbo-urethral glands and the arteries of the bulb. *In the female*, the urethra is closer to the symphysis and the **arteries of the bulbs** accompany the vagina. The internal pudendal arteries and the dorsal nerves of the penis or clitoris pierce the membrane anterolaterally [Figs. 230, 231]. The urethral orifice in the membrane is large enough to permit urethral distention.

Dissection

Separate the perineal membrane from the pubic arch on the side from which the crus of the penis (clitoris) was removed. Carefully reflect the membrane medially. This exposes a thin sheet of muscle consisting of the **sphincter urethrae** anteriorly and the **deep transverse perineal muscles** posteriorly, but they are difficult to dissect and differentiate from each other.

Follow the **internal pudendal artery** forwards (with the dorsal nerve of the penis or clitoris) in this deep perineal space and through the perineal membrane to its division into the deep and dorsal arteries of the penis or clitoris. Find and trace the artery of the bulb.

In the male, look for the **bulbo-urethral gland** posterolateral to the urethra on the superior surface of the deep transverse perineal muscle.

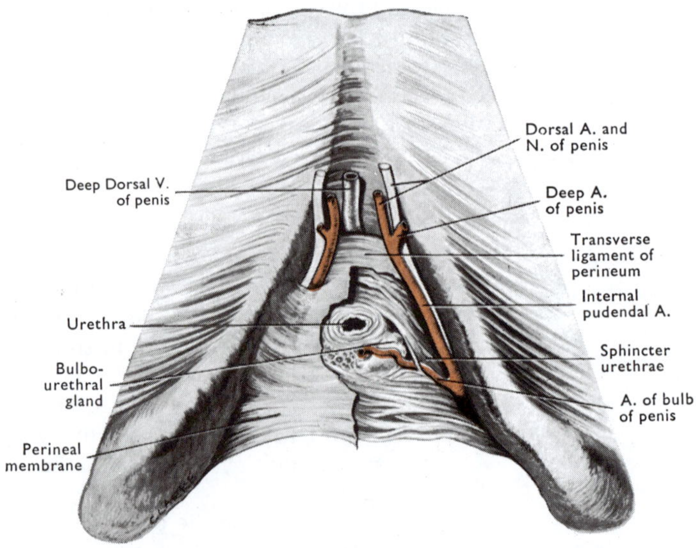

Fig. 230. A deep dissection of the male perineum. The penis has been removed, the urethra cut across, and the left half of the perineal membrane removed to expose sphincter urethrae and the artery to the bulb.

Deep perineal space

This space, between the perineal membrane and the superior fascia of the urogenital diaphragm, contains the sphincter urethrae, the deep transverse perineal muscles, and the bulbo-urethral glands in the male. These form the urogenital diaphragm with the enclosing layers of fascia. The space is traversed by the urethra and vagina, and transmits the internal pudendal vessels and the dorsal nerves of the penis or clitoris.

The **sphincter urethrae** consists of transverse muscle fibres which arise from the medial surface of the inferior pubic ramus. *In the male*, the fibres pass medially to unite with the opposite fibres in a median raphe anterior and posterior to the urethra. Adjacent to the urethra, the muscle fibres pass circularly around it. The most posterior fibres are the **deep transverse perineal muscle.** *In the female*, the arrangement is the same, but the posterior fibres are attached to the vaginal wall. **Nerve supply:** minute branches of the perineal nerve. **Action:** this is the *voluntary sphincter of the urethra* composed of striated muscle fibres.

The membranous part of the urethra in the male is the least distensible part. It is 1 cm long and is continuous above with the prostatic part through the superior fascia of the urogenital diaphragm, and below with the spongy part of the urethra through the perineal membrane [Fig. 244]. It is lined with columnar epithelium.

Female urethra

This tube is 4–5 cm long and 6 mm wide. It is very dilatable, and extends from the neck of the bladder through the pelvic cavity and the urogenital diaphragm, to open immediately anterior to the vaginal orifice [Fig. 236]. Throughout its length it is attached to the anterior wall of the vagina. Most of the lining is stratified squamous or columnar epithelium, and a number of small mucous glands open into it.

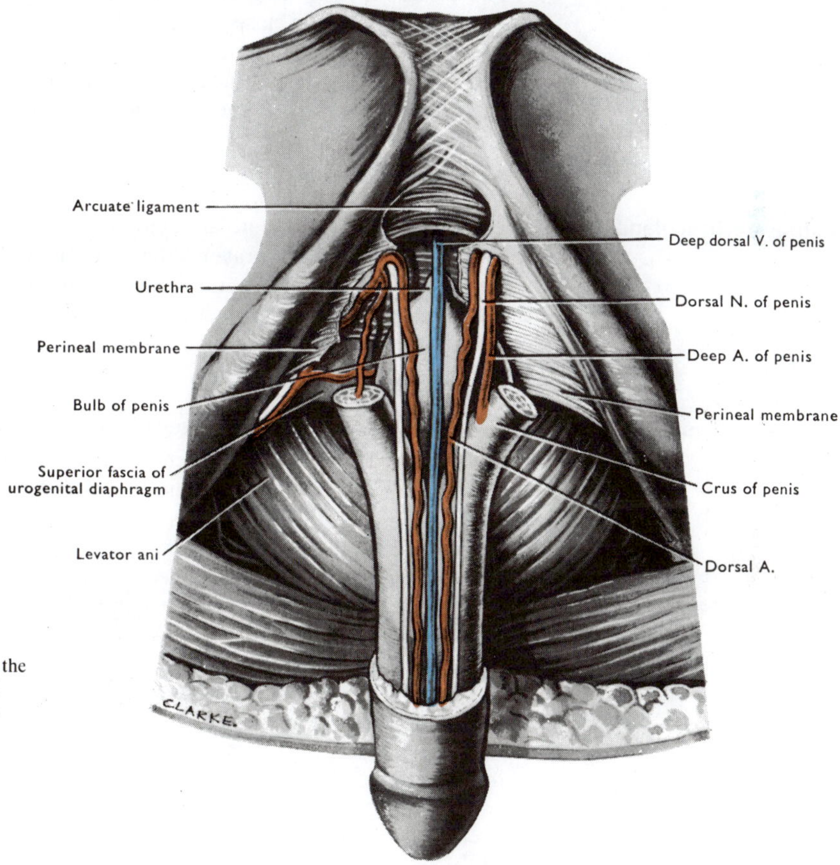

Fig. 231. A dissection to show the pubic symphysis and the dorsal vessels and nerves of the penis.

Internal pudendal artery

This artery arises in the pelvis from the internal iliac artery. It enters the gluteal region through the greater sciatic foramen, and leaves it with the pudendal nerve through the lesser sciatic foramen to enter the ischiorectal fossa in the **pudendal canal**. It enters the deep perineal space at the posterior border of the perineal membrane, and runs forwards with the dorsal nerve of the penis or clitoris; 1–2 cm from the pubic symphysis it pierces the perineal membrane either before or after dividing into dorsal and deep arteries of the penis or clitoris [Fig. 230].

Branches

For inferior rectal, perineal, and posterior scrotal or labial see pages 203 and 204.

The **artery of the bulb** arises in the posterior part of the deep perineal space. It passes medially, inferior to the sphincter urethrae, supplying it and the bulbo-urethral gland in the male. Then piercing the perineal membrane it enters the corpus spongiosum (or bulb of the vestibule) and supplies it [Fig. 230].

The **deep artery of the penis or clitoris** enters the crus and supplies the corpus cavernosum.

The **dorsal artery** passes anterosuperiorly on to the dorsum of the penis or clitoris [Fig. 231].

Pudendal nerve
[S. (1), 2, 3, 4]

It arises from the sacral plexus in the pelvis, and emerges through the lower part of the greater sciatic foramen. It enters the lesser sciatic foramen on the sacrospinous ligament, and giving off the **inferior rectal nerve** [p. 203] runs in the pudendal canal dividing into the perineal nerve and the dorsal nerve of the penis (clitoris).

The **perineal nerve** passes with the internal pudendal artery to the posterior margin of the urogenital diaphragm. Here it gives off two **posterior scrotal** or **labial nerves** [p. 204], and divides into small terminal branches. These enter the superficial and deep perineal spaces to supply the contained muscles and the bulb of the penis or of the vestibule.

The **dorsal nerve of the penis** or **clitoris** runs in the pudendal canal and in the deep perineal space close to the pubic arch. It gives a branch to the crus of the penis or clitoris, and then runs with the dorsal artery of the penis or clitoris [Fig. 231] sending branches round the side of that organ to its ventral surface. It thus supplies all the skin and the glans.

The pudendal nerve also carries some of the **autonomic nerve fibres** to the erectile tissue of the penis or clitoris.

Bulbo-urethral glands

These small glands lie posterolateral to the membranous urethra in the male [Fig. 230]. The long ducts traverse the perineal membrane with the urethra, and enter its spongy part a short distance further distally [Figs. 245, 246]. The cells of these glands are markedly pleomorphic and seem to secrete a number of substances responsible for some of the physical characteristics of seminal fluid.

Lymph vessels of perineum

These numerous and important vessels cannot be demonstrated by dissection. Lymph from all the perineal structures, including the inferior parts of the anal canal, vagina, and urethra, drain to the **medial superficial inguinal lymph nodes**. Lymph from the upper parts of these tubes drains superiorly into the pelvis [Fig. 255] together with some deep vessels which drain along the internal pudendal vessels and the deep dorsal vein of the penis.

It is important to remember that enlargement of the medial superficial inguinal lymph nodes may be the first sign of infection in the perineum, and also that the *testicular lymph vessels drain via the spermatic cord to the lumbar lymph nodes*, though the skin and fascial layers of the **scrotum** drain to the superficial inguinal lymph nodes.

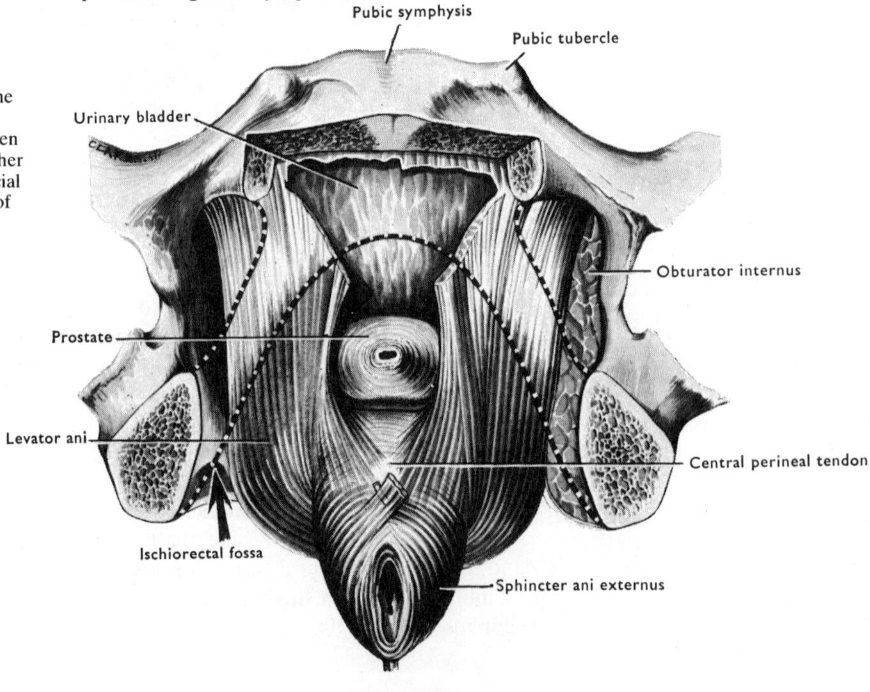

Fig. 232. A dissection of the levator ani muscles in the male. The perineum has been tilted forwards; the ischial rami and the inferior rami and parts of the bodies of the pubic bones (broken lines) have been removed together with the contents of the superficial and deep perineal spaces and of the ischiorectal fossae.

Dissection

Remove the exposed muscle of the deep perineal space and then the superior fascia of the urogenital diaphragm. Remove the fat and fascia to expose as much as possible of the perineal surface of **levator ani** [Fig. 232]. Note that the anterior part of this muscle has a free medial border which is separated from its fellow by a gap anterior to the insertion of its most medial fibres into the central tendon of the perineum. Confirm that the gap transmits the urethra in the male or the urethra and vagina in the female. Note that some of the fibres which pass to the central perineal tendon, turn round the posterior vaginal wall and form a partial sphincter for it. In the male, the prostate lies on the medial margins of the levator ani muscles with its apex projecting downwards in the gap between them. These parts of the levator ani muscles are known as the **levator prostatae.**

Trace the more posterior fibres of levator ani to the sides of the anal canal, deep to the external sphincter. Some of the fibres of the levator join the longitudinal muscle layer and extend to the perianal skin. Confirm the origin of levator ani from the fascia covering the obturator internus muscle. Note that each levator ani muscle forms a continuous sheet with the corresponding sacrospinous ligament [p. 190]. The right and left sheets are united where the levator ani muscles are inserted into the central perineal tendon, anal canal, and anococcygeal ligament. Thus they form a fibromuscular floor for the pelvis—the **pelvic diaphragm.** This floor is deficient anteriorly where the two levator ani muscles separate, but this gap is filled by the urogenital diaphragm inferior to the levator ani muscles.

Retropubic space

This is the space between the anterior surface of the bladder and the pelvic surface of the pubic bones and symphysis. It is filled with loose, fatty connective tissue, the **retropubic pad of fat**, which extends posterolaterally on the sides of the bladder as far as the ureters. Posterior to the bodies of the pubic bones, the space is limited inferiorly by the strong puboprostatic ligaments (pubovesical or, more accurately, pubo-urethral in the female) which pass to the neck, i.e. lowest part of the bladder and to the base, i.e. upper part of the prostate (or urethra in the female). Superiorly the space is continuous with the loose extraperitoneal tissue which extends up the anterior abdominal wall to the level of the umbilicus, between the lateral umbilical ligaments. This arrangement permits the bladder to expand superiorly between the anterior abdominal wall and its peritoneum.

Dissection

Push a finger inferiorly between the bladder and the pubis till the resistance of the puboprostatic or pubovesical ligaments is felt. Carry the finger round the side of the bladder and note the presence of loose connective tissue here also. Place a finger in the ischiorectal fossa, and note that a finger in the pelvic cavity is separated from it by the levator ani muscle and its fascia. As far as possible, explore the relation of pelvic cavity to ischiorectal fossa and perineum by passing the fingers forwards and backwards. Try to define the extent of the puboprostatic (pubovesical) ligaments by palpation in this way.

The pelvic viscera

Ovaries

[Figs. 216, 233, 248]

These pinkish-white, ovoid structures measure approximately 3 cm long, 1.5 cm wide, and 1 cm thick. Between them they usually produce one ripe **ovum** per menstrual cycle. This develops in a small cyst or **follicle** which ruptures approximately at the middle of the menstrual cycle, and releases the ovum into the peritoneal cavity. The remaining lining cells of the follicle then develop into a **corpus luteum**. This produces progestogens which complete the preparation of the uterine lining (**endometrium**) for the implantation of the fertilized ovum. If the ovum is not fertilized, the corpus luteum degenerates towards the end of the menstrual cycle, and is gradually replaced by a fibrous scar (**corpus albicans**). Thus the originally smooth surface of the ovary becomes puckered with scars. In women after the menopause, the entire ovary shrinks following the loss of stimulation by pituitary gonadotrophic hormones.

Each ovary lies near the lateral wall of the pelvic cavity in a slight depression between the ureter posteromedially, the external iliac vein laterally, the obturator nerve posterolaterally, and the uterine tube in the free margin of the broad ligament anteriorly [Fig. 233]. The extremity of the **uterine tube** curves round the lateral end of the ovary and is attached to it by one or more of the **fimbriae** [Fig. 215]. The ovary is attached to the superior surface of the broad ligament by a very short peritoneal fold (**mesovarium**) through which the ovarian vessels enter its **hilus**. The medial extremity of the ovary is attached to the uterus by the **ligament of the ovary**. When the **appendix vermiformis** is pelvic in position, it may be very close to the right ovary.

In pregnancy the broad ligament and ovary are carried superiorly with the expanding uterus. When it subsequently contracts in the postpartum period, the ovary may return to a site other than that described above.

Vessels and nerves

Each **ovarian artery** arises from the aorta below the renal artery. It descends on the posterior abdominal wall, crosses the external iliac artery, and enters the lateral part of the broad ligament (suspensory ligament of the ovary). It sends branches through the mesovarium to the ovary, and continues medially in the broad ligament to supply the uterine tubes and anastomose with the uterine artery.

The **veins** leave the hilus as a **pampiniform plexus** on the artery. A single ovarian vein is formed near the superior aperture of the pelvis. The right vein ascends to the inferior vena cava, the left to the left renal vein.

The **lymph vessels** unite with those from the uterine tube and the fundus of the uterus, and ascend with the vein to end in lumbar lymph nodes from the bifurcation of the aorta to the level of the renal vessels.

Structure

Make a cut into the ovary and note its dense stroma. In a young individual it contains follicles in various stages of development and many large, scattered germ cells (oogonia) which can only be seen under the microscope and which

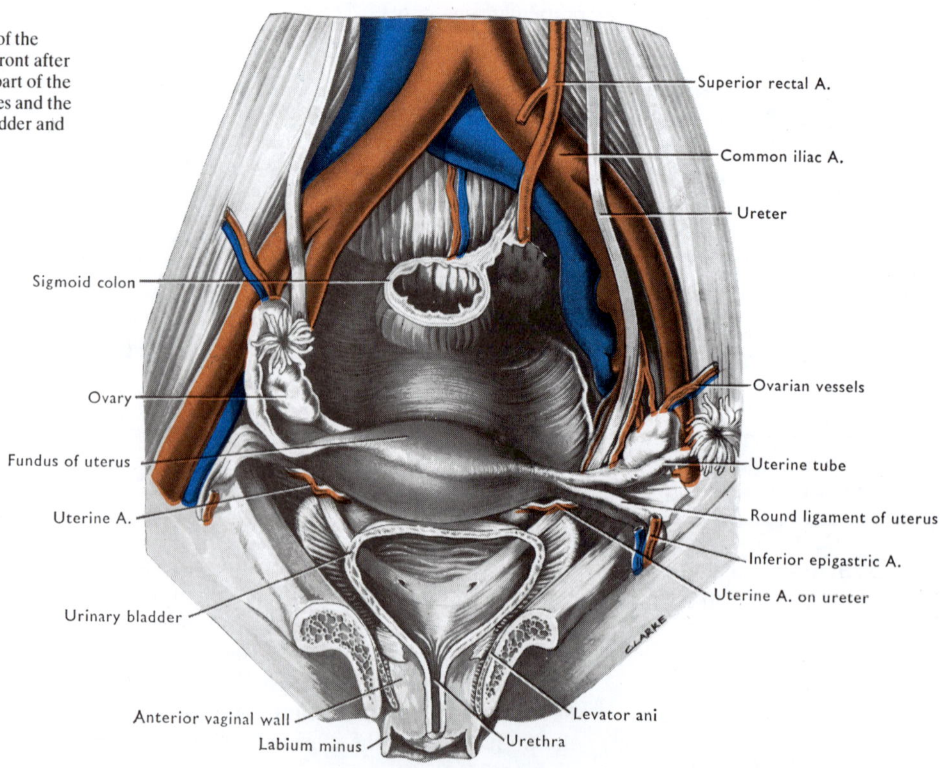

Fig. 233. A dissection of the female pelvis from the front after removal of the greater part of the bodies of the pubic bones and the anterior parts of the bladder and urethra.

may develop into follicles. The surface of the ovary is covered by a cubical epithelium ('germinal epithelium') which is continuous with the flattened mesothelium of the peritoneum at the mesovarium.

Uterine tubes

[Figs. 215, 233, 249]

Each tube, approximately 10 cm long, is narrow as it passes through the wall of the uterus (**uterine part**) to join the narrow **isthmus** of the tube (2–3 cm long) in the free edge of the broad ligament at the junction of the fundus and body of the uterus. The isthmus is continuous laterally with the expanded and slightly convoluted **ampulla** which forms most of the remainder of the tube, and passes towards the lateral pelvic wall. Here it rises out of the superior surface of the broad ligament on a short mesentery, and curving over the lateral extremity of the ovary, expands into the funnel-shaped **infundibulum**. This opens into the peritoneal cavity with a fringe of finger-like processes (**fimbriae**) some of which, the **ovarian fimbriae**, are attached to the ovary. Near the time of ovulation, the tube becomes turgid and the infundibulum expands medially over the ovary. Thus the discharged ovum is easily carried into the tube by the action of the ciliated columnar epithelium covering the fimbriae and lining the mucous membrane of the tube. The fimbriae are continuous with the numerous *longitudinal folds of mucous membrane* that virtually fill the infundibulum and ampulla.

Dissection

Open one uterine tube longitudinally. Note the folds of its mucous membrane, the thinness of its wall, and the variations in its internal diameter. Trace the ovarian vessels to the ovary and uterine tube, and follow them to their origins and terminations. Note the course of the ovarian artery in the broad ligament and its anastomosis with the uterine artery near the uterus.

The ovum is fertilized in the ovarian end of the uterine tube, and development begins as it slowly passes to the uterus. If delayed, the ovum may adhere to the tube and burrow into the wall. Unlike the uterus, the tube is too thin-walled to withstand the invading ovum, and rupture of the tube occurs with severe intraperitoneal bleeding—one cause of acute abdominal emergency in women of childbearing age. This is the commonest type of **ectopic gestation**. Very rarely a fertilized ovum may escape into the peritoneal cavity and may then implant in the peritoneal surface of any of the pelvic viscera or walls.

Vessels

The blood vessels are branches of the ovarian and uterine vessels. The lymph vessels join those of the ovary and pass to the lumbar nodes.

Ligament of ovary

[Fig. 249]

This band of connective tissue and smooth muscle extends from the medial end of the ovary to the superior surface of the junction of the uterine tube and uterus. It forms a ridge on the superior surface of the broad ligament.

Round ligament of uterus

[Figs. 215, 233]

This consists of the same tissue as the ligament of the ovary. It arises from the tubo-uterine junction opposite the attachment of the ligament of the ovary. The round ligament passes to the side wall of the pelvis, forming a ridge on the inferior surface of the broad ligament. It then sweeps forwards, immediately deep to the peritoneum, to the deep inguinal ring. Here it hooks round the lateral side of the inferior epigastric vessels, traverses the inguinal canal, and spreads out to its attachment in the labium majus.

The ligament of the ovary and the round ligament of the uterus together represent the remains of the **gubernaculum** in the embryo [p. 260]—a structure partly responsible for the descent of the testis to the scrotum in the male. In the female, the continuity of the gubernaculum is broken by the persistence of the ducts which form the uterus and uterine tubes but which disappear in the male. This prevents the gubernaculum from drawing the ovary from its original position in the upper abdomen to the labium majus (the homologue of the scrotum). Instead, the ovary is first drawn down into the greater pelvis and remains there in the child till the pelvis enlarges to accommodate the urinary bladder and uterus which are abdominal organs until that stage [Fig. 238]. Very rarely the ovary may descend into the inguinal canal or even be carried to the labium majus.

Pelvic parts of the ureters

[Figs. 215, 217, 233, 254]

Half of the 25-cm-long ureter lies in the pelvis and half in the abdomen. Each ureter crosses the origin of the external iliac artery, and runs postero-inferiorly on the front of the internal iliac artery, deep to the peritoneum of the lateral wall of the pelvis. In the female, it is postero-inferior to the ovary. At the level of the ischial spine, it curves anteromedially above levator ani. *In the female*, it passes beside the **lateral fornix of the vagina**, inferior to the broad ligament and to the **uterine artery** turning superiorly into that ligament. *In the male*, it remains in contact with the peritoneum until it is separated from it by the ductus deferens a short distance before it reaches the posterosuperior angle of the bladder, the same point as in the female.

In both sexes, the ureters pass obliquely through the bladder wall in an inferomedial direction, to open at the corresponding superolateral angle of the **trigone of the bladder** [Fig. 234].

Dissection

Remove the peritoneum from the superior surface of the bladder, stopping short of the depths of the uterovesical pouch in the female. Identify and follow the median umbilical ligament [Fig. 239] from the apex of the bladder. Remove the fat from the retropubic space and from the paravesical fossae. Displace the apex of the bladder posteriorly and expose the puboprostatic or pubovesical ligaments.

In the male, trace the ductus deferens and ureter to the base of the bladder on both sides. In the female, expose the ligament of the ovary, the round ligament of the uterus, and the ureter on the side on which the uterine tube was opened. In following the ureter in the female, identify the uterine artery crossing above the ureter at the side of the vaginal fornix.

Make an incision through the bladder wall along the junction of the superior and inferolateral surfaces on both sides [Fig. 239]. Carry these to the lateral extremities of the base, then fold back the superior wall of the bladder and examine the internal surface [Figs. 233, 234].

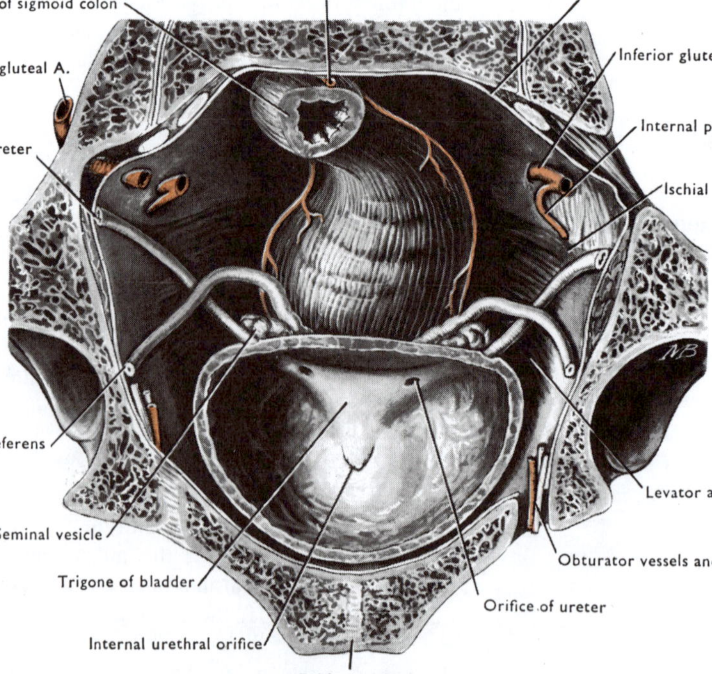

Fig. 234. Some of the contents of the male lesser pelvis seen from above and in front.

Internal surface of urinary bladder

The internal surface of the contracted bladder is ridged to a variable degree by folds of mucous membrane, some of which cover protuberant bundles of interlacing muscle fibres, especially in the hypertrophied bladder. On the posterior wall is a smooth triangular area—the **trigone of the bladder** with its inferior angle at the median **internal urethral orifice** and a small, obliquely placed **ureteric orifice** at each of its superolateral angles. The last two orifices are joined by a well-defined **interureteric fold** which forms the superior margin of the trigone.

Orifices of ureters

Pass a fine seeker into each ureteric orifice. It passes obliquely through the bladder wall into the corresponding ureter. As a result, any increase in intravesical pressure (due to contraction of the vesical muscle as in urination) presses the walls of the intramural parts of the ureters together and prevents the pressure in the bladder being transmitted to the ureters and kidneys. This is an important feature, because raised pressure in the ureters and pelves of the kidneys, if continued, can rapidly cause irreversible damage to the kidneys.

Internal urethral orifice

This is a Y-shaped slit at the inferior angle of the trigone. In the male, the mucous membrane is bulged forwards (uvula of the bladder) between the posterior limbs of the Y by the median lobe of the prostate gland which immediately underlies this part of the trigone.

Pubic symphysis

This is the joint which unites the two hip bones anteriorly. The articular surfaces of the pubic bones are covered with hyaline cartilage, and united by a **disc** of fibrous tissue which is similar to an intervertebral disc but has a central slit-like cavity. The disc is surrounded by ligaments. Anteriorly the ligament is very strong and is fused superficially with the abdominal aponeuroses. Inferiorly, it forms the strong arcuate ligament—a curved band which rounds off the apex of the pubic arch and extends along the inferior pubic rami. The deep dorsal vein of the penis or clitoris enters the pelvis between the arcuate and transverse perineal ligaments [p. 208].

The pubic symphysis permits a small amount of movement between the hip bones, and absorbs shocks transmitted from the femora. In common with many other tissues, the disc contains more tissue fluid in the later stages of pregnancy, and may permit a slight increase in range of movement in childbirth.

Dissection

Expose the superior, anterior, and arcuate parts of the superficial ligament of the pubic symphysis. Near the arcuate ligament, some fibrous bundles arise from the antero-inferior part of the symphysis, and pass with the dorsal vein of the clitoris to the urethra. This is the inferior part of the **pubo-urethral ligament** which stabilizes the urethra in the female.

In the male, make a median section through the penis, opening the entire length of the spongy part of the urethra. Examine the internal surface of the urethra. Note any recesses or lacunae in its dorsal wall, especially at the proximal end of the fossa navicularis [Fig. 121] in the glans penis. Identify the intrabulbar fossa [Fig. 222] and the opening of the membranous part of the urethra. Pass a metal rod through the urethra into the bladder, from the external orifice in the female, or from the opening of the membranous part in the male.

Cut through the pubic symphysis in the median plane, and extend the incision into the urethra by cutting down on the metal rod. Remove the metal rod and continue the median incision to the anterior surfaces of the sacrum and coccyx. In the perineum, this incision should pass through the middle of the central perineal tendon, anal canal, and anococcygeal ligament. In the pelvis it should divide the bladder through the internal urethral orifice, then pass either through the uterus and vagina or between the two deferent ducts, and divide the rectum longitudinally. Make a median dorsal saw cut through the fourth and fifth lumbar vertebrae, the sacrum, and coccyx to meet the knife cut through the soft tissues. Avoid carrying the saw into the soft tissues of the pelvis.

Separate the two halves of the pelvis, wash out the rectum and vagina with a jet of water, and examine the cut surfaces of all the tissues [Figs. 235, 236].

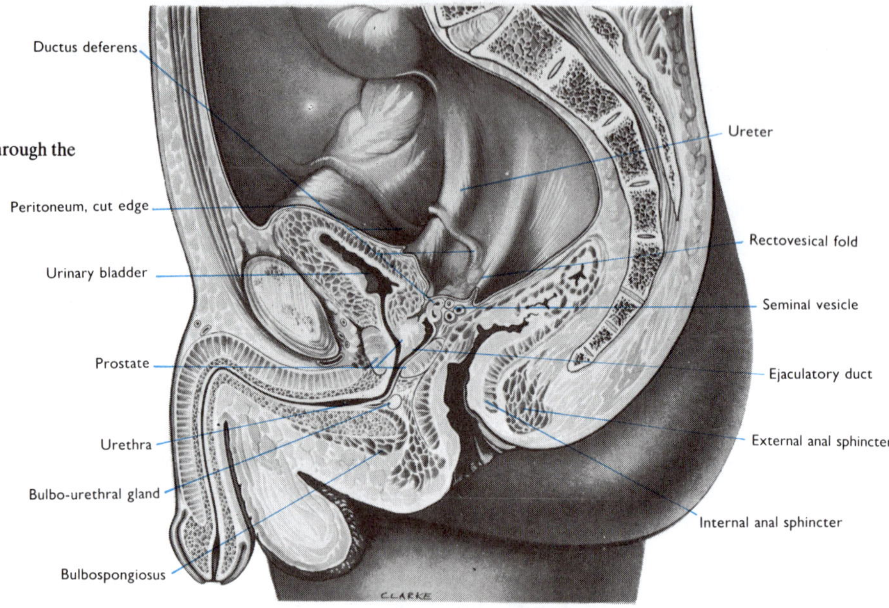

Fig. 235. A section through the male pelvis.

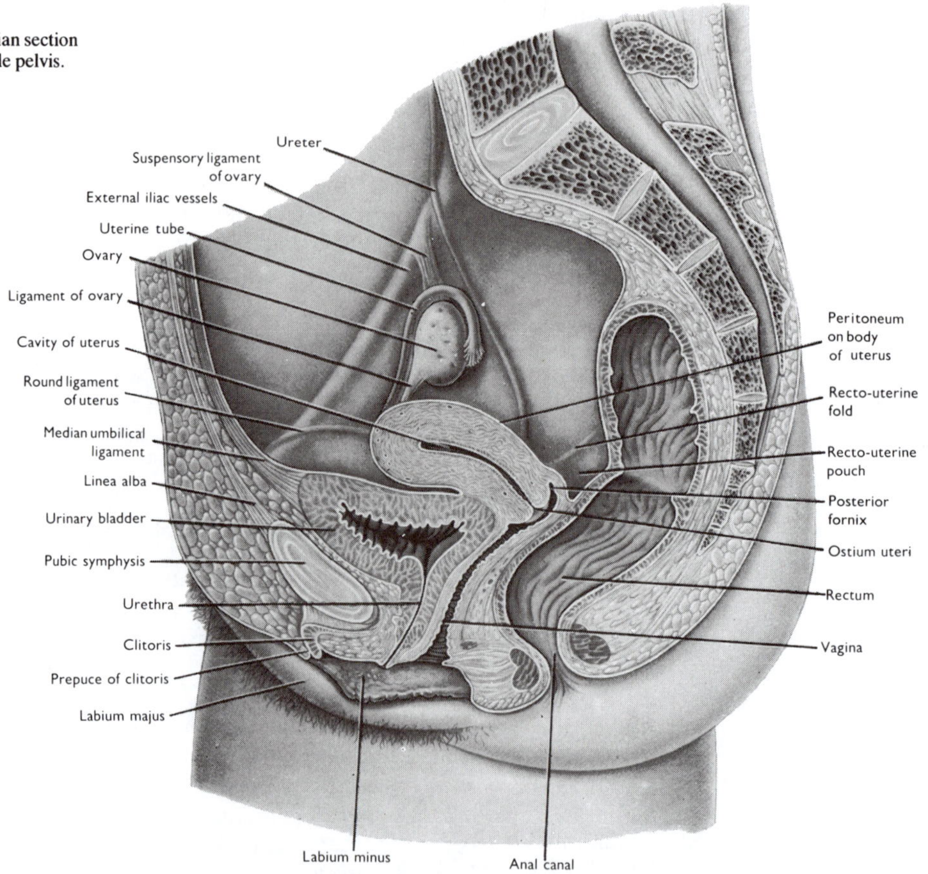

Fig. 236. A median section through the female pelvis.

Urinary bladder

[Figs. 217, 234–242, 245, 246, 290A]

This muscular urine store, when empty, lies in the antero-inferior part of the lesser pelvis. Its superior surface is covered with **peritoneum** which is reflected near the posterior border of the bladder on to the junction of the body and cervix of the uterus in the female (uterovesical pouch) or over the superior surfaces of the deferent ducts in the male. The bladder lies relatively free in the surrounding loose extraperitoneal tissue except at its inferior part (**neck**) which is held firmly by the **puboprostatic** (male) or **pubovesical** (female) **ligaments**. Thus it is free to expand superiorly in the extraperitoneal tissue of the anterior abdominal wall, stripping the peritoneum from the transversalis fascia—a feature which permits the introduction of instruments into the distended bladder through the anterior abdominal wall without involvement of the peritoneal cavity.

In the child [Fig. 238] the bladder is an abdominal organ even when empty. It begins to enter the enlarging pelvis at six years of age, but is not entirely a pelvic organ till after puberty.

Shape

The empty bladder has the shape of a three-sided pyramid with its apex anteriorly [Fig. 239], but becomes spherical when distended [Fig. 237]. The apex is continuous with the **median umbilical ligament** posterior to the upper margin of the pubic symphysis. This ligament is the fibrous remnant of the

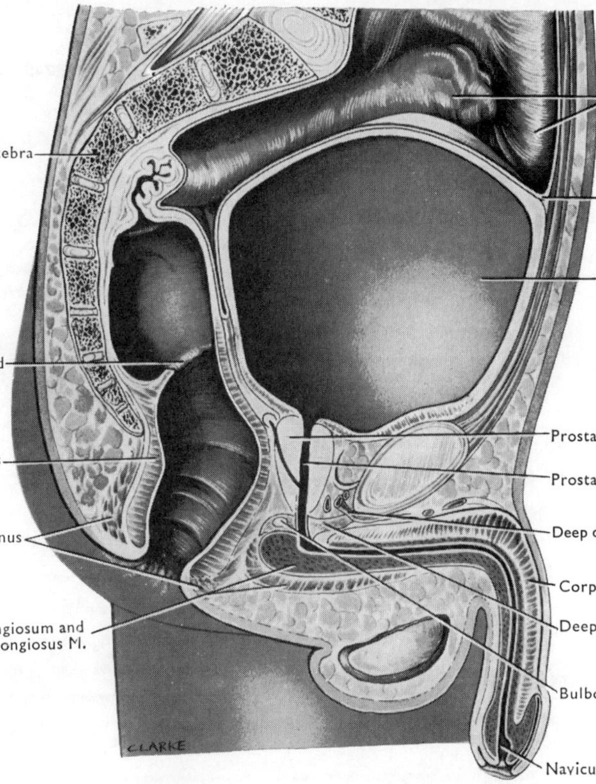

Fig. 237. A section through the male pelvis. The urinary bladder and rectum are distended. Note that the peritoneum is removed from the lower part of the anterior abdominal wall by the distended bladder.

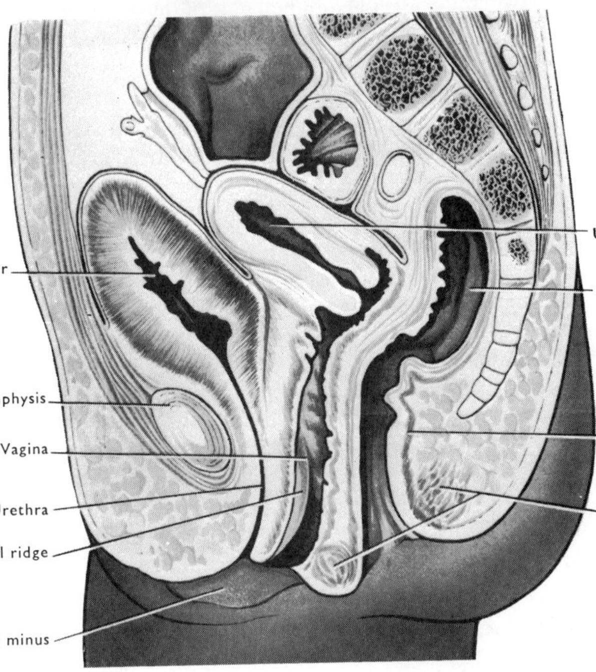

Fig. 238. A median section through the lower abdomen and pelvis of a new-born female child. Note that the urinary bladder and uterus lie in the abdomen.

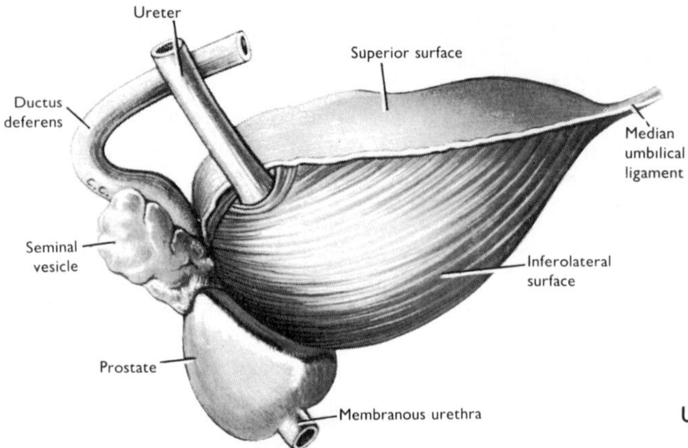

Fig. 239. A lateral view of the urinary bladder, prostate, and seminal vesicle. The bladder is nearly empty.

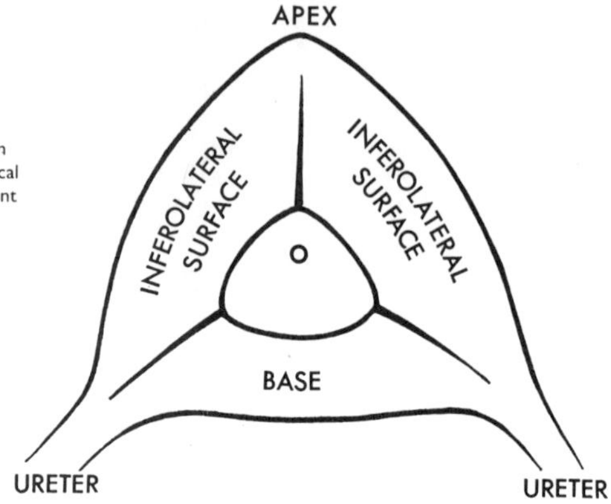

Fig. 240. A diagram of the urinary bladder as seen from below. The enclosed area marks the position of the prostate.

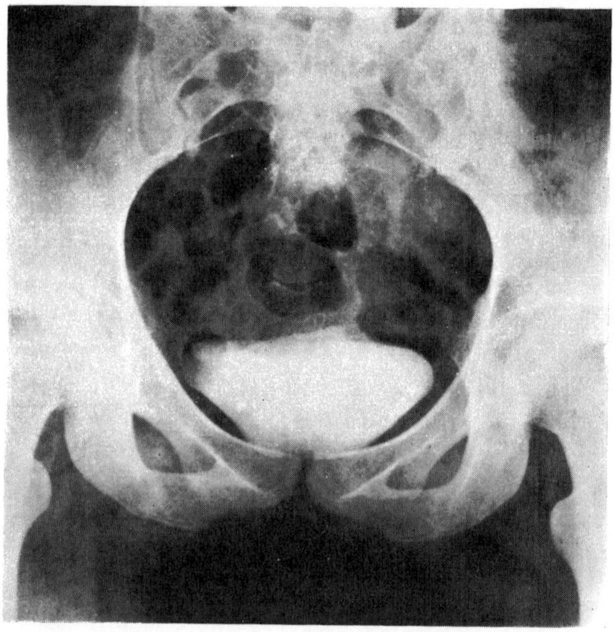

Fig. 241. A radiograph of the female pelvis to show the urinary bladder filled with contrast medium. Note the pyramidal shape of the partly distended bladder.

intra-abdominal part of the **allantois**—a tubular structure which extends from the bladder into the umbilical cord in the embryo. It may remain patent in part, or rarely throughout its length. In the latter case, urine may be discharged through the umbilicus when the umbilical cord is cut at birth.

The triangular **base** (or **fundus**) of the bladder faces postero-inferiorly. It is applied to the genital septum (and its contents) which separates the bladder from the rectovesical (or recto-uterine) pouch and rectum.

The sides of the pyramid are the two **inferolateral surfaces** and the **superior surface** [Figs. 239, 240]. The inferolateral surfaces lie on the retropubic fat, parallel to the levator ani muscles, and form one wall of the retropubic space. They meet at a blunt edge (posterior to the pubic symphysis) which slopes postero-inferiorly from the apex to meet the inferior angle of the base at the most inferior part or neck of the bladder. Here it is continuous with the urethra [Figs. 235, 236].

The base (or fundus) and the superior surface are continuous at the posterior border. The ureters join the bladder at the lateral ends of this border. *In the female*, the base is in contact with the cervix of the uterus and the upper part of the vagina. *In the male*, the two seminal vesicles, with the ampullae of the deferent ducts between them, cover all but a small median part of the base immediately below the posterior border [Fig. 242].

Structure of bladder

The muscle layer is thick. It consists of bundles of smooth muscle running in many directions [see p. 163]. Towards the neck, they come together to form a ring that surrounds the uppermost part of the urethra, the **involuntary sphincter of the bladder**. Other muscle fibres run radially into this region, and tend to pull open the urethral orifice when they contract on micturition. *In the female*, the muscle at the neck of the bladder is continuous with that of the urethra; *in the male*, it is continuous with the muscular stroma of the prostate gland.

The **mucous membrane** is lined with transitional epithelium which is urine-proof and capable of considerable stretching. The underlying connective tissue is loose and inelastic, and so becomes wrinkled when the bladder contracts except over the trigone where the epithelium is more firmly bound to the muscle and tends to remain smooth.

Dissection

Pull the half bladder medially and expose the structures on its lateral aspect—the obliterated umbilical artery and its superior vesical branches passing to the bladder, the obturator vessels and nerve, and the superior part of levator ani.

In the male, follow the **ductus deferens** to the base of the bladder. Separate it from the adjoining **seminal vesicle,** and follow both to the base of the prostate [Fig. 242]. Note the visceral pelvic fascia descending from these structures to form the posterior fascial sheath of the prostate (the **rectovesical septum**). Follow this fascia inferiorly to the superior fascia of the urogenital diaphragm on the side where the diaphragm is intact.

Find the **deep dorsal vein of the penis** entering the pelvis anteriorly. It joins the plexus of veins in the angle between the bladder and the prostate [Fig. 244]. Follow the prostatic fascia on to the back of the pubic bone and symphysis as the puboprostatic ligament.

Pull the bladder and prostate medially to expose the medial margin of levator ani immediately inferolateral to the prostate (**levator prostatae muscle**). The urethra and apex of the prostate descend to the urogenital diaphragm through the gap between the medial margins of the levator ani muscles.

The prostate is a firm structure which is traversed by the urethra and is separated from the rectum only by the rectovesical septum.

The upper and lower parts of the **prostatic urethra** lie at an angle to each other. Immediately inferior to the angle, a small hillock (**seminal colliculus**) projects forwards from a median, posterior ridge (**urethral crest** [Fig. 246]) which extends the length of the prostatic urethra with a groove on each side of it, the **prostatic sinus**. On the apex of the colliculus is the small opening of a blind, median pouch (**prostatic utricle**) which extends posterosuperiorly into the prostate. It is the remnant of the structure which forms the vagina in the female. On each side of the utricle is the smaller opening of an **ejaculatory duct**. Pass a fine seeker into the latter opening. It enters either the ductus deferens or the seminal vesicle for they unite in the ejaculatory duct near the base of the prostate [Fig. 245]. Find the beginning of the ejaculatory duct and trace it through the posterior part of the prostate.

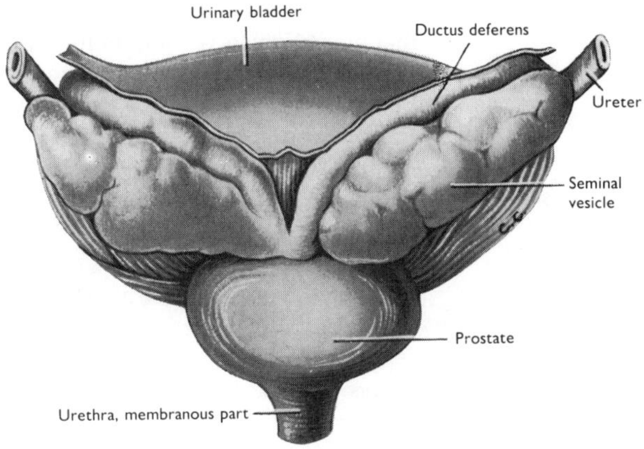

Fig. 242. The posterior surfaces of the urinary bladder, prostate, and seminal vesicles.

Ductus deferens

[Figs. 217, 234, 242, 254]

This thick-walled, muscular duct of the testis and epididymis has already been traced from the inferior pole of the testis through the spermatic cord and inguinal canal to the deep inguinal ring [pp. 100, 106]. Here it leaves the other constituents of the spermatic cord, and runs over the external iliac vessels to the lateral wall of the lesser pelvis, immediately external to the peritoneum. It then crosses the ureter near the posterolateral angle of the bladder [Fig. 235], turns medially on the base of the bladder, superior to the seminal vesicle, and bends inferiorly medial to the vesicle, expanding into a sacculated **ampulla** [Fig. 242]. This is enclosed with the vesicle in the upper part of the **rectovesical septum**. The ductus then narrows rapidly and joins the duct of the seminal vesicle to form the **ejaculatory duct** immediately posterior to the neck of the bladder.

The thick **muscular wall** of the ductus deferens makes it readily palpable in the spermatic cord. This smooth muscle is heavily innervated with autonomic nerve fibres to ensure rapid contraction and discharge of the contained spermatozoa and secretions.

Seminal vesicle

[Figs. 222, 239, 242, 243, 290A]

This is a sacculated tube, approximately 15 cm long, with short distended branches. It is folded upon itself to form a piriform structure and is bound to the base of the bladder by the fascia of the rectovesical septum. The vesicle extends superolaterally from its narrow duct posterior to the neck of the bladder to the entry of the ureter into the bladder. It lies below the ductus deferens and lateral to its ampulla.

The seminal vesicle is not a store for spermatozoa. It produces a secretion which is mixed in the ejaculatory duct with the spermatozoa from the ductus deferens by the synchronous contraction of the muscle of both structures. The alkaline secretion of the vesicle contains fructose, mucus, and a coagulating enzyme. The vesicle and the ampulla of the ductus deferens have the same structure, and its thick secretion seems to be concerned with the nutrition of the spermatozoa.

Ejaculatory duct

[Fig. 245]

Each of these ducts is formed by the union of the ductus deferens with the duct of the seminal vesicle close to the median plane and immediately posterior to the neck of the bladder. It passes antero-inferiorly through the upper, posterior half of the prostate and along the side of the prostatic utricle, to open into the prostatic urethra on the seminal colliculus at the side of the utricle. The wall of the ejaculatory duct is formed by columnar epithelium and a thin layer of circular and longitudinal muscle.

Prostate

[Figs. 232, 235, 239, 243, 245, 246, 291]

This gland resembles a compressed, inverted cone, approximately 3 cm from apex to base, and 3.5 cm across the base. The complex glandular elements are buried in a firm, dense fibromuscular **stroma** which is directly continuous with the smooth muscle of the neck of the bladder at the base of the prostate. A peripheral groove between the base of the prostate and the bladder lodges part of the **prostatic plexus of veins**, and has the **ejaculatory ducts** entering it posteriorly.

The **apex** of the prostate projects inferiorly between the medial margins of the levator ani muscles, and rests on the superior fascia of the urogenital diaphragm which is continuous with the fascial sheath of the prostate. The **urethra** emerges from the prostate immediately anterosuperior to the apex.

The convex **inferolateral surfaces** of the prostate are clasped by the medial margins of the levator ani muscles (levator prostatae). These two surfaces meet in the rounded **anterior surface** which lies behind the lower part of the pubic symphysis.

The **posterior surface** of the prostate is nearly flat. It is easily palpated by a finger in the rectum because only the rectovesical septum intervenes [Fig. 253] and the prostate is firm. The prostate has a thin **capsule** of fibromuscular tissue, but is also enclosed in a loose **sheath** of visceral pelvic fascia which is separated from the capsule at the front and sides by the **prostatic venous plexus**. The plexus drains the prostate, the bladder, and the deep dorsal vein of the penis [Fig. 244].

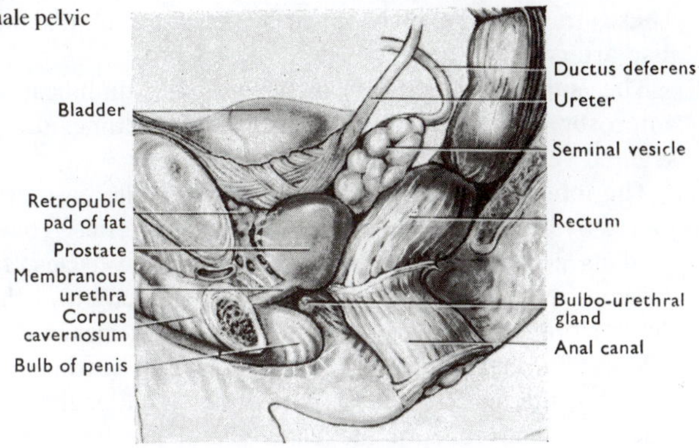

Fig. 243. Dissection of male pelvic organs from the left side.

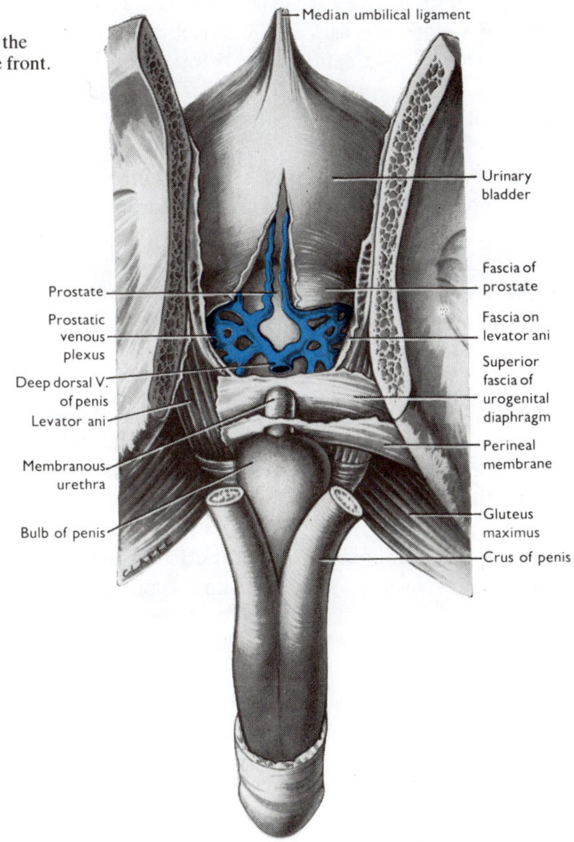

Fig. 244. A dissection of the retropubic space from the front.

Structure

The glandular part of the prostate develops as a considerable number of minute tubular outgrowths of the prostatic part of the urethra. These form the **ducts** of the numerous separate elements which make up the prostate, but only those that arise from the posterior part of the urethra form glands of any size. Thus the major ducts enter the prostatic sinuses, and most of the glandular tissue lies in the posterior and lateral parts of the prostate.

The **median lobe** of the prostate is the part that lies posterior to the urethra above the ejaculatory ducts. Superiorly, it is in direct contact with the inferior part of the trigone of the bladder, and bulges it upwards to produce the **uvula of the bladder**. Laterally, there is no separation of the median lobe from the remainder of the prostate which is arbitrarily divided into **right** and **left lobes** by the urethra.

The prostatic **secretion** is a watery, opalescent fluid which contains acid phosphatase and protein. It is discharged into the urethra by contraction of the muscular stroma at ejaculation. The size and activity of the prostate and seminal vesicles are controlled by sex hormones. Thus both develop rapidly at puberty. Hypertrophy of the prostate is a common cause of obstruction of the urethra in elderly men.

Blood and lymph vessels of bladder, prostate, seminal vesicles, and deferent ducts

These structures are all supplied by three irregular branches of each internal iliac artery [p. 232].

The **superior vesical** branches of the umbilical arteries supply the anterosuperior parts of the bladder and sometimes the superior parts of the seminal vesicles and ductus deferens.

The **inferior vesical arteries** pass towards the base of the bladder and are joined by branches from the middle rectal arteries. They supply the prostate (and its contained structures), the seminal vesicles, the ampullae of the deferent ducts, and the greater part of the length of these ducts through a slender branch which accompanies each—**arteries of the deferent ducts**.

Veins corresponding to the arteries drain to the internal iliac veins. In addition, the anterosuperior part of the bladder may drain to the external iliac vein, and veins of the bladder and prostate, together with the deep dorsal vein of the penis, drain through the prostatic plexus to the **inferior vesical veins**. These drain to the internal iliac veins, and communicate through the **lateral sacral veins** and pelvic sacral foramina with the **internal vertebral venous plexuses** in the vertebral canal [Fig. 205]. Thus the blood they transmit may ascend either through the inferior vena cava or through the veins of the vertebral column. This vertebral route is thought to be responsible for the dissemination of prostatic cancer cells to the vertebral bodies or even to the skull.

The **lymph vessels** drain to the external iliac nodes from the superior parts, to the internal iliac nodes from the inferior parts. Some vessels from the region of the neck of the bladder pass directly to sacral or common iliac nodes.

The **nerve supply** of the pelvic viscera is from the inferior hypogastric (pelvic) plexuses. These contain sympathetic, parasympathetic, and sensory nerve fibres.

Puboprostatic and pubovesical ligaments

These fibro-elastic condensations of pelvic fascia contain some smooth muscle. They pass from the back of the bodies of the pubic bones, close to the median plane, to the anterior surface of the sheath of the prostate and the neck of the bladder in the male, or to the neck of the bladder and the urethra in the female. They are united across the median plane by a thin fascial layer, and extend laterally to fuse with the fascia over the medial margins of the levator ani muscles. They are important structures in maintaining the position of the bladder, prostate, and urethra. *In the female*, the upper part of the S-shaped urethra is convex anteriorly because of the attachment of the pubo-urethral ligament. Inferiorly, the urethra curves forwards below the pubic symphysis, and is held there by a **pubo-urethral ligament** which arises from the antero-inferior part of the symphysis.

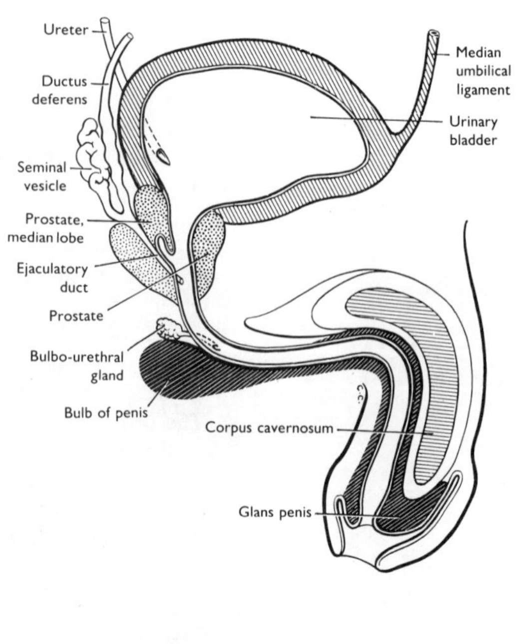

Fig. 245. A diagram of the bladder, urethra, and penis.

Male urethra

[Figs. 222, 235, 245, 246; p. 263]

The parts of this tube have been described [p. 201], and the entire length has been opened. The urethra consists of a layer of fibro-elastic tissue and smooth muscle lined with a vascular **mucous membrane**, predominantly with a stratified columnar epithelium. Superior to the prostatic utricle, the epithelium is transitional, while it is stratified squamous in the navicular fossa. The mucous membrane is pitted by a number of minute recesses (**urethral lacunae**) which face distally, and it contains many small mucous glands.

Prostatic part

It is approximately 3 cm long, and pierces the prostate from its base to a point just anterosuperior to its apex. It is the widest and most dilatable part of the urethra, and is concave anteriorly. A narrow, median ridge (**urethral crest**) with a groove (**prostatic sinus**) on each side, extends inferiorly on the posterior wall from the internal urethral orifice to a rounded eminence (**seminal colliculus**) on the crest about the middle of the prostatic part. The crest then rapidly diminishes and is absent in the membranous part.

Fig. 246. A dissection of the urinary bladder and urethra from the front in the male. The contents of the deep perineal space have been removed except for the membranous urethra.

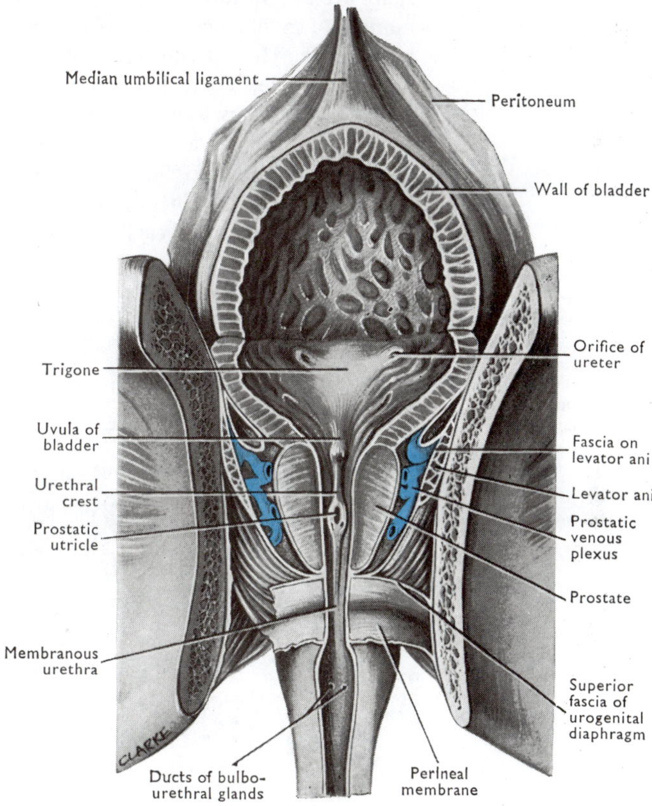

The **seminal colliculus** has three small openings on it—the median prostatic utricle with a slit-like **ejaculatory duct** on each side. The numerous **ducts of the prostate gland** open in the prostatic sinuses.

The **prostatic utricle** (approximately 1 cm long) is a blind sac which extends posterosuperiorly into the prostate, and is wider than its aperture. It represents the remains of the fused parts of the **paramesonephric ducts** of the embryo which form the vagina in the female.

Membranous part

This is the narrowest, shortest (1 cm), and least dilatable part of the urethra. It pierces the superior and inferior fasciae of the urogenital diaphragm, and is surrounded by the sphincter urethrae between them.

Immediately below the inferior fascia of the urogenital diaphragm (perineal membrane), the urethra inclines forwards and enters the corpus spongiosum obliquely, leaving its anterior wall uncovered for a short distance. It is this part which may be ruptured in attempting to pass a bougie into the membranous part before the tip has reached the correct position.

Spongy part

This long part (16 cm) begins on the upper surface of the bulb of the penis. At first it bulges backwards forming the **intrabulbar fossa** [Fig. 222] and then passes longitudinally through the corpus spongiosum. In the glans penis, it expands dorsoventrally to form the slit-like **fossa navicularis**. This has a fold of mucous membrane in the posterior part of its roof against which the tip of a bougie or catheter may catch [Fig. 121].

Vessels and nerves

The urethra shares in the nerve, blood, and lymph supply of the prostate, urogenital diaphragm, and penis. Most of the lymph drains to the internal iliac nodes, but some passes to the deep inguinal nodes from the distal spongy part.

Female urethra

[Figs. 233, 236, 247; p. 262]

The female urethra is equal in length (4 cm) to the prostatic and membranous parts in the male. It is wider and more dilatable in the female, and is lined by transitional, and stratified columnar and squamous epithelia from above downwards. The mucous membrane contains mucous glands and is pitted by small **urethral lacunae** which face inferiorly. On each side of the urethra are a number of small mucous glands supposed to be homologous with the prostate in the male. Their **para-urethral ducts** open near the margin of the external urethral orifice. There is a considerable layer of **smooth muscle** much of which is formed by loops descending from the bladder wall.

The female urethra is S-shaped when seen from the side. The superior part, corresponding to the prostatic urethra is convex anteriorly; the inferior part curves forwards below the pubic symphysis. Each part is held in a position by a **pubo-urethral ligament** [p. 222] which also supports the anterior vaginal wall to which the urethra is closely applied [Fig. 247].

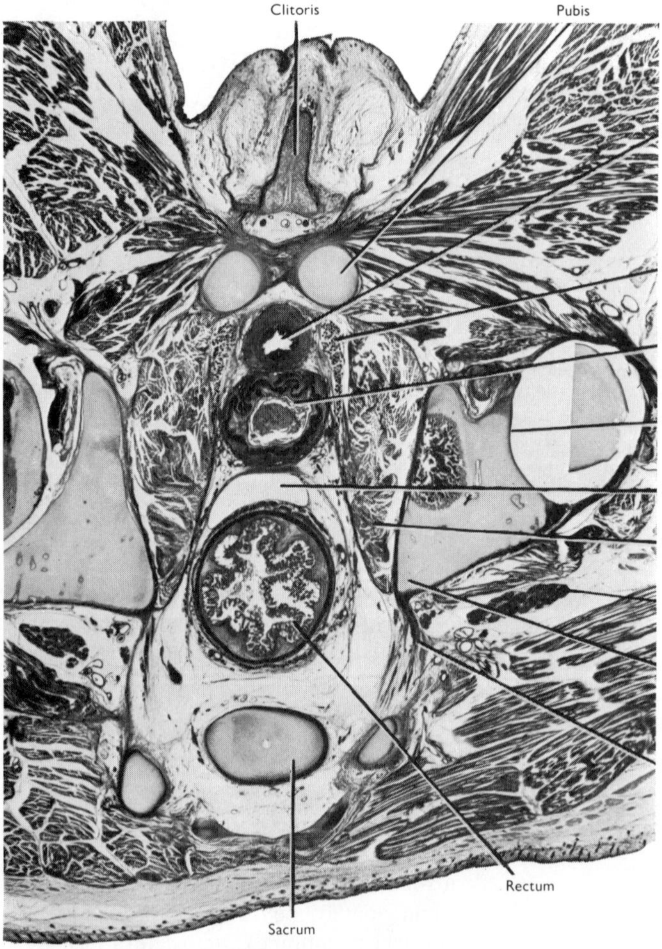

Fig. 247. A horizontal section through the lesser pelvis of a seven-month female human fetus.

Vessels

The blood supply is from the vaginal and internal pudendal vessels. Lymph vessels pass to the sacral and internal iliac nodes; a few pass to the inguinal nodes with the other lymph vessels of the vulva.

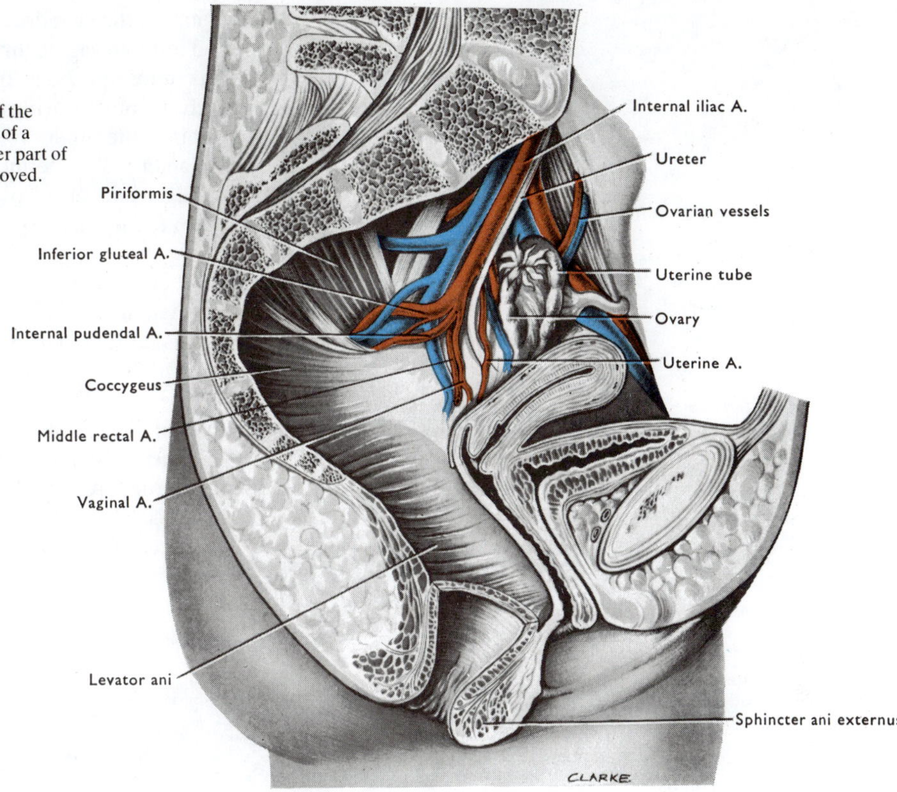

Fig. 248. A dissection of the structures in the left half of a female pelvis. The greater part of the rectum has been removed.

Dissection

Lift the divided **uterus** and confirm that the body is covered with peritoneum on its superior and inferior aspects, and is, therefore, free to move. Compare this with the fixity of the **cervix** which is only covered with peritoneum on the posterosuperior surface of that part which lies outside the vagina (**supravaginal part**), and which is attached to the lateral pelvic wall by the thick base of the broad ligament, the most posterior part of which passes to the sacrum—the **uterosacral ligament**. The part of the cervix which projects into the vagina through its upper anterior wall is surrounded on all sides by a narrow, slit-like part of the vaginal cavity, the **fornices of the vagina**.

If there is no fat in the upper, thin part of the broad ligament, transilluminate it and attempt to see the remnant of the mesonephric duct and tubules (the epoophoron [Fig. 249]) of the embryo. This is sometimes visible between the ovary and the uterine tube. It corresponds to the efferent ductules of the testis and the epididymis which degenerate in the female.

Note the position and examine the interior of the vagina. Compare the laxity of the tissue which separates it from the rectum with the dense tissue which binds it to the bladder, urethra, and central perineal tendon. Confirm the attachment of the bladder and urethra to the pubis by the pubovesical and pubo-urethral ligaments. Note how the urethra could be bruised against the pubis by the fetal head during childbirth.

Uterus

[Figs. 233, 248, 250; p. 262]

This thick-walled, firm, muscular organ has a narrow lumen surrounded by a mucous membrane (endometrium) which is firmly bound to the muscle (myometrium). The endometrium contains simple tubular glands that reach into the innermost layer of the muscle. In the body of the uterus, the endometrium undergoes cyclical changes induced by ovarian hormones. If pregnancy does not occur, each cycle ends with the menstrual flow produced by the breakdown and discharge of all but the outermost layer of a thickened endometrium, which is then reconstituted, new epithelium growing from the bases of the glands to cover its internal surface.

The uterus is 7–8 cm long. Nearly half of the cylindrical neck or **cervix** (2.5 cm in diameter and length) is inserted into the vagina through the uppermost part of its anterior wall. The cervix joins the body of the uterus at the **isthmus**—a slight constriction which is only obvious prior to the first pregnancy. The body expands from this to the fundus (5 cm wide and 2.5 cm thick) in the free edge of the broad ligament. The uterine tubes pass laterally from the sides of the fundus, and the **ligaments** of the ovaries and the round ligaments of the uterus are attached to the uterus respectively superior and inferior to the uterotubal junction.

The uterus overlies the posterior part of the superior surface and the upper part of the base of the bladder. Thus when the bladder is empty, the uterus is tilted forwards (*anteversion* of the uterus) at right angles to the vagina and to the plane of the superior aperture of the lesser pelvis [Fig. 248]. Also the body is slightly bent downwards (*anteflexion* of the uterus) at the isthmus on the firmer, more fibrous cervix [Fig. 236]. The body of the uterus, enclosed between the layers of the **broad ligament**, is freely mobile. Thus as the bladder fills, the uterus is raised, and may be forced back till it lies in line with the vagina when the bladder is fully distended: it is then said to be *retroverted*. In certain pathological conditions, the uterus may be permanently retroverted, and even bent backwards on itself at the isthmus—a condition known as *retroflexion*.

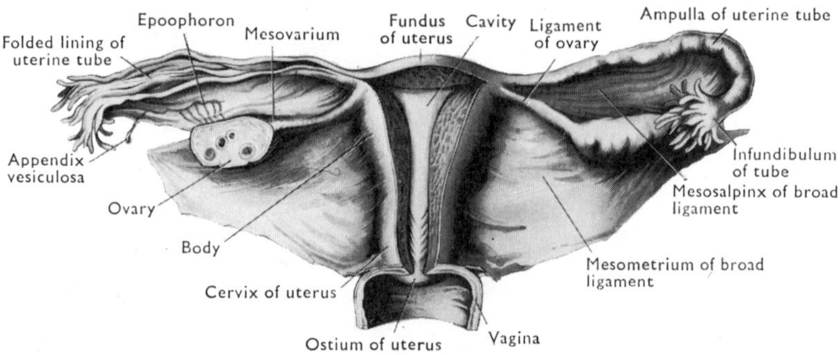

Fig. 249. The posterosuperior surface of the broad ligament and associated structures. The vagina, uterus, and left uterine tube have been opened, and the left ovary is sectioned parallel to the broad ligament.

Cervix

The **vaginal part** of the cervix, lying within the uppermost part of the vagina, is covered on its external surface by the stratified squamous epithelium of the vagina. This epithelium is continuous with the simple columnar lining of the uterus just within the centrally placed ostium uteri. Peripherally, the epithelium arches off the cervix on to the vaginal wall, thus surrounding the **fornix of the vagina** which encircles the cervix. For descriptive purposes, the fornix is artificially divided into anterior, posterior, and right and left lateral fornices. The anterior fornix is shallow [Fig. 248].

The posterosuperior surface of the **supravaginal part** of the cervix and the adjacent posterior vaginal fornix are the only parts of these structures covered with peritoneum. The antero-inferior surface of the cervix is directly in contact with the upper part of the base of the bladder [Fig. 248].

The **canal of the cervix** is spindle-shaped. It is continuous anterosuperiorly with the cavity of the body of the uterus without any demarcation, except in the pregnant uterus where the cervix remains small and is not dilated until parturition. In the later stages of pregnancy the **isthmus** is elongated to form the *lower uterine segment*. Inferiorly the canal of the cervix opens into the vagina through the **ostium uteri**—a narrow, transverse slit with a short anterior and long posterior lip. In nullipara, the endometrium of the cervix is folded like the fronds of a palm leaf (**plicae palmatae**). It contains numerous tubular, branched **glands**, the ducts of which may be occluded so that the glands become distended with secretion and give rise to cysts in the cervix (Nabothian follicles). The endometrium of the cervix plays no part in the changes of menstruation.

The cervix, unlike the body of the uterus, is held in position by a number of structures which are principally condensations of fascia and some smooth muscle in the base of the broad ligament. The main mass surrounds the uterine artery (**transverse ligament of the cervix**). It passes from the cervix and lateral fornix on each side to the corresponding lateral wall of the pelvis. A similar condensation in each recto-uterine fold forms the **uterosacral ligaments**. Thus the cervix tends to remain in position while the body of the uterus expands upwards in pregnancy.

Body of uterus

The inferior or **vesical surface** of the uterus is nearly flat. The **uterovesical pouch of peritoneum** extends between it and the bladder to the junction of the body and cervix. Here the peritoneum on the uterus is reflected on to the posterior margin of the upper surface of the bladder. The pouch is empty unless the uterus is retroverted when a coil of intestine may lie in it.

The convex superior or **intestinal surface** of the uterus is covered with peritoneum. This extends posteriorly over the supravaginal part of the cervix and posterior fornix of the vagina to the recto-uterine pouch [Fig. 236] which contains loops of ileum and sigmoid colon.

Attached to the uterus on each side is the broad ligament with the uterine vessels passing between its layers.

The **cavity of the uterus** is a mere triangular slit between the intestinal and vesical walls. The uterine tubes enter the angles in the fundus, the apex is continuous with the cervical canal.

Vessels of uterus

These are the **uterine arteries** and veins which enter the broad ligament beside the lateral fornices of the vagina, superior to the ureters [Fig. 250]. They pass along the sides of the uterus, and turn laterally in the broad ligament to anastomose with the ovarian arteries close to the uterine tube. Large branches pass into the muscle of the uterus, and running within it, send smaller vessels into the **endometrium** to give separate supplies to the external and internal parts of that mucous lining. The arteries supplying the internal layers of the endometrium (which are involved in menstruation) are coiled arteries. The presence of the large vessels within the muscle wall of the uterus ensures closure of these vessels when the uterus contracts at parturition. When the placenta is torn away from the internal surface of the uterus and discharged, it leaves a large raw area from which severe haemorrhage can occur if uterine contraction is not maintained.

The **lymph vessels** pass by a number of routes [Fig. 255]. (1) From the cervix, body, and fundus they pass laterally through the broad ligament (occasionally interrupted by small para-uterine nodes in the broad ligament) to the external iliac nodes. (2) From the fundus they also pass with the ovarian lymph vessels to the lumbar nodes; a few passing along the round ligaments of the uterus to the superficial inguinal nodes. (3) From the cervix to the internal iliac and sacral nodes.

The **nerves** of the uterus come from the inferior hypogastric plexus. Many of the postganglionic parasympathetic nerve fibres arise in large pelvic ganglia close to the cervix.

Vagina

[Figs. 236, 248, 250; p. 262]

This tube descends antero-inferiorly from its posterior fornix to open into the vestibule between the labia minora. It passes between the medial borders of the two levator ani muscles, and pierces the urogenital diaphragm with the sphincter urethrae muscle in it. The anterior wall is 7.5 cm long and is in contact with the longer (9 cm) posterior wall, which extends above the cervix to the posterior fornix. The cervix projects into a slightly enlarged part of the cavity of the vagina, and separates the two walls.

The **anterior wall** is in contact with the base of the bladder and the terminal parts of the ureters. It is tightly bound to the neck of the bladder and to the urethra, and thus to the pubis through the pubovesical and pubo-urethral ligaments.

The **posterior fornix** is covered with peritoneum. Thus injuries to this part of the vagina may involve the peritoneal cavity. Inferior to this, only loose areolar tissue separates the **posterior wall** from the lowest part of the rectum, a feature which allows the vaginal wall to separate from the rectum and protrude through the vaginal orifice when the cervix descends from its normal position in prolapse of the uterus. This can only happen if the **central perineal tendon** is stretched or torn (thus removing its support from the

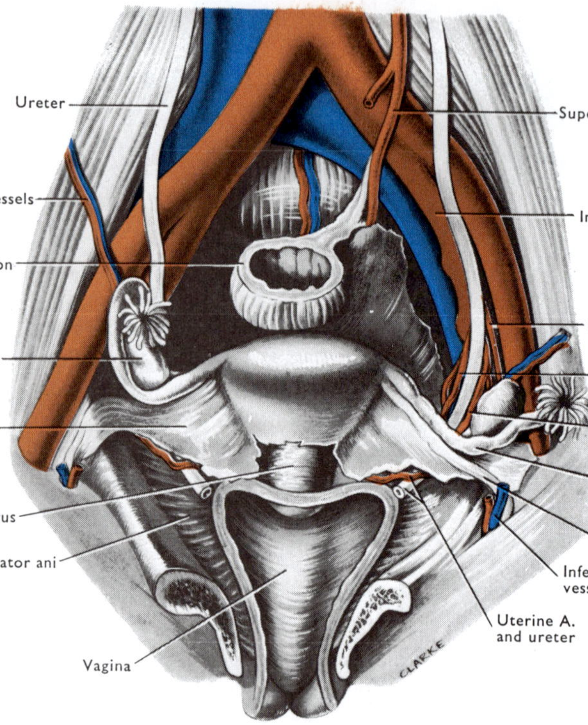

Fig. 250. A dissection of the female pelvis from the front. The uterus has been displaced backwards, and the bladder, urethra, and anterior wall of the vagina removed.

lowest part of the posterior wall) and the **ligaments of the cervix** are stretched—both common results of childbirth.

In the region of the **lateral fornices**, the narrow **lateral walls** give attachment to the base of the broad ligament where it contains the uterine vessels and ureters. Pulsations of the uterine arteries may be felt through the lateral fornices in the living. Inferiorly, the lateral walls are in contact with the levator ani muscles, the urogenital diaphragm, and the great vestibular glands and bulb of the vestibule.

Vessels of vagina

A **vaginal artery** (corresponding to the inferior vesical in the male) supplies it on each side, and is supplemented by twigs from the uterine, middle rectal, and arteries of the bulbs of the vestibule. The **veins** form submucous and adventitial plexuses. The submucous are so thin-walled and numerous as to resemble erectile tissue, and are liable to be distended and varicose. The veins drain with the arteries.

The **lymph vessels** of the upper part drain with the uterine vessels to the internal (and external) iliac nodes. The middle part drains with the vaginal vessels to the internal iliac nodes. The inferior part drains either to the sacral and common iliac nodes, or with the vessels of the vulva to the superficial inguinal nodes [Fig. 255].

Structure

This highly distensible tube is lined with the mucous type of stratified squamous epithelium, with an elastic areolar layer which contains many veins, a few lymph follicles, but no glands. The muscle layer contains bundles of longitudinal and circular smooth muscle, but without definite layers. At the margin of the orifice of the vagina, the mucous membrane may extend inwards as a circumferential fold, **the hymen**. Rarely this may be a complete membrane which prevents the discharge of the menstrual flow at puberty. More usually an incomplete ring, the hymen is torn at childbirth and remains as the **carunculae hymenales** [p. 198].

Dissection

Confirm the relation of the peritoneum to the upper two-thirds of the **rectum** [p. 229]. Examine the mucous membrane of the rectum, noting its transverse folds, and then strip some of it from the upper part. Note the relative laxity of the submucosa (less obvious in fixed than in fresh tissue) and look for evidence of the submucous venous plexus. Expose part of the circular muscle layer.

Find the **superior rectal artery**. Trace it on to the posterior surface of the upper part of the rectum, and follow its branches downwards on the posterolateral surfaces to the lowest part of the rectum [Fig. 252]. Strip the remaining peritoneum and fascia from the external surface of the rectum to expose the outer, longitudinal layer of muscle.

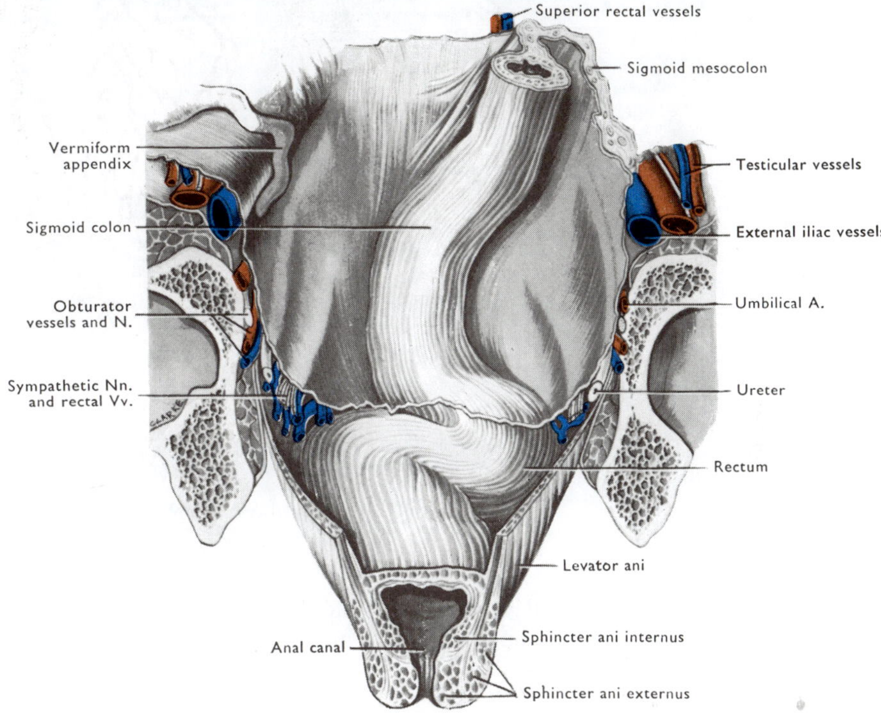

Fig. 251. A dissection of the rectum from the front.

Rectum

[Figs. 234, 236, 251, 252]

The rectum begins as the continuation of the sigmoid colon on the pelvic surface of the third piece of the sacrum. It is approximately 12 cm long, and first follows the curve of the sacrum and coccyx. It then runs antero-inferiorly to the central perineal tendon, lying on the **anococcygeal ligament** and the parts of the levator ani muscles passing to that ligament. It ends by turning postero-inferiorly as the **anal canal**, 2–3 cm from the tip of the coccyx, and immediately posterior to the **central perineal tendon** and to the apex of the prostate in the male. The lower part, frequently more distended than the remainder, is known as the **ampulla**.

In spite of its name, the rectum is not straight. In the sagittal plane it follows the curve of the sacrum and coccyx [Fig. 236]. In the coronal plane it is S-shaped with an increasing curvature inferiorly [Fig. 251].

Peritoneum covers the front and sides of the upper third of the rectum, and gradually passing forwards, turns off the front of the rectum at the junction of its middle and lower thirds to form the floor of the **rectovesical** or **recto-uterine pouch** and pass on to the back of the bladder (male) or the posterior fornix of the vagina (female). Thus the upper two-thirds of the rectum are in contact anteriorly with coils of sigmoid colon and ileum. The lower third is separated, *in the male*, from the base of the bladder by the seminal vesicles and deferent ducts and from the prostate by the rectovesical septum, *in the female*, from the vagina by loose areolar tissue.

The **recto-urethralis muscle** consists of some weak bundles of longitudinal rectal muscle which pass forwards to the apex of the prostate *in the male* [Fig. 253], or to the back of the vagina *in the female*, as an extension of its insertion into the central perineal tendon.

Posteriorly, the rectum has a branch of the superior rectal artery on each side, and is separated only by a layer of pelvic fascia from the sacrum, coccyx, and anococcygeal ligament in the median plane, and on each side from the muscles attached to these—piriformis, coccygeus, and levator ani. Between

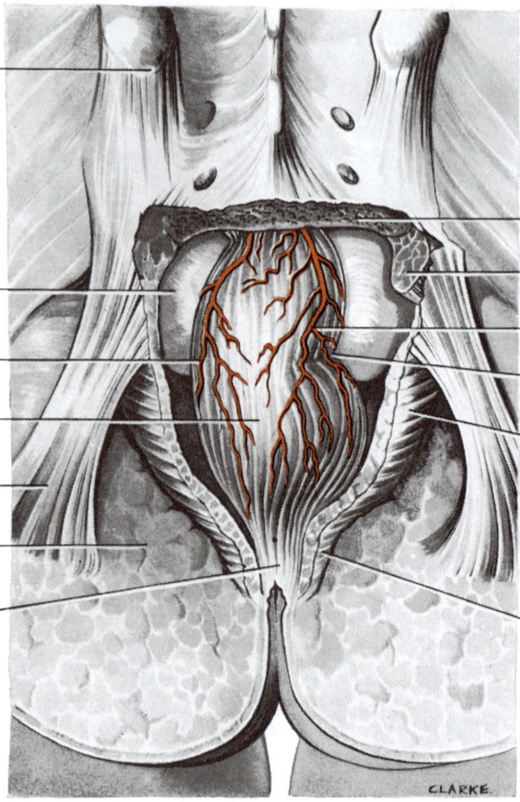

Fig. 252. A dissection of the rectum from behind.

these structures and the pelvic fascia are the median sacral vessels, a sympathetic trunk on each side and the ganglion impar on the coccyx. Lateral to these are the lateral sacral vessels and the lower sacral and coccygeal nerves.

Laterally, the rectum is in contact with the peritoneum superiorly, and inferiorly with the fat and fascia over coccygeus and the levator ani muscles. Some of this fascia, condensed around the middle rectal artery, passes to the fascial sheath of the rectum and helps to hold it in position.

Rectal and vaginal examinations

In the male, a finger in the rectum may be used to palpate the posterior surface of the prostate, or the seminal vesicles and terminal parts of the deferent ducts superior to the prostate. *In the female*, the firm cervix may be palpated through the rectal and vaginal walls. The cervix and body of the uterus may also be examined by bimanual palpation with two fingers in the vagina and a hand on the anterior abdominal wall. This method also allows palpation of the ovaries through the lateral fornices, particularly if the ovaries are enlarged.

Dissection

Examine the lining of the **anal canal**. Identify, if possible, the junction of the mucous membrane and skin, usually below the middle of the canal. The **mucous membrane** is thrown into a number of longitudinal folds (anal columns) which are united inferiorly by small, horizontal, semilunar folds (anal valves). These enclose small pockets of the mucous membrane (anal sinuses). From the anal orifice, the canal is lined first by true skin, and then by modified skin devoid of hair follicles and glands. At the valves, the epithelium becomes columnar, but this may not occur until nearer the rectum.

When these structures have been identified, strip the mucous membrane and skin from a sector of the anal canal. Identify the thickened part of the circular muscle layer forming the internal sphincter of the anus. Note that the anal valves lie at the middle of the sphincter. Follow the circular muscle superiorly into continuity with that of the rectum.

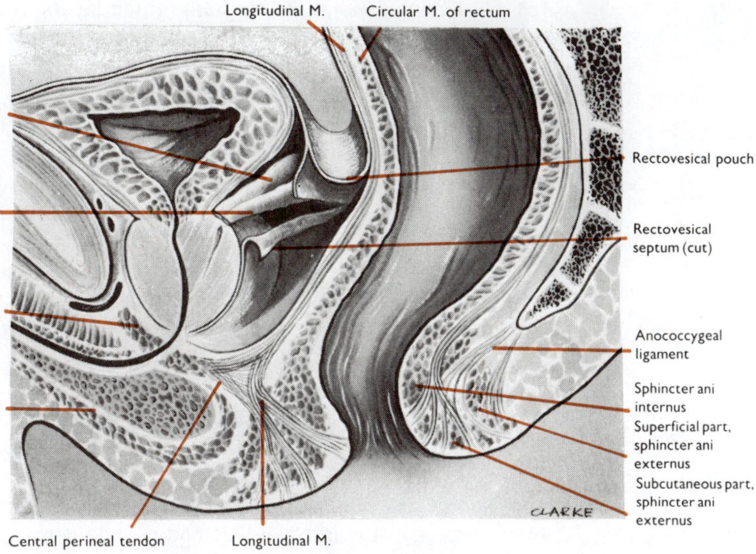

Fig. 253. A median section of the male pelvis.

Anal canal

This terminal part of the large intestine is approximately 4 cm long. It descends postero-inferiorly between the anococcygeal ligament and the central perineal tendon in the median plane. It is surrounded by the internal and external sphincter of the anus and the levator ani muscles, and has the ischiorectal fossae lateral and inferior to the levator ani muscles. It ends at the anus.

The **internal sphincter** consists of a thickening of the circular smooth muscle of the intestine around the upper two-thirds of the anal canal. The **external sphincter** [p. 202] surrounds the lower two-thirds of the anal canal. Thus it overlaps the internal sphincter and the fibres of levator ani which pass to the wall of the canal between them. The **puborectales** (see below) also act as a sphincter. They sweep round the sides and posterior aspect of the anorectal junction, and pulling this anteriorly, increase the angle between the rectum and anal canal. Some of the more *vertical fibres of the levator ani muscles* pass in to join the longitudinal muscle of the intestine and run with it through the external sphincter to the perineal skin, thus anchoring the longitudinal muscle and levator ani inferiorly. **Longitudinal muscle** bundles of the rectum pass forwards into the central perineal tendon and to the apex of the prostate or posterior vaginal wall (**recto-urethralis** [Fig. 253]).

Structure of rectum and anal canal

The **rectum** is surrounded by a fascial layer internal to the pelvic fascia. The smooth **muscle** is in outer longitudinal and inner circular layers. The longitudinal layer is of more uniform thickness than in the colon, the taeniae coli having given way to anterior and posterior longitudinal thickenings. These help to maintain the flexures of the rectum.

The **submucous layer** is formed of loose areolar tissue which allows the mucous membrane to slide freely on the muscle. It contains an extensive, asymmetrical **plexus of veins** which links the superior (inferior mesenteric) and inferior (internal pudendal) rectal veins. When distended, this plexus forms haemorrhoids (piles) especially on the left lateral and right anterior and posterior segments.

The **mucous layer** is thick. The columnar epithelial lining contains large numbers of goblet cells, and forms numerous simple tubular glands which extend into a connective tissue layer rich in lymphocytes and plasma cells. In the **ampulla**, some **deep glands** extend into the submucosa, and may even penetrate the muscle. The mucosa is so loosely connected to the muscle layer that it may prolapse through the anus with the dilated submucous veins. The mucosa is raised into three **transverse folds**, one opposite the concavity of each rectal flexure. These folds include the mucous, submucous, and some of the muscle layers of the rectal wall. The right fold is largest and lies at the level of the rectovesical (or recto-uterine) pouch. The other two are approximately 4 cm above and below it.

The **anal canal** has the same three layers as the rectum in its upper two-thirds, but the lower third is lined by skin. It is surrounded by the sphincter layers described above. The mucous layer forms a series of longitudinal ridges (**anal columns**) which are united to each other inferiorly by horizontal folds (**anal valves**) near the mucocutaneous junction (see above). These form a series of small pockets (**anal sinuses**) each at the inferior end of a groove between two ridges. The anal valves are liable to be torn by the passage of a hard faecal mass, thus allowing infection to spread into the wall of the anal canal (fissure *in ano*).

The **anal valves** lie at the level formerly occupied by the anal part of the **cloacal membrane**. In the embryo this temporarily closes the anal end of the alimentary canal, and if it persists, leads to the condition known as imperforate anus.

Vessels

There are five anastomosing **rectal arteries:** one superior rectal (from the inferior mesenteric); two middle rectal (from the internal iliac); two inferior rectal (from the internal pudendal in the ischiorectal fossa). The **veins** form submucous and adventitial plexuses. They drain along the corresponding arteries to the internal iliac and portal veins.

Lymph vessels [Fig. 255] (1) From the lower part of the anal canal and surrounding perianal skin run forwards to the medial **superficial inguinal lymph nodes**. (2) From the upper part of the anal canal lymph vessels either drain across the ischiorectal fossa with the inferior rectal blood vessels, or ascend with the middle rectal vessels to the **internal iliac nodes**. (3) Others pass from the rectum to the **sacral** and **common iliac lymph nodes**. (4) Some ascend with the inferior mesenteric vessels to **inferior mesenteric** and **lumbar nodes**.

The vessels of the lesser pelvis

Dissection

Pull the pelvic viscera away from the pelvic walls and follow the internal iliac vessels and their branches and tributaries [Figs. 248, 254]. If necessary remove the veins to get a clearer exposure of the arteries. Note any parts of the hypogastric plexus that are exposed with the vessels.

Superior rectal artery

This is the continuation of the inferior mesenteric artery. It begins on the middle of the left common iliac artery and, descending in the medial limb of the sigmoid mesocolon, divides into two branches on the third piece of the sacrum. These branches descend first on the back and then on the sides of the rectum. Each then divides into three or four branches which pierce the muscle layers at regular intervals on the circumference of the rectum, and descend in the submucosa to the anal canal where they anastomose with branches of the inferior (and middle) rectal arteries.

The **superior rectal vein** accompanies the artery to become the inferior mesenteric vein where it joins the sigmoid veins. It drains the rectal venous plexuses and other pelvic plexuses which anastomose with them (see below).

Internal iliac artery
[Figs. 248, 254]

In the adult this is the smaller of the two branches of the common iliac artery, though it is larger in the fetus when it transmits blood to the placenta through the umbilical artery. At birth the umbilical arteries are tied, and rapidly degenerate into fibrous cords to the level of the last persistent branch, the superior vesical artery.

The internal iliac is the artery of the walls and contents of the pelvis except those parts supplied by the inferior mesenteric, ovarian, and median sacral arteries. The arrangement of its visceral branches is very variable.

The artery begins medial to psoas major and anterior to the sacro-iliac joint, at the level of the lumbosacral intervertebral disc. It passes posteriorly into the lesser pelvis medial to the external iliac vein and the obturator nerve, and immediately lateral to the pelvic peritoneum. It lies between the ureter

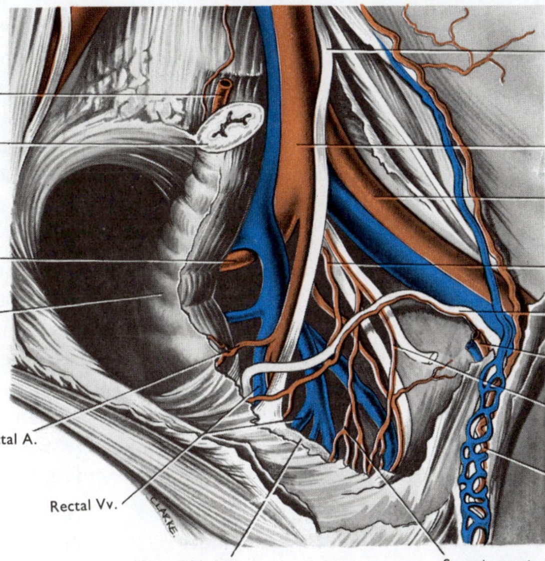

Fig. 254. The structures on the lateral wall of the male pelvis. These are exposed by retracting the bladder and rectum and removing the peritoneum and extraperitoneal fat.

inferiorly and the internal iliac vein superiorly and usually ends in anterior and posterior divisions at the upper margin of the greater sciatic notch.

Branches to pelvic walls

Posterior and posterolateral walls

Posterior division

1. The **superior gluteal artery** passes backwards between the lumbosacral trunk and the ventral ramus of the first sacral nerve to traverse the uppermost part of the greater sciatic foramen, superior to piriformis, with the corresponding vein and the superior gluteal nerve.

2. The **iliolumbar artery** ascends deep to psoas and divides into (a) an iliac branch which runs laterally on the abdominal surface of iliacus and (b) a lumbar branch which ascends posterior to psoas to supply it and quadratus lumborum. It may form the fifth lumbar artery. The corresponding vein joins the common iliac vein.

3. **Lateral sacral arteries** two on each side, descend in front of the pelvic sacral foramina through which they send branches to the sacral nerves, the contents of the sacral canal [p. 192], and to the muscles and skin overlying the dorsal sacral foramina.

Anterior division

4. The **inferior gluteal artery** passes postero-inferiorly between the ventral rami of the first and second sacral nerves to enter the gluteal region below piriformis and beside the sciatic nerve.

Anterolateral wall

The **obturator artery** passes antero-inferiorly with the obturator nerve and vein through the obturator canal to the adductor compartment of the thigh. In the pelvis it gives small branches to surrounding structures including a pubic branch which anastomoses with the corresponding branch of the inferior epigastric artery [p. 103] on the pelvic surface of the body of the pubis. This anastomosis may replace part or all of the obturator artery (**accessory obturator artery**) and may be accompanied by an abnormal obturator vein.

Floor

The **internal pudendal artery** descends anterior to piriformis and the sacral plexus, leaves the pelvis through the lowest part of the greater sciatic foramen and, passing over the posterior surface of the ischial spine, enters the perineum through the lesser sciatic foramen.

Branches to pelvic viscera

1. The **umbilical artery** passes antero-inferiorly between the bladder and the lateral wall of the pelvis. It gives two or three superior vesical branches to the bladder, ureter, and ductus deferens (sometimes) and, losing its lumen, runs from the anterior part of the pelvis through the extraperitoneal tissue of the anterior abdominal wall to the umbilicus as the lateral umbilical ligament. The umbilical vein does not accompany the artery but ascends from the umbilicus to the liver in the fetus and persists as the ligamentum teres of the liver after birth.

2. The **inferior vesical artery** (vaginal artery in the female) runs forwards to the base of the bladder, supplies its postero-inferior part, the seminal vesicle, and prostate, and sends the long, slender **artery of the ductus deferens** on that structure to the testis.

The **vaginal artery** supplies the vagina, the postero-inferior part of the bladder, and the pelvic part of the urethra.

3. The **uterine artery** [Fig. 250] may be separate or may arise from the vaginal, umbilical, or middle rectal arteries. It passes along the root of the broad ligament to the lateral vaginal fornix. Here it turns anterosuperiorly, *above the ureter*, to run a tortuous course along the lateral margin of the uterus. It supplies the superior part of the vagina, the uterus, and part of the uterine tube. It ends by anastomosing with the corresponding **ovarian artery** in the broad ligament.

In the base of the broad ligament, the uterine artery is surrounded by a condensation of connective tissue (the **transverse ligament of the cervix**) which helps to hold the cervix in position by attaching it to the lateral pelvic wall.

4. The **middle rectal artery** is a small branch which passes medially to the rectum. It supplies branches to the rectum and to the vagina or seminal vesicle and prostate, and anastomoses with the other rectal arteries.

Pelvic hernia

The branches of the internal iliac artery that leave the pelvis all pierce the pelvic fascia. These are points of relative weakness which occasionally permit the formation of herniae along the gluteal or obturator arteries.

Median sacral artery

This small vessel, originally the caudal part of the aorta, arises from the posterior surface of the aorta immediately above the bifurcation. It descends on the vertebral column, in the median plane, to end in a series of arteriovenous anastomoses in the cellular **coccygeal body**, on the front of the coccyx. It gives rise to the fifth lumbar arteries, sends twigs to the back of the rectum, and anastomoses with the lateral sacral arteries.

Veins of pelvis

[Figs. 248, 254]

The venous drainage of the pelvis is through the internal iliac veins, though blood also passes by the **superior rectal, median sacral**, and **ovarian veins**, and by the **internal vertebral venous plexus** which communicates through the pelvic sacral foramina.

The internal iliac vein is posterosuperior to the artery, and receives tributaries which correspond to its branches, except for the **umbilical** and **iliolumbar veins** which drain respectively into the liver and the common iliac vein. The superior gluteal vein is the largest tributary, except in pregnancy when the uterine veins greatly exceed it.

Pelvic venous plexuses

The veins of the pelvis form a number of important, intercommunicating plexuses which are difficult to dissect.

The **rectal venous plexuses** lie on the surface of the rectum and in its submucosa. They drain through the **superior, middle**, and **inferior rectal veins**, and hence form a route of communication between the portal and systemic venous systems. Thus blockage of the portal vein can lead to distention of these plexuses, though this most commonly occurs without portal obstruction. When distended to form haemorrhoids, the submucous plexus may cause prolapse of the rectal mucosa through the anus. Since the rectal plexuses communicate with the other pelvic plexuses, they may be distended whenever pelvic blood flow is increased, e.g. in pregnancy and, to a lesser degree, in menstruation.

In the male, the **vesical venous plexus** is principally found on the base of the bladder around the seminal vesicles, deferent ducts, and the ends of the ureters. It drains through the **inferior vescial veins** to the **internal iliac veins**, and also along the rectovesical fold to the anterior surface of the sacrum. Thence it may drain either through the pelvic sacral foramina with tributaries from the rectum to the **internal vertebral venous plexus**, or through the lateral sacral veins to the **internal iliac vein**. The size of the internal vertebral venous plexus is such that it can form an alternative route for all the blood in the inferior vena cava when this vein is obstructed.

The **prostatic venous plexus** lies on the front and sides of the prostate within its fascial sheath. It receives the deep dorsal vein of the penis, and drains into the vesical venous plexus.

In the female, the **vesical plexus** surrounds the pelvic part of the urethra and the neck of the bladder. It receives the dorsal vein of the clitoris, and drains into the vaginal plexuses. These lie on the sides of the vagina and in its mucosa. They communicate with the uterine and rectal plexuses, and drain mainly through the **vaginal veins**.

The **uterine plexuses** lie principally at the sides of the uterus between the layers of the broad ligament. They drain through the **uterine veins** accompanying the uterine arteries, but they also communicate through the broad ligament with the pampiniform plexus, and thus drain partly with the **ovarian veins**.

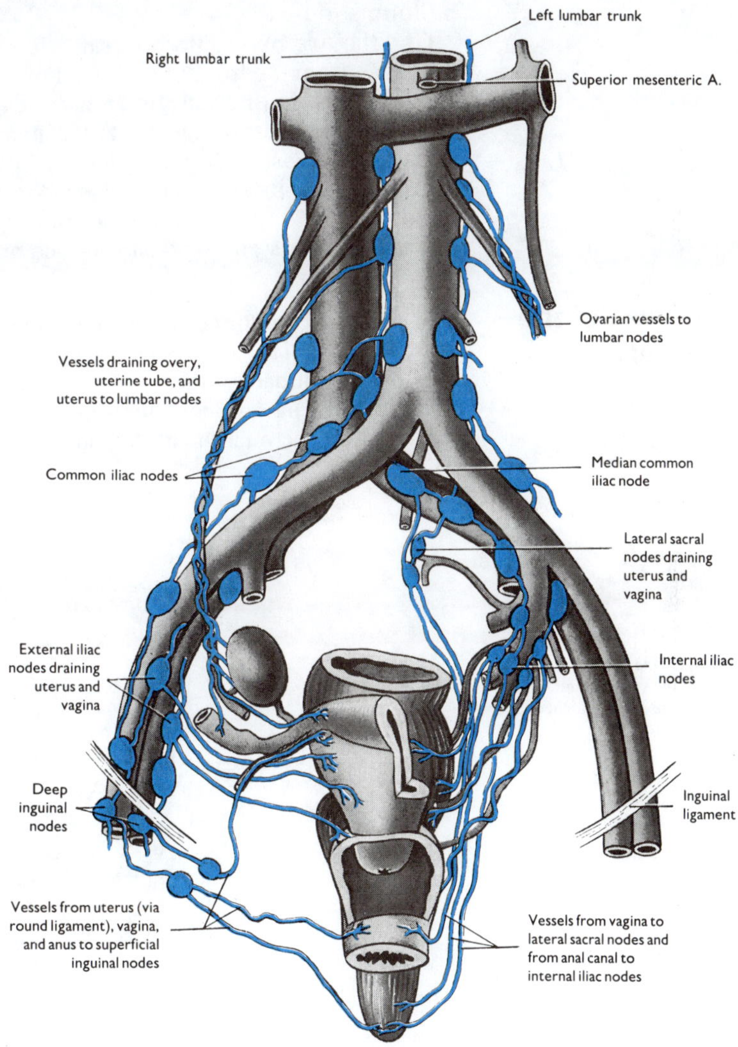

Fig. 255. A diagram of the lymph vessels and nodes of the female pelvis and abdomen.

Lymph nodes and vessels of pelvis
[Figs. 200, 255]

These are numerous and difficult to demonstrate especially in the aged.

The **external iliac nodes** [p. 178] not only drain lymph from the lower limb and abdominal wall, but also receive direct vessels from the bladder and prostate, or uterus.

The **internal iliac nodes** lie along the artery and its branches. They receive lymph from all the pelvic contents, and from the deeper structures in the perineum (internal pudendal), gluteal region, and back of the thigh (superior and inferior gluteal vessels). Like the external iliac nodes, they drain to the **common iliac nodes** [Fig. 289B].

The **sacral nodes** lie along the median and lateral sacral arteries. They drain the dorsal wall of the pelvis, and also the rectum, neck of the bladder, and prostate, or cervix of the uterus. They drain to the common iliac nodes.

In addition to these groups, small nodes lie in the broad ligament and in the fascial sheaths of the bladder and rectum.

Dissection

Find the sympathetic trunks as they enter the pelvis. Trace them to their termination in the **ganglion impar** on the coccyx. Note that the sacral splanchnic branches are small, and that the **grey rami communicantes** are the largest branches. One of these passes to each sacral ventral ramus as it emerges through the pelvic sacral foramen.

If the **superior hypogastric plexus** can be found anterior to the common iliac vessels, follow it to the **inferior hypogastric plexus** in the pelvis. Find the branches (**pelvic splanchnic nerves**) which pass to this plexus from the ventral rami of the second to fourth sacral nerves.

Expose the lumbosacral trunk and each of the five sacral ventral rami in turn. Follow them inferolaterally to the sacral plexus on the piriformis muscle.

Find the two nerves (to quadratus femoris and obturator internus) that arise from the front of the sacral plexus, and follow them till they leave the pelvis through the greater sciatic foramen. Lift the sacral plexus forwards and expose its terminal branches—the sciatic and pudendal nerves. Then find the branches that arise from the dorsal surface of the plexus (see below). Trace the **fourth sacral ventral ramus.** Part of it joins the fifth and the coccygeal nerve to form the coccygeal plexus on the pelvic surface of coccygeus.

The nerves of the lesser pelvis

Lumbosacral trunk

This is a thick cord formed from the entire ventral ramus of the fifth lumbar nerve [Fig. 289B] and the descending part of the fourth. It descends obliquely over the lateral part of the sacrum into the pelvis, posterior to the pelvic fascia. It then passes above the superior gluteal vessels across the pelvic surface of the sacro-iliac joint, to join the sacral ventral rami on the front of piriformis.

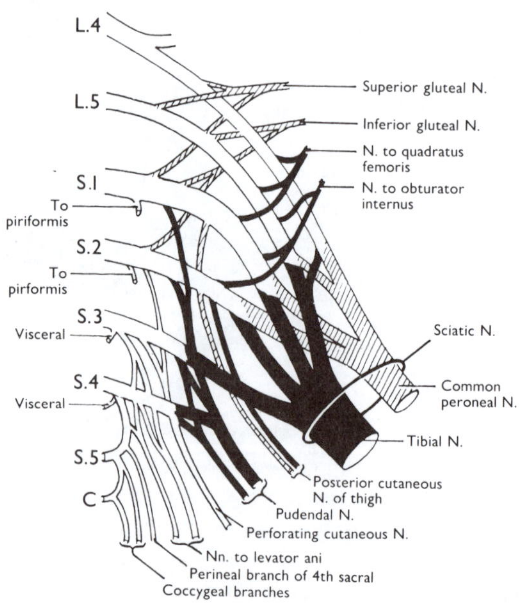

Fig. 256. A diagram of the sacral and coccygeal plexuses. Ventral divisions of the ventral rami, black; dorsal divisions, cross-hatched. See also Fig. 203.

Sacral and coccygeal ventral rami

The upper four sacral ventral rami emerge through the pelvic sacral foramina; the fifth and coccygeal pierce the sacrospinous ligament and coccygeus, respectively above and below the transverse process of the coccyx. The first and second sacral ventral rami are large, the remainder diminish rapidly in size from above downwards.

The lumbosacral trunk and the **first sacral ventral ramus** are separated by the superior gluteal vessels. Both cross the pelvic surface of the **sacro-iliac joint** before uniting on piriformis, so both may be involved in pathological changes in this joint. The first sacral ventral ramus is separated from the

second by the inferior gluteal vessels. All these ventral rami, together with the third and part of the fourth sacral, converge on the lower part of the greater sciatic foramen, between piriformis and the pelvic fascia, to form a solid, triangular mass of nerve fibres and connective tissue—**the sacral plexus**. This splits into a smaller, medial, **pudendal nerve** and a larger, lateral, **sciatic nerve**; other branches arise from the dorsal and pelvic surfaces of the plexus. The internal pudendal vessels descend over the front of the plexus, while the rectum overlaps the ventral rami from the third downwards. The inferior part of the fourth sacral ventral ramus descends to the coccygeal plexus on the surface of coccygeus.

Each ventral ramus receives a **grey ramus communicans** from the sympathetic trunk, and gives rise to certain branches before uniting in the plexus. (1) Twigs to piriformis from the first and second. (2) Irregular branches from the others to coccygeus and levator ani. (3) The **pelvic splanchnic nerves** are slender branches from the second and third, or third and fourth, sacral ventral rami to the inferior hypogastric plexus. They consist of **preganglionic parasympathetic nerve fibres** that are distributed to peripheral parasympathetic ganglia which innervate the pelvic viscera, the descending and sigmoid parts of the colon, and the external genitalia.

Terminal branches of the sacral plexus

The **sciatic nerve** (L. 4, 5; S. 1, 2, 3) forms on the front of piriformis, and leaves the pelvis through the lower part of the greater sciatic foramen. In the back of the thigh it divides into tibial and common peroneal nerves. Occasionally, when this division occurs in the pelvis, the common peroneal pierces piriformis as it leaves the pelvis: a circumstance which makes it possible to demonstrate the origin of the tibial nerve from ventral divisions of the ventral rami, and the common peroneal from their dorsal divisions (cf. femoral and obturator nerves).

The **pudendal nerve** (S. (1), 2, 3, 4) arises by separate branches from these ventral rami. It leaves the pelvis between piriformis and coccygeus, and hooks round the sacrospinous ligament to enter the perineum.

Nerves arising from pelvic surface of plexus

The **nerve to quadratus femoris** (L. 4, 5; S. 1) passes out of the pelvis anterior to the sciatic nerve.

The **nerve to obturator internus** (L. 5; S. 1, 2) leaves the pelvis between the sciatic and pudendal nerves and follows the latter into the ischiorectal fossa.

Nerves arising from dorsal surface of plexus

The **superior gluteal nerve** (L. 4, 5; S. 1) arises above piriformis and accompanies the superior gluteal vessels.

The **inferior gluteal nerve** (L. 5; S. 1, 2) and the **posterior cutaneous nerve of the thigh** (S. 1, 2, 3) arise partly by the same roots. They leave the pelvis either immediately posterior or medial to the sciatic nerve.

The **perforating cutaneous nerve** (S. 2, 3) descends on piriformis and coccygeus. It may then pierce coccygeus or pass between it and levator ani to reach and pierce the sacrotuberous ligament and gluteus maximus. It supplies gluteal skin.

The **perineal branch of the fourth sacral nerve** descends on coccygeus, pierces it, and appears in the posterior angle of the ischiorectal fossa at the side of the coccyx by passing deep to the sacrotuberous ligament. It runs on the perineal surface of levator ani to supply the external anal sphincter and the surrounding skin.

Coccygeal plexus
(S. 4, 5; Co.)

This minute plexus on the pelvic surface of coccygeus supplies that muscle and part of levator ani. It pierces coccygeus and supplies skin from the coccyx to the anus.

Obturator nerve
(L. 2, 3, 4)
[Figs. 204, 254]

This nerve is formed in the substance of psoas from the ventral divisions of the second to fourth lumbar ventral rami. It descends through psoas, emerges from its medial aspect deep to the common iliac vessels, and crosses the margin of the superior aperture of the lesser pelvis, lateral to the internal iliac vessels and the ureter. It then runs antero-inferiorly on obturator internus, in front of the obturator vessels, and leaves the pelvis through the obturator canal. In the lesser pelvis, it lies postero-lateral to the **ovary** (and may be involved in pathological changes in this organ), and is then crossed by the attachment of the broad ligament.

Autonomic nerves of pelvis

The sympathetic trunks

The trunks descend in the pelvis between the bodies of the sacral vertebrae and the pelvic sacral foramina, and unite in the median **ganglion impar** on the coccyx. They lie posterior to the pelvic fascia and to the peritoneum superiorly, and to the rectum below the third piece of the sacrum.

There are four sacral ganglia on each trunk and the common ganglion impar.

Branches

(1) Grey rami communicantes to all the sacral and coccygeal ventral rami. (2) Small branches to the median sacral artery. (3) **Sacral splanchnic nerves** to the inferior hypogastric plexus from the upper ganglia and to the rectum from the lower ganglia. (4) Twigs to the coccygeal body from the ganglion impar.

Inferior hypogastric plexuses [Fig. 202]

The **superior hypogastric plexus** descends into the pelvis, and divides into two inferior hypogastric (pelvic) plexuses. Each of these surrounds the corresponding internal iliac artery, and receives small branches from the upper sacral ganglia of the sympathetic trunk. The main plexus divides into subsidiary plexuses along the branches of the internal iliac artery (principally its visceral branches). These plexuses communicate with each other and receive branches from the **pelvic splanchnic nerves**. Small ganglia are found in these plexuses and their extensions.

Visceral plexuses

These are extensions of the inferior hypogastric plexuses on the walls of the pelvic viscera. (1) The **rectal plexus** receives a contribution from the inferior mesenteric plexus, and sends ascending **parasympathetic fibres** into that plexus and along the wall of the large intestine to its sigmoid and descending parts. (2) The **vesical plexus** is continuous with that over the deferent ducts, seminal vesicles, and prostate. The **prostatic plexus** sends **cavernous nerves** along the membranous urethra to the penis. (3) The **uterine** and **vaginal plexuses** accompany the corresponding arteries. The vaginal plexus supplies the urethra and sends **cavernous nerves** to the bulbs of the vestibule and to the clitoris.

Muscles of the lesser pelvis

Dissection

Define the attachment of piriformis to the sacrum, and follow it to the greater sciatic foramen, or to the greater trochanter of the femur if the gluteal region has been dissected already. Identify the **ischial spine** [Fig. 208] and the fibres of coccygeus and levator ani that are attached to it [Fig. 259]. Turn the bladder, prostate (or uterus and vagina), and rectum medially, and expose the superior surface of **levator ani.** Take particular care posteriorly where the muscle is thin. Trace its fibres inferomedially to their insertion. With a finger in the ischiorectal fossa, determine the origin of the muscle from the ischial spine to the pelvic surface of the body of the pubis, across the fascia covering obturator internus. Identify the free, medial border of the muscle by removing the lateral attachment of the puboprostatic (pubovesical) ligament from the fascia covering levator ani.

Piriformis

This conical muscle passes inferolaterally from its origin on the pelvic surface of the sacrum [Fig. 257]. It enters the gluteal region through the greater sciatic foramen, below the sacro-iliac joint, and crosses the posterior surface of the hip joint to be inserted into the tip of the greater trochanter of the femur. **Nerve supply:** twigs from the ventral rami of the first and second sacral nerves. **Action:** it is one of the short muscles that help to stabilize the hip joint. It can act as a lateral rotator of the extended femur, or an abductor when it is flexed.

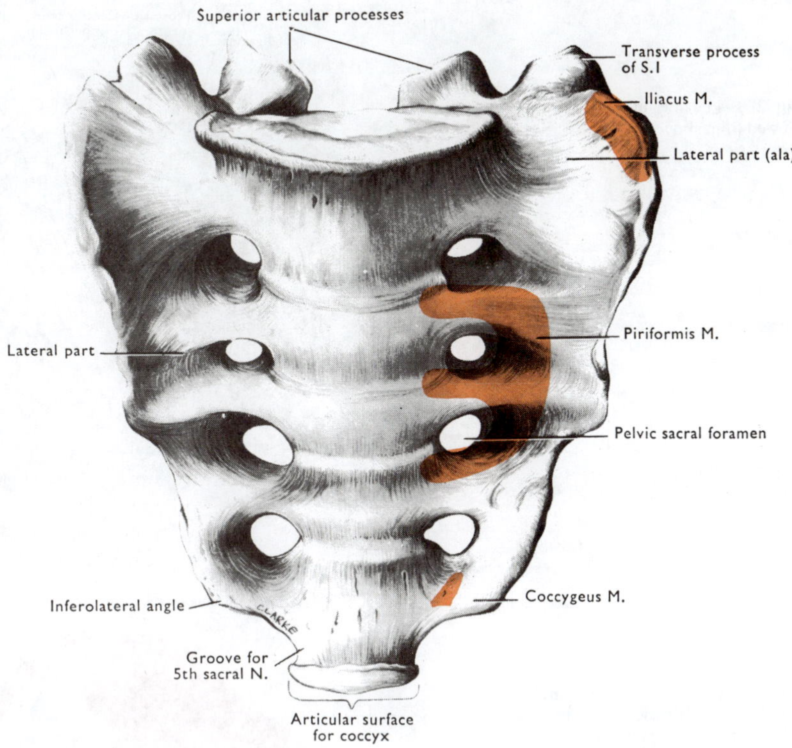

Fig. 257. The pelvic surface of the sacrum.

Coccygeus

This is the muscular anterior part of the sacrospinous ligament. It passes from the ischial spine to the lateral margins of the coccyx and the last piece of the sacrum. It is parallel to the inferior margin of piriformis (but is separated from it by the structures leaving the pelvis inferior to that muscle), and is edge to edge with the posterior border of levator ani. Thus it forms the lowest part of the posterior wall of the lesser pelvis and the posterior part of the muscular **pelvic diaphragm**, formed mainly by levator ani. In many mammals, coccygeus and levator ani are concerned mainly with movements of the tail. With the loss of this organ in man, coccygeus is virtually replaced by ligamentous tissue, and levator ani takes on the important role of supporting the pelvic floor in the erect posture. **Nerve supply:** the lower sacral ventral rami. **Action:** it may assist the sacrospinous ligament in supporting the pelvic contents. It can only produce minor movements of the coccyx.

Levator ani

[Figs. 221, 231, 232, 246, 248, 251]

These thin, curved sheets of muscle together form the gutter-like floor of the lesser pelvis, and separate it from the ischiorectal fossae.

Each muscle has a long, linear *origin* from the pelvic surface of the body of the pubis to the ischial spine. Between these two points, each arises from a **tendinous arch** (thickening) of the fascia covering obturator internus. The two muscles converge, and are *inserted* together into the central perineal tendon, the anal canal, the anococcygeal ligament, and the coccyx. The anterior fibres of both pass horizontally backwards below the prostate (**levator prostatae**) and bladder (or beside the vagina—**pubovaginalis**) to the central perineal tendon, separated by a gap which transmits the urethra (and vagina). The posterior fibres run inferomedially. Those that join the **anal canal** pass between the internal and external anal sphincters with the longitudinal smooth muscle layer to the perianal skin. Those that pass to the anococcygeal ligament and coccyx lie inferior to the terminal part of the rectum and support it.

The **puborectalis part** of the muscle arises from the pubis and passes posteriorly inferior to the other fibres. It loops round the side and posterior surface of the anorectal junction, and fusing with the corresponding fibres of the opposite muscle, forms a U-shaped sling on the junction.

Nerve supply: the perineal surface receives fibres from the inferior rectal

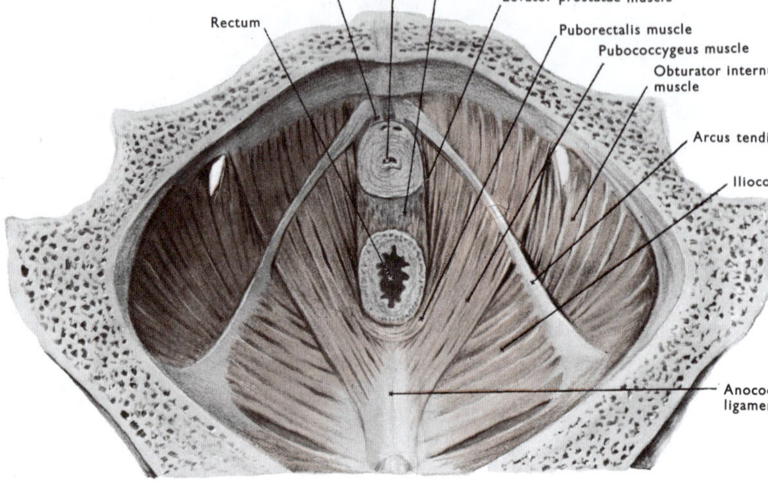

Fig. 258. Levator ani muscles viewed from above.

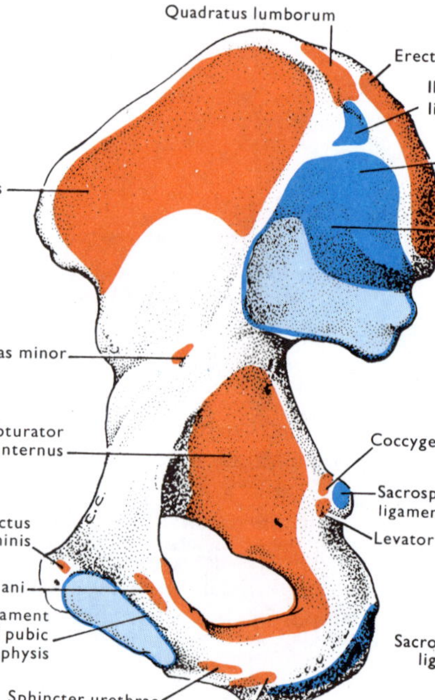

Fig. 259. The medial aspect of the right hip bone. Muscle attachments, red; ligamentous attachments, blue.

nerve, the pelvic surface from the ventral rami of the lower sacral and coccygeal nerves.

Actions: the two levator ani muscles act together to raise the pelvic diaphragm. This assists the muscles of the abdominal wall to compress the abdominal contents, e.g. in forced expiration, coughing, vomiting, urination, and in fixing the trunk for strong movements of the upper limbs. The fibres that are inserted into the central perineal tendon support the prostate or the posterior wall of the vagina, and together with the bulbospongiosus muscles act as an incomplete **sphincter of the vagina**. The fibres that are inserted into the anal canal and central perineal tendon pull the canal over the descending mass of faeces. The **puborectalis** pulls the anorectal junction forwards. This increases the angle between the rectum and the anal canal and prevents the passage of faeces from the rectum into the canal. *In childbirth*, the whole muscle supports the head of the fetus during dilatation of the cervix, and the anterior part may be torn as the head passes through the vagina, thus reducing the support of the posterior vaginal wall unless the tear is repaired.

Dissection

When the levator ani muscles have been fully dissected, separate them from their origins to expose the obturator fascia. Remove the fascia from obturator internus, and identify the pudendal canal and its contents in the lower part of the fascia, above the attachment of the sacrotuberous ligament. Expose this attachment, and follow the fibres of obturator internus to the lesser sciatic notch. Lift its tendon from the notch, and identify the bursa between it and the bone.

Obturator internus [Fig. 291]

This thick, fan-shaped muscle covers most of the side wall of the lesser pelvis. It arises from the obturator membrane, the margins of the obturator foramen (except at the obturator sulcus), and a wide area between the obturator foramen and the greater sciatic notch [Fig. 259] medial to the acetabulum. The fibres converge postero-inferiorly on a strong tendon which hooks round the lesser sciatic notch, and runs laterally over the posterior surface of the hip joint to the medial aspect of the greater trochanter. In the last part of its course it is accompanied by the **gemelli**. **Nerve supply:** a special nerve from the sacral plexus [p. 237]. **Action:** it helps to stabilize the hip joint and acts as a lateral rotator of the femur in the erect position, but abducts it when the hip joint is flexed.

Obturator fascia

This is the dense layer of fascia covering the pelvic surface of obturator internus. It fuses with the periosteum at the margins of the muscle except: (1) at the obturator sulcus where it turns over the anterior surface of the muscle to form the floor of the obturator canal for the obturator vessels and nerve; (2) postero-inferiorly where it unites with the falciform process of the sacrotuberous ligament [Fig. 262].

Most of the levator ani muscle arises from the thickened **tendinous arch** of this fascia between the body of the pubis and the ischial spine. Inferior to this, the fascia forms the lateral wall of the ischiorectal fossa, and splits to form the pudendal canal medial to the ischial tuberosity.

The joints of the pelvis

The sacrum, coccyx, and hip bones make up the pelvis. The five pieces of the sacrum are fused together and are joined to the coccyx by the **sacrococcygeal joint** [p. 242]. The sacrum lies posterosuperiorly between the two hip bones. On each side, the lateral part of the sacrum articulates with the ilium at a **sacro-iliac joint**. These synovial joints are maintained by strong **interosseous** and **dorsal sacro-iliac ligaments**, but the sacrum and coccyx are also held in position relative to the hip bones by the **sacrotuberous** [p. 190] and **sacrospinous** [p. 190] **ligaments** [Fig. 261]. Anteriorly the hip bones are united in the **pubic symphysis** [p. 215]. Superiorly the sacrum is joined to the remainder of the vertebral column by the **lumbosacral joints**, supported by the iliolumbar ligaments.

Dissection

The iliolumbar and dorsal sacro-iliac ligaments have already been partly exposed [p. 190]. Complete the exposure of these structures by removing any remnants of the thoracolumbar fascia and the erector spinae muscles from the dorsal surface of the sacrum and fifth lumbar vertebra. Identify the **ventral sacro-iliac ligament** on the pelvic surface of the sacro-iliac joint. If fusion between the lateral part of the sacrum and the ilium has not occurred, cut through the ligament and open the joint by bending the sacrum backwards against the ilium. Note the thinness of the ventral sacro-iliac ligament. The cartilage-covered joint surfaces are irregular and so closely fitted as to leave very little possibility of movement. Strip off the dorsal sacro-iliac ligaments to expose the interosseous sacro-iliac ligaments which lie deep to them. Divide the interosseous ligaments and separate the sacrum from the ilium. Examine the joint surfaces again.

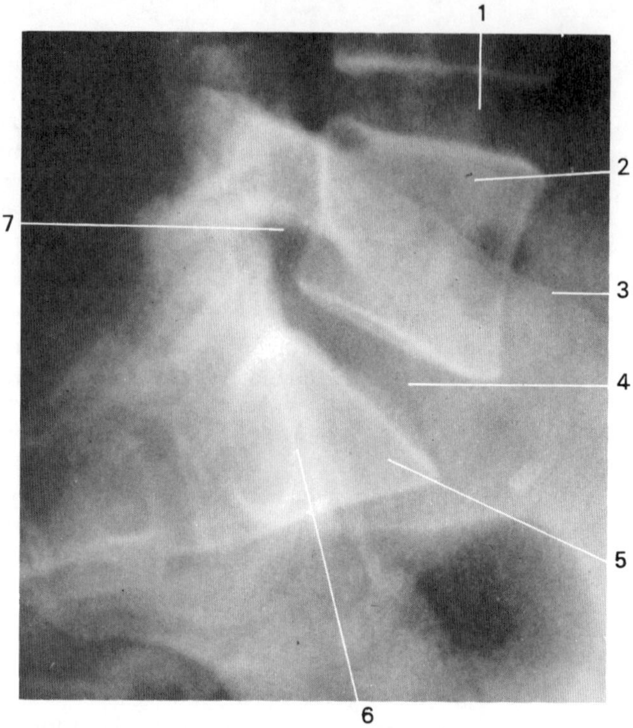

Fig. 260. Lateral radiograph of the lumbosacral region. Note wedge shape of lumbosacral intervertebral disc.
1. Intervertebral disc between 4th and 5th lumbar vertebra.
2. Body of 5th lumbar vertebra.
3. Iliac crest.
4. Lumbosacral intervertebral disc.
5. Body of 1st sacral vertebra.
6. Surfaces of lateral parts of sacrum overlapping first sacral vertebral body.
7. Intervertebral foramen for 5th lumbar nerve.

Lumbosacral joints

These joints are similar to those between the lumbar vertebrae [p. 79] but the lumbosacral **intervertebral disc** is more wedge-shaped than the others to take up the considerable angulation between the adjacent surfaces of the fifth lumbar vertebra and the sacrum [Figs. 90, 260]. The *stability* of this articulation is increased by: (1) the widely spaced articular processes; (2) the strong *iliolumbar ligaments* [p. 190; Fig. 310].

This articulation has a number of variations which may give rise to symptoms. The fifth lumbar vertebra or its transverse processes may be fused on one or both sides with the sacrum (*sacralization*), or the transverse process may articulate with the lateral part of the sacrum. The first sacral vertebra may be partly or completely separated from the remainder of the sacrum (*lumbarization*). The normal **sacral hiatus** may extend superiorly into the upper part of the sacrum or lumbar region (*spina bifida*), thus weakening the neural arch of the fifth lumbar vertebra. Rarely, the spine, laminae, and inferior articular processes of the fifth lumbar vertebra are separate from the remainder of the vertebra. This condition allows the body of the fifth lumbar vertebra to slide forwards on the sloping superior surface of the sacrum (spondylolisthesis).

The sacrococcygeal joint has a thin intervertebral disc and ligaments corresponding to the anterior and posterior longitudinal ligaments of the other intervertebral joints. The sacral and coccygeal cornua and transverse processes are also linked by ligaments which may ossify. Coccygeal joints are present in young subjects, but they ossify early.

Sacro-iliac joint

This very strong synovial joint is responsible for transmitting the weight of the body to the hip bones, and consequently has little movement. The sacrum is wedged between the iliac bones so that the cartilage on the uneven **auricular surfaces** of both bones is firmly coapted and held in position by powerful **interosseous** and **dorsal sacro-iliac ligaments**.

The weight of the body tends to drive the base of the sacrum downwards between the hip bones, thus tightening the sacro-iliac ligaments and drawing the articular surfaces close together. The same force tends to tilt the apex of the sacrum upwards, moving the sacrum around a horizontal, transverse axis, for which the auricular areas form a segment of the circumference. This tilting is resisted by the sacrotuberous and sacrospinous ligaments [p. 190] acting as shock absorbers.

The **ventral sacro-iliac ligament** is a thin ribbon of transverse fibres

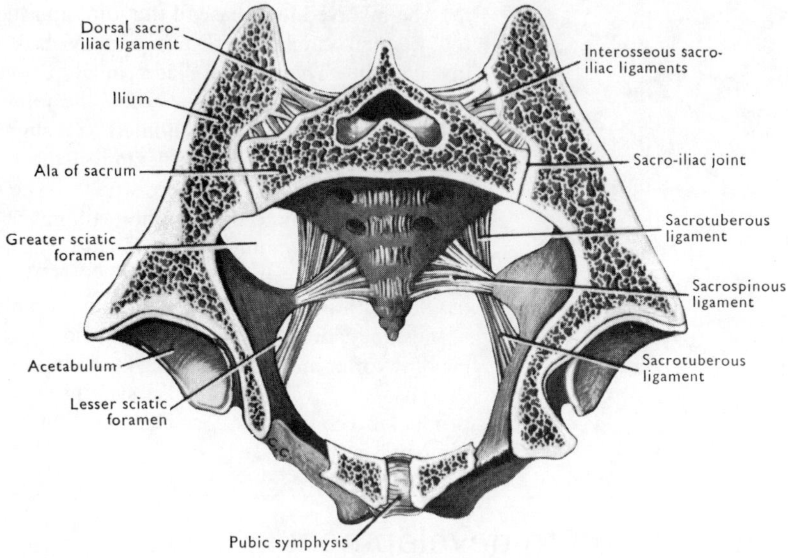

Fig. 261. An oblique section through the lesser pelvis to show the ligaments and sacro-iliac joints.

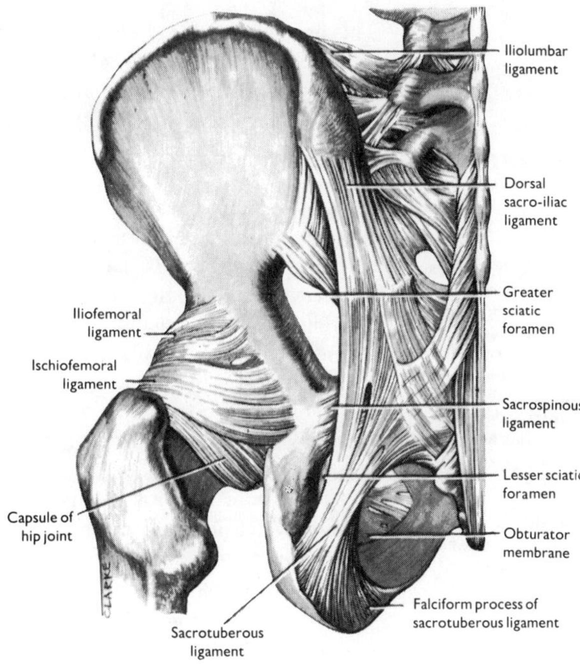

Fig. 262. Dorsal view of the pelvic ligaments and the hip joint.

between the convex margins of the articular surfaces. It does little more than close the abdominopelvic surface of the joint.

The interosseous sacro-iliac ligaments are very strong. They unite the wide, rough areas that adjoin the concave margins of the auricular surfaces [Figs. 302, 308, 309], and close the sacro-iliac joints dorsally.

The dorsal sacro-iliac ligaments are immediately superficial to the interosseous ligaments and are fused with them. They consist of: (1) short transverse fibres that pass from the ilium to the first and second tubercles of the lateral crest of the sacrum; (2) a longer, more vertical band from the posterior superior iliac spine to the third and fourth tubercles, which blends with the medial edge of the sacro-tuberous ligament.

Posteriorly the joint is covered by the erector spinae and gluteus maximus muscles. The skin dimple marking the position of the posterior superior iliac spine lies at the level of the middle of the joint, while the posterior inferior spine marks the posterior and most superficial part of the joint.

The abdominal surface of the joint is covered by psoas and iliacus, with the **obturator** and **femoral nerves** close to it. The pelvic surface is crossed by the **lumbosacral trunk** and the **first sacral ventral ramus**. Any of these nerves may be involved in disease of the joint and thereby give rise to pain which is felt in their cutaneous distribution [Vol. 1, Fig. 218], not at the site of involvement. The internal iliac vein and the superior gluteal vessels are also in contact with the pelvic surface of the joint.

Movement at the joint is limited to a slight rotation around a horizontal axis towards the end of full flexion of the trunk on the hip joints, e.g. in touching the toes with the knees straight. The main function is to prevent the direct transmission to the vertebral column of forces suddenly applied to the feet, e.g. when landing from a height. The resilience of the sacrotuberous ligament cushions the shock [Fig. 99 (C)]. The joint may become partly ossified with increasing age, especially in males.

In some animals, and possibly also in man, the sacro-iliac ligaments become softer and more yielding in the later stages of pregnancy. They share this property with the pubic symphysis and sacrococcygeal ligaments, producing a combined effect which facilitates the passage of the fetus through the pelvis at term.

Introduction to development

This brief section is not intended to cover all aspects of development but is designed as an introduction to those parts which help with an understanding of the arrangement of body structures and of those areas where development is essential to the appreciation of structural defects which are of profound clinical importance.

The early human embryo

The early embryo consists of a double-layered disc formed by the apposition of two fluid-filled, epithelial sacs [Fig. 263 (A)] (the **amnion** formed by ectoderm and the **yolk sac** formed by entoderm) surrounded by a layer of cells (**extra-embryonic mesoderm**) and suspended within a larger sac (the **chorion**) by a rod of extra-embryonic mesoderm (**connecting stalk**) which connects the amnion/yolk sac complex from the future tail end of the embryo to the internal surface of the chorion formed by a separate layer of extra-embryonic mesoderm. This lines the epithelial surface of the chorion (**trophoblast**) and forms the chorion with it. The space between the amnion/yolk sac complex and the chorion is the extra-embryonic coelom.

As the embryo grows it bulges away from the margin of the disc into the amnion which forms a water bath in which the embryo can float and which enlarges with the embryo to fill the entire chorion [Fig. 263 (B)]. Ventrally the amnion forms the covering of the **umbilical cord** by wrapping together the connecting stalk, the part of the yolk sac which is not taken into the embryo, and a diverticulum of the yolk sac (**allantois**) which protrudes into the connecting stalk. This growth process relegates the original margin of the embryonic disc to the ventral surface of the embryo where it forms the edge of the umbilical orifice with the umbilical cord attached to it [Fig. 263 (B)]. It also results in the extra-embryonic coelom being obliterated except in the umbilical cord close to its attachment to the embryo.

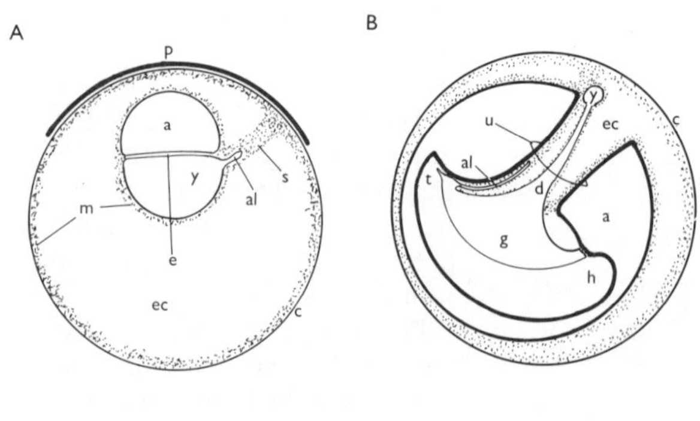

Fig. 263. Diagrams of two stages in the early development of the human embryo to show how the embryonic disc in (A) bulges up into the expanding amniotic cavity (B) thus forming the umbilical cord on its ventral aspect. In this early stage the amnion expands more rapidly than the chorion and so obliterates the space (extra-embryonic coelom) which initially separates the amnion/yolk sac complex from the chorion except in the umbilical cord where it persists long enough to permit the development of the midgut loop [Fig. 136] within the base of the cord until there is room in the abdomen for it to return. This happens when the relative size of the liver decreases as its importance as a blood-forming organ diminishes with the formation of bone marrow (8–10 weeks of intra-uterine life).
a. Amniotic cavity.
al. Allantois.
c. Chorion.
d. Duct (vitello-intestinal) connecting the intra-embryonic and extra-embryonic parts of the yolk sac.
e. Embryonic disc.
ec. Extra-embryonic coelom.
g. Gut tube (intra-embryonic yolk sac).
h. Head of embryo.
m. Extra-embryonic mesoderm.
p. Final placental site.
s. Connecting stalk.
t. Tail of embryo.
u. Umbilical cord.
y. Yolk sac.
For details of the intra-embryonic changes during this procedure see Fig. 266.

Implantation and placenta

By the stage of development shown in Fig. 263 (A) the trophoblast has come into contact with the lining of the uterus (endometrium) and has digested it in such a way that the entire chorion and its contents (chorionic vesicle, all of which developed from the fertilized ovum) are buried in the endometrium which closes over and separates it from the uterine cavity. The digestion of the endometrium includes the vessels adjacent to the chorionic vesicle which is, therefore, bathed in maternal blood and forms a diffusion membrane through which material can be absorbed into and excreted from the chorionic vesicle. At first the entire surface of the chorionic vesicle forms this diffusion membrane and increases its area of contact with maternal blood by the outgrowth of branched **chorionic villi**. However, as the chorionic vesicle increases in size and bulges towards the uterine cavity, the endometrium on this surface thins, loses its large blood supply, and can no longer support an active diffusion membrane. As a result, the area concerned with this process becomes reduced to that facing the highly vascular endometrium between the chorionic vesicle and the uterine muscle from which blood vessels enter the endometrium. Thus the diffusion area forms a discoid placenta [Fig. 263] on the embryonic pole of the chorionic vesicle. The **placenta** consists of masses of closely packed chorionic villi suspended in a lake of circulating maternal blood with some villi anchoring the chorion to the intact, deeper layers of the endometrium which separate it from the uterine muscle. The remainder of the chorion loses its villi and becomes smooth.

The **trophoblast** cells also function as an endocrine gland. They produce many substances including **gonadotrophins** which first maintain the corpus luteum of the ovary and later replace its functions in preventing the onset of menstruation which would otherwise lead to the abortion of the chorionic vesicle.

The chorionic layer of the extra-embryonic mesoderm rapidly forms blood vessels which link up with those being formed in the embryo (see below) so that an early circulation of embryonic blood in the chorionic villi is established. This **circulation** from the embryo remains entirely separate from the maternal circulation through the placenta and acts as a transport mechanism between the embryo and the chorion. Leakage of embryonic or fetal blood cells into the maternal circulation is an accident which causes the production by the mother of antibodies to the fetal cells which can lead to

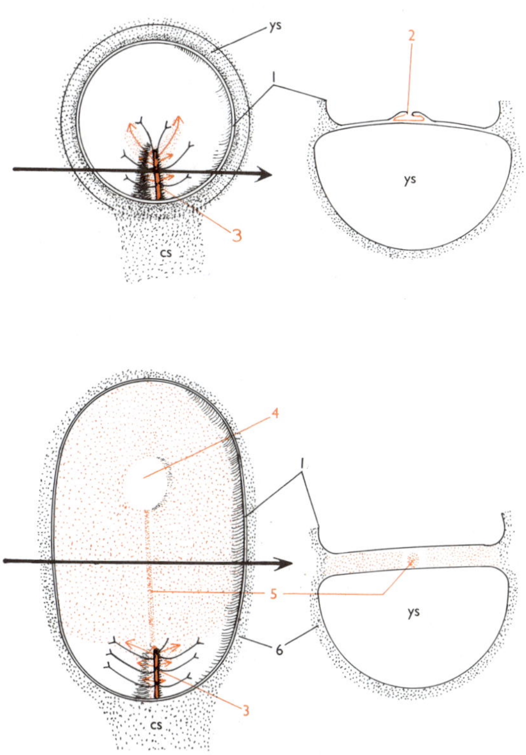

Fig. 264. Diagrammatic surface views (left) and transverse sections (right, at the levels of the large arrows) of two stages in the development of the embryonic disc to show the formation of the intra-embryonic mesoderm (red). The small, black/red arrows show the direction of movement of the ectoderm through the primitive streak to extend between the ectoderm and the entoderm as mesoderm. As the embryonic disc grows in length away from the primitive streak, the mesoderm tucked forwards from the primitive streak in the midline forms the notochord. In the surface views, the ectoderm is shown as transparent.
1. Cut edge of amnion.
2. Ectoderm becoming mesoderm at primitive streak.
3. Primitive streak.
4. Buccopharyngeal membrane, ectoderm and entoderm only.
5. Notochord.
6. Extra-embryonic mesoderm.
cs. Connecting stalk.
ys. Yolk sac.

their destruction and the death of the fetus when such antibodies cross the placenta into the fetal circulation.

The early establishment of the embryonic circulation is essential if growth is to take place. This is achieved by formation of mesoderm within the embryonic disc by a linear infolding of the ectoderm towards the entoderm at the caudal end of the disc [Fig. 264] as a median groove (**primitive streak**). Here the ectodermal layer moves downwards towards the entoderm and spreads outwards separating the ectoderm and entoderm except at the **buccopharyngeal membrane** (future oral orifice) [Fig. 264] and later at the **cloacal membrane** (future anal and urogenital orifices) which is formed in exactly the same way as the buccopharyngeal membrane by the last of the meosderm to be produced growing caudally around each side of the membrane (where ectoderm and entoderm are left in contact) and meeting beyond it.

The **intra-embryonic mesoderm** so formed is basically in two layers because of the infolding of the expanding ectodermal layer. Towards the edge of the disc the two layers separate, one attached to the ectoderm (body wall) the other to the roof of the yolk sac [Figs. 265, 266 (A)]. The space between these layers is the **intra-embryonic coelom** which will become the pericardial, pleural, and peritoneal cavities. Laterally this cavity breaks through into the extra-embryonic coelom but anteriorly, where the two halves of the intra-embryonic coelom meet in front of the buccopharyngeal membrane, the peripheral mesoderm forms a solid bar (**septum transversum**) separating this part of the coelom (later pericardial cavity) from the extra-embryonic coelom and uniting ectoderm and entoderm. Thus the intra-embryonic coelom forms a U-tube [Fig. 265, arrow].

Embryonic vessels

Embryonic vessels are formed from **blood islands**. These proliferating clumps of cells appear in the mesoderm of the chorion, connecting stalk, and yolk sac. As the clumps grow, the outer cells become flattened to form an endothelial layer and the inner cells, separating from each other, form primitive blood cells. Coalescence of these islands leads to the formation of an interconnected mesh of capillary vessels and, in the embryonic disc, the production of two longitudinal vessels extending from the septum transversum to the connecting stalk in the mesoderm of the yolk sac [Fig. 265]. Where they lie inferior to the transverse limb of the coelomic tube [Fig. 265] they develop contractile elements in their walls which milk the contained blood caudally by serial contraction—low-pressure, simple peristaltic pumps, the **heart tubes**. Caudal to this the longitudinal vessels communicate with the

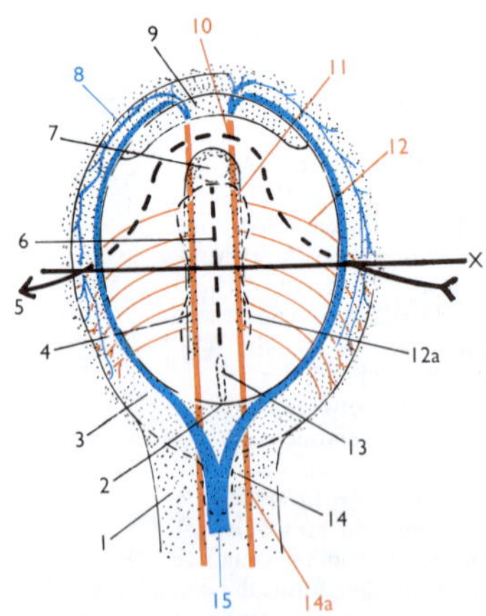

Fig. 265. A diagrammatic surface view of the embryonic disc with the amnion cut away and the ectoderm shown as though transparent. Mesoderm, black dots except where it is separated into two layers to enclose the intra-embryonic coelom and where the somite mesoderm lies, clear. Red, heart tube and arteries. Blue, veins.

1. Connecting stalk.
2. Cut edge of amnion.
3. Extra-embryonic mesoderm on yolk sac.
4. Intermediate mesoderm.
5. Head of arrow passing through intra-embryonic coelom.
6. Notochord.
7. Buccopharyngeal membrane.
8. Vitelline vein.
9. Septum transversum.
10. Heart tube.
11. Aorta.
12. Vitelline artery.

12a. Edge of neural plate.

13. Primitive streak.
14. Allantois.

14a. Umbilical artery.

15. Umbilical vein.

X. Plane of section shown in Fig. 266 (A).

yolk sac and chorionic plexuses and these communications become the **vitelline** (yolk sac) and **umbilical** (chorionic or allantoic) **arteries**—as yet only simple endothelial tubes. Blood entering the vitelline plexuses flows forwards to join the heart tubes at the septum transversum (**vitelline veins** [Fig. 265]) and that in the chorionic plexus returns along the connecting stalk as an umbilical vein which splits at the caudal extremity of the disc into right and left **umbilical veins** skirting the disc in the mesoderm of the body wall and separated from the vitelline vessels by the continuity of the intra-embryonic and extra-embryonic coeloms [Fig. 266 (A)]. At the septum transversum they communicate with the vitelline veins and together enter the cranial end of each heart tube. Considerably later, as the body wall mesoderm develops, a plexus is formed in it which communicates with the longitudinal arteries **(aortae)** leading from the heart tubes and forms a third circulation. This drains through the **cardinal veins** to enter the venous end of the heart through the septum transversum which forms a link between the body wall, vitelline, and umbilical systems of veins [Fig. 268].

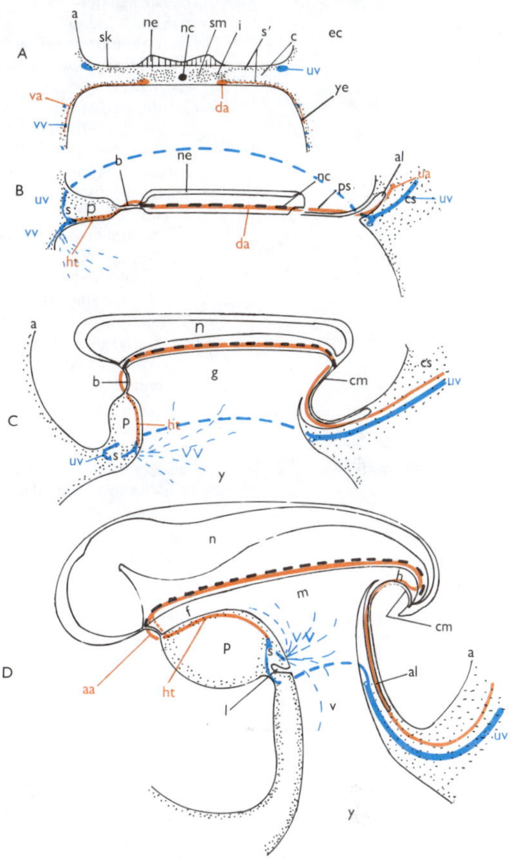

Fig. 266. (A) Diagrammatic transverse section of the embryo shown in Fig. 265 along the line X in Fig. 265.
(B) Median section (diagrammatic, longitudinal) of the embryo shown in Fig. 265. The blood vessels which lie on one side of the median plane are projected on to it to show their positions.
(C and D) Diagrammatic median development of the embryo to show the change in position of its parts when it bulges into the amniotic cavity. Both are shown in the same way as (B).
a. Amnion.
aa. First pharyngeal arch artery. The broken line caudal to this represents the developing second pharyngeal arch artery.
al. Allantois—diverticulum of yolk sac
b. Buccopharyngeal membrane.
c. Intra-embryonic coelom continuous laterally with extra-embryonic coelom.
cm. Cloacal membrane.
cs. Connecting stalk.
da. Aorta. Part which becomes dorsal aorta in (D).
ec. Extra-embryonic coelom.
f. Foregut tube.
g. Intra-embryonic part of yolk sac.
h. Hindgut.
ht. Heart tube.
i. Intermediate mesoderm.
l. Liver outgrowth from caudal end of foregut.
m. Midgut.
n. Neural tube—central nervous system.
nc. Notochord.
ne. Neural plate—neural ectoderm.
p. Pericardial part of coelom—pericardial cavity.
ps. Primitive streak.
s. Septum transversum.
s'. split, lateral mesoderm.
sk. Skin ectoderm.
sm. Somite mesoderm.
ua. Umbilical artery.
uv. Umbilical vein.
v. Vitello-intestinal duct.
va. Vitelline (yolk sac) artery.
vv. Vitelline veins.
y. Yolk sac.
ye. Yolk sac entoderm.

Reversal of embryo

As the embryo bulges into the amniotic cavity (see above) the head (which arises caudal to the buccopharyngeal membrane) and the tail (which arises cranial to the cloacal membrane) grow respectively forwards and backwards away from the margin of the embryonic disc so that the extreme anterior and posterior parts of the disc are turned on to the ventral aspect of the embryo and their directions reversed [Fig. 266]. Thus the septum transversum comes to lie caudal to the pericardial cavity and the veins enter the caudal ends of the heart tubes from it. The originally straight, longitudinal vessels (aortae) of the embryo are now bent on themselves as they lie beside the buccopharyngeal and cloacal membranes forming **arch arteries** at the sides of these membranes. The heart tubes now run cranially dorsal to the pericardial cavity on the part of the yolk sac which has been drawn cranially by the forward growth of the head to produce the **foregut** tube [Fig. 266]. During this process, a median thickening of the ectoderm overlying the notochord and the unsplit mesoderm has formed the **neural ectoderm** or **plate** [Figs. 266, 267] which therefore extends from the buccopharyngeal to the cloacal membrane. Near the middle of the embryo (future cervical region) the edges of the neural plate fold dorsally on the midline of the plate and, approaching each other, fuse to turn the plate into a **neural tube** [Fig. 267]. At the same time, the skin ectoderm, with which the neural plate is continuous, fuses with its fellow and separates the neural tube from the surface. The cells which lie at the junction of skin and neural ectoderms remain as a **neural crest** dorsal to the neural tube. This process of closure extends headwards and tailwards, the last parts of the tube to close being close to the buccopharyngeal and cloacal membranes.

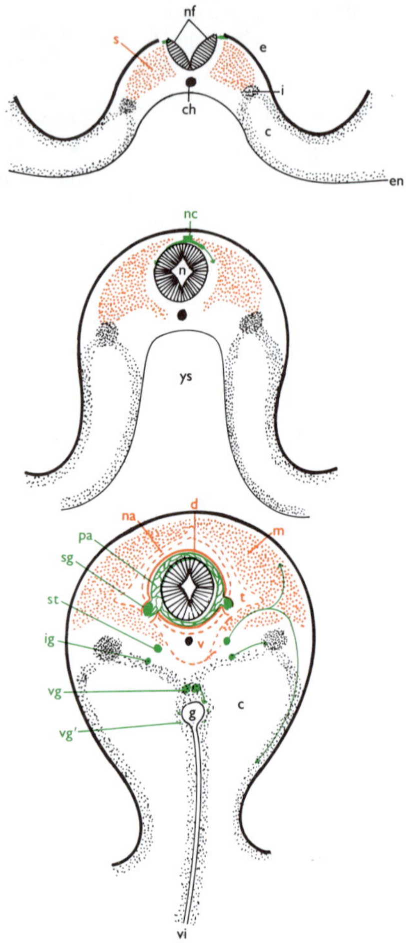

Fig. 267. Diagrams of transverse sections through three embryos at different stages of development to show the closure of the neural tube, the formation of the neural crest and some of its derivatives (green), and the somites and their main derivatives (red).
c. Intra-embryonic coelom.
ch. Notochord.
d. Dura mater.
e. Skin ectoderm.
en. entoderm—wall of yolk sac.
g. Gut tube—intra-embryonic entoderm.
i. Intermediate mesoderm.
ig. Sympathetic ganglion for intermediate mesoderm—also forms suprarenal medulla.
m. Long muscles of back.
n. Neural tube.
na. Neural arch of vertebra.
nc. Neural crest.
nf. Neural folds.
pa. Pia-arachnoid (leptomeninges).
s. Somite.
sg. Spinal ganglion (sensory cells).
st. Sympathetic trunk (body wall autonomic supply).
vg. Sympathetic ganglion for viscera.
vg'. Parasympathetic ganglion for viscera.
vi. Vitello-intestinal duct. Unites intra-embryonic and extra-embryonic parts of yolk sac and normally disappears.

As the neural plate folds posteriorly, the medial, unsplit mesoderm extends dorsally beside it and breaks up into a series of blocks (**somites**) lying in a row on each side of the neural tube. The somites extend dorsally between the skin and neural crest to separate them and ventrally to surround the notochord and the neural tube [Fig. 267]. The part of each somite nearest to the neural tube forms the dura mater; external to this it produces the vertebral column and the long muscles of the back in the spinal region [Fig. 267]. Part is also believed to form the dermis of the skin.

The migratory cells of the **neural crest** form a considerable number of structures including the **leptomeninges** (pia-arachnoid), cells of sensory and autonomic ganglia [Fig. 267], the suprarenal medulla, sheath cells of peripheral nerves, and the pigment-forming dendritic cells of the skin.

The heart and great vessels

As the embryo bulges into its amniotic cavity, the two heart tubes, now running cranially on the foregut tube from the septum transversum to the buccopharyngeal membrane, slide ventrally towards each other and, fusing, sink into the pericardial cavity carrying some of the foregut mesoderm as a dorsal mesentery [Fig. 268] which rapidly disappears leaving the single heart tube suspended across the pericardial cavity with full freedom of movement. This ventral displacement moves the vitelline veins and their confluence with the other veins (**sinus venosus**) from the gut tube into the septum transversum [Fig. 268] where the sinus forms the caudal extremity of the heart tube. At its cranial end the heart tube is continuous with a short arterial stem (**ventral aorta**) from which the right and left arch arteries pass around the sides of the buccopharyngeal membrane into the parts of the original aortae dorsal to the foregut tube—the **dorsal aortae**. Subsequently four other arteries are developed joining the ventral to the dorsal aortae caudal to the original arch artery [Fig. 268]. These pharyngeal (or branchial) arch arteries correspond to the gill arteries of the fish and like them are arteries of the foregut which lie in pharyngeal arches (Vol. 3) corresponding to the gill bars of the fish.

Fig. 268. Diagrammatic median section through the anterior end of an embryo at a later stage of development than that shown in Fig. 266 (D). As in that figure, the blood vessels are projected on to the median plane to show their relative positions. Arteries, umbilical vein, and heart contents—red. Vitelline and cardinal veins—blue. Entoderm—green. Inset, transverse section through heart tube.

1. Anterior cardinal vein.
2. Common cardinal vein.
3. Vitelline (superior mesenteric) artery.
4. Dorsal aorta.
5. Posterior cardinal vein.
6. Umbilical artery.
7. Umbilical vein.
8. Vitelline (portal) vein.
9. Liver outgrowth.
10. Liver in septum transversum.
11. Endothelium of heart.
12. Endocardial tissue.
13. Muscle of heart.

13a. Transitory dorsal mesentery of heart.

14. Ventral aorta dividing into pharyngeal arch arteries. The sixth sends a long descending pulmonary artery on the foregut tube.
15. Ectodermal mouth—stomodaeum.
16. Head of embryo.

a. atrium.
b. bulbus cordis.
s. sinus venosus.
v. ventricle.

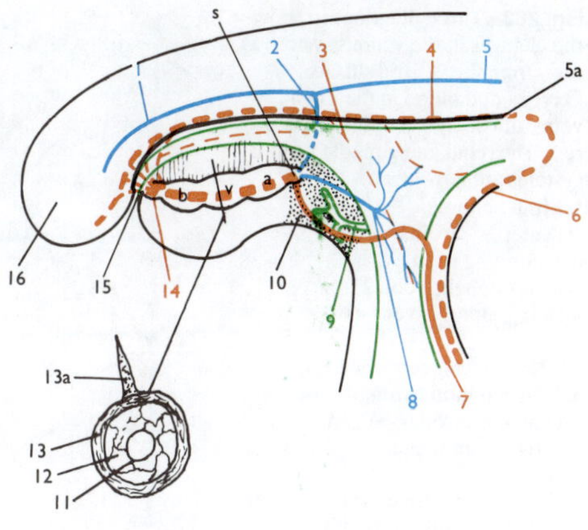

However, they do not break into gill capillaries though the most caudal of them (number 6, so-called because of a transitory vessel (No. 5) between it and the fourth) sends a long descending branch on the foregut to the lung bud developing dorsal to the septum transversum—the **pulmonary artery**. Subsequently, as the lung is carried cranially with the growing head, the lung root ascends into the concavity of the sixth arch artery so that the pulmonary artery becomes a short branch (see below).

A series of changes takes place in the veins, the heart, and the arteries at the same time but each is dealt with separately in this brief account. The changes lead to the development of the veins mainly on the right side and the arteries mainly on the left together with the division of the single heart tube into two parallel channels arranged in series, one concerned with the **pulmonary circulation**, the other with the **circulation (systemic)** to the body. However, the establishment of a functioning pulmonary circulation to replace the respiratory function of the placenta does not take place till after birth, hence certain temporary valvular and bypass arrangements are necessary to maintain the intra-uterine circulation while preparing for the sudden changes which have to take place at birth. These are the ductus venosus, the foramen ovale, and the ductus arteriosus (see below) all of which are temporary openings which close at birth to establish the postnatal circulation.

Veins

Fig. 269 shows three stages in the **development of the venous system** as seen from the ventral surface. The three separate venous systems, yolk sac or vitelline (gut tube or future portal venous system), umbilical or placental (temporary antenatal), and the body wall (systemic), each has its own symmetrical system of veins (vitelline, umbilical, cardinal) and all three drain into the sinus venosus at the septum transversum.

The first change [Fig. 269 (B)] is due to the outgrowth from the caudal end of the foregut of a liver diverticulum [Fig. 268]. This splits the vitelline and umbilical veins into the **liver sinusoids** in the septum transversum thus forming the portal and hepatic veins from part of the vitelline system. At the same time the right umbilical vein atrophies and the left develops a direct communication (**ductus venosus**) to the hepatic veins to form the most cranial part of a future inferior vena cava. The ductus ensures that the oxygenated placental blood reaches the heart without passing through the liver sinusoids particularly at a time when the liver is the main blood-forming organ—a function which seems to require low oxygen tension— before a significant amount of bone marrow has been produced by the ossification process starting about the eighth week of intra-uterine life.

Both posterior cardinal veins are replaced, except their most caudal parts (internal iliac veins), by a para-aortic, azygos venous system which receives the body wall veins. At first this system is symmetrical and drains into the common cardinal vein on each side. However, a ventral communication with the liver sinusoids on the right side at the level of the renal veins gives this system a direct communication to the hepatic veins. This becomes the main

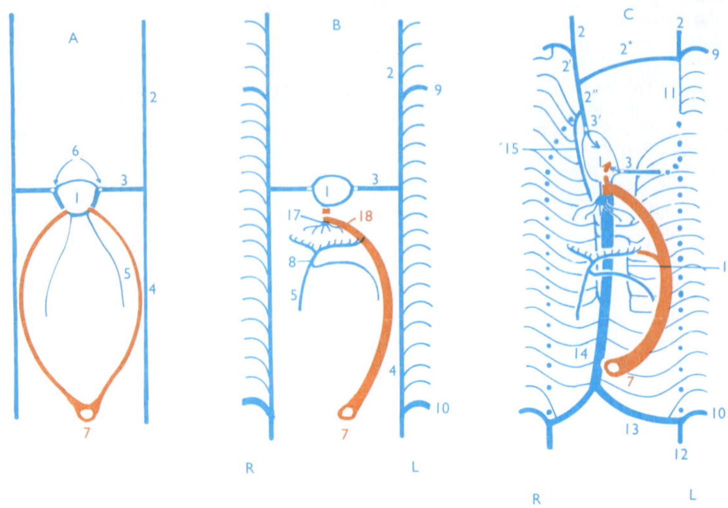

Fig. 269. Three diagrams to show the changes in the venous system as seen from the ventral surface. Oxygenated blood in the umbilical veins and ductus venosus is shown red. The renal and gonadal venous systems are not shown.
1. Sinus venosus.
2. Anterior cardinal vein (2′, part forming right brachiocephalic vein; 2″, part forming superior vena cava with 3′).
2*. Left brachiocephalic vein.
3. Left common cardinal vein (becoming coronary sinus).
3′. Right common cardinal vein.
4. Posterior cardinal vein.
5. Vitelline (yolk sac or gut) vein.
6. Positions where nodal tissues will develop and from which impulse for cardiac contraction arises, in C they have become the sino-atrial and atrioventricular nodes.
7. Umbilical vein.
8. Portal vein.
9. Subclavian vein.
10. External iliac vein.
11. Left superior intercostal vein.
12. Internal iliac vein.
13. Left common iliac vein.
14. Inferior vena cava.
15. Azygos vein.
16. Hemiazygos vein.
17. Hepatic veins.
18. Ductus venosus.

route of drainage for the caudal part of the body [Fig. 269 (C)]—the **inferior vena cava**—and takes over the system on the left by means of transverse anastomoses posterior to the aorta (left lumbar veins and the right part of the **left common iliac vein**) and by a single, large, transverse anastomosis anterior to the aorta where the inferior vena cava turns forwards towards the liver (right part of **left renal vein**). Cranial to this, a variable number of the same postaortic anastomoses carries blood from the left azygos system (hemiazygos) through the azygos vein to the right common cardinal vein so that the left azygos loses its drainage to the left common cardinal vein. The caudal part of the inferior vena cava and the midsection of the left renal vein (all that remains of a transitory **left inferior vena cava**) are parts of the azygos system. Hence they are continuous respectively with the caudal ends of the azygos and hemiazygos veins where the inferior vena cava turns forwards. At this level also each receives the gonadal veins—a symmetrical arrangement which appears asymmetrical.

Superior vena cava

Cranial to the heart a major ventral anastomosis (left brachiocephalic vein) develops between the left and right anterior cardinal veins at the level of the left subclavian vein. This drains the left anterior cardinal to the right. Consequently (a) the left anterior cardinal vein loses its connection with the left common cardinal vein; (b) its part caudal to the subclavian vein drains upwards as the left superior intercostal vein; and (c) the left common cardinal vein, now isolated from the cardinal system, remains in its original, transverse, atrioventricular (see below) position as the coronary sinus. On the other hand the right common cardinal vein is displaced cranially, brought into line with the right anterior cardinal vein, and moves its entry to the superior extremity of the right atrium as a result of the forward displacement of the anterior cardinal veins with the head and upper limbs. Hence it forms the caudal part of the vertical superior vena cava and the right nodal tissue (**sino-atrial node** [Fig. 269]), similarly displaced, lies at the entry of the superior vena cava removed from its atrioventricular position which the left node still retains at the entry of the coronary sinus (**atrioventricular node**).

As a result of these changes, the inferior vena cava (containing the oxygenated placental blood—ductus venosus) enters the right atrium from below while the superior vena cava (containing only deoxygenated blood) enters from above and on a more anterior plane [Fig. 60]—an essential element in the separation of the two streams. The inferior vena cava contains a large element of deoxygenated blood. Hence the embryo and fetus have poorer oxygenation of their arterial blood than in postnatal life—a situation partly mitigated by the higher concentration of red blood cells and the oxygen dissociation curve of fetal haemoglobin.

Heart

The straight heart tube, formed by the fusion of two separate tubes, extends across the pericardial cavity from the sinus venosus in the septum

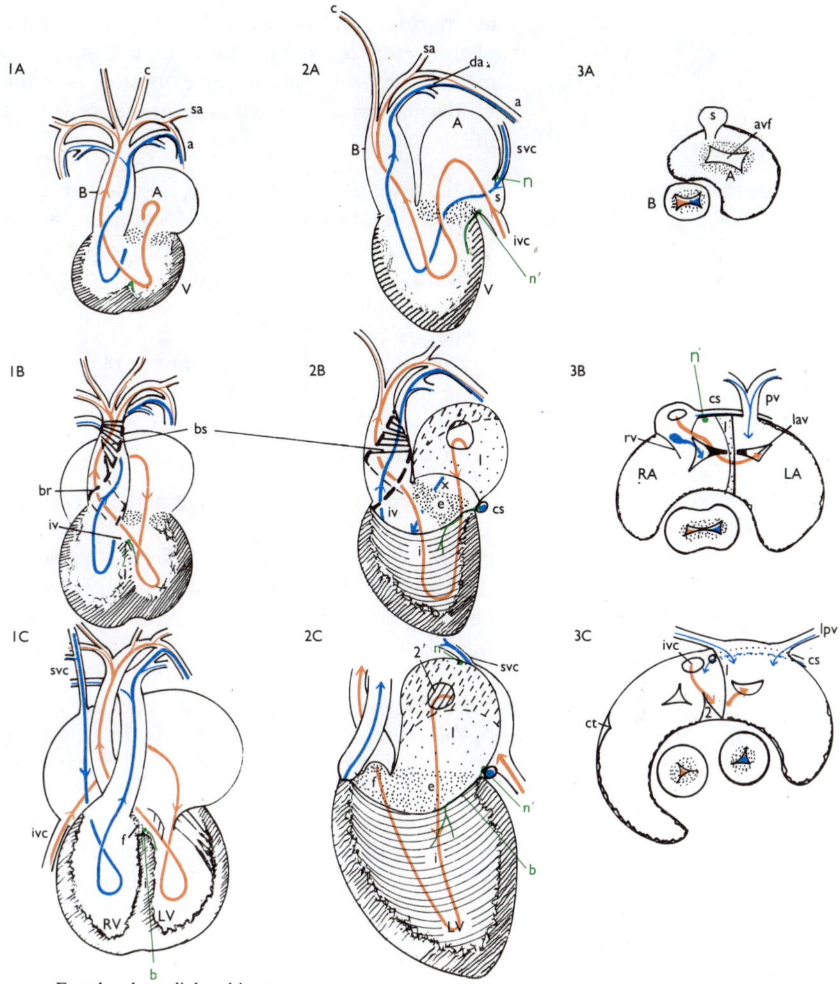

Fig. 270. Diagrams of three stages in the development of the heart to show its division into right and left channels and the establishment of the definitive intra-uterine circulation.
1. Anteroposterior views with ventricle coronally sectioned.
2. Views from the left with atrium and ventricle sagitally sectioned to the left of their septa in B and C.
3. Horizontal sections through the atrium and bulbus seen from above.
In 1B and 2B the interrupted lines in the bulbus indicate the positions of the major bulbar ridges which are shown fused internally in the upper bulbus. In 2B and 3B the endocardial cushions have fused separating the atrioventricular foramen into right and left parts, the septum primum has not yet closed the foramen primum (x) and a foramen secundum has appeared in its upper part (not visible in 3B though inferior vena caval blood is shown passing through it at a higher level). In 2B the position where the septum secundum will appear later is shown though it would not be present at this stage. It is seen through a transparent septum primum in 2B and 2C. For the arteries see Figs. 271 and 272. Red, direction of flow of inferior vena caval blood containing oxygenated blood from the placenta; blue, direction of flow of deoxygenated superior vena caval blood together with pulmonary and coronary sinus venous blood; green, positions of the nodal tissues, the atrioventricular bundle, and some of its branches.
A. Atrium.
B. Bulbus.
LA. Left atrium.
LV. Left ventricle.
RA. Right atrium.
RV. Right ventricle.
V. Ventricle.
a. Dorsal aorta.
avf. Atrioventricular foramen.
b. Atrioventricular bundle.
br. Major bulbar ridge.
bs. Bulbar septum forming.
c. Common carotid artery.
cs. Coronary sinus.
ct. Crista terminalis.
da. Ductus arteriosus.
e. Fused endocardial cushions.
f. Forward extension of fused endocardial cushions to meet bulbar septum and close interventricular foramen—membranous interventricular septum.
i. Muscular interventricular septum.
iv. Interventricular foramen.
ivc. Inferior vena cava.
lav. Left atrioventricular orifice.
lpv. Left pulmonary vein.
n. Right (sino-atrial) node.
n′. Left (atrioventricular) node.
pv. Pulmonary vein.
rv. Right venous valve.
s. Sinus venosus.
sa. Subclavian artery.
svc. Superior vena cava.
x. Foramen primum of atrium about to be closed by septum primum.
1. Septum primum of atrium.
2. Septum secundum of atrium.
2′. Septum secundum of atrium seen through foramen secundum in septum primum.

transversum to the ventral aorta close to the buccopharyngeal membrane. It is a simple endothelial tube surrounded by a layer of jelly-like **endocardial tissue** enclosed by a muscle layer [Fig. 268]. Contractions start at the sinus venosus (where the nodal tissue will later develop [Fig. 269]) and spread along the tube milking the contained blood into the ventral aorta. The endocardial tissue makes the muscle contraction effective and prevents the reflux of blood. Very shortly the tube develops three swellings [Fig. 268], atrium, ventricle, and bulbus cordis in that order, from the sinus venosus to the ventral aorta.

The heart tube begins to fold [Figs. 28–31, 270] by the loss of the dorsal wall of the ventricle and the ventral wall of the atrium. At the same time the sinus venosus moves into the pericardial cavity to lie in the atrioventricular sulcus with the transversely placed common cardinal veins because of the loss of the ventral wall of the atrium [Fig. 270 (2A)]. This brings the sinus into direct contact with both atrium and ventricle—an arrangement which would produce synchronous contraction of both if the sinus impulse were able to spread through the muscle. This is avoided by the development of a **fibrous**

atrioventricular (AV) ring which separates sinus and atrial muscle from that of the ventricle except where the left nodal tissue is developing as a delay mechanism and sending an extension into the ventricular muscle (**atrioventricular bundle**) which ensures the spread of the delayed sinus impulse to the ventricle.

Endocardial tissue

At the level of the AV fibrous ring there is considerable proliferation of the endocardial tissue to form endocardial cushions which project into the AV orifice and will form the AV valves. In the ventricle, the endocardial tissue is converted to muscle (which thickens its wall) and is directly continuous with the ventricular surface of the endocardial cushions. For bulbar endocardial tissue see below.

The folding of the heart is not in the sagittal plane but places the bulbus anteriorly and to the right with the atrium behind it and to the left [Fig. 270 (1A)] with the ventricular cavity running transversely between the atrioventricular and bulbar orifices.

Atrium

The atrium expands to the right and partly surrounds the bulbus carrying the sinus venosus with it so that the opening between them (which has a vertically placed valve with right and left flaps—the **venous valves** [Fig. 270 (3)]) lies to the right of the midline. Subsequently a single, median, pulmonary vein enters the dorsal surface of the atrium through the persisting venous part of the dorsal mesocardium lying between and to the left of the two venae cavae [Fig. 31]. As the atrium expands, the sinus venosus together with the pulmonary vein and its tributaries are absorbed into the right and left halves of the atrium respectively forming the smooth-walled, posterior parts of the atrium into which four separate pulmonary veins open to the left with the venae cavae and coronary sinus to the right. On the right, the smooth-walled area is limited by the remains of the right venous valve—the **crista terminalis**—and the valves of the inferior vena cava and coronary sinus. The left valve flap fuses with the interatrial septum.

Interatrial septum

The atrium is divided by the formation of a valvular septum which only permits the flow of blood from its right to left halves. The first part to form is the thin **septum primum** (I) which grows downwards from the posterosuperior wall of the atrium between the sinus venosus and the pulmonary vein towards the AV opening. As it approaches the AV orifice, (a) the anterior and posterior endocardial cushions fuse [Fig. 270 (3B)] and separate the orifice into right and left parts, (b) the septum breaks down in its superior part to form a new communication (**foramen secundum** (II)—**foramen I** being the original continuity) between the two halves of the atrium, and then (c) closes foramen I by uniting with the fused parts of the endocardial cushions. Considerably later a **second septum** (II) is formed. This grows downwards and backwards from the anterosuperior wall of the atrium to the right of septum I towards the inferior vena cava but does not reach the endocardial cushions or the inferior vena cava. It ends in a free margin which covers foramen II [Fig. 270 (2C)]. This rigid septum directs the inferior vena caval blood towards septum I which is ballooned to the left so that the blood passes through foramen II into the left atrium. This oblique route between the two septa is the **foramen ovale**. Septum II also separates the superior vena caval blood from foramen II so that it passes directly to the right AV orifice anterior to the other stream.

Before birth there is very little flow of blood through the pulmonary vessels (see below) so virtually all the venous blood reaching the heart enters the right atrium. Hence the pressure in this atrium is higher than in the left keeping septum I displaced to the left and the foramen ovale open. After birth (1) the volume of blood entering the left atrium from the pulmonary veins equals that entering the right and (2) the left atrium has to work harder to distend the thicker left ventricular wall. Hence the left atrial pressure rises higher than that in the right and keeps septum I pressed against septum II and the foramen ovale closed. However, if septum I fails to close foramen I or septum II fails to cover foramen II so that an interatrial foramen is present which the pressure differences cannot close, some left atrial blood will pass into the right atrium and be recirculated through the lungs. This blood is lost to the systemic circulation so that the patient may suffer from oxygen depletion even becoming blue (cyanosed) and excessively breathless on exercise. Equally, any venous anomaly which produces an excessive flow of blood to the right atrium at the expense of the left will maintain patency of the foramen ovale with a right to left shunt continuing (see Cardiovascular anomalies).

Interventricular and bulbar septa

Initially there is a single ventricle which transmits blood from left to right into the bulbus [Fig. 270 (1A)]. As the ventricle enlarges, the right and left expand separately leaving a muscular interventricular septum between them and the original ventricular channel as an **interventricular foramen** through which the left ventricle discharges its blood to the bulbus cordis [Fig. 270 (1B)] while the right ventricle discharges its blood vertically into the bulbus. These two streams of blood impinge on each other to produce a spiral flow through the bulbus [Fig. 270], that from the right ventricle passing anterior to that from the left as they enter the bulbus. This spiral flow sculptures the bulbar endocardial tissue into four (two major and two minor) **spiral ridges**. The major ridges fuse from the ventral aorta towards the ventricles producing first an internal division of the bulbus and later, as its walls invaginate the spiral septum, a separation into independent vessels—the ascending aorta and the pulmonary trunk. This internal spiral septum is shown partly formed in Fig. 270 (B) with complete separation in Fig. 270 (C). The septum divides the ventral aorta so that the sixth arch arteries are connected to the pulmonary trunk and the other persisting arch arteries (see below) to the aorta.

At the ventricles, the bulbar septum meets the muscular interventricular septum anteriorly but arches above the right ventricle to form the supraventricular crest between the right AV orifice and the infundibulum of that ventricle. It also leaves the aortic orifice lying posterior and to the left of the infundibulum above the interventricular septum—its final position if the interventricular foramen is not closed. The persisting **interventricular foramen**, which becomes progressively smaller relative to the size of the heart as that organ grows, is closed by the forward growth of the fused endocardial cushions along the interventricular septum to fuse with the bulbar septum and to form the right, antero-inferior wall of the lowest part of the left ventricular outflow (aortic vestibule) separating it from the right ventricle. The endocardial cushions form only membrane; hence this becomes the major part of the **membranous interventricular septum**. Posteriorly [Fig. 270 (2B, 2C,e)] the fused endocardial cushions form part of the interventricular wall. Because the interatrial septum meets the fused endocardial cushions to the left of the interventricular septum, the upper part of this area separates the left ventricle from the right atrium—**membranous AV septum**—while a narrow strip below the septal cusp of the right AV valve and immediately above the AV bundle [Fig. 270] is the membranous interventricular septum.

Valves

The endocardial cushions form the AV valves by excavation of their ventricular surfaces while the continuity of this surface with the inner ventricular muscular layer (trabeculae carneae) produces the **chordae tendineae** and the **papillary muscles.**

The aortic and pulmonary valvules are formed by excavation at the valvular level of the three bulbar ridges produced in each vessel by the division of the bulbus [Fig. 270 (3B, 3C)]; elsewhere the ridges disappear.

The great arteries

The five **arch arteries** (1, 2, 3, 4, and 6) which are formed symmetrically on each side of the developing pharynx (cranial part of the foregut) and which unite the ventral and dorsal aortae, have been mentioned above. The first and second disappear early on both sides leaving a plexus of vessels out of which the external carotid arteries develop. On both sides, the part of the dorsal aorta between the third and fourth arteries (**ductus caroticus**) disappears as (a) it becomes a backwater between the cranially directed third arch artery which is carried forwards with the growing head and the caudally directed fourth and (b) the intersegmental body wall branches of this part of the aorta (akin to intercostal and lumbar arteries further caudally) are

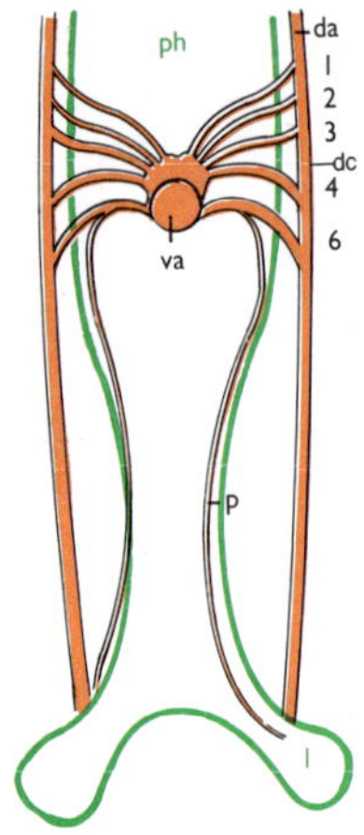

Fig. 271. A diagram to show the arrangement of the pharyngeal (branchial) arch arteries and their relation to the foregut tube at an early stage in development. At no time are all these arteries present together, the first and second disappearing before the sixth is formed. Compare with Fig. 272 to see how the foregut tube and its lung buds change their relationship to the arteries and the pulmonary artery progressively shortens as the head grows forwards carrying the gut tube with it. The same movement accounts for the changing relationship of the nerves of the pharyngeal arches to their arteries, e.g. recurrent laryngeal nerve, the nerve of the sixth arch which originally supplies the larynx when it lies at the level of that artery.
da. Dorsal aorta.
dc. Part of dorsal aorta which becomes ductus caroticus and is lost (cf. Fig. 272).
l. Lung bud.
p. Pulmonary artery.
ph. Pharynx.
1–6. The pharyngeal arch arteries.

replaced by other longitudinal arteries (vertebral, cervical, etc. which are the main arteries of the neck [Fig. 57, Vol. 3]), branches of the enlarged seventh intersegmental artery which supplies the developing upper limb—the subclavian.

On the right side the dorsal aorta also disappears from the point of entry of the fourth arch artery to the point of junction of the two dorsal aortae to form a single vessel. This leaves the fourth arch artery to end in the subclavian artery and the left dorsal aorta to take over the intersegmental and bronchial branches of the missing right artery. The distal part of the right sixth arch artery also disappears so that it ends in its pulmonary branch.

On the left side all three arches persist, the third forming the common and internal carotid arteries, the fourth the aortic arch, and the sixth the left pulmonary artery and **ductus arteriosus**.

The division of the ventral aorta and bulbus directs (a) the left ventricular blood (containing oxygenated placental blood) through the third and fourth arch arteries to the head, neck, and upper limbs with only a small quantity entering the descending aorta and (b) the right ventricular deoxygenated blood through the sixth arch arteries mainly to the descending aorta through the ductus arteriosus. Because of this relative separation of the two outflows, the part of the dorsal aorta between the origin of the left subclavian artery and the ductus arteriosus is usually much narrower than the rest and may remain so after birth—**coarctation of the aorta**. (For other cardiovascular anomalies see below.)

The passage of the right ventricular output through the ductus arteriosus rather than through the pulmonary arteries is due to contraction of a **hypertrophied muscular layer in the pulmonary arteries** before birth. This contraction is maintained by low oxygen tension but is released when the oxygen tension rises with the first breath after birth. This leads to (1) the sudden establishment of a pulmonary circulation; (2) a drop in pulmonary arterial pressure with consequent flow of blood from the aorta through the ductus arteriosus to the pulmonary arteries until the ductus closes during the first 24–48 hours after birth by muscular contraction; (3) a rise in left atrial pressure and closure of the foramen ovale due to the entry of pulmonary venous blood in quantity; (4) after the ductus closes the lowered pressure of the right ventricular output leads to a loss of right ventricular muscle. Clearly children born in conditions of low oxygen tension may not establish an adequate pulmonary circulation because of the continued contraction of the pulmonary arterial muscle which will not lose its hypertrophied state as it normally would. See also patent ductus arteriosus.

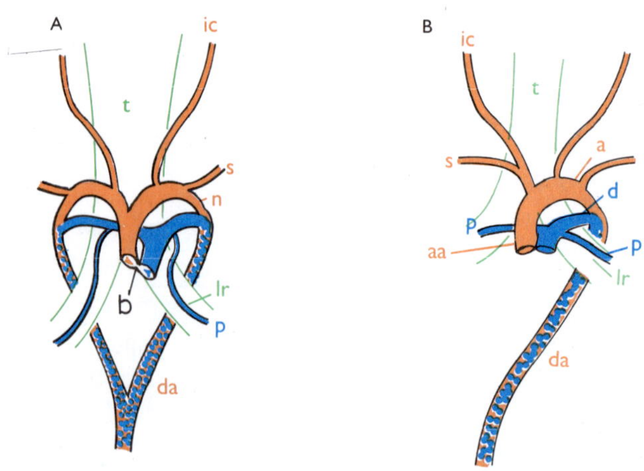

Fig. 272. Diagrams of the arrangement of the pharyngeal arch arteries at two stages in development subsequent to the loss of the first and second of these arteries. (A) shows the situation after the loss of the ductus caroticus on both sides but before the loss of the right dorsal aorta caudal to this [cf. Fig. 271]. (B) shows the situation which persists until birth when the ductus arteriosus begins its closure.
a. Arch of aorta.
aa. Ascending aorta.
b. Dividing bulbus cordis.
d. Ductus arteriosus.
da. Dorsal aorta.
ic. Internal carotid artery.
lr. Lung root.
n. Narrow segment of aorta between fourth and sixth arch arteries.
p. Pulmonary artery.
s. Subclavian artery.
t. Trachea.

The intra-embryonic coelom and lung

The transverse limb (pericardial cavity) of the original U-shaped, intra-embryonic coelom [Fig. 265] is bent downards as the embryo bulges up into the amniotic cavity. On both sides the pericardial cavity is continuous with the caudal part of the coelom through a narrow **pericardioperitoneal channel** which is lateral to the foregut tube and dorsomedial to the lateral part of the septum transversum which projects into the channel and has in its edge the **common cardinal vein** and the **phrenic nerve** which arises from the spinal medulla at this fourth cervical level. It is at this level that the foregut begins to divide into a dorsal oesophagus and a ventral **laryngotracheal tube** [Fig. 273 (C)] from which the lung buds grow laterally towards the edge of the septum transversum. As they do so, this edge splits into two ridges with a groove (definitive **pleural cavity**) between them [Fig. 273 (F)]. The cranial ridge (**pleuropericardial membrane**) contains the common cardinal vein and the phrenic nerve while the caudal ridge is the **pleuroperitoneal membrane**. The lung enters the groove which expands into the body wall between the membranes to accommodate it. Meanwhile the head growing forwards carries the larynx and trachea with it so that the lung moves cranially to lie dorsal to the pericardial cavity and the pleuropericardial membrane becomes a horizontal shelf between the pleural cavity dorsally and the pericardial cavity ventrally [Fig. 273 (G, H)]. The separation of the pleural and pericardial cavities arises from fusion of the edge of the pleuropericardial membrane with the anterior surface of the corresponding lung root in which lie the pulmonary veins [Fig. 273 (I)]. This fusion occurs at a time when veins of the embryo are little more than endothelial tubes; hence the right pulmonary veins may fuse with the common cardinal vein and an anomalous pulmonary venous drainage to the right atrium is established. This may also happen on the left side and usually results in a persistence of the upper part of the left superior vena cava (left superior intercostal vein) which drains to the left brachiocephalic vein. Very occasionally it may drain to the coronary sinus (see venous development). Thus all the pulmonary venous blood may drain to the right atrium.

Fig. 273 (I) shows the further extension of the pleural cavity within the body wall as the lungs grow forwards to surround the heart and pericardial cavity forming the fused mediastinal pleura and pericardium from an extended pleuropericardial membrane which contains the phrenic nerve on both sides and the superior vena cava on the right.

The pleuroperitoneal membrane is also extended as the lung expands within the body wall. Immediately medial to the free edge of this membrane lies the oesophagus in its dorsal and ventral (septum transversum) mesenteries. Closure of the pleuroperitoneal channel occurs due to fusion of this edge with these mesenteries thus completing the diaphragm. Fig. 273 (C) shows that the original pericardioperitoneal channel (later divided into pleuropericardial and pleuroperitoneal channels as the two membranes are formed) lies immediately anterior to the intermediate mesoderm which forms the kidneys and suprarenals caudal to the diaphragm. Hence any persistent **pleuroperitoneal channel** lies beside the oesophagus but separated from it by the paramedian part of the diaphragm formed by its mesenteries (essentially the crura) and anteromedial to the suprarenal and kidney. Such an aperture can lead to **congenital diaphragmatic hernia** on the left but is unlikely to do so on the right because of the mass of liver filling that side of the upper abdomen. The normal **diaphragm** therefore consists of the two pleuroperitoneal membranes peripherally, the mesenteries of the oesophagus on each side of the midline posteriorly, and the septum transversum in a median position anteriorly—the **central tendon**—pierced by the inferior vena cava and the phrenic nerves.

Cardiovascular anomalies

Venous

These are very numerous at the periphery but are not usually significant. The most significant anomaly is **abnormal pulmonary venous drainage** of either or both lungs (a) to the superior vena cava or (b) to the portal vein because the lungs are part of the foregut tube which initially has a venous plexus continuous with that on the foregut in the abdomen. In either case, the reduced or absent venous input to the left atrium maintains the *patency of the foramen ovale*. In (a) this leads after birth to completely deoxygenated blood passing from the inferior vena cava into the left atrium and systemic circulation. Hence the infant is born apparently normal but becomes cyanosed (blue) when the umbilical vein is tied (loss of oxygenated placental blood in the inferior vena cava). Such an infant depends for its oxygen supply on any mixing of the two streams of venous blood in the right atrium because the pulmonary venous blood mostly passes from the superior vena cava into

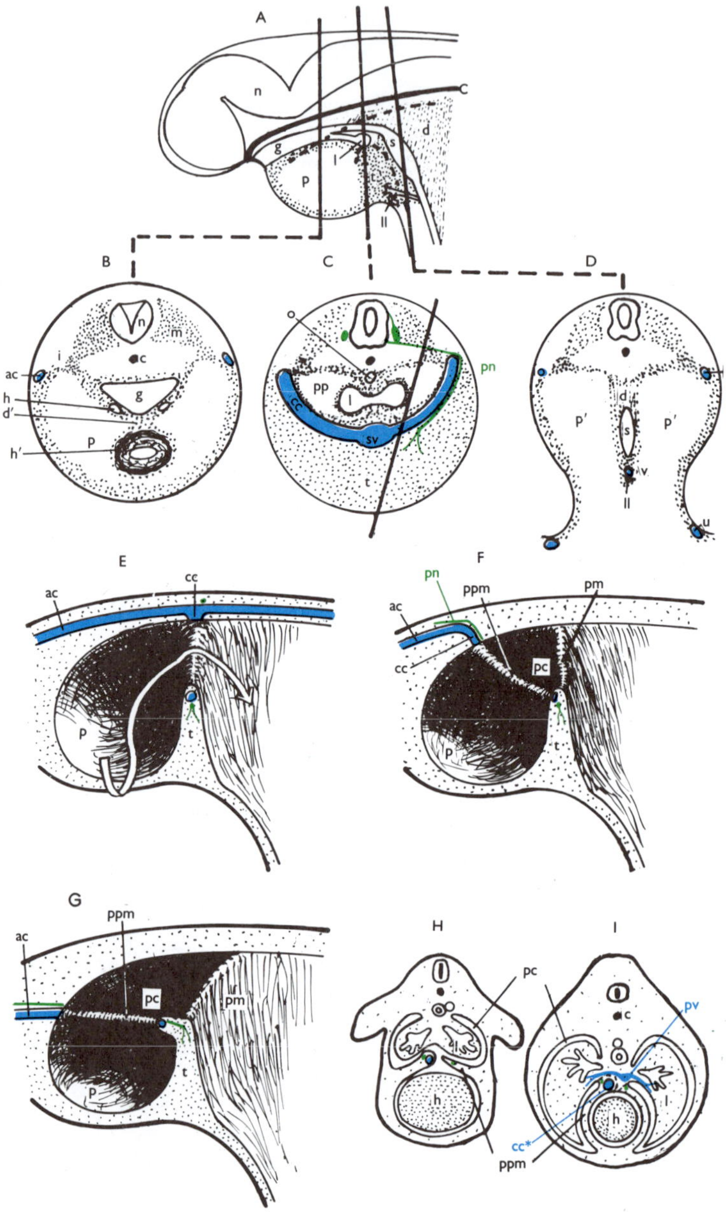

Fig. 273. Diagrams to show the division of the original U-shaped coelomic cavity into pericardial, pleural, and peritoneal cavities by the growth of the pleural cavity into the dorsolateral part of the septum transversum and its extension into the substance of the body wall.

(A) Median section through the cephalic part of a human embryo (Fig. 266 (D)]. The interrupted line indicates the continuity of the pericardial part of the coelom with the peritoneal part caudal to the septum transversum through the pericardioperitoneal channel.

(B, C, and D) are transverse sections at the levels of the lines passing through (A) to which they are attached by interrupted lines. In (B), the original positions of the heart tubes and their position in the pericardial cavity after fusion and before the loss of the dorsal mesocardium are both shown.

(E, F, and G) are views of the lateral part of the section indicated by the line drawn through (C) and viewed from the medial side. They show the splitting of the dorsolateral part of the septum transversum to accommodate the pleural cavity, its extension into the body wall, and its displacement cranially with the lung to lie dorsal to the pericardial cavity from which it is partially separated by the pleuropericardial membrane until the edge of that membrane fuses with the lung root immediately posterior to it. They also show the placing of the common cardinal vein and the phrenic nerve in the pleuropericardial membrane. The arrow in (E) passes across the pericardial cavity and through the pericardioperitoneal channel.

(H and I) show the position of the lungs (not shown in E, F, or G) relative to the pleuropericardial membrane as seen in a transverse section along the leader line ppm in G (H) and the position after the pleural cavity and lung have completed their invasion of the body wall (extending both pleuropericardial and pleuroperitoneal membranes) and the edge of each pleuropericardial membrane (right and left) has fused with the corresponding lung root (interrupted lines in I).

ac. Anterior cardinal vein.
c. Notochord.
cc. Common cardinal vein.
cc.* Superior vena cava.
d. Dorsal mesentery.
d'. Dorsal mesocardium.
g. Foregut (pharynx).
h. Heart tube (original position).
h'. Fused heart tubes in pericardial cavity.
i. Intermediate mesoderm.
l. Lung.
ll. Liver outgrowth (bile-duct).
m. Somite mesoderm.
n. Neural tube.
o. Oesophagus.
p. Pericardial cavity.
p'. Peritoneal cavity.
pc. Pleural cavity.
pm. Pleuroperitoneal membrane.
pp. Pleuroperitoneal channel.
ppm. Pleuropericardial membrane.
pn. Phrenic nerve.
pv. Pulmonary vein.
s. Stomach.
sv. Sinus venosus.
t. Septum transversum.
u. Umbilical vein.
v. Ventral mesentery—part of septum transversum.

the right ventricle and back to the lungs. In (b) there is less cyanosis as indeed there is less when only one lung is involved but the foramen ovale remains patent in all cases.

Low-pressure system defects

These consist of varying degrees of failure to form a normal interatrial septum. The effects are described above (p. 252). A patent foramen ovale may be a compensation for another defect as in anomalous pulmonary venous drainage.

High-pressure system defects

1. *Failure of the septa* to separate the ventricles or their outflow tracts (interventricular or bulbar septal defects with right/left communication) or failure of the ductus arteriosus to close. All such anomalies prevent the

development of a low-pressure pulmonary system side by side with a high-pressure systemic system and ensure continuing high pulmonary pressure. This rapidly leads to pathological changes in the pulmonary arterial system as well as causing right ventricular hypertrophy (which makes the angular cardiac shadow of a chest radiograph into a globular one) which leads to right ventricular failure.

2. *Uneven division of the bulbus* so that one vessel is abnormally small (stenosis) or even closed (atresia). When this affects the **aorta** and is severe it is often incompatible with antenatal survival. Since the pulmonary circulation has no significant function before birth, fetuses can survive pulmonary atresia. In extreme cases there is an inevitable **interventricular septal defect** because ventricles have to discharge through the aortic channel. The last part of the interventricular septum to form is usually deficient [Fig. 270 (2C, f)]. This places the aortic orifice over the interventricular septum (sometimes called dextroposition) and leads to right ventricular hypertrophy because of the communication with the high-pressure systemic system and/or the resistance encountered in the stenosed pulmonary trunk or infundibulum. This relatively common complex (**tetralogy of Fallot**) is basically a pulmonary stenosis. In less severe degrees where the interventricular septum is completed the right ventricular hypertrophy overcomes the effect of the stenosis for a while but there is eventual right ventricular failure.

In **pulmonary atresia** the only direct supply to the lungs is through the **ductus arteriosus**. If this remains open after birth, a pulmonary circulation is established. If the ductus closes, then the only possible supply to the lungs is through the bronchial arteries which anastomose with the pulmonary arteries in the lungs. These may become enormously enlarged and extremely fragile but can sustain a reduced pulmonary circulation. In either case the pulmonary circulation is inefficient because the blood delivered to the lungs is a mixture of deoxygenated and oxygenated blood as is that eventually delivered to the systemic circulation through the common aorta. Except in severe cases the infant is likely to survive but suffers from a greater or lesser degree of oxygen lack which reduces activity and produces cyanosis when it is undertaken, in addition to the eventual ventricular failure.

3. If the bulbus is not placed to the right in the folding of the heart tube but lies centrally, then each ventricle discharges vertically through it and a straight bulbar septum forms causing the left ventricle to discharge into the pulmonary arteries and the right ventricle into the aorta. This **transposition of the great vessels** leads to two separate, closed circulations—pulmonary and systemic. In intra-uterine life the ductus arteriosus permits the transfer of oxygenated blood to the aorta though it passes caudally rather than cranially to head and neck and upper limbs so that the new-born infant may be blue in this area though a normal pink in its caudal parts. As the ductus closes after birth, no oxygenated blood can reach the systemic circulation and severe cyanosis develops which is fatal unless, as a temporary measure, the foramen ovale is torn open to permit some left atrial blood to enter the right atrium and the systemic circulation to maintain the child until definitive surgery can be undertaken.

4. **Coarctation**. This narrowing of the aorta, usually between the left subclavian origin and the entry of the ductus arteriosus but sometimes in adjacent parts, may be so extreme that the ductus arteriosus is the only supply to the lower parts of the body. In these cases the colour difference may be obvious at birth though there is usually the development of a collateral circulation between the subclavian arteries and the aorta or its branches inferior to the coarctation, i.e. between the internal thoracic arteries and (a) the aorta through the anterior and posterior intercostal arteries and (b) through the epigastric arteries to the external iliac arteries. Also through the highest intercostal arteries anastomosing with their more caudal fellows from the aorta.

In all but the most minor cases a difference in blood pressure is measurable in the upper and lower limbs and the enlarged intercostal arteries may notch the ribs sufficiently for this to be seen in radiographs.

Development of the midgut

This is not dealt with in any more detail than that shown in Figs. 136, 175, and 180 and the associated notes in the text because it is not usually associated with abnormalities of great clinical significance. The **caecum**, originally placed close to the liver, may remain in a high position and not descend into the right iliac fossa. Rotation of the midgut may be reversed so that a mirror image of the usual arrangement can take place (**situs inversus**), or there may be no rotation such that the large intestine lies in the lower abdomen and the small intestine in the upper abdomen. Similarly those parts of the intestine which lose their mesenteries by adhesion to the posterior abdominal wall (duodenum, ascending colon, and descending colon) may fail to adhere so that they retain a greater or lesser amount of their mesenteries, a situation most common in the ascending colon.

Development of the caudal part of the foregut in the abdomen, though helpful in understanding the arrangement of the structures in the upper abdomen, is not usually associated with major abnormalities but requires a description of developmental stages which can add to the complexity rather than clarifying the anatomy in the area of the omental bursa.

Development of the hindgut and urogenital system

When the embryo bulges into the amniotic cavity and the tail grows away from the embryonic disc, the allantois and the adjacent part of the yolk sac are carried tailwards with the cloacal membrane and reversed in much the same way as the foregut is carried headwards with the growing head [Fig. 266]. This produces the **infra-umbilical part of the anterior abdominal wall** between the caudal margin of the original disc (caudal edge of the umbilical orifice) and the cloacal membrane. Initially the **allantois** (entoderm) is in contact with the ectoderm throughout this length [Fig. 266 (D)] but the last part of the mesoderm to be formed by the primitive streak grows around the sides of the cloacal membrane, separates allantois and ectoderm [Fig. 275 (A)], and forms the muscles, connective tissues, etc. of this part of the abdominal wall thereby restricting the cloacal membrane to the caudoventral surface of the **cloaca**—the chamber which is common to the hind gut tube and the allantois [Fig. 275].

As the embryo narrows towards its tail, the intermediate mesoderm comes to lie lateral to the cloaca [Fig. 274] and extends round the cloacal membrane into the infra-umbilical anterior abdominal wall in much the same way as it surrounds the buccopharyngeal membrane at the head end. However, there is no split mesoderm beyond this and so no cavity corresponding to the pericardial cavity is formed.

Kidneys

Between the buccopharyngeal and cloacal membranes the intermediate mesoderm forms a series of kidneys on each side. In the future cervical region it produces a series of rudimentary nephridia—the **pronephros**. These segmental cell strands represent the nephridia of invertebrates and, like them, are attached to the surface of the coelomic cavity. These non-functional rudiments join together laterally to form a cord of cells (**pronephric duct**) which passes tailwards in the intermediate mesoderm to the cloaca—a very short distance at this stage. Caudal to the pronephros, **mesonephric tubules** develop in the intermediate mesoderm. These short, coiled tubes extend laterally from an aortic glomerulus to link up with and canalize the pronephric duct (now the **mesonephric duct**) to the cloaca. Such tubules are numerous in each segment and form further caudally as the embryo elongates, the cranial tubules degenerating as more caudal tubules are formed. In this way this **mesonephros** (middle kidney) moves caudally. It is not certain that the mesonephros is functional in man though it certainly is in animals where the placental diffusion membrane is much thicker, e.g. the pig.

Caudal to the mesonephros a dorsal diverticulum of the mesonephric duct grows into the intermediate mesoderm which condenses over its expanded end. The diverticulum is the **ureteric bud** and the condensation the **metanephrogenic mesoderm**. Together they form the third and final kidney—the **metanephros**—and its duct system. The stem of the diverticulum forms the **ureter;** the expanded end the **pelvis of the kidney**, the major and minor

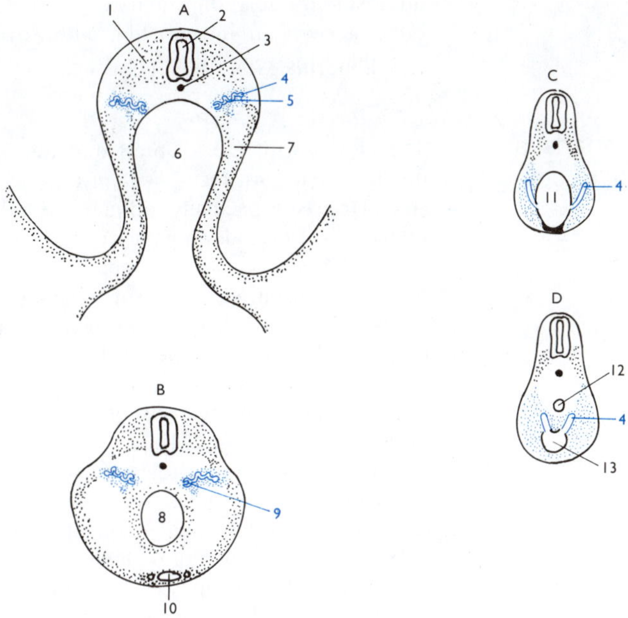

Fig. 274. Diagrammatic transverse sections to show the relationship of intermediate mesoderm to the midgut (A), the cranial hindgut (B), and the cloaca (C) in an early human embryo. (D) shows the same region as (C) after the formation of the urorectal septum.
1. Somite.
2. Neural tube.
3. Notochord.
4. Mesonephric duct.
5. Mesonephric tubule.
6. Midgut.
7. Intra-embryonic coelom.
8. Hindgut (cephalic part).
9. Mesonephric glomerulus.
10. Allantois.
11. Cloaca.
12. Rectum.
13. Urogenital sinus.

calyces, and the **collecting tubules** of the kidney [p. 171] by repeated branching. The collecting tubules link up with the **nephrons** formed from the metanephrogenic cap in a series of progressively more superficial generations while the kidney continues to grow, the oldest surviving nephrons being those closest to the medulla of the kidney (**juxtamedullary glomeruli**) which have their loops of Henle descending furthest into the medulla.

The earlier branches of the ureteric bud obtain separate caps of metanephrogenic mesoderm. Each of these develops into a separate lobule partly fused with its fellows but outlined on the surface by a groove which makes the fetal and early postnatal kidney lobulated. As growth continues the lobules coalesce completely and the kidney usually develops a smooth external surface.

The repeated divisions of the ureteric bud may start before it reaches the metanephrogenic cap; this leads to a **bifid ureter** which may start close to the mesonephric duct so that each part later opens separately into the urinary bladder (see below).

Failure of union of the nephrons with the collecting ducts may be a cause of severe **congenital cystic kidney** which destroys that organ before birth. The more usual congenital cystic kidney is not due to failure of fusion but is part of a more widespread cystic disease which can involve the liver and lungs where there is no question of fusion of separately formed parts. In this case the individual may survive for a normal span or may develop renal failure at any age because of the loss of excretory units which have become cystic.

Once formed the metanephros slowly ascends relative to the other viscera from its pelvic origin. It does so dorsal to the mesonephros and developing gonad and within the mesoderm which later forms the fascial envelope of the abdomen (transversalis, pelvic, iliac, and diaphragmatic fascia) splitting it to form the **renal fascia**. It also obtains a new blood supply at each level (internal iliac, common iliac, and aorta—a series of branches). Hence it is not uncommon for it to have an **accessory renal artery** passing to its lower pole—a remnant of an earlier main artery. During ascent the kidney rotates so that its sinus moves from an anterior to an anteromedial position. This is not possible if the two metanephrogenic caps (which are relatively close together when first formed) fuse at their caudal ends producing a **horse-shoe kidney**. The median part of such a fused kidney ascends anterior to the aorta and impinges on the inferior mesenteric artery so that its ascent is arrested at this level—the right and left ureters emerging from the right and left anterior surfaces.

The ureteric bud or the metanephrogenic cap may fail to develop on one or both sides—unilateral or bilateral **renal agenesis**. Unilateral agenesis is of interest to the surgeon who may be called upon to remove a diseased kidney; bilateral cases are incompatible with extra-uterine life unless action is taken to replace the renal functions.

Cloaca, gonads, and urogenital ducts

The cloaca with the allantois and the hindgut entering its cranial end is divided by the **urorectal septum** into ventral (**urogenital sinus**) and dorsal (rectal) parts respectively continous with these two structures. This septum of intermediate mesoderm passes craniocaudally between the allantois and the hindgut to reach the cloacal membrane which is depressed below the surface by the proliferation of the surrounding mesoderm. The **cloacal membrane** breaks down as the septum reaches it to form two separate orifices (urogenital and anal) the anal in the depths of an ectodermal pit, the proctodaeum (cf. stomodaeum in Vol. 3). The mesonephric ducts are carried medially in the urorectal septum to open into the dorsal aspect of the urogenital sinus [Fig. 274].

The base of the allantois expands to form the **urinary bladder** and the urogenital sinus elongates. As a result, the mesonephric ducts are taken into its wall until ureters and mesonephric ducts open together [Fig. 275 (B)]. Subsequent absorption of both ducts leads to the ureters entering the base of the bladder while the mesonephric ducts continue to join the urogenital sinus [Fig. 275 (C)]. Thus much of the epithelium of the base of the bladder (**trigone**) and of the posterior wall of the urogenital sinus is formed from these ducts which are derived from mesoderm (intermediate) while the remainder is derived from the entoderm of the cloaca and allantois.

Clearly the urorectal septum may fail to form either in part or altogether. This is probably the result of failure of the caudal mesoderm to be produced. It produces a persistent communication between the hindgut and the urinary system and is commonly associated with varying degrees of **ectopia vesicae**—a condition in which the cloacal membrane is not restricted to its usual area by the formation of the mesoderm of the anterior abdominal wall (infra-umbilical— see above) but extends to the umbilicus on the allantois [Fig. 266]. In this case the extended cloacal membrane breaks down so that the posterior walls of allantois, urinary bladder, and urethra form the midline anterior abdominal wall below the umbilicus and have urinary and genital ducts (see below) opening on this area as well as the rectum (incomplete or absent urorectal septum). All the elements normally superficial to these structures, e.g. pubic symphysis, penis (or clitoris), and paramedian muscles, etc., being absent. In lesser degrees of ectopia vesicae there may be an opening from the urethra or urinary bladder on the infra-umbilical anterior abdominal wall (see epispadias).

Each **gonad** develops as a swelling on the posterior abdominal wall anteromedial to the mesonephros and beside the mesentery of the hindgut. Both receive large cells (primordial germ cells) which migrate from the entoderm of the hindgut and are believed to form the strands of cells (**sex cords**) which develop in the gonads. Shortly after this a further duct (**paramesonephric**) is formed on each side. It arises as an outpouching of the coelomic cavity at the cranial end of the mesonephros and grows caudally along the mesonephric duct to the caudal pole of the mesonephros. Here it crosses in front of the mesonephric duct into the cephalic extremity of the urorectal septum in which it passes medially to fuse with its fellow and form the median **uterovaginal canal**. This descends in the midline to end blindly on the posterior wall of the urogenital sinus between the openings of the mesonephric ducts [Figs. 275 (C)]. The paramesonephric ducts therefore open into the coelomic cavity at their cranial ends and, where they cross the mesonephric ducts, each is attached to that duct and to the caudal pole of the gonad by a condensation of mesoderm (**gubernaculum**) which descends on the posterior abdominal wall and passes through the developing inguinal canal to spread out in the subcutaneous tissues between the opening of the urogenital sinus and the groin. This condensation plays a part in the descent of the gonad.

Up to this point the development is the same in all embryos but subsequently diverges in the two sexes.

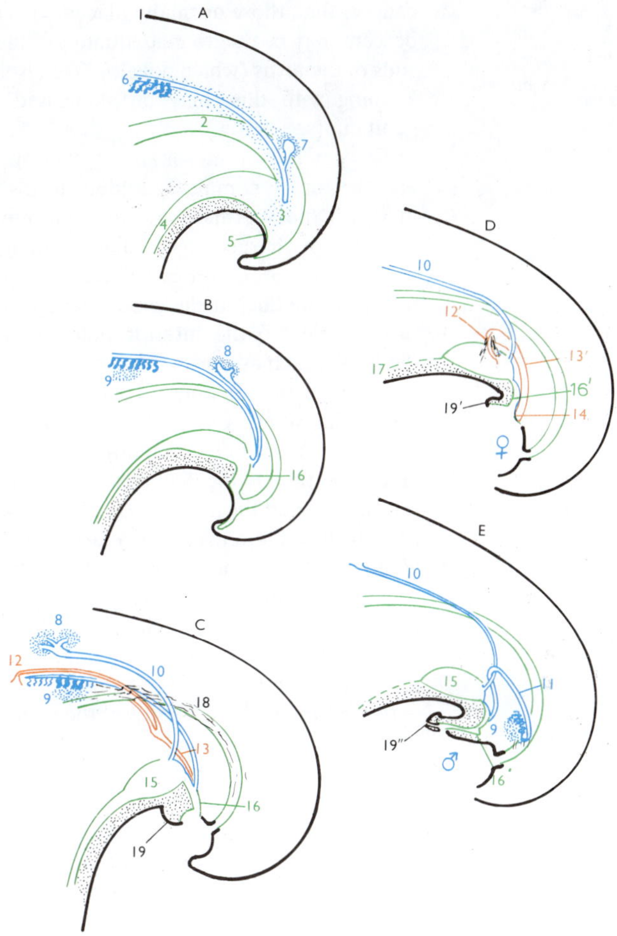

Fig. 275. Diagrams of the development of the cloaca and urogenital system as seen from the median plane in the caudal half of the embryo. Bilateral organs are seen on one side only. (A), (B), and (C) show the indeterminate stages of development common to both sexes. (D) shows the development in the female and (E) that in the male. In (E) the testis is displaced posteriorly to avoid confusion with the process of urethral closure. Black—ectoderm, gubernaculum, and mesoderm of the infra-umbilical anterior abdominal wall (dots). Green—entoderm. Blue—mesonephric tubules and duct, gonad, intermediate mesoderm, ureteric bud, ureter, and the parts of the genital system formed from these ducts. red—paramesonephric ducts and their derivatives.

1. Ectoderm.
2. Hindgut.
3. Cloaca.
4. Allantois.
5. Cloacal membrane.
6. Mesonephros.
7. Ureteric bud covered by nephrogenic mesoderm.
8. Metanephros.
9. Gonad.
10. Ureter.
11. Ductus deferens.
12. Paramesonephric duct.
12′. Uterine tube.
13. Uterovaginal canal.
13′. Vagina.
14. Hymen.
15. Urinary bladder.
16. Urogenital sinus.
16′. Definitive urethra.
17. Urachus.
18. Gubernaculum.
19. Genital tubercle.
19′. Clitoris.
19″. Penis.

In the male, the paramesonephric ducts fail to develop and gradually disappear leaving only their abdominal (**appendix testis**, p. 108) and urogenital sinus (**prostatic utricle**) ends [Fig. 275 (E)]. The sex cords of the testis continue to develop and gradually form the **seminiferous tubules** and, by extension posteriorly, the **rete testis**, while the surface of the testis forms a dense layer of fibrous tissue—the tunica albuginea. Some of the mesonephric tubules adjacent to the testis lose their glomeruli and link to the rete testis to become the **efferent ductules** of the testis while those cephalic and caudal to this degenerate or remain as the **appendix of the epididymis** (cranial tubules) and **aberrant ductules** cranial and caudal (**paradidymis**) to the testis. With the degeneration of the paramesonephric ducts each gubernaculum is attached only to the testis and the mesonephric duct (now **ductus deferens**). As the embryo grows and the gubernaculum does not, the testis is displaced caudally along the posterior abdominal wall anterior to the ascending metanephros and its ureter. Both testis and gubernaculum project into the peritoneal cavity and are adherent to the peritoneum. Thus the peritoneum on the anterior surface of the shortening gubernaculum is carried down through the inguinal canal with the gubernaculum forming the **processus vaginalis** ahead of the arrival of the testis at the inguinal canal [Fig. 115]. Later the testis descends along the posterior wall of the processus to a scrotal position where the processus forms the **tunica vaginalis**, though the testis may end in the groin, the perineum, or the inguinal canal because of the diffuse ending of the gubernaculum. Normally the testis reaches a scrotal position at the time of birth but can usually be displaced upwards along the processus vaginalis to the inguinal canal. Subsequently the processus normally disappears leaving the tunica vaginalis isolated from the peritoneal cavity but the processus may persist and form the basis for an oblique inguinal hernia [p. 102]. The testis may fail to enter the processus and remain an abdominal organ. Such **abdominal testes** are sterile and have a much higher incidence of testicular cancers than those normally placed. It is thought that the failure of complete descent may be due to inadequate production of androgens by the interstitial cells of the testis (which develop from isolated pieces of the sex cords) and, in keeping with this, may be associated with feminization of the external genitalia (see below).

The part of the mesonephric duct applied to the testis elongates rapidly and, becoming complexly folded, forms the **epididymis**—an elongated tube in which the spermatozoa can continue their maturation and from which some are discharged on ejaculation though most ripe spermatozoa are stored in the ductus deferens. Since the gubernaculum is attached to the mesonephric duct at the caudal pole of the testis, the epididymis runs from the superior to the inferior pole of the testis where it joins the ductus deferens which ascends in the spermatic cord behind the testis and processus vaginalis to the abdomen. Here it hooks over the ureter to descend to the urogenital sinus. Close to its entry into the urogenital sinus the ductus develops a lateral diverticulum which forms a convoluted tube—the **seminal vesicle**—lateral to the ductus deferens on the base of the urinary bladder. The terminal part of the mesonephric duct which is common to the seminal vesicle and ductus deferens is the **ejaculatory duct** and is buried in a mass of glandular tissue formed by multiple outgrowths from all surfaces of the urogenital sinus—the **prostate**. Subsequently the number of these outgrowths is reduced and the definitive glandular elements arise mainly from the posterior surface of the urogenital sinus in this part which becomes the prostatic urethra.

In the female, the sex cords of the ovary break up into small clusters and no tunica albuginea is formed. The mesonephric ducts and tubules degenerate, though remnants of them may be found between the cranial (lateral in the adult) ends of the ovaries and the cervix of the uterus in the substance of the broad ligament (epoophoron and paroophoron adjacent to the ovary). These, like similar remnants in the male, may give rise to cysts because they are formed of an epithelium which can begin to secrete fluid.

The **paramesonephric ducts** continue to develop, the cervix and body of the **uterus** arising from the upper part of the uterovaginal canal and the parts of each duct to the point of attachment of the gubernaculum. Superior to this each duct forms a uterine tube, so the **gubernaculum**, failing to shorten, remains as the **ligament of the ovary** and the **round ligament of the uterus** both of which are attached to the uterotubal junction.

The development of the **vagina** is uncertain though it seems most likely that the inferior part of the urogenital sinus is everted on to the perineum as the **vulva** so that the urogenital sinus (urethra) and lower uterovaginal canal (vagina) reach the surface separately, the vagina now ending blindly superior to the posterior vulva while the urethra opens immediately anterior to it. If this is the correct view, the **female urethra** corresponds to the part of the prostatic urethra above the entry of the ejaculatory ducts in the male, the **para-urethral glands** which develop as outgrowths of the female urethra correspond to the prostate, and the **hymen** represents the separating membrane between the end of the fused uterovaginal canal and the urogenital sinus—a membrane which normally breaks down in both male and female but which may persist as an imperforate hymen and not be recognized until puberty when there is no apparent menstrual discharge.

Anomalies of the genital system are relatively common because they do not, of themselves, lead to death of the embryo, fetus, or child. However, they can cause major problems at puberty if not recognized and properly dealt with as soon after birth as possible.

The major anomalies of the female genital tract arise out of failure of fusion of the elements of the uterus and/or vagina. Thus there may be a median cervix but the uterus is represented by two separate and usually small horns, each continuous with a uterine tube (**bicornuate uterus**). Such horns are usually incompatible with pregnancy and are often associated with multiple other anomalies. The vagina may also be double in whole or in part. There may be agenesis of one or both ovaries as may also occur with the testis in the male.

External genitalia

Early in development the mesoderm surrounding the opening of the urogenital sinus proliferates on its cranial margin to form the **genital tubercle** (future penis or clitoris) and at the sides to form the **genital (labioscrotal) swellings**. As the genital tubercle grows forwards it carries the anterior wall of the lowest part of the urogenital sinus on its inferior (ventral) surface as a **urethral groove**. The margins of the groove project inferiorly as the urethral folds especially at the sides of the opening of the urogenital sinus. In the female, the urethral folds persist as the **labia minora** and the genital swellings lateral to them as the **labia majora**. In the male, the urethral folds come together posteriorly and fuse below the opening of the urogenital sinus as the genital swellings, increasing in size to accommodate the testes, meet inferior to this and fuse to form the **scrotum**—the lines of fusion forming the scrotal and perineal septa. Fusion of the margins of the urethral groove extends forwards to form the penile urethra as far as the ventral edge of the glans. The terminal part of the male urethra is formed by an ingrowth of epithelium at the tip of the glans. This tunnels through the glans to meet the urethral groove on the ventral surface and, as this ectodermal rod canalizes, the extremity of the urethral groove closes so that the urethra opens on the apex of the glans penis.

The differences between the sexes are principally due to hormones secreted by the gonads. Hence any inadequacies of these hormones may lead to intermediate forms of external genitalia. In the male, failure of the urethral folds to fuse together with failure of descent of the testes and a small penis may make the external genitalia have a female appearance but there is no vaginal opening or hymen. In lesser degree the urethral folds may fail to fuse anteriorly so that there is a urethral opening on the ventral surface of the penis (**hypospadias**) very often close to the glans penis and representing a failure of the terminal urethra to form properly. The opening may be anywhere between this point and the perineum. Very uncommonly there may be **epispadias** where the urethra opens on the dorsal surface of the root of the penis. This is probably a limited form of ectopia vesicae (see above) with the genital tubercle (essentially a bilateral structure) growing across the opening of a slightly extended cloacal membrane.

In the female, the clitoris may be large giving the appearance of a rudimentary penis and the urethral folds may fuse at least posteriorly simulating a severe hypospadias. Hence the individual may be classified as male until menstruation occurs through the 'urethral' orifice in the anterior perineum, it having been assumed that there was no uterus or vagina and that the individual had undescended testes.

Tables of nerves, muscles, and movements of the trunk

Table **1**

Approximate levels of structures in the trunk

It should be appreciated that all the horizontal levels given in this table are subject to considerable variation: (a) because certain organs, e.g. heart, lungs, liver, stomach, spleen, and kidneys, move with respiration and with changes in position (erect or recumbent, flexed or extended); (b) in normal individuals of different physical types; (c) in the cadaver as compared with the living. In the cadaver, the recumbent position, combined with relaxation of the diaphragm and the elastic recoil of the lungs, leads to abnormally high levels.

The table gives the various structures in order from above downwards, together with structures on the anterior and posterior surfaces of the body at corresponding levels. Where an internal structure lies vertically between two superficial structures on the same surface, it is so placed in the table. It is important to note that the vertical height of any part of the table is determined by the number of internal structures listed and not by the vertical height of that part of the body.

Anterior surface	Internal structure	Posterior surface: Vertebral body	Posterior surface: Spine	Other
1–3 cm superior to med. ⅓ of clavicle	Apex of lung	T.1	C.7–T.1	
	Arch of subclavian A.			
	Brachiocephalic trunk, bifurcation	T.2		
Sternoclavicular joint	Brachiocephalic Vv. formation			
1st chondrosternal joint	Aortic arch, upper margin	T.3	T.2	
	Superior vena cava, formation			
	Trachea, bifurcation	T.4	T.3	Scapula, med. end of spine
	Azygos V. arch			
	Lung, apex of lower lobe			
	Lung, upper margin of root			
2nd chondrosternal joint	Aortic arch, ends of	T.5	T.4	
Sternal angle	Sup. mediastinum, inf. border			
	Pulmonary trunk, bifurcation			
	Pericardium, superior margin	T.6		
3rd chondrosternal joint	L. atrium, superior margin		T.5	
	Pulmonary valve			
	Superior vena cava, end of	T.7		
	Aortic valve			
4th chondrosternal joint	Lung, lowest part of root		T.6	
	L. atrioventricular orifice			
5th chondrosternal joint	R. atrioventricular orifice			
	L. lung, cardiac notch			
	R. dome of diaphragm			
6th chondrosternal joint	Liver, highest part			
7th chondrosternal joint	Inferior vena cava in diaphragm	T.8		
	L. dome of diaphragm		T.7	Scapula, inf. angle
	Stomach, fundus			
	R. ventricle, inf. margin	T.9		
Xiphoid process			T.8	
5th intercostal space within midclavicular line	Apex of heart			
	Spleen, superior limit			
	Diaphragm, oesophageal orifice	T.10	T.9	
	Gastro-oesophageal junction		T.10	
	Lung, lower limit, paravertebral			
	L. kidney, superior limit	T.11		
	Diaphragm, aortic orifice	T.12	T.11	
	Pleura, lower limit paravertebral			
	Duodenum, superior part			
	Coeliac trunk and ganglia			
	Spleen, inferior limit			
	L. colic flexure			
	Sup. mesenteric A. origin			
	Portal V. formation	L.1	T.12	Transpyloric plane
	Hilus of kidney, upper			

Anterior surface	Internal structure	Posterior surface		Other
		Vertebral body	Spine	
9th costal cartilage, midclavicular	Fundus of gall-bladder		L.1	
	End of spinal medulla			
	Bile-duct, end of Duodenojejunal flexure	L.2		
	Colon, R. flexure		L.2	
	Duodenum, horizontal part			Costal margin midaxillary line
	Kidney, lower pole	L.3		
	Inf. mesenteric A. origin		L.3	
Umbilicus	Aorta, bifurcation	L.4	L.4	Highest point iliac crest
	Appendix vermiformis, root			
			S.1	
Ant.sup. iliac spine	Common iliac A. bifurcation Midpoint of ureter	S.1		Sacral promontory
	Dural sac, inferior end		S.2	Post.sup. iliac spine
	Ischial spine Midpoint of hip joint Cervix of uterus			
Pubic symphysis, anterosuperior surface	Urinary bladder, superior surface if empty Ureters enter bladder	Coccyx		

Table **2**

Actions of trunk muscles

Flexion

1. Against resistance, e.g. raising head and shoulders from the supine position.
   Rectus abdominis.
   Psoas major.
   External oblique.
   Internal oblique.
2. With gravity.
   Erector spinae acting excentrically.

Lateral flexion

1. Against resistance.
   Oblique muscles of abdomen acting unilaterally.
   Quadratus lumborum of same side.
   Psoas of same side.
   Erector spinae of same side.
   Latissimus dorsi if arm fixed [Vol. 1].

With gravity; same muscles of opposite side acting excentrically.

Extension

Erector spinae.

Rotation

1. To right.
   L. external oblique acting with R. internal oblique.
2. To left.
   R. external oblique acting with L. internal oblique.

Inspiration = increasing intrathoracic volume.

1. *In quiet respiration.*
   Diaphragm increases vertical extent of thorax by lowering its dome (see accessory muscles).
   Scalene muscles of neck raise the first and second ribs [Vol. 3].
   External intercostal muscles slide upper ribs forwards on lower ribs of each space. This raises the ribs and increases the space between them. Only upper muscles active in quiet or moderate respiration; lower muscles involved in forced respiration.
   Accessory muscles.
   Vertical posterior fibres of **internal** and **external oblique muscles**, and **quadratus lumborum** hold down the lowest ribs so that the contraction of the diaphragm can be effective in lowering its dome.
2. *In forced respiration.*
   Sternocleidomastoid raises sternum.
   Pectoralis major and **minor** help to raise the ribs, especially if the scapula and arm are elevated by levator scapulae and trapezius. Serratus anterior may also assist.
   Erector spinae extends trunk. This separates the ribs anteriorly and increases the distance between the first rib and the pubic symphysis, thereby enlarging both thorax and abdomen.

Expiration = decreasing intrathoracic volume.

1. *By lowering the ribs.*
   Gravity and elastic recoil of the lungs in quiet respiration.
   In more forceful respiration.
   External and **internal oblique muscles** acting from the hip bone with **quadratus lumborum** draw down the ribs.
   Internal and **innermost intercostals** and **subcostals**, acting from below, slide upper ribs backwards on lower ribs, and thus lower and approximate the ribs. Though rectus abdominis is capable of lowering the sternum and costal cartilages, it is not so used except in violent expiratory effort associated with trunk flexion (see erector spinae under inspiration).
   In moderate respiration and in other types of controlled expiration, e.g. singing, the diaphragm and external intercostal muscles may be active in the early phases of expiration. This prevents too rapid expulsion of air by the elastic recoil of the lungs distended with air.
2. *By elevation of the relaxed diaphragm.*
   Elastic recoil of the lung alone in quiet respiration.
   Abdominal compression in more forceful respiration, or when it is necessary to maintain a steady flow of expiratory air as the elastic recoil of the lung diminishes.
   External and **internal oblique muscles** and **transversus abdominis**. In forceful expiration against resistance, e.g. in asthma, this may raise the intra-abdominal pressure sufficiently to cause discharge of urine (stress incontinence) if sphincter urethrae is not contracted. *In all cases where contraction of the abdominal muscles causes raised intra-abdominal pressure, it is accompanied by contraction of the perineal muscles.*

3. *In coughing and sneezing.*
   These sudden, violent expirations use the same muscles as in forced expiration (with the addition of **latissimus dorsi**), but the air passages are closed by approximation of the vocal folds in the larynx (closure of the glottis) till the intrathoracic and intra-abdominal pressure has reached a high level. The vocal folds are then separated (opening the glottis) so that the air is discharged through the mouth (coughing) or nose (sneezing).

Vomiting

The muscles used in this action are those used in coughing, except that there is no build-up of intrathoracic pressure since it is the diaphragm and **abdominal muscles** that contract. The stomach does not contract but is rhythmically compressed. The airway is normally closed during vomiting. Perineal muscles also contract.

Urination against resistance, defecation, and parturition

In all of these actions, the expulsion is assisted to a greater or lesser degree by the contraction of the *abdominal muscles*. When these contractions are mild, they are associated with diaphragmatic contraction so that costal respiration can continue. When powerful, they are always associated with closure of the glottis and a build-up of intrathoracic as well as intra-abdominal pressure by contraction of the expiratory muscles without expulsion of air from the lungs. The end of the expulsive activity is marked by the expiration of the air previously held under pressure in the lungs.

In any strenuous activity, e.g. lifting heavy weights, pushing, pulling.

Expiratory muscles of thorax and abdomen are powerfully contracted against a closed glottis, together with perineal muscles, and flexor and extensor muscles of the trunk. This turns the trunk into a rigid structure on which the limbs can work, but also produces very high pressures within it. In this action, as in all other actions which raise intra-abdominal pressure, the lower fibres of **internal oblique** and **transversus abdominis** which arch over the inguinal canal to fuse in the **conjoint tendon**, close down on the spermatic cord and reduce the chance of the high intra-abdominal pressure producing an inguinal hernia.

In this action, as in powerful extension of the flexed vertebral column, the compressive force applied to the vertebral column is very considerable and the pressures within the **intervertebral discs** rise accordingly. Any weakness of the anulus fibrosus may result in protrusion of the nucleus through it. This most usually occurs posteriorly towards the spinal nerve in the intervertebral foramen because of the relative thinness of the anulus in this region. It is made much more likely if the vertebral column is flexed when the compression forces are applied, because the posterior part of the anulus is then stretched.

Transverse sections and CT scans of the trunk

It is the conventional arrangement to view CT and ultrasound scans from below. Hence the following illustrations are of the lower surfaces of trunk sections so as to fit with the accompanying CT scans. A. Anterior; P. posterior; L. left; R. right.

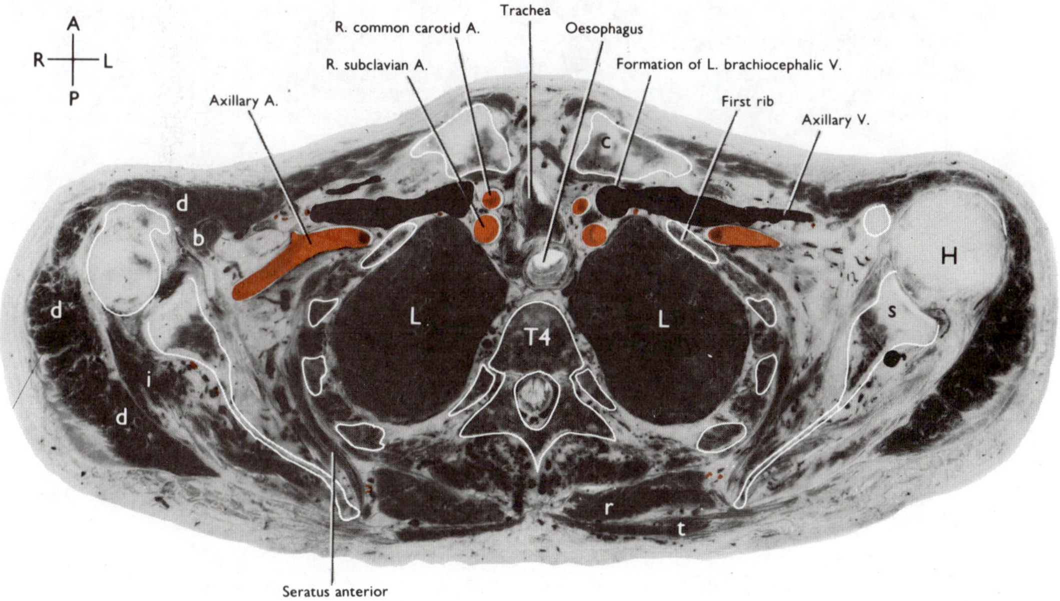

Fig. 276. Section through the fourth thoracic vertebral body (T4) and the sternoclavicular joints. The junction of the subclavian and internal jugular veins is present on both sides.

b. Short head of biceps and coracobrachialis.
C. Clavicle.
d. Deltoid.
H. Head of humerus.
L. Lung.
i. Teres minor.
r. Rhomboid major
S. Scapula.
t. Trapezius.

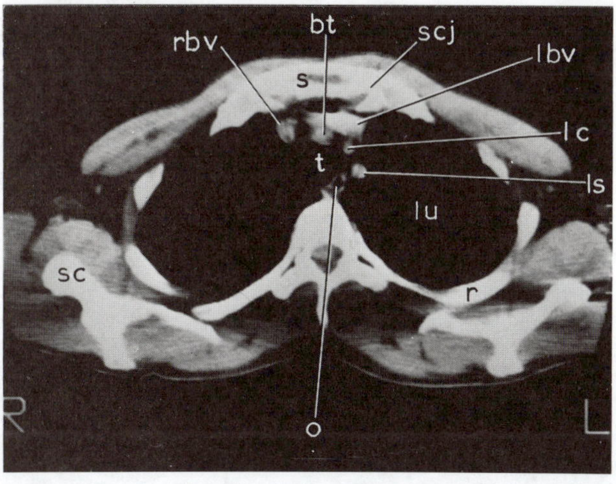

Fig. 276A. A CT scan through the lower parts of the sternoclavicular joints. The level is similar anteriorly to that in Fig. 276 but falls just below the bifurcation of the brachiocephalic trunk and the formation of the brachiocephalic veins posteriorly. This type of scan can show the presence of abnormal masses (tumours, abscesses, or cysts) in the mediastinum either by their own density or by the displacement of surrounding structures. If dense, such masses will also be visible in the lung areas but are made more obvious if a different density of scan is used as in Fig. 277A.

bt. Brachiocephalic trunk.
lbv. Left brachiocephalic vein.
lc. Left common carotid artery.
ls. Left subclavian artery.
lu. Lung.
o. Oesophagus.
r. Rib (4th).
rbv. Right brachiocephalic vein.
s. Sternum.
sc. Scapula.
scj. Sternoclavicular joint.
t. Trachea.

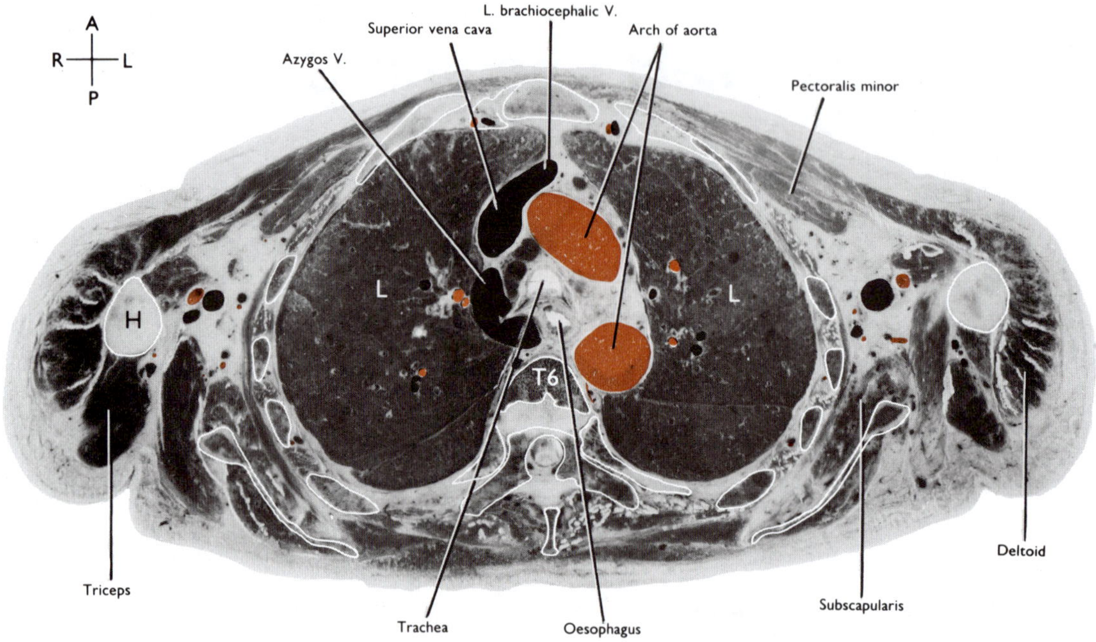

Fig. 277. Section through the lower parts of the sixth thoracic vertebra (T6) and manubrium sterni. The oblique fissure is visible in both lungs, and tracheal lymph nodes are present on both sides of the trachea. The origin of the brachiocephalic trunk from the aortic arch is immediately posterior to the left brachiocephalic vein. In this and the other sections, the plane is not horizontal, but passes downwards as well as backwards.
H. Humerus.
L. Lung.

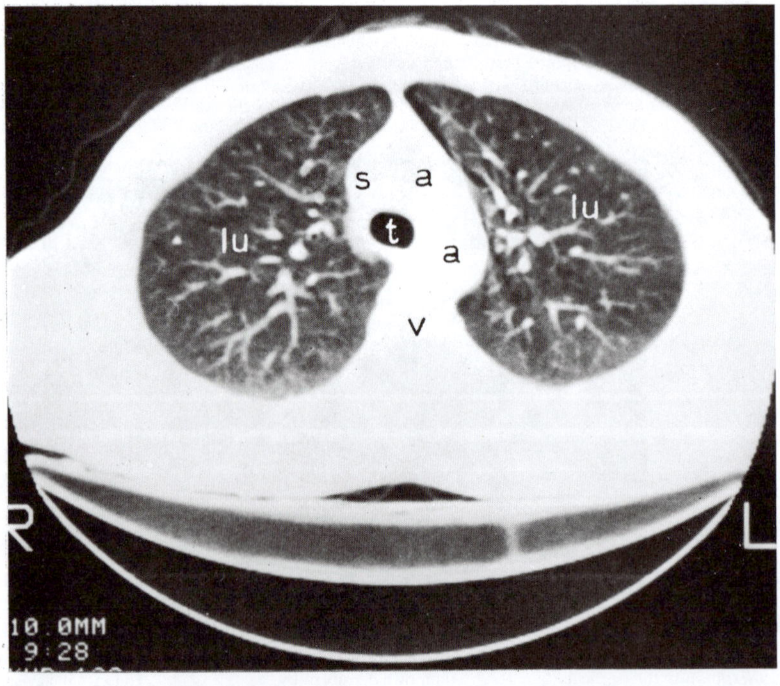

Fig. 277A. A CT scan at the level of the aortic arch exposed to show vessels in the lung fields.
a. Aortic arch.
lu. Lung.
s. Superior vena cava.
t. Trachea.
v. Vertebral body.

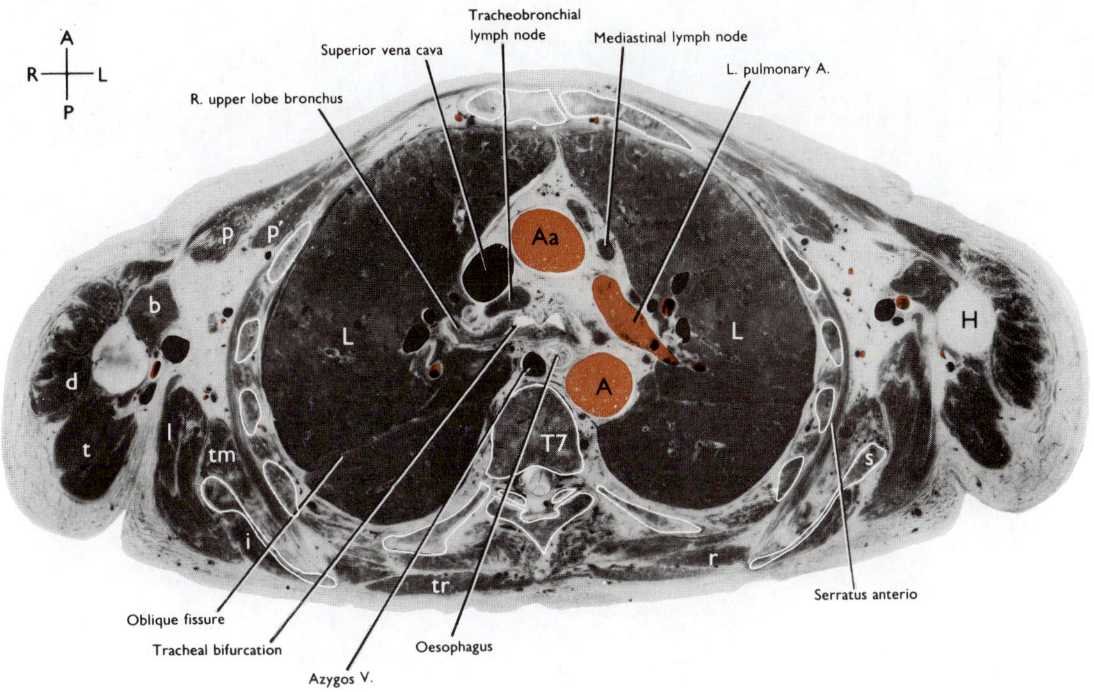

Fig. 278. Section through the seventh thoracic vertebra (T7) and the manubriosternal synchondrosis.
A. Descending aorta.
Aa. Ascending aorta.
b. Biceps and coracobrachialis.
d. Deltoid.
H. Humerus.
i. Infraspinatus.
L. Lung.
l. Latissimus dorsi.
p. Pectoralis major.
p′. Pectoralis minor.
r. Rhomboid major.
s. Scapula.
t. Triceps.
tm. Teres major.
tr. Trapezius.

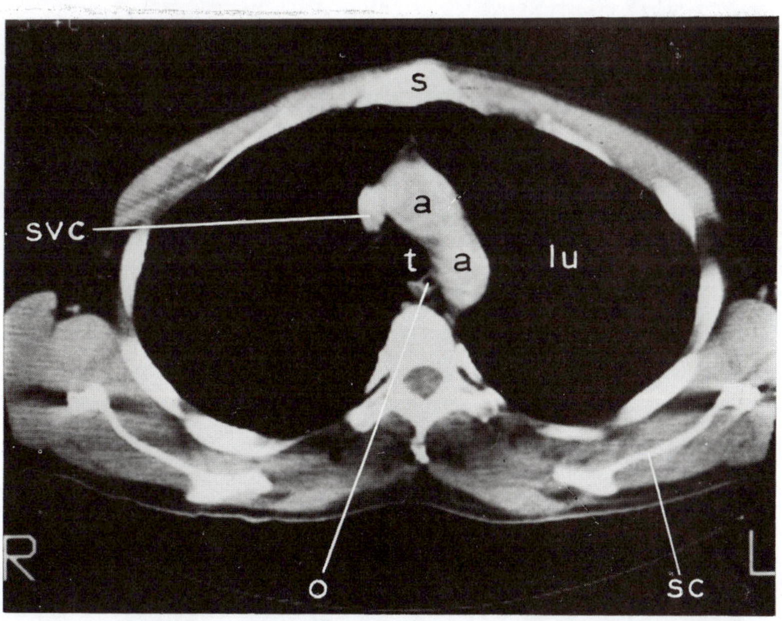

Fig. 278A. A CT scan at the level of the aortic arch to show the mediastinal contents.
a. Aortic arch.
lu. Lung [cf. Fig. 277A].
o. Oesophagus.
s. Sternum.
sc. Scapula.
svc. Superior vena cava.
t. Trachea.

It is easy to see how dilatation of the aorta (aneurysm) can be seen directly in such a scan as this when its presence may only have been guessed at from the clinical signs shown by the patient. It can also be differentiated from an adjacent mass by introducing contrast into the artery which would show it unchanged in diameter.

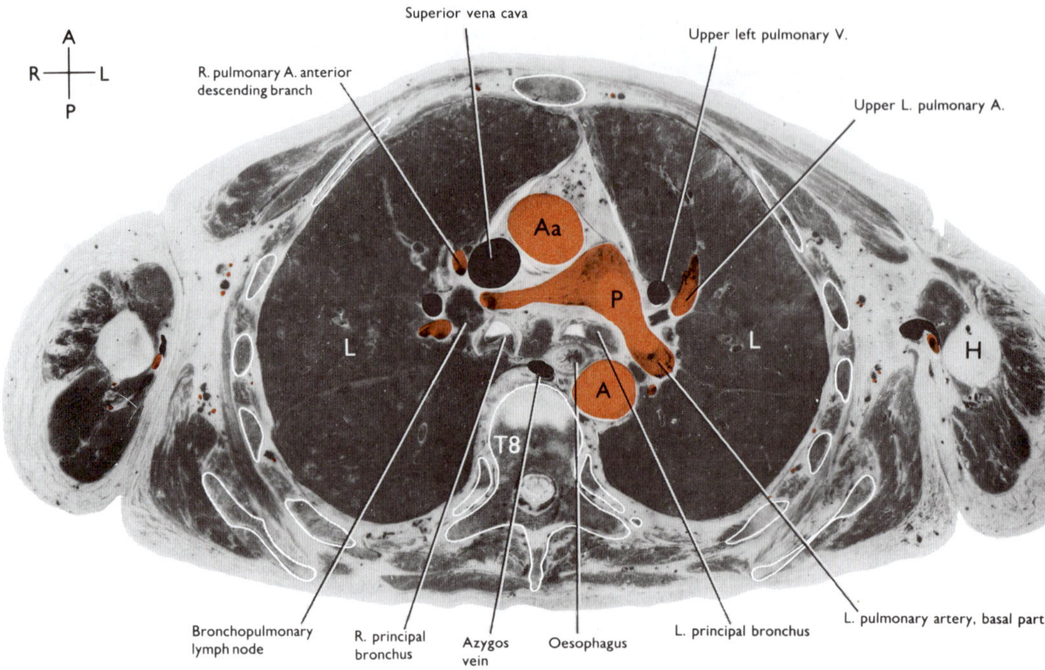

Fig. 279. Section through the eighth thoracic vertebra (T8) and the bifurcation of the pulmonary trunk. A tracheobronchial lymph node lies between the two principal bronchi.

A. Descending aorta.
Aa. Ascending aorta.
H. Humerus.
L. Lung.
P. Bifurcation of pulmonary trunk.

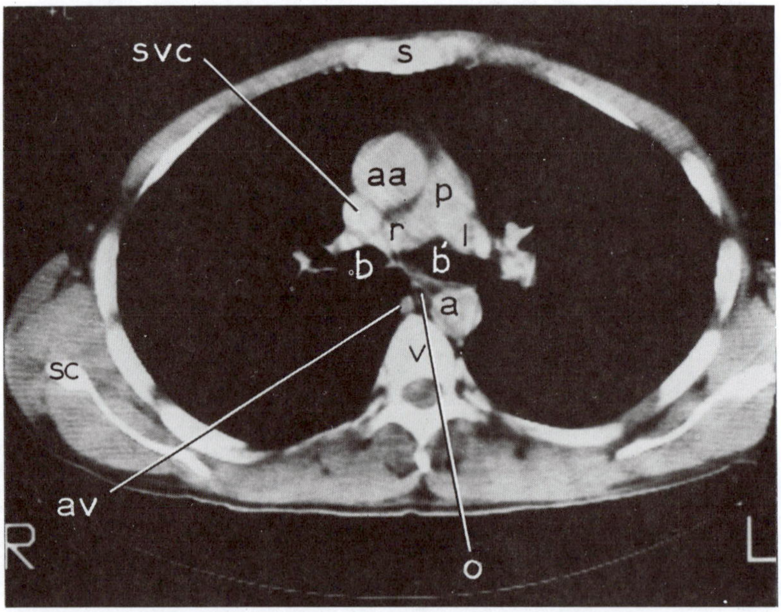

Fig. 279A. A CT scan through the bifurcation of the pulmonary trunk. [cf. Fig. 280A].
a. Descending aorta.
aa. Ascending aorta.
av. Azygos vein.
b and b′. Right and left principal bronchi.

l. Left pulmonary artery.
o. Oesophagus.
p. Pulmonary trunk.
r. Right pulmonary artery.
s. Sternum.
sc. Scapula.
svc. Superior vena cava.

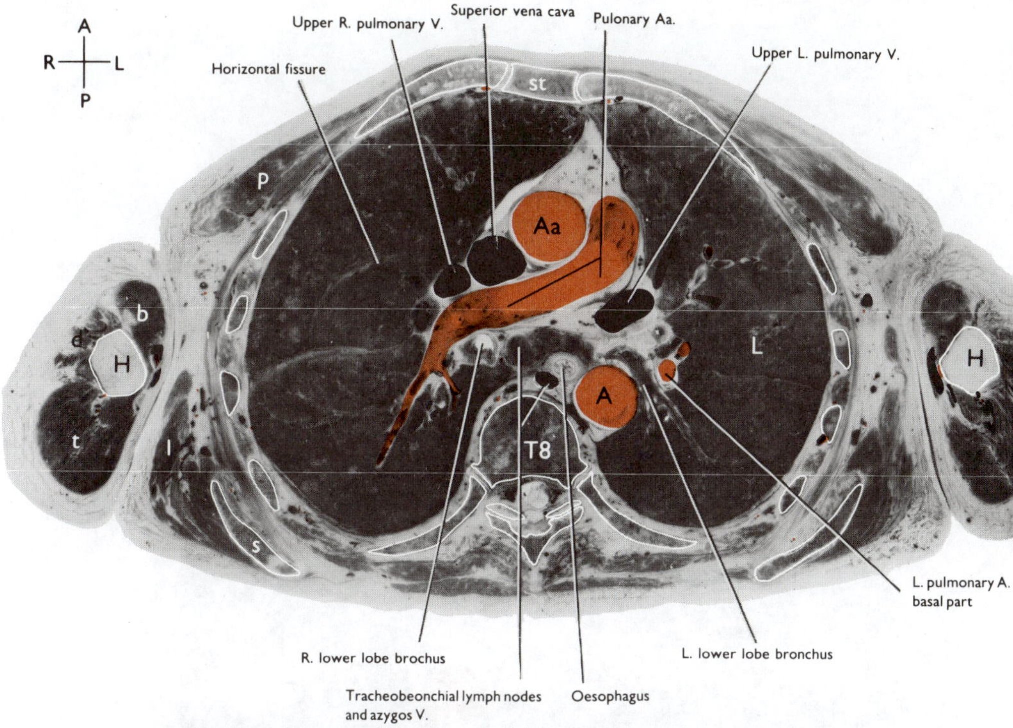

Fig. 280. Section through the body of the eighth thoracic vertebra (T8) and the third sternocostal articulation. The entire length of the right pulmonary artery and the beginning of its branch to the lower lobe of the right lung are shown.
A. Descending aorta.
Aa. Ascending aorta.
b. Biceps and coracobrachialis.
d. Deltoid.
H. Humerus.
L. Lung.
l. Latissimus dorsi.
p. Pectoralis major.
s. Scapula.
st. Sternum.
t. Triceps.

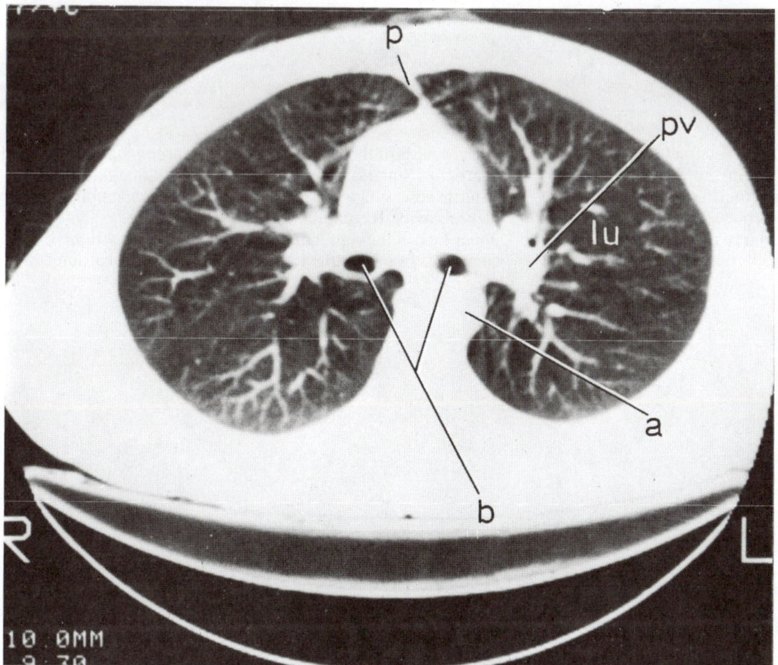

Fig. 280A. A CT scan at the same level as Fig. 280 at an exposure level to show intrapulmonary structure.
a. Descending aorta.
b. Principal bronchi.
lu. Lung.
p. Right and left pleurae in costomediastinal recesses.
pv. Pulmonary vessels.
The size of the white area caused by the pulmonary vessels in the hilus of the lung is increased if the lymph nodes here are enlarged by disease thus adding to the solid tissue in the lung root.

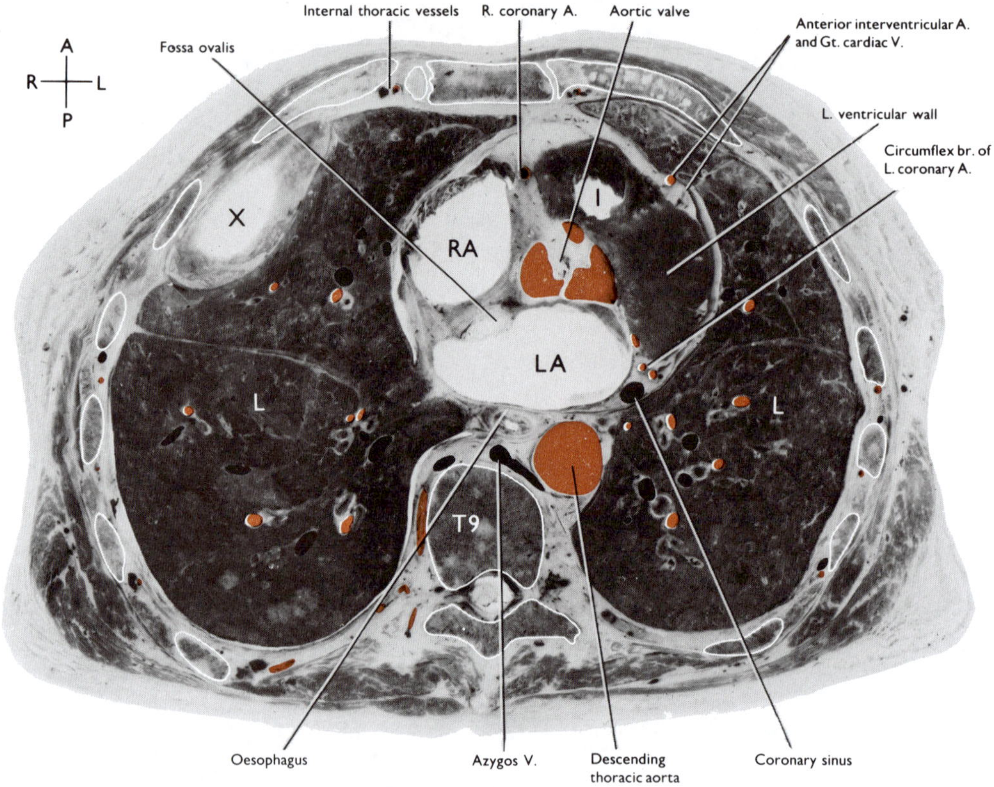

Fig. 281. Section through the body of the ninth thoracic vertebra (T9) and the fourth sternocostal joint. The section shows the relative positions of the chambers of the heart, particularly the atria and the outflow parts of the right and left ventricles. X marks the position of a sterile abscess closed off from the pleural cavity. It compresses the upper lobe of the right lung. The circumflex branch of the left coronary artery is branching to give a left marginal branch.
I. Infundibulum of right ventricle.
L. Lung.
LA. Left atrium.
RA. Right atrium.

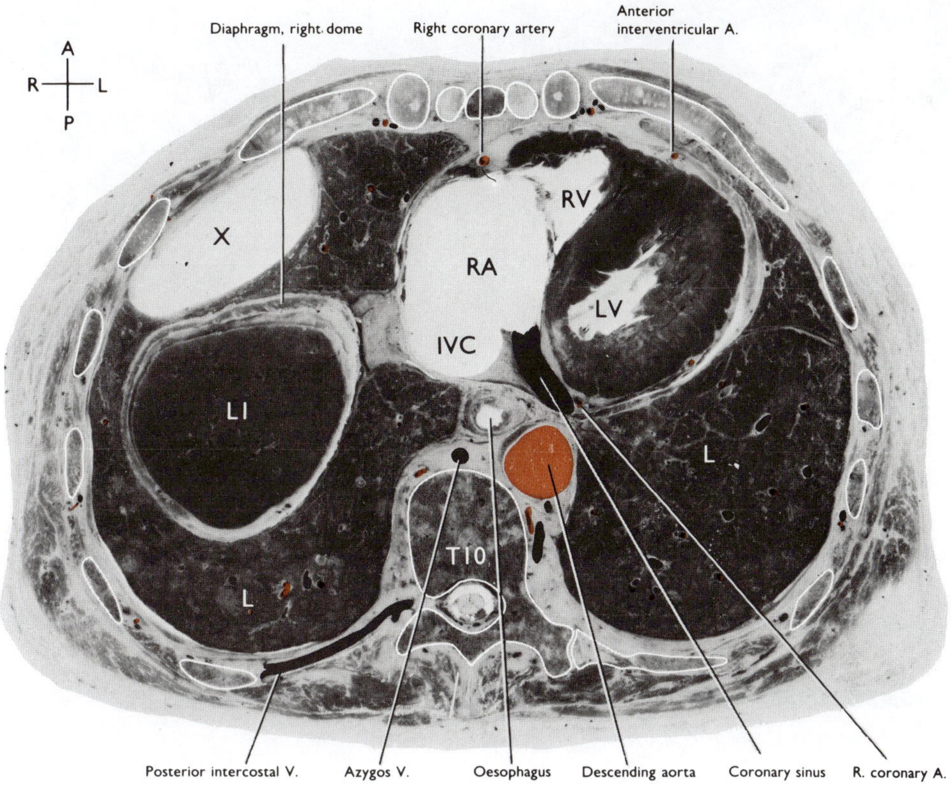

Fig. 282. Section through the tenth thoracic vertebral body (T10) and the seventh sternocostal joint. It also shows the entry of the inferior vena cava (IVC) and the coronary sinus into the right atrium, the right dome of the diaphragm and the liver applied to it. For X see legend to Fig. 281.
IVC. Inferior vena cava opening into right atrium.
L. Lung.
LI. Liver.
LV. Left ventricle.
RA. Right atrium.
RV. Right ventricle.

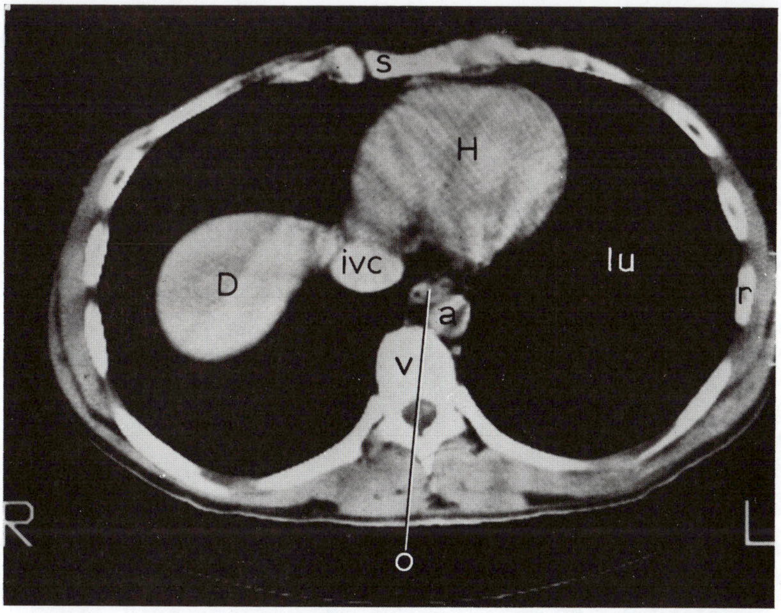

Fig. 282A. A CT scan through the upper part of the right dome of the diaphragm.

a. Descending aorta.
D. Dome of diaphragm and right lobe of liver.
H. Heart.
ivc. Inferior vena cava.
lu. Lung.
o. Oesophagus.
r. Rib.
s. Sternum.
v. Vertebral body.

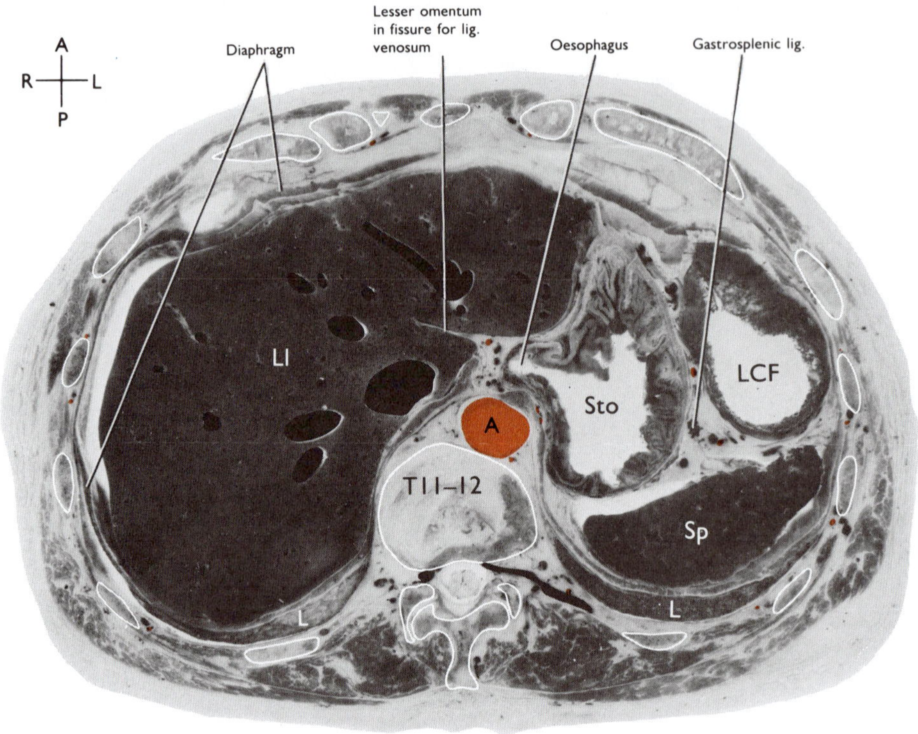

Fig. 283. Section through the intervertebral disc between the eleventh and twelfth thoracic vertebrae (T11–12) and the xiphoid process. The left lobe of the liver is unusually thick and pushes the stomach to the left and forwards. The left colic flexure is also higher than usual so that it lies anterior to the greater part of the vertical extent of the spleen. Note the lung in the costodiaphragmatic recess of the pleural cavity.

A. Descending aorta.
IVC. Inferior vena cava.
L. Lung.
LCF. Left colic flexure.
LI. Liver.
Sp. Spleen.
Sto. Stomach.

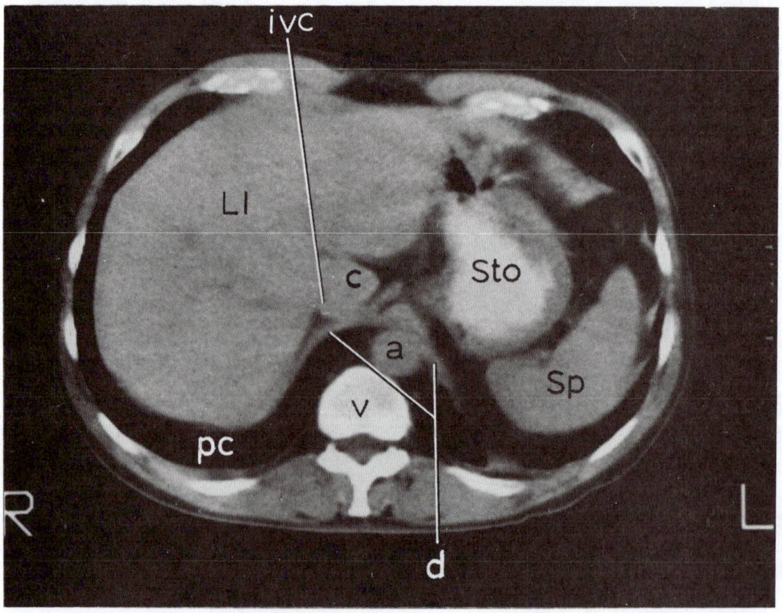

Fig. 283A. A CT scan at T.11 vertebral body.

a. Descending thoracic aorta.
c. Caudate lobe of liver.
d. Diaphragm.
ivc. Inferior vena cava.
Ll. Right lobe of liver.
pc. Pleural cavity.
sp. Spleen.
sto. Stomach.
v. T.11 vertebral body.

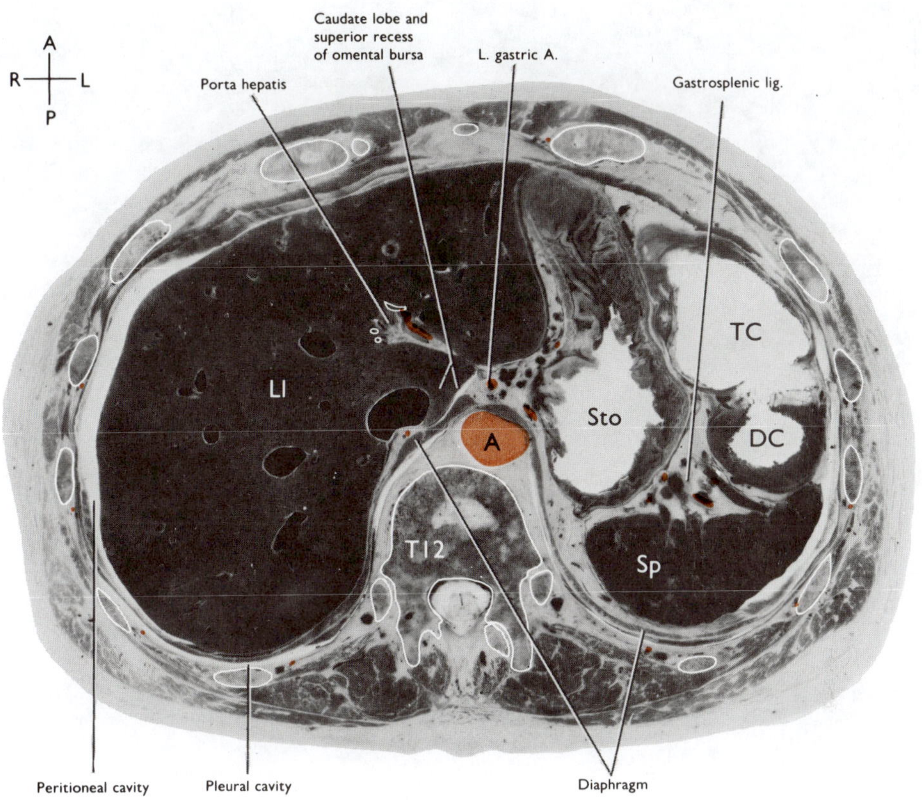

Fig. 284. Section through the body of the twelfth thoracic vertebra (T12) and the tip of the xiphoid process. Tributaries of the hepatic ducts are outlined in white. The lesser omentum passes into the fissure for the ligamentum venosum in the liver between the left and caudate lobes of the liver.
A. Descending aorta.
DC. Descending colon.
IVC. Inferior vena cava.
LI. Liver.
Sp. Spleen.
Sto. Stomach.
TC. Transverse colon.

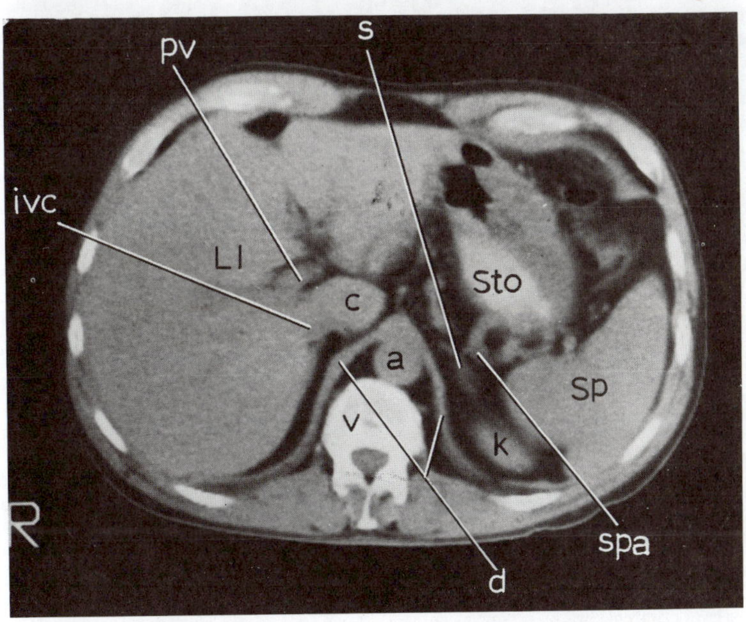

Fig. 284A. A CT scan at the level of T. 11/12 vertebrae.
a. Descending thoracic aorta.
c. Caudate lobe of liver.
d. Diaphragm.
ivc. Inferior vena cava.
k. Left kidney.
Ll. Right lobe of liver.
pv. Portal vein.
s. Left suprarenal.
sp. Spleen.
spa. Splenic artery.
sto. Stomach.
v. Vertebral body adjacent to disc.

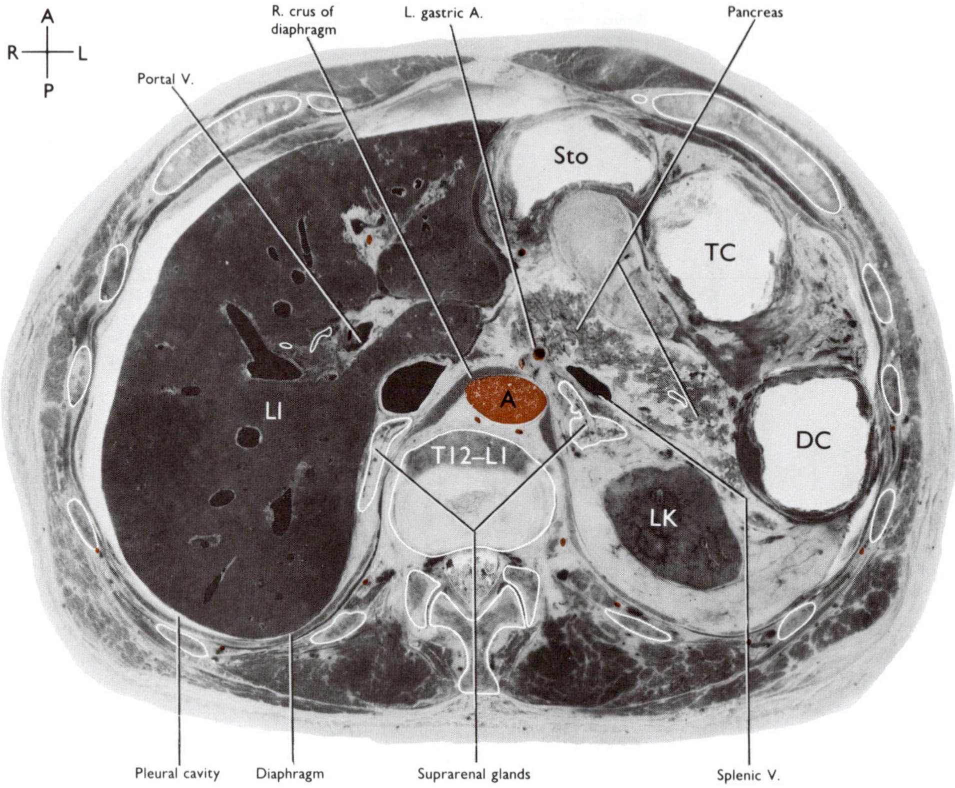

Fig. 285. Section through the intervertebral disc between the twelfth thoracic and first lumbar vertebrae (T12–L1). The suprarenal glands, the pancreatic duct, and the tributaries of the hepatic ducts are outlined in white.

The common stem of the inferior phrenic arteries lies immediately posterior and to the right of the left gastric artery. The left crus of the diaphragm lies on the left posterior surface of the aorta.

A. Descending aorta.
DC. Descending colon.
IVC. Inferior vena cava.
LI. Liver.
LK. Left kidney.
Sto. Stomach.
TC. Transverse colon.

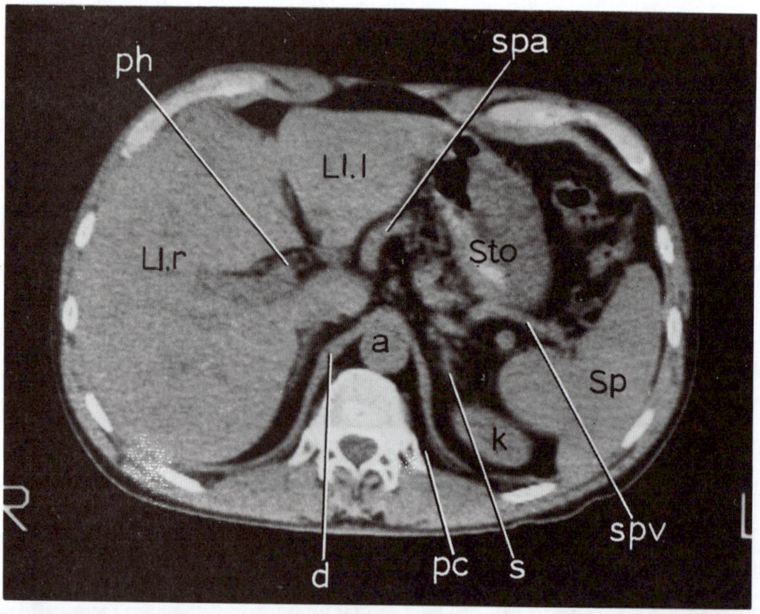

Fig. 285A. A CT scan through the upper part of the twelfth thoracic vertebra—a level slightly below that shown in Fig. 285.
a. Thoracic aorta.
d. Diaphragm.
k. Left kidney.
Ll.l. Left lobe of liver.
Ll.r. Right lobe of liver.
pc. Pleural cavity (pointer ends beside head of twelfth rib).
ph. Porta hepatis.
s. Left suprarenal.
sp. Spleen.
spa. Splenic artery.
spv. Splenic vein.
sto. Stomach.

In this scan, as in all others, distortion of the normal anatomy can uncover the presence of abnormal masses (cancers, abscesses, or cysts) which may be directly visible even in the substance of organs such as the liver or spleen even if they have only a slight difference in density from its tissue. Such information may permit a decision about the applicability or otherwise of surgery in a particular case without the need to open the abdomen or thorax.

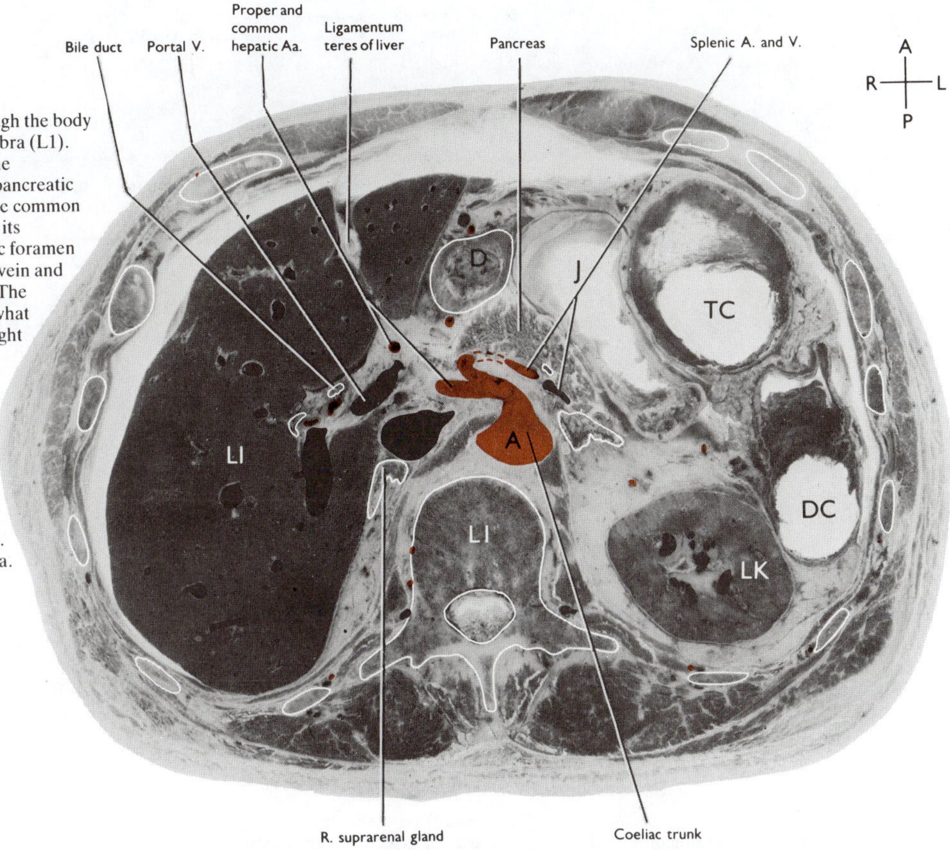

Fig. 286. Section through the body of the first lumbar vertebra (L1). Outlined in white are the suprarenal glands, the pancreatic duct, the duodenum, the common hepatic duct and one of its tributaries. The epiploic foramen lies between the portal vein and the inferior vena cava. The kidneys are both somewhat lower than usual, the right especially so, and both suprarenal glands are separated from their respective kidneys by a considerable amount of perirenal fat.

A. Descending aorta.
D. Duodenum.
DC. Descending colon.
IVC. Inferior vena cava.
J. Jejunum.
LI. Liver.
LK. Left kidney.
TC. Transverse colon.

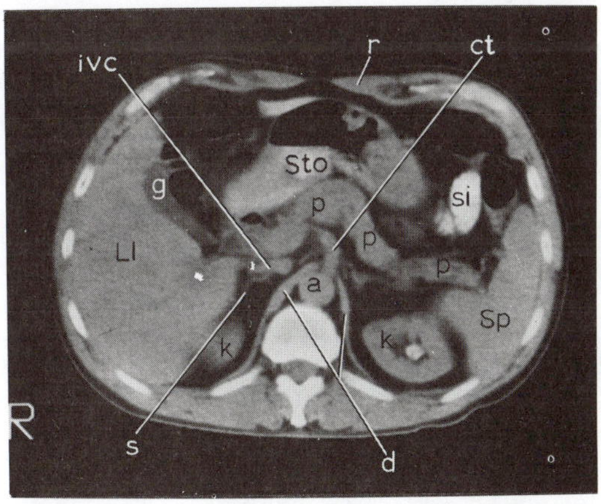

Fig. 286A. A CT scan through the lowest part of the twelfth thoracic vertebra.

A scan such as this can demonstrate the presence of a cancer in the head of the pancreas which might only have been suspected because of blockage of the bile-duct in the head of the pancreas showing as jaundice (seen as yellowing of the sclerae or skin). It might also show a distended gall bladder with gall stones or evidence of an enlarged spleen—all potential indicators of the cause of the jaundice—and permit a decison as to the appropriate treatment.

a. Abdominal aorta.
ct. Coeliac trunk.
d. Crura of diaphragm.
g. Gall bladder.
ivc. Inferior vena cava.
k. Kidneys.
Ll. Right lobe of liver.
p. Pancreas.
r. Rectus abdominis.
s. Right suprarenal.
si. Small intestine.
sp. Spleen.
sto. Stomach.

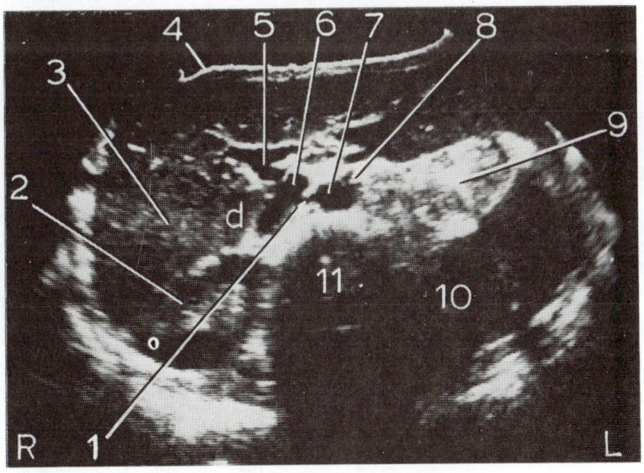

Fig. 286B. Ultrasound, transverse scan of upper abdomen. The shape of the abdomen is distorted by this technique which depends on reflection of ultrasound waves from surfaces. The slice produced in this way is seen from below.

This type of scan, though more difficult to read because of its distortion of the normal anatomical picture of a CT scan, does not expose the individual to X-rays and so is particularly useful when repeated investigations are necessary or the area to be seen contains tissues which are very X-ray sensitive, e.g. the ovaries in the pelvis or an embryo or fetus *in utero*. It is understood that ultrasound has no damaging effect on tissues which are sensitive to X-rays.

1. Common hepatic artery.
2. Right kidney.
3. Liver, right lobe.
4. Skin.
5. Portal vein branching.
6. Inferior vena cava.
7. Aorta.
8. Coeliac trunk branches—left gastric and splenic.
9. Stomach between left lobe of liver and left kidney.
10. Left kidney.
11. Vertebral body.

d. Duodenum.

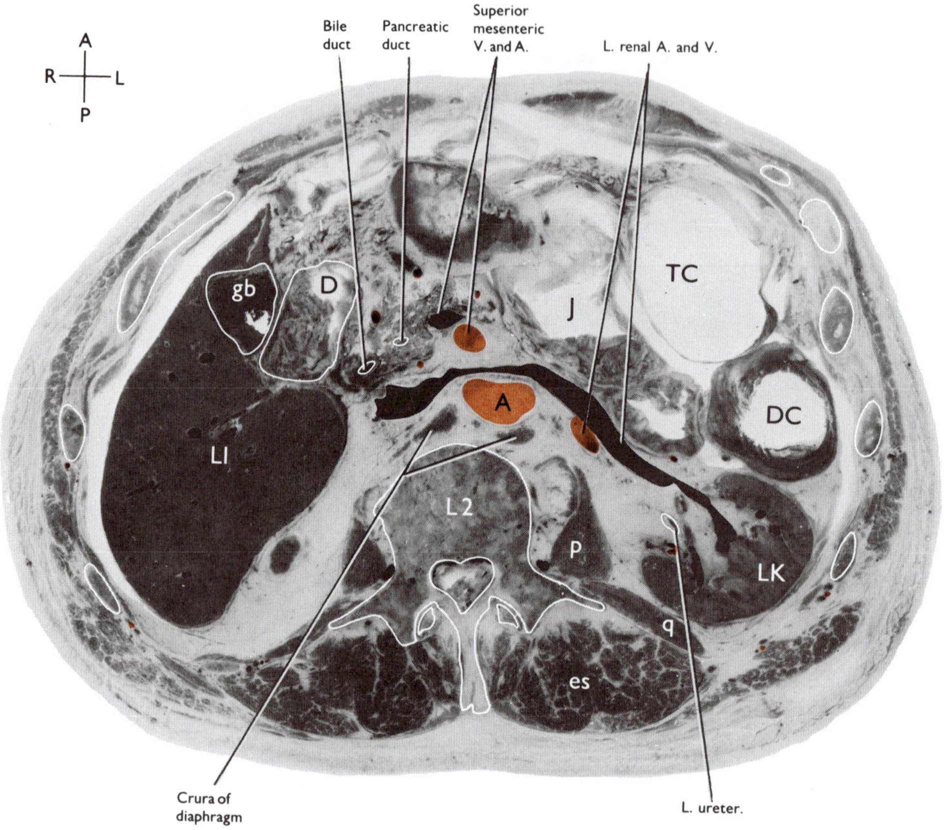

Fig. 287. Section through the second lumbar vertebral body (L2). Outlined in white are the left ureter, the pancreatic and bile-ducts, the duodenum, and the gall-bladder. The two ducts lie in the head of the pancreas to the right of the superior mesenteric vessels. The entire length of the left renal vein is seen. A large superior pancreaticoduodenal artery lies on the pancreas beside the duodenum. The crura of the diaphragm are clearly seen.
A. Descending aorta.
D. Duodenum.
DC. Descending colon.
es. Erector spinae.
gb. Gall-bladder.
IVC. Inferior vena cava.
J. Jejunum.
LI. Liver.
LK. Left kidney.
p. Psoas.
q. Quadratus lumborum.
TC. Transverse colon.

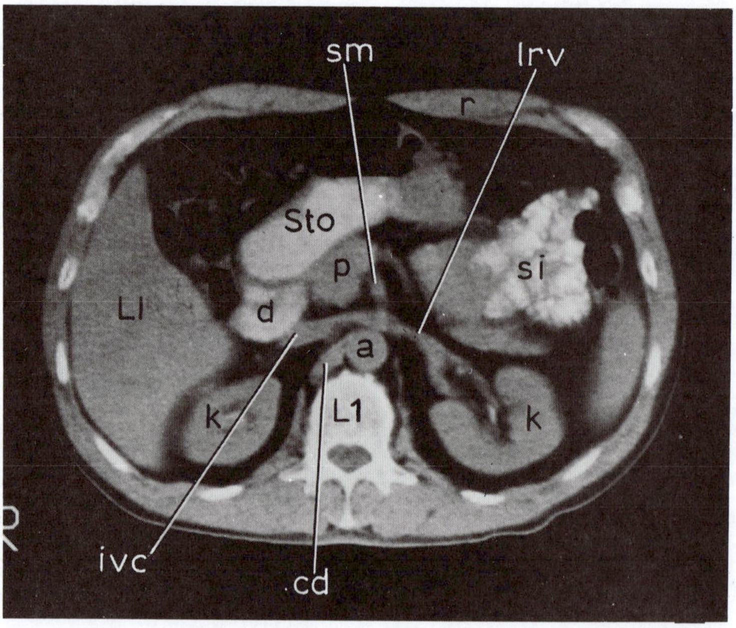

Fig. 287A. A CT scan at the level of the first lumbar vertebra.
a. Abdominal aorta.
cd. Right crus of diaphragm.
d. Duodenum.
ivc. Inferior vena cava.
k. Kidney.
L1. First lumbar vertebral body.
Ll. Right lobe of liver.
lrv. Left renal vein.
p. Pancreas (head).
r. Rectus abdominis.
si. Small intestine.
sm. Superior mesenteric artery.
Sto. Stomach.

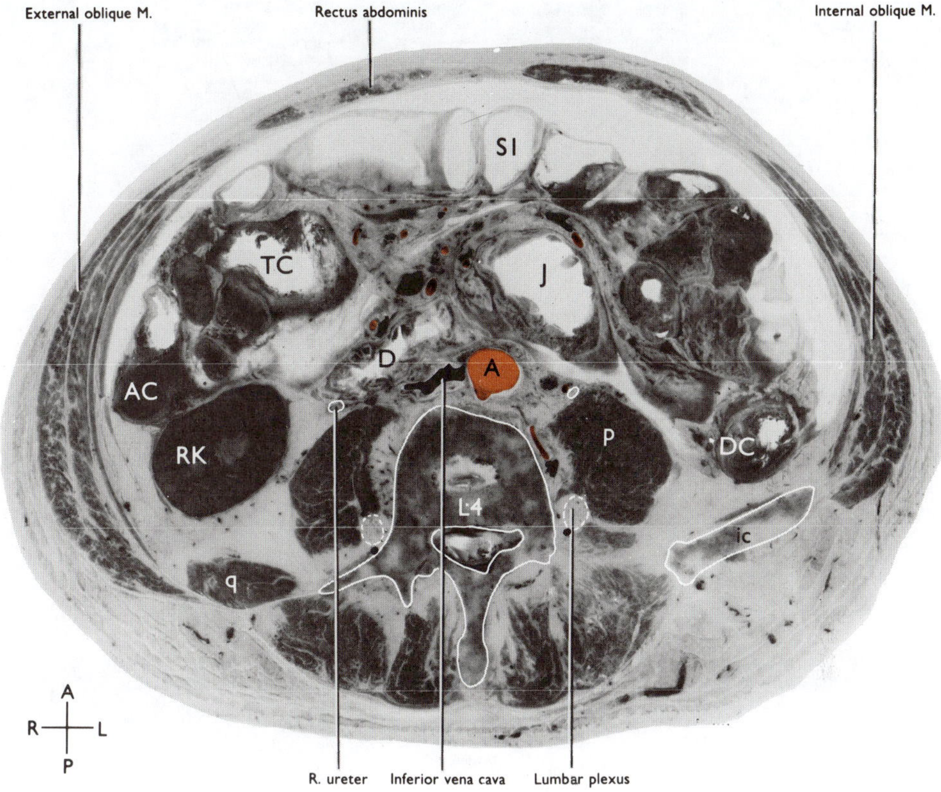

Fig. 288. Section through the body of the fourth lumbar vertebra (L4). Outlined in white are the ureters and parts of the lumbar plexuses (broken line). The inferior mesenteric vessels lie close to the left ureter. Branches of the superior mesenteric vessels are present in the mesentery running to several parts of the small intestine which have been sectioned.
A. Descending aorta.
AC. Ascending colon.
D. Duodenum.
DC. Descending colon.
ic. Iliac crest.
J. Jejunum.
p. Psoas.
q. Quadratus lumborum.
RK. Right kidney.
SI. Small intestine.
TC. Transverse colon.

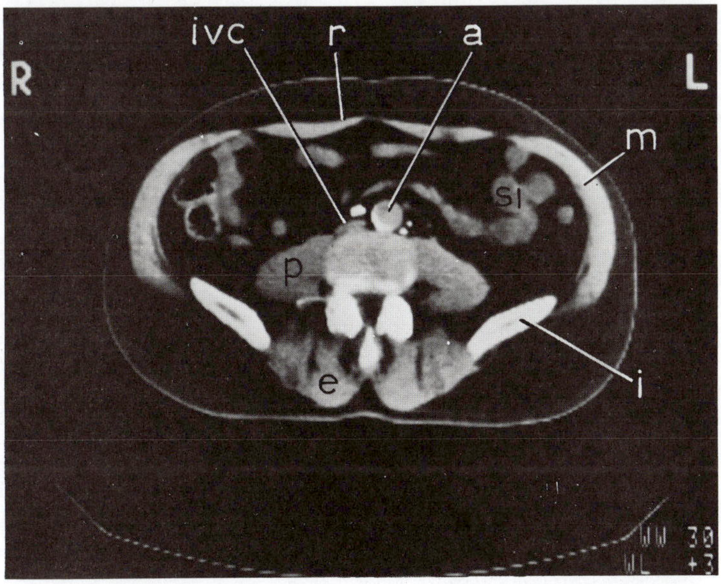

Fig. 288A. A CT scan at the upper level of the iliac crests.
a. Aorta.
e. Erector spinae.
i. Ilium.
ivc. Inferior vena cava.
m. Muscles of abdominal wall.
p. Psoas.
r. Rectus abdominis.
si. Small intestine.

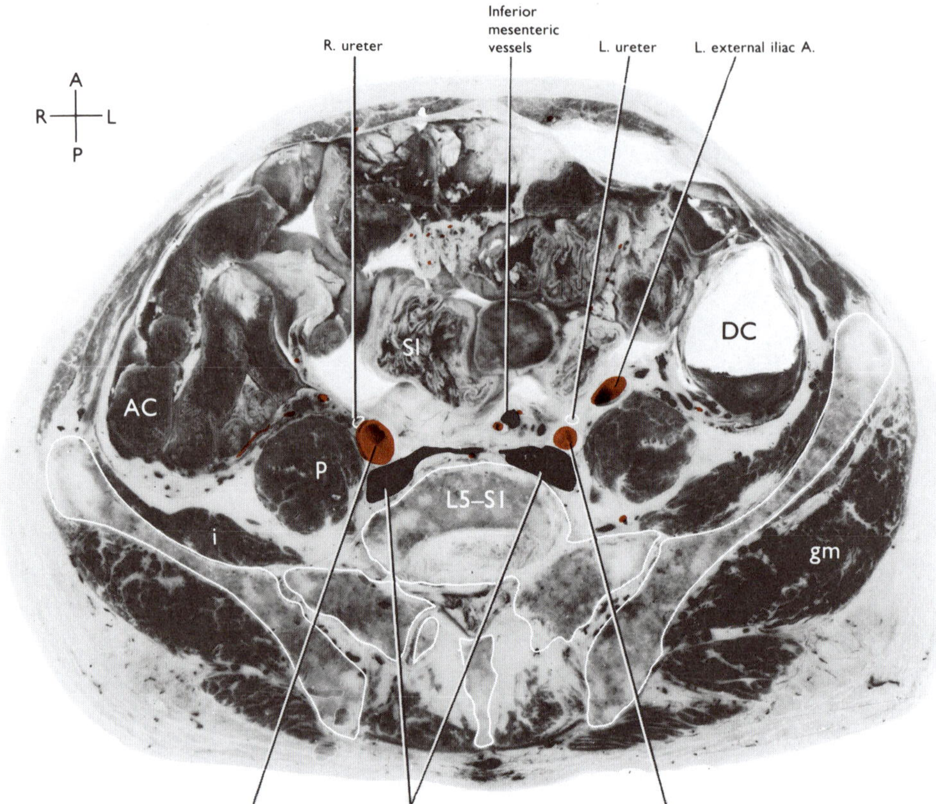

Fig. 289. Section through the lumbosacral intervertebral disc (L5–S1) just below the formation of the inferior vena cava by the union of the two common iliac veins. Outlined in white are the ureters, the left on the internal iliac artery, the right on the common iliac artery. This difference indicates the slight obliquity of the sections, the right side of the body (left side of the illustration) being cut at a slightly higher level than the left.

AC. Ascending colon.
DC. Descending colon.
i. Iliacus.
gm. Gluteus maximus.
p. Psoas.
SI. Small intestine.

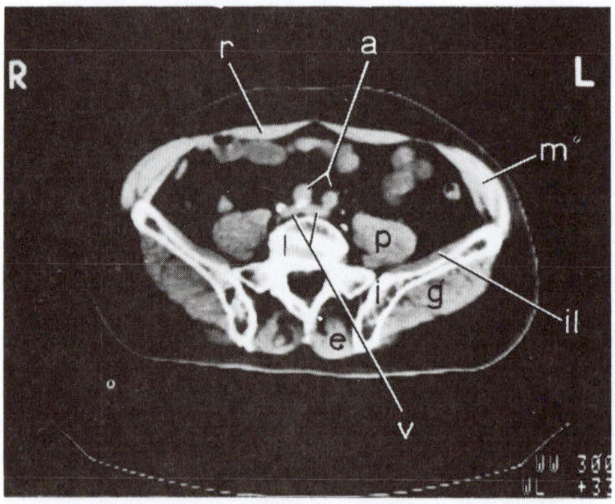

Fig. 289A. A CT scan through the level of the anterior superior iliac spines.

a. Common iliac arteries.
e. Erector spinae muscle.
g. Gluteus medius.
i. Ilium.
il. Iliacus muscle.
l. Lumbosacral joint.
m. Muscles of abdominal wall.
p. Psoas muscle.
r. Rectus abdominis muscle.
v. Common iliac veins.

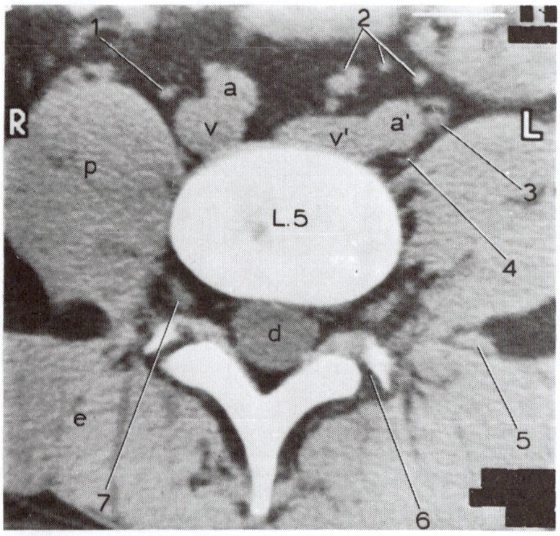

Fig. 289B. Electronically enlarged CT scan through the lower part of the fifth lumbar vertebra. This shows the type of detail which can be obtained due to the minor differences in X-ray absorption by fat (darker areas) and other tissues.

a and a′. Right and left common iliac arteries.
d. Dural sac containing the cauda equina.
e. Erector spinae.
p. Psoas muscle.
v and v′. Right and left common iliac veins.

1. Right ureter.
2. Common iliac lymph nodes.
3. Left ureter.
4. Sympathetic trunk.
5. Femoral nerve.
6. Lumbosacral synovial joint between articular processes (zygopophysial joint) the light area immediately anterior to this is the ligamentum flavum.
7. Fifth lumbar ventral ramus passing to lumbosacral trunk.

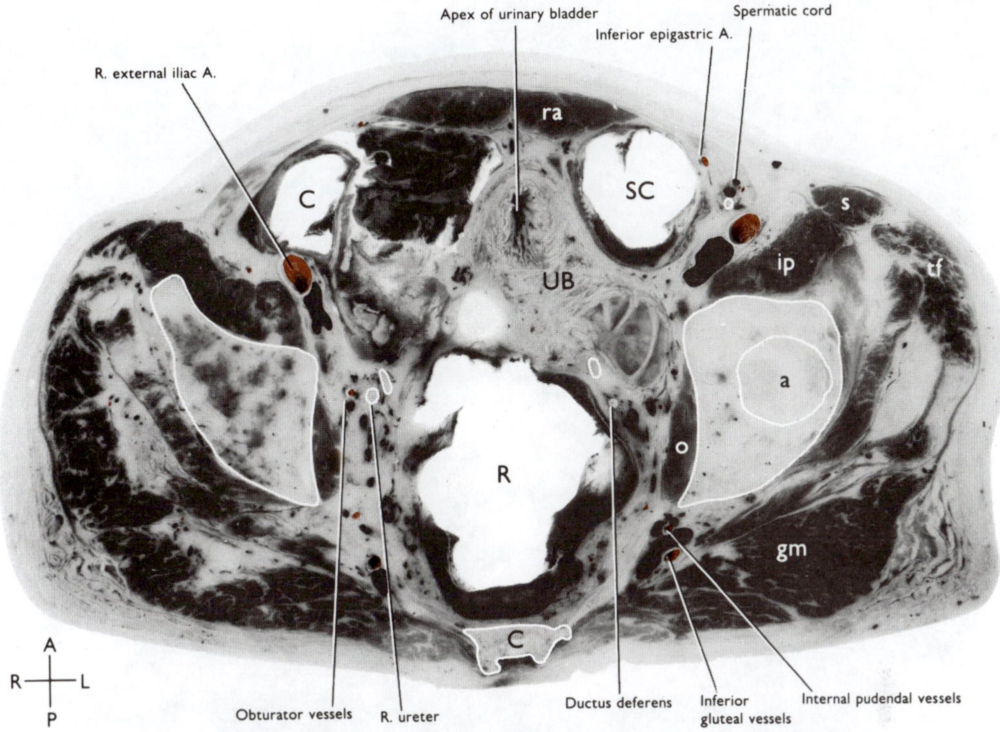

Fig. 290. Section through the coccyx, the upper part of the left hip joint, and the superior surface of the urinary bladder (left side and apex). Outlined in white is each ureter and ductus deferens. The right ductus deferens (left side of illustration) lies immediately anteromedial to the right ureter, the left is in the spermatic cord. The left inferior gluteal and internal pudendal vessels lie immediately posterior to the sacrospinous ligament, the spine of the ischium lying below the level of the section.

a. Head of femur in acetabulum.
C. Caecum.
C. Coccyx.
gm. Gluteus maximus.
ip. Iliopsoas.
o. Obturator internus.
R. Rectum (distended).
ra. Rectus abdominis.
s. Sartorius.
tf. Tensor fasciae latae.
U.B. Urinary bladder.
SC. Sigmoid colon.

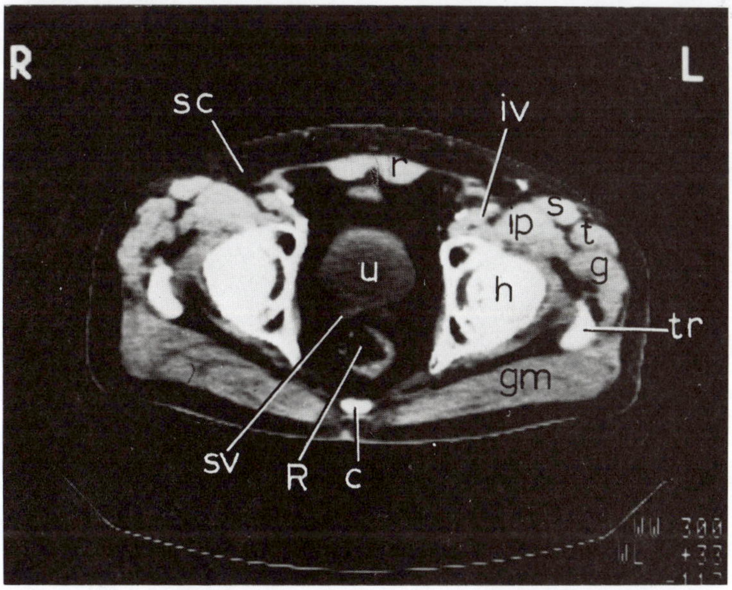

Fig. 290A. A CT scan through the level of the centres of the hip joints.

c. Coccyx.
g. Gluteus minimus.
gm. Gluteus maximus.
h. Head of femur in acetabulum.
ip. Iliopsoas muscle.
iv. External iliac vessels.
R. Rectum.
r. Rectus abdominis.
s. Sartorius.
sc. Spermatic cord.
sv. Seminal vesicle.
t. Tensor fasciae latae.
tr. Greater trochanter.
u. Urinary bladder.

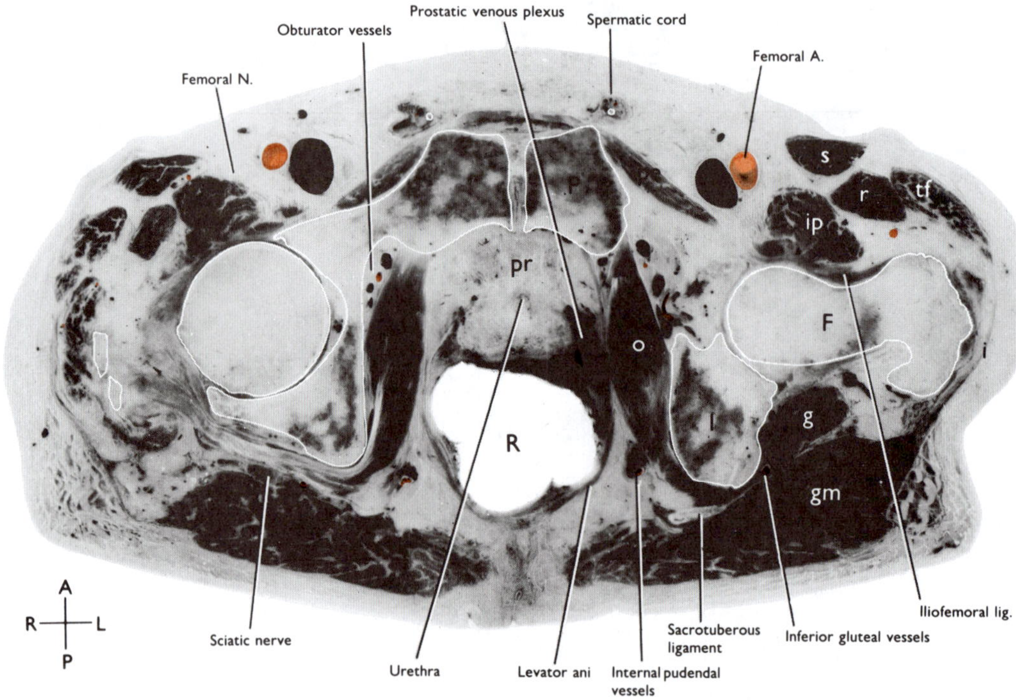

Fig. 291. Section through the pubic symphysis and the two hip joints. The left hip joint appears incomplete because the section passes through the acetabular notch. The entire length of the obturator internus is shown on the right side of the body, its tendon lying posterior to that of obturator externus as it approaches its insertion. The ductus deferens is outlined in white in each spermatic cord.

g. Gemellus inferior.
gm. Gluteus maximus.
ip. Iliopsoas.
o. Obturator internus.
P. Body of pubic bone.
pe. Pectineus.
pr. Prostate gland.
r. Rectus femoris.
R. Rectum (distended).
s. Sartorius.
tf. Tensor fasciae latae.

The bones of the thorax, vertebral column, and pelvis

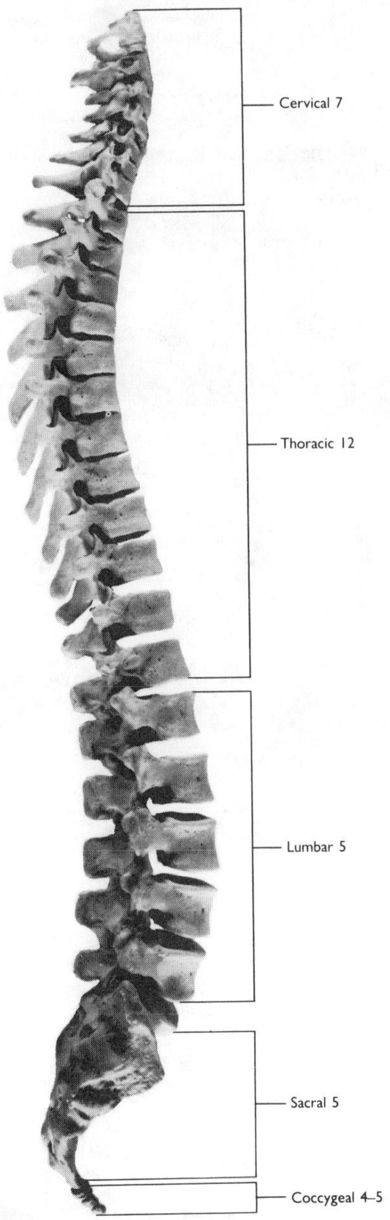

Fig. 292. The right surface of the vertebral column.

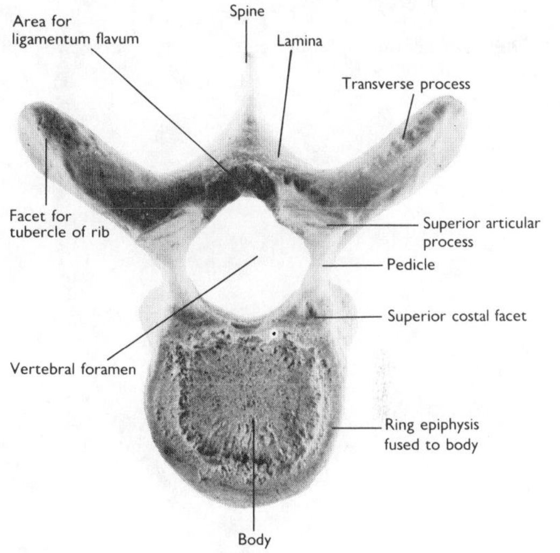

Fig. 293. The superior surface of the seventh thoracic vertebra.

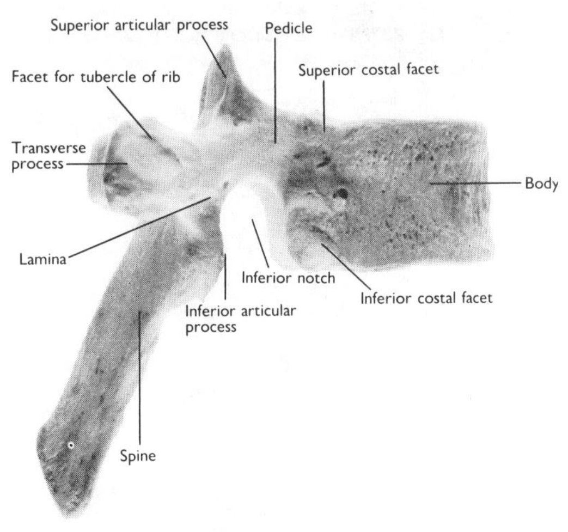

Fig. 294. The right surface of the seventh thoracic vertebra.

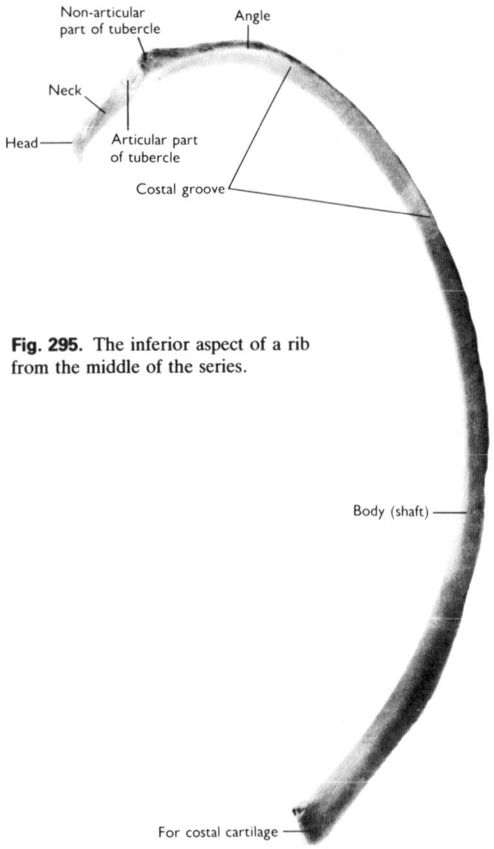

Fig. 295. The inferior aspect of a rib from the middle of the series.

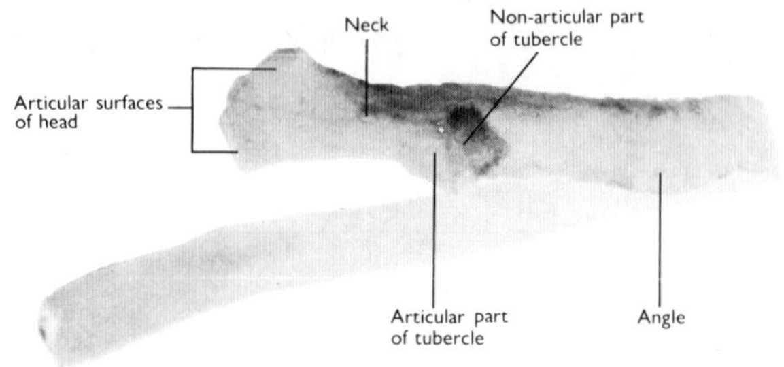

Fig. 296. The sixth right rib seen from behind.

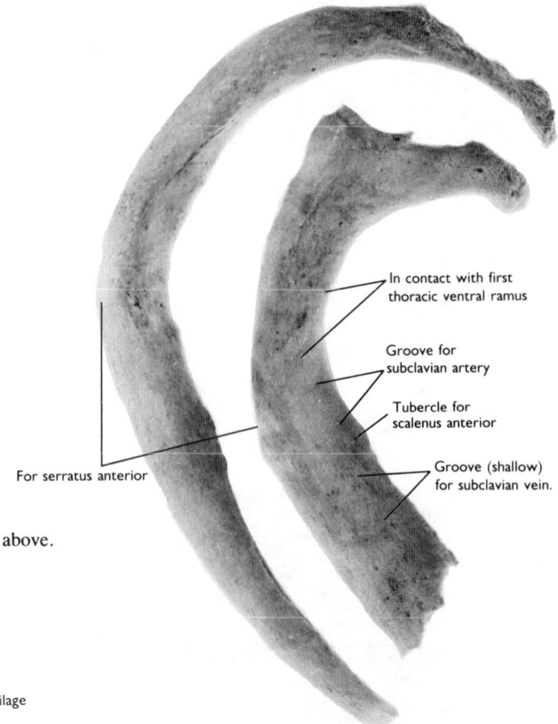

Fig. 297. First and second right ribs as seen from above.

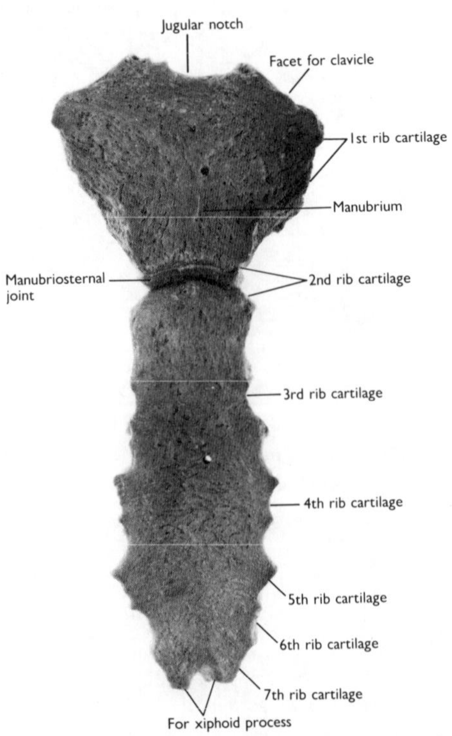

Fig. 298. Sternum (anterior view). The xiphoid process is missing.

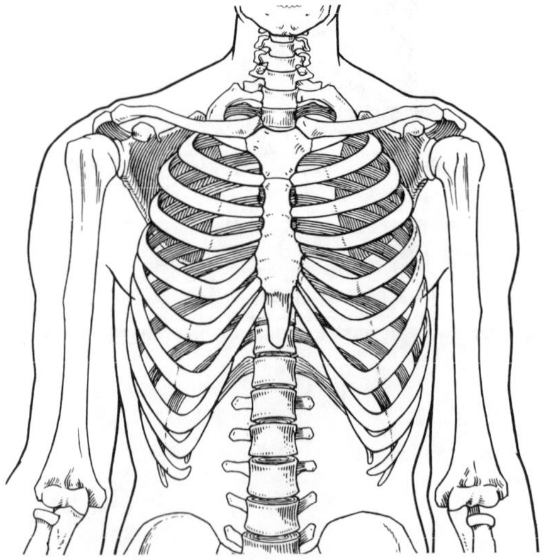

Fig. 299. Front of portion of skeleton showing thorax.

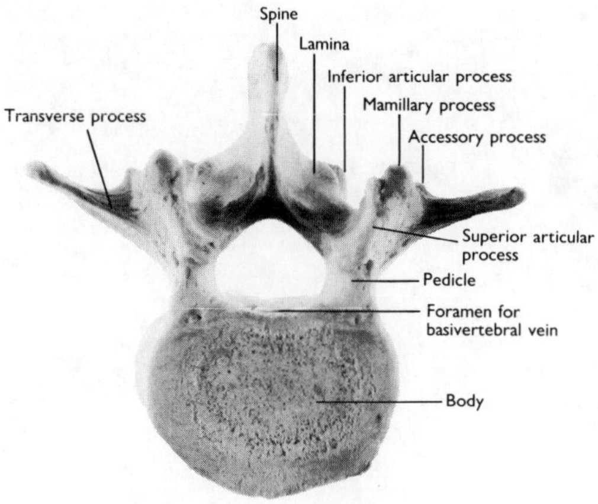

Fig. 300. The superior surface of the third lumbar vertebra.

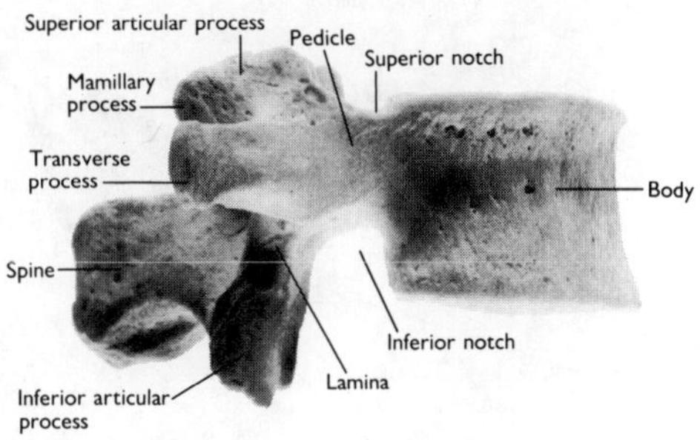

Fig. 301. The right surface of the third lumbar vertebra.

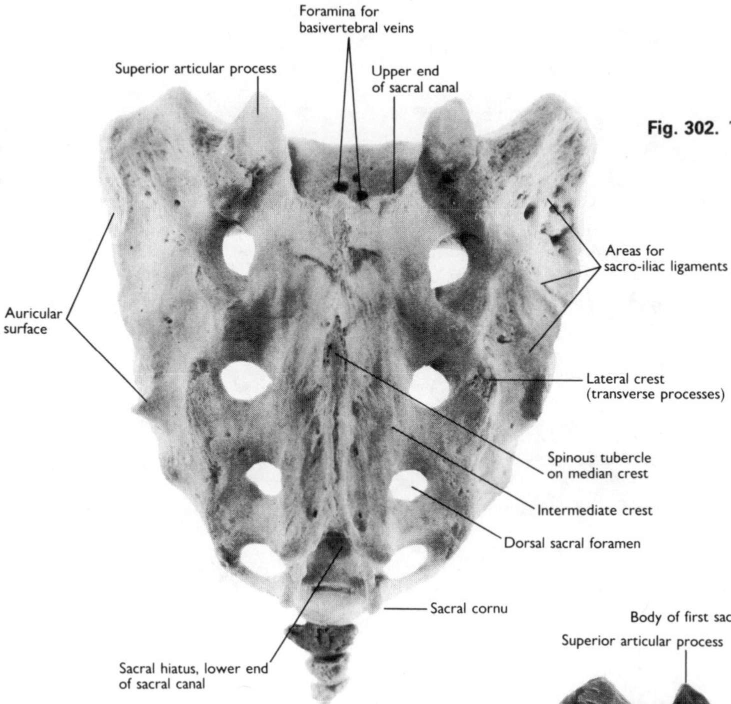

Fig. 302. The sacrum and coccyx (dorsal surface).

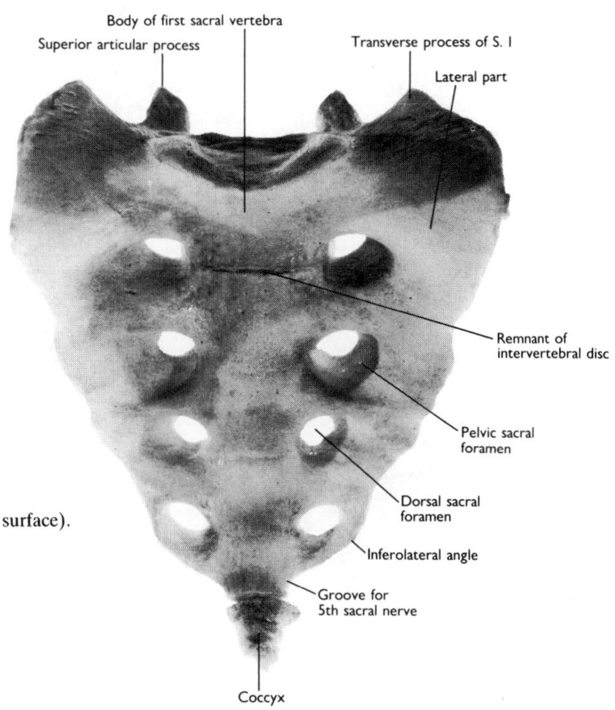

Fig. 303. The sacrum and coccyx (pelvic surface).

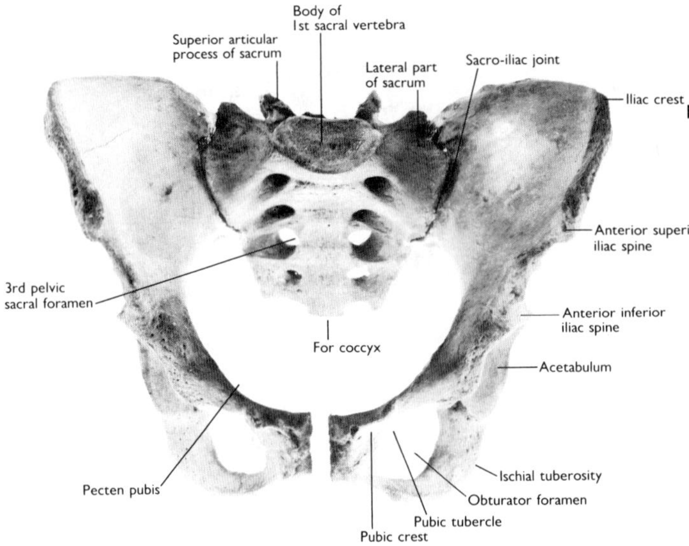

Fig. 304. The female pelvis seen from in front.

Fig. 305. The male pelvis seen from in front without coccyx.

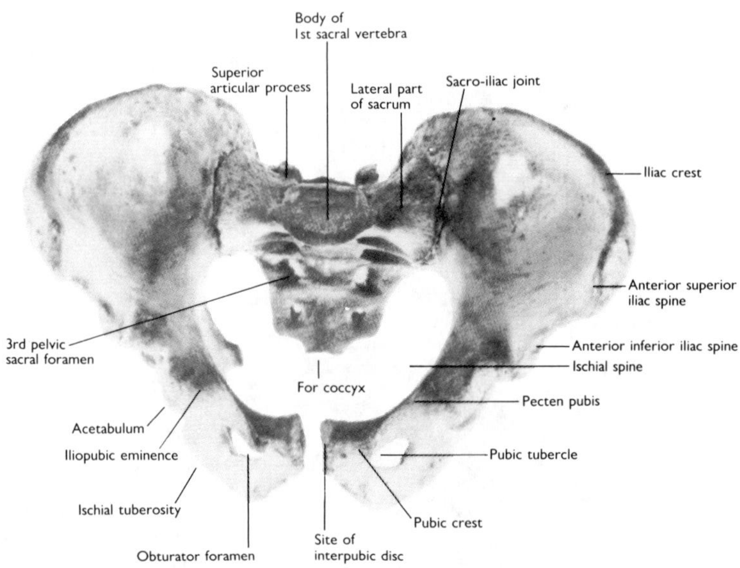

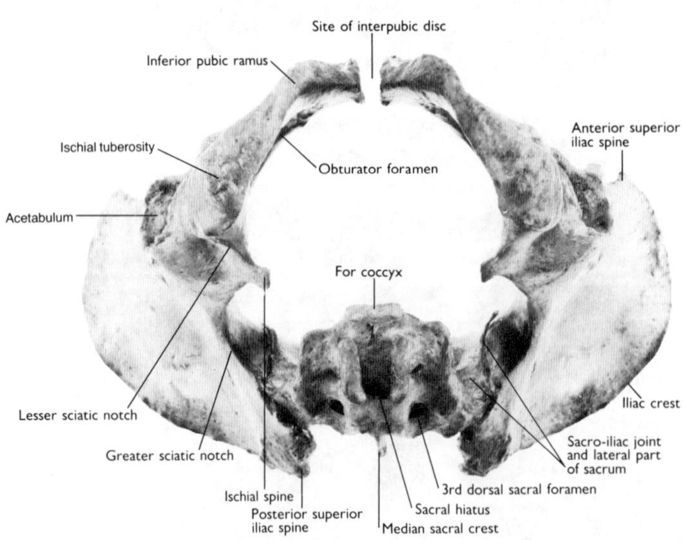

Fig. 306. The inferior aperture of the male pelvis without coccyx.

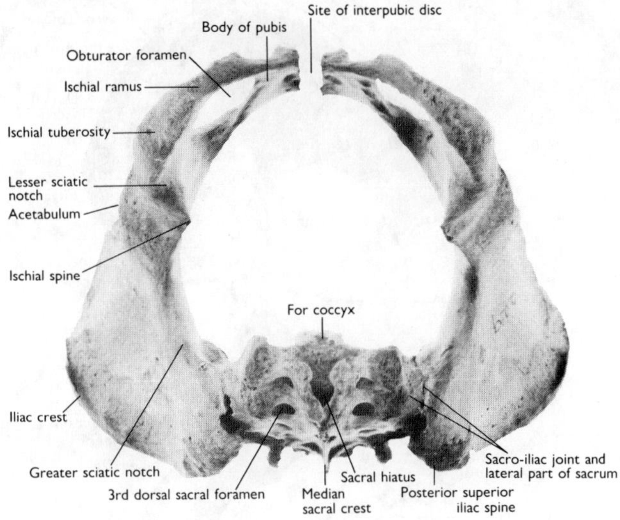

Fig. 307. The inferior aperture of the female pelvis without coccyx.

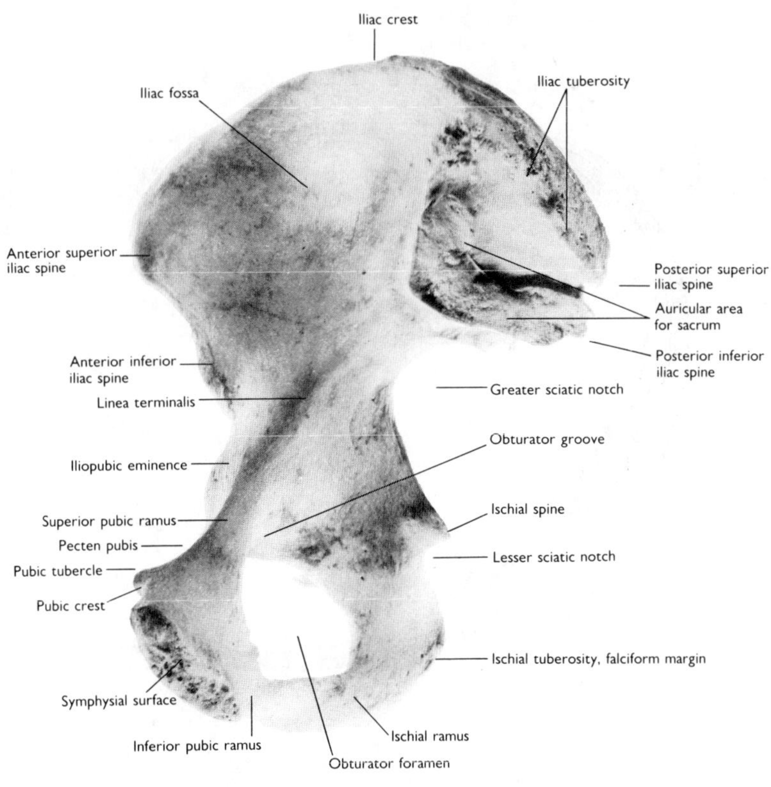

Fig. 308. The right hip bone from the medial side.

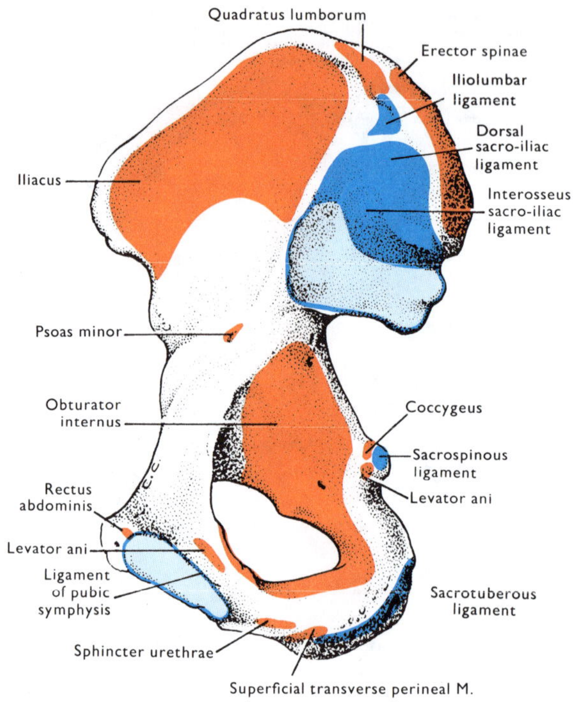

Fig. 309. The medial aspect of the right hip bone. Muscle attachments, red; ligamentous attachments, blue.

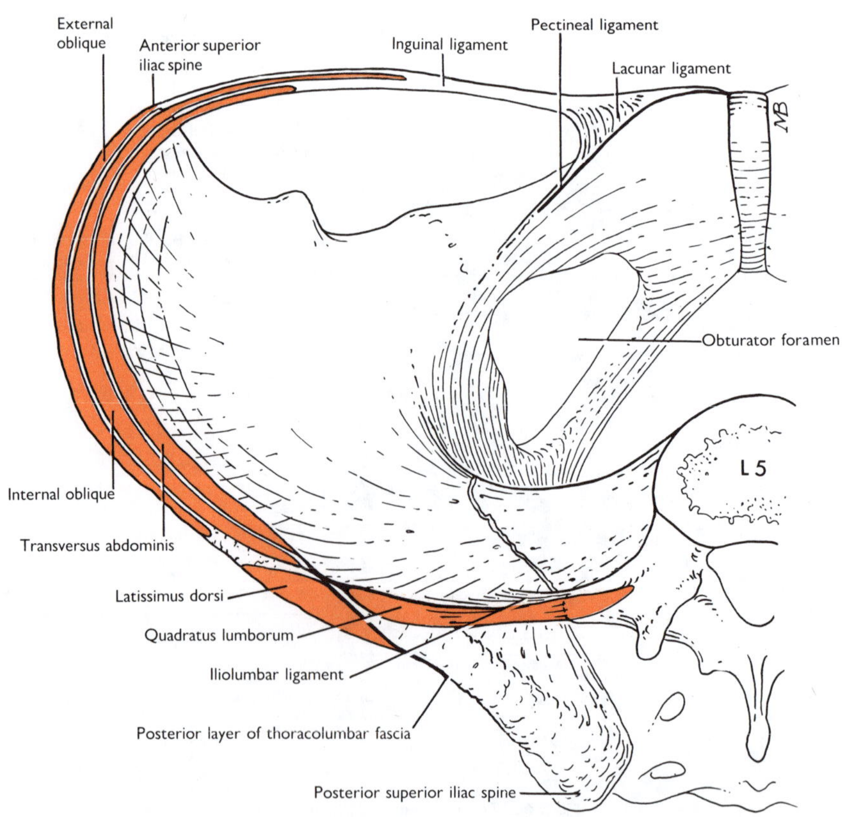

Fig. 310. The bony pelvis and fifth lumbar vertebra seen from above.

Index

References to tables are denoted by an asterisk (*) after the page number. Figures are indicated by a dagger (†). **Bold** type denotes the principal entries.